Clinical Skills

D1594201

'It is purely a matter of skill,
Which all may attain if they will'

The Yeomen of the Guard, Act 2 (W. S. Gilbert).

Clinical Skills

A System of Clinical Examination

SECOND EDITION

EDITED BY IAN A. D. BOUCHIER, MD, FRCP, FRCPE

Professor of Medicine, University of Dundee; Honorary Consultant Physician, Ninewells Hospital and Medical School, Dundee

AND JOHN S. MORRIS, MD, FRCP

Consultant Physician and Gastroenterologist, Bridgend General Hospital, Glamorgan

1982

W. B. Saunders Company Ltd

London · Philadelphia · Toronto

W. B. Saunders Company Ltd: 1 St Anne's Road
Eastbourne, East Sussex BN21 3UN

West Washington Square
Philadelphia, PA 19105

1 Goldthorne Avenue
Toronto, Ontario M8Z 5T9

British Library Cataloguing in Publication Data

Bouchier, Ian A. D.
  Clinical skills. — 2nd ed.
  1. Diagnosis
  I. Title II. Morris, John S.
  616.07 '5   RC71

ISBN 0-7216-1893-6

Printed at The Lavenham Press Limited, Lavenham, Suffolk, England.

Print No: 9 8 7 6 5 4 3 2 1

Contributors

IAN A. D. BOUCHIER, MD, FRCP, FRCPE, Professor of Medicine, University of Dundee; Honorary Consultant Physician, Ninewells Hospital and Medical School, Dundee.

P. G. CAMPBELL, MA, BM, MRCP, MRCPsych, MPhil, *formerly* Senior Lecturer, Royal Free Hospital School of Medicine, University of London; Honorary Consultant, Royal Free Hospital and Friern Hospital, London.

STEWART CLARKE, MD, FRCP, Consultant Physician, Royal Free Hospital and Brompton Hospital, London.

H. L. F. CURREY, MMed (Cape Town), FRCP, Professor of Rheumatology, The London Hospital Medical College, University of London; Honorary Consultant in Rheumatology, The London Hospital, London.

D. EMSLIE-SMITH, MD, FRCP, FRCPE, Reader in Medicine, University of Dundee; Honorary Consultant Physician, Ninewells Hospital and Medical School, Dundee.

W. FRAIN-BELL, MD, FRCPE, Honorary Senior Lecturer in Dermatology, University of Dundee; Consultant Dermatologist, Ninewells Hospital and Medical School, Dundee.

W. M. HAINING, FRCSE, Consultant Ophthalmologist, Ninewells Hospital and Medical School, Dundee.

C. W. H. HAVARD, MA, DM, FRCP, Consultant Physician and Endocrinologist, Royal Free Hospital and Royal Northern Hospital, London.

A. V. HOFFBRAND, DM, FRCP, MRCPath, Professor of Haematology, Royal Free Hospital School of Medicine, University of London; Honorary Consultant Haematologist, Royal Free Hospital, London.

J. A. R. LENMAN, MB, ChB, FRCPE, FRSE, Reader in Neurology, University of Dundee; Honorary Consultant Neurologist, Ninewells Hospital and Medical School, Dundee.

JOHN S. MORRIS, MD, FRCP, *formerly* Lecturer in Medicine, Royal Free Hospital School of Medicine, University of London; Consultant Physician and Gastroenterologist, Bridgend General Hospital, Glamorgan.

J. E. PETTIT, MD, FRCPA, MRCPath, Associate Professor of Haematology, University of Otago Medical School, Dunedin, New Zealand.

GERALD RUSSELL, MD, FRCP, FRCPE, FRCPsych, Professor of Psychiatry, Institute of Psychiatry, London; Honorary Consultant, Moresley and Bethlem Royal Hospital, London.

WILLIAM KINNEAR STEWART, MD, FRCP, FRCPE, Senior Lecturer in Medicine, University of Dundee; Honorary Consultant Physician, Ninewells Hospital and Medical School, Dundee.

Contents

Preface to the First Edition

At a time when the clinician has available a vast array of laboratory and radiological techniques to aid in making a diagnosis, it requires emphasis that the art and skill of examining the patient remain the basis for competent medical practice. The modern methods of patient examination have been accepted for at least 100 years; the basic techniques are described adequately in a number of distinguished books. What, therefore, is the advantage of another textbook dealing with the method of the clinical examination?

While the techniques of history taking and performing a physical examination are well established, we believe that the understanding and interpretation of symptoms and signs do alter with progress in medical knowledge. For example developments in cardiology have enabled sophisticated interpretations of cardiac function to be made from bedside auscultation of the heart. On the other hand there is a degree of disenchantment with the traditional methods for examining the chest which can produce misleading information and clinicians rely greatly upon chest radiographs and pulmonary function tests. Similarly the emphasis placed upon aspects of a patient's history will vary as our knowledge and understanding of diseases alter. More and more the emphasis will be to recognise from the history certain early features of illness. Thus just as textbooks on disease will evolve and require updating, so will those texts which deal with the examination of the patient. We hope that in this new contribution to the medical literature we have presented both the traditional and established techniques of history taking and examination while at the same time presenting modern concepts of the significance of the symptoms and signs.

Distinguished scholars have commented previously that the clinical examination forms the basis for the effective practice of medicine. It is our belief that there can be no double standards for the clinical method: there can be no 'introductory' text; there must not be one method of clinical examination for junior students and another for seniors. The principles and techniques of the examination are the same regardless of the maturity of the student. The way to elicit a physical sign will not change with the age or experience of the examiner, but the interpretation of a symptom or sign will. For this reason we hope that this book will be read with profit by students not only at the commencement of their clinical training but also during the course of the undergraduate years and even in preparation for postgraduate examinations.

Inevitably there will be differences of opinion over the best methods which may be employed in the clinical examination; not all experts agree on how to palpate or appreciate temperature differences. Rather than obscure these differences and present a rigid approach we have included some of the various techniques which are in common usage. It is for the individual to adopt the method which suits him best and thereafter, by thought and practice, to sharpen his own technique so that it becomes an effective tool for obtaining valid clinical information.

Psychiatric and psychological illnesses are becoming more frequent in clinical practice and the clinician, whatever his discipline, should be able to assess the mental and emotional status of his patient. We hope that the fairly detailed section on the psychiatric examination will fulfil this need.

Frequently the practitioner is required to evaluate the function of an organ or system. The process, which starts with the bedside examination, is completed by radiological and laboratory tests. In order to present a comprehensive picture of how this exercise is undertaken in practice, we have included a brief summary, at the end of each chapter, of what further procedures are available to investigate the function of various organs. In contrast to the detail of the clinical evaluation, these side room and special investigations are given in the merest outline.

We would wish to express our gratitude to our numerous colleagues who contributed by making many helpful suggestions and who provided material for inclusion in the book. Mr David Inglis of W. B. Saunders was a constant support and guided the book to its final production with considerable expertise.

Ian A. D. Bouchier
John S. Morris

Preface to the Second Edition

The preparation of a second edition of *Clinical Skills* has provided us with the opportunity to introduce a number of changes. Dr W. Haining has contributed a section on the examination of the eye, there is a new chapter devoted to the skin written by Dr W. Frain-Bell, and the psychiatric examination has been expanded to include the topical and important problem of alcohol abuse. Furthermore we have included new tables, deleted a number of figures which proved to be unsatisfactory and included a set of new figures. The purpose of the book remains unchanged, to provide a comprehensive account of the clinical examination for both undergraduates and postgraduates. The reader should learn not only how to examine a patient but also the mechanism and significance of symptoms and signs.

We thank the contributors who have adapted so well to the task and have assimilated the spirit of the book. We are particularly grateful to The Upjohn Company, who generously have made available to us the colour prints from their text on ophthalmology; their inclusion has greatly enhanced the section on funduscopy. Mr David Inglis and his staff at W. B. Saunders have continued to provide understanding support, skilful advice and guidance, and to them we offer our grateful appreciation.

Ian A. D. Bouchier
John S. Morris

1 The Medical Interview

I. A. D. Bouchier

Patients usually consult doctors because they feel unwell or because they have a problem for which they require help. The medical interview serves as the basis for the patient—doctor interaction and is fundamental to the practice of medicine. Normally the interview commences with the patient recounting his awareness that matters are not right with certain parts of his body or with his mental functions. These expressions of disordered function are known as *symptoms.* The next stage in the interview is the undertaking of a physical examination of the patient during which the doctor attempts to detect and define alterations in the structure or function of a particular organ or body system; that is, to elicit *physical signs.* It is on the basis of the symptoms and signs that a diagnosis is made and therapy is instituted.

HISTORY TAKING

An accurate medical history is essential if a diagnosis is to be formulated and the patient understood as an individual. The art of obtaining a detailed history can be learnt with training and experience. It is the most important part of the interview, for it is recognised that the process of making a diagnosis is hindered considerably by the absence of an accurate history. Indeed, there are many diseases which are diagnosed solely on the basis of an adequate history, for example angina pectoris or epilepsy.

The aim of the history is to build up a comprehensive picture of the patient as an individual, the circumstances of his illness, and his environment. At the conclusion of the history it should be possible to evaluate both the disease and the illness. It is useful to distinguish between the two. The *disease* is no more than a diagnostic label permitting the classification of the abnormal physical and mental processes at work, for example, myocardial infarction. The *illness* describes the effects of a particular disease upon an individual. Thus the effects of a myocardial infarct will differ from one patient to another depending upon age, severity of the infarct, social circumstances, and the patient's own reaction to his disease. The clinician should be aware of the patient's reaction to his illness if problems are to be anticipated and correct decisions made regarding management. By the end of the initial interview the clinician should have begun to understand his patient as a unique person with an individual reaction to his disease and with ensuing problems which are peculiar to him.

Patient—Doctor Relationship

It is fundamental to an effective therapeutic relationship that the physician establishes rapport with his patient. This basis of a sound relationship is developed during the medical interview. Rapport is the end result of complex psychological mechanisms involving both patient and clinician. By consulting a doctor the patient is indicating, consciously or unconsciously, his willingness to place himself in a position of dependence upon a doctor. For some patients this role is difficult to accept and their attitudes can hinder the development of rapport. With care and skill the doctor can develop the relationship into one of trust and understanding, of benefit not only to the patient but to the doctor himself. The clinician must be sympathetic but not sentimental; he should be moral but not a moralist. At no time should the patient feel that the clinician is being contemptuous or disapproving of him. The patient seeks understanding from his doctor who can be warm and honest but nevertheless can still be critical. However, it is important that any criticism is muted and carefully handled so that the patient does not feel rejected. It is under such circumstances that a relationship of trust can be developed and the patient will become sufficiently secure to discuss his uncertainties and problems, thereby enabling his doctor to achieve a more complete understanding of the illness.

Many factors influence the doctor—patient relationship: the social, cultural and educational background of both the patient and the clinician; the previous medical experiences of the patient; the age of the clinician and his attitudes towards the patient. Considerable differences in cultural background lead to difficulties in interpreting symptoms, particularly when these are a manifestation of a psychosomatic disorder. The difficulties of managing the psychological ailments of an immigrant are well recognised and they are compounded when there is a language barrier as well. Much patience and tolerance is required during history taking and this is extended into the physical examination. Particular care must be taken to make the patient feel at ease and understand what will be done and what is expected of him. Any explanation of the illness and instructions about therapy become difficult in these circumstances.

The age of the doctor is seldom a barrier to developing rapport. A few elderly patients find it difficult to accept a youthful doctor, but a calm, gentle and serious approach usually wins co-operation and approval.

The attitude of the clinician towards his patient is of great importance. Personal problems and prejudices can impinge upon a medical relationship making for an unduly critical or unsympathetic approach. Thus the doctor who grew up in a home in which alcoholism was a problem may find himself emotionally unable to manage alcoholic patients. Emotional reactions to a patient can undoubtedly cloud judgement — for example the new resident who examined a young woman with purpura and splenomegaly and avoided making the diagnosis of leukaemia because he did not wish the young patient to have this disease. Close identification with the patient may bring on the one hand an unreasonable sense of guilt should the patient die and on the other an emotional involvement which may be trying or even dangerous. Care must be taken at all times that a satisfactory relationship does not undergo an erotic transference. The clinician must recognise that this can occur both on his part and the part of his patient and he must develop protective methods for dealing with the situation.

Frequently patients are curious about the doctor: 'Are you married?', 'Have you any children?'. A satisfactory rapport does not require any exchange of personal or initimate details with the clinician. The clinician should not be discomforted or discouraged by a display of emotion from the patient which can often be a means of developing rapport. It is of benefit to the patient to be able to cry during the interview. Anger or dissatisfaction with the clinician may also be expressed and in the face of such a reaction the doctor should adopt a calm and understanding approach. The reasons for the patient's reaction should be sought. Little is gained and much lost if the doctor counteracts aggressively.

The patient—doctor relationship takes place not only at a verbal level. With perception, training and experience it is possible to appreciate that communication can take place at an emotional level. Such thought processes which are expressed and perceived in this way can have an important bearing upon the clinical history and the clinician must be on the alert to this unspoken channel of communication. Thus the patient who presents with vague abdominal pain may have serious domestic problems which he cannot bring himself to discuss openly. However, the clinician may sense that there are other problems than abdominal discomfort and can gently direct the patient towards this traumatic area. He must develop an appreciation of the different levels of communication thereby enabling him to recognise problems and conflicts which the patient has been unable to introduce freely himself. Patients may be aware of certain problems but may not feel able to introduce them directly. The difficulties, for example marital or personal, may be hinted at, the clues may be introduced into the history but the patient will expect the doctor to recognise this and himself introduce the stressful topic.

Non-verbal communication may take the form of *static cues*, which remain unaltered during the consultation, for example dress, hair style, cleanliness, condition of the hands and body posture; and *dynamic cues*, which are behavioural in nature, such as gaze, eye focus and facial movements. Information derived from non-verbal communication is used by the doctor in determining the kind of person who is ill, the relative importance of physical or psychological factors in the illness, and even decisions on management. The patient too, will use and interpret the behaviour of the doctor and the way in which he speaks, to form an opinion of the doctor, whether concerned and sympathetic or stern and forbidding.

Patients have differing concepts of and make different demands upon their doctor. Some require that the doctor should be a warm person, readily available at all times, bright, and communicative; others wish their medical attendant to be more reserved, even austere, and are happy not to spend time in idle conversation. Some patients want to have their illness explained in great detail, others profess to the reverse, claiming that they prefer to be kept in relative ignorance. It is the task of the clinician to evaluate the reaction of a patient to the illness and to the doctor—patient relationship. The doctor cannot change his basic personality nor need he alter his underlying philosophy, but he should be adaptable. He must judge what the patient expects of him as an individual, and then decide to what extent he can or will accommodate himself. Such important evaluations and decisions are made at the time of the initial medical interview and developed further during subsequent visits.

General Procedure for Obtaining a History

The medical interview should be conducted in a quiet, relaxed atmosphere and be as unhurried as possible. Naturally the ideal is not always possible and different circumstances may demand a modification of the basic technique. The method of taking a history from a shocked patient who has a myocardial infarct will be different from that used for the ambulant patient seen in the consulting rooms complaining of chest pain. Similarly, the busy family doctor will need to adapt his interview according to the circumstances and his knowledge of his patients.

It is important that the doctor starts by putting his patients at ease. For many patients a visit to the doctor is mildly stressful and for some it causes extreme anxiety. It is improbable that a full history will be obtained or any rapport established if the patient, or the doctor, is tense. The doctor's greeting should be friendly and relaxed, and the interview should be conducted within an atmosphere of calm efficiency. The patient will rapidly sense any impatience by the doctor and this will severely inhibit communication.

On first being seen the patient is greeted by the doctor who introduces himself if he is unknown to the patient. If the patient is being seen as a referral then the doctor should mention that he has had a letter or telephone call from the patient's own doctor. Questions are then asked about why the patient is seeking medical advice and what the major symptoms are. Such questions have to be put carefully and it is best to avoid asking 'What is wrong with you?' for it may provoke the reply 'I don't know; that is for you to find out'. A more satisfactory approach is 'What are you complaining of?'; or 'In what way do you feel that things are not right?'; or 'Your doctor says you have been troubled by . . .'.

Within the broad context of a history is is possible to group certain events together thereby conferring order to the history and permitting ready analysis. In the first instance a distinction is made between the account of the illness as volunteered in an uninterrupted manner by the patient; there is a second stage when the patient is asked specific questions about his health. It is convenient to group these questions according to the body systems and this part of the history is known as the System Review. The material obtained during the eliciting of the medical history can also be arranged according to a Present History: the immediate complaints which have led to the consultation; as a Past History: previous medical events in the patient's life; and then those details of the patient and his way of life which provide insight into the patient as a person, as Family History, Social History and Personal History.

The patient should recount his history uninterrupted and in his own way. Every patient presents his complaint differently. Some are loquacious, others brief, and others reticent. During the initial phase of the interview the patient is encouraged to speak freely with the minimum of interruption from the clinician. Premature interruption or questioning at this stage disturbs the train of thought and can seriously inhibit free flow of thought. A perceptive clinician will be aware when an injudicious interruption has prevented the emergence of emotionally charged material of some importance and frequently such information is not produced subsequently. The occasional nod or gesture may be all that is required to indicate the attention of the doctor and ensure that the patient goes on talking. With experience a limited amount of guidance can be given mainly to ensure that one particular symptom is reasonably fully described before the next is produced. The clinician can also gently direct the patient towards aspects of the history thought to be more meaningful. During the interview there may be pauses or longer intervals of silence. These are of significance and the patient should not be hurried through them; nor should they make the doctor feel ill at ease. The patient can be helped by gentle encouragement such as 'what happened then?' or 'and so' or 'go on'.

This phase of the interview may last from five to ten minutes during which time a number of important and unimportant facts will be presented. Many patients recount their symptoms in no specific order with no attention to severity or time. The clinician will need to listen to a full account of the symptoms before a pattern emerges. It will be possible then to arrange the complaints into a more orderly form and questions can be directed towards individual symptoms. Patients are discouraged from using medical terminology or recounting their symptoms in terms of a diagnosis: 'It is angina which is bothering me' or 'I have had a stomach ulcer for years and the pain is getting me down'. Such statements should not be accepted on face value but the patient questioned to determine whether the symptom-complex fits with the diagnosis proferred. Similarly symptoms should be recorded by neutral medical terms, avoiding any aetiological or pathogenetic implications such as 'the patient complained of pleuritic pain'; rather the complaint of 'chest pain worse on breathing or coughing' should be documented.

Characterisation of Symptoms

The majority of symptoms can be defined according to the following features: character, severity, time relationship, precipitating and aggravating factors, relieving factors, and associated manifestations. When the complaint is one of pain then the site of discomfort must be described.

Character

This is a description of the symptoms, for example pain or dizziness or diarrhoea. Pain can be described in various ways: throbbing, burning, dull, sharp, crushing, stabbing. Most patients find it difficult to give a clear description of pain. Certain types of pain are characteristic, such as the 'crushing' chest pain of myocardial infarction or the 'stabbing' pain of pleurisy. The character of the stool can be described according to its colour and consistency. Sputum may be clear, coloured, or blood-stained.

Severity

Pain may vary from being little more than an itch to discomfort of unbearable severity. A patient who has diarrhoea should be asked about the frequency of the stools as well as the quantity. Generally symptoms are graded as mild, moderate or severe.

Time relationship

The precise onset of symptoms can often be of diagnostic value. Pain induced by exertion and relieved by rest suggests ischaemia, for example of the myocardium or of the calf muscle; chest pain aggravated by coughing and deep breathing suggests pleurisy although similar pain can occur from spinal nerve irritation. The relationship of abdominal pain to defaecation is a feature of the irritable bowel syndrome. The circumstances under which a patient becomes dizzy are of much significance; dizziness upon suddenly standing suggests postural hypotension, on coughing suggests cough syncope while patients with cervical spondylosis and vertebrobasilar insufficiency may become dizzy if they turn the head sharply. The duration of a symptom is recorded as well as whether it is persisting unchanged or becoming better or worse.

Precipitating and aggravating factors

This defines the circumstances under which the symptom occurs. Patients with allergic rhinitis may only sneeze and have nasal stuffiness at certain times of the year. A patient with intermittent claudication will only develop calf pain after he has walked a specific distance.

Relieving factors

The way in which a patient obtains relief from a symptom can have diagnostic significance. For example, the pain of angina pectoris can be relieved by rest and by trinitrin tablets, peptic ulcer pain is often helped by antacid preparations.

Associated manifestations

It is not uncommon for one symptom to occur regularly as part of a group of symptoms. Thus dyspnoea together with cough and frothy sputum suggests left-sided heart failure. The association of diarrhoea and flushing occurs in the carcinoid syndrome.

The association of various symptoms by the clinician is a fundamental step in formulating a diagnosis or differential diagnosis. To do so requires an understanding of disease. With experience the interviewer will recognise certain symptoms as being indicative of particular disorders and specific questions can be asked to bring out any characteristic associations. Thus a patient who complains of weight loss may on further questioning admit to excessive perspiration, heat intolerance and irritability which will suggest hyperthyroidism. The patient with pruritus vulvae may on questioning describe excessive thirst and polyuria which should suggest diabetes mellitus and a monilial infection. The association of abnormal olfactory or auditory phenomena followed by loss of consciousness will suggest temporal lobe epilepsy.

Site

Patients can usually describe the place where they experience pain or feel a lump. However, at times the description is vague and this applies particularly to pain. Patients may be unable to locate the precise site of pain and describe whether it is superficial or deep. Similarly, patients are encountered who bring up blood-stained material but are unable to say whether this was coughed up (haemoptysis) or vomited (haematemesis).

Personal Significance of Symptoms

The patient recounts his symptoms to the doctor as experiences which worry him. Sometimes they serve as a means of communicating a need for help and may not represent disordered bodily function. Especially when their significance or severity is uncertain, it can be helpful to enquire about the effects his symptoms have had on his daily life, the amount of disability they cause him and the extent to which they have affected his work, his leisure pursuits and his social and sexual relationships. Perhaps they are charged with personal meaning for him or for close relatives, so that they are thought to signify cancer, heart disease, madness or some other dreaded consequence which he is reluctant to mention. Often, particularly when symptoms are chronic, it may be important to enquire why the patient presents with them now, rather than, say, last month or last year. All sorts of extraneous factors such as a threat of marital separation, recent disease in a friend or a change of general practitioner may come to light as the reason for the patient seeking medical help when he does. It is often useful for the doctor to ask the patient directly what he fears is wrong with him.

System Review

The systemic enquiry can take place after the patient has volunteered the presenting symptoms. It is convenient at this stage to
follow with questions about the symptoms and about the various
body systems. Another technique is to follow the present history
with questions about the past history and leave the system review
until the end of the interview.

During the systemic enquiry the patient is asked specific
questions about the function of the various systems. In order to
avoid unduly influencing the patient's answers leading questions
must be avoided. Questions must be posed in such a way as not to
suggest an answer. When asking about dyspnoea the question is
asked 'Do you sleep well?' or 'Can you manage the day's work
satisfactorily?' rather than 'Do you wake up short of breath?' or
'Do you get breathless when you work?'. If the answers are in the
negative then it is reasonable to ask a more direct question. Patients
may be asked direct questions demanding a straight 'yes' or 'no'
answer. Such questions should not be confused with leading
questions which are couched in such a way as to suggest an answer
to the patient.

It is a matter of individual preference how this phase of the
examination is conducted. In many ways the simplest method is to
group the questions according to functioning systems: cardio-
respiratory, gastrointestinal, etc. Another technique is to start at
the head and work according to anatomy: headache, hearing,
vision, swallowing, palpitations, oedema. A list of the questions
usually asked during the systematic enquiry is given later in this
chapter. Regardless of the method developed, the essential point is
that by the end of the interview all the important questions have
been asked.

Past History

The previous history is an account of all the medical events in the
patient's life until the presentation of the current illness. It is not
always easy to make a clear separation between the present illness
and any previous illnesses, but this is not important for in many
ways the distinction is artificial. The patient presenting with
dyspnoea and oedema may have had chest pain suggestive of a
myocardial infarct some three weeks before. Since these two

episodes are probably related they could well be included together in the presenting history. Similarly, the event of a gastric resection for cancer of the stomach some six months previously in a patient presenting with abdominal pain and swelling could be regarded as relating to the presenting complaint and not as the past history. However, there is the danger of making misleading associations and linking two events which are unrelated.

It is preferable to enquire about past illnesses after the main complaints have been given and the system review obtained. Patients may believe that the doctor is not paying attention to what really matters and they can become antagonistic. A patient presenting with abdominal pain may not see the logic of being asked questions about his health many years before. It is better to encourage the patient to give an account of his current symptoms before enquiring about his previous medical history.

All medical events in the patient's past should be recorded: major illnesses, infections, operations, accidents, allergies, immunisations and pregnancies. The patient is given the opportunity to volunteer the information but direct questioning is usually necessary. Patients should be asked to give precise dates and places for events. Where necessary the names of doctors and hospitals should be obtained so that events can be verified. It is frequently valuable to obtain a copy of previous medical records. It is common to encounter patients who have undergone an operation but who have no clear idea why the operation was undertaken and what was done.

A full history of immunisations is required from children. Previous events of relevance in childhood include the health of the mother during pregnancy, the nature of labour and the nature of the neonatal period including crying, cyanosis, vomiting and convulsions. Growth and development are recorded: age of sitting, standing, walking, talking, eruption of teeth.

A complete obstetrical history is necessary and may have a direct bearing upon the current illness. It is of diagnostic value to obtain a history of severe postpartum haemorrhage in a woman suspected of panhypopituitarism; recurrent mild jaundice of pregnancy is encountered in some women who develop cholestatic jaundice when taking the contraceptive pill. The dates of all deliveries and miscarriages in pregnant patients should be recorded.

The precise detail of the information sought in the past history depends to a large extent upon the circumstances. In an elderly patient it is impractical and unnecessary to obtain a complete account of previous illnesses, many of which may be trivial. Likewise a detailed obstetric history is uncontributory to the medical background of an elderly female. The amount of information about past events that is looked for will depend upon a number of factors: the age of the patient, the nature of illness and the circumstances under which the interrogation is being conducted.

Drug History

A complete drug history is becoming increasingly important. It is necessary to know the drugs being taken and the precise dose. When there is any doubt it is helpful to consult the family doctor or the hospital. Many drugs cause or contribute to disease: anti-inflammatory drugs and gastrointestinal bleeding, methyldopa and chronic liver disease, phenothiazine derivatives and a neurological syndrome of extrapyramidal dysfunction. The administration of one drug often modifies the effects of another. Phenobarbitone, by inducing the drug-metabolising enzymes in the liver, can increase the rate of metabolism of phenylbutazone or dicoumarol. Both salicylates and phenylbutazone potentiate the effects of warfarin, tolbutamide and chlorpropamide. Thiazide diuretics potentiate antihypertensive agents, and by causing potassium depletion precipitate the toxic side-effects of digitalis.

Adverse reactions to drugs should be enquired about, particularly penicillin which is an important cause of potentially fatal anaphylactic reactions. Patients will very often use the term 'allergy' in a loose and inaccurate manner. If a drug has been used for a long time the patient may well forget that he is taking it if asked about pills or medicines. It is often helpful to ask specifically about laxatives, aspirin, night sedation or the contraceptive pill.

Personal and Social History

At this stage of the interview sufficient rapport should have been established to enable the patient to be relaxed and confident enough to speak freely about himself, his work and his reaction to his disease. It is at this stage that the clinician formulates his opinion of the patient as an individual. What is the patient's occupation? How much does he enjoy his work? What are his relations with his colleagues or workmates? Previous occupations are important because they may provide a clue to the diagnosis and also because they give an indication of the patient's stability. A patient with chronic lung disease may have been exposed in the past to industrial hazards such as silica, asbestos, beryllium or iron oxide.

It is necessary to ask about alcohol and smoking habits, sporting activities and hobbies. The history of alcohol intake is notoriously inaccurate particularly when obtained from a patient with alcohol abuse. Rather than asking for the daily or weekly consumption of alcohol, an impression of the quantity of alcohol consumed may be gained from asking how much is spent on alcoholic drinks over a week. Even so, the assessment may be difficult and close relatives should be questioned. Relationships between the patient and his family should be explored but the extent of the questioning will depend upon the circumstances of the interview and a more detailed account is required when there is the possibility of an emotional illness or evidence suggesting a past history of a psychiatric disorder. Information is needed about the economic circumstances and housing and diet are important. Children are asked about their relationship with siblings, friends and teachers. If both parents work it is necessary to determine who looks after the children. Such information is essential if the mother is to be admitted to hospital.

Some attempt should be made to gauge the patient's reaction to his illness: does he accept it or is he depressed or resentful?

Family History

The exact place of the patient in the family is established. Normally it is necessary to know the state of health of the parents, siblings, the spouse and children. In the event of a death the age and the cause of death is recorded. A family history of a particular illness may provide the clue to the diagnosis, for example haemophilia, polyposis coli, Huntington's chorea. Where the question of an hereditable disease arises a much more detailed family history is necessary and information is sought about the health of first- and second-degree relatives. A family tree detailing the affected members is constructed (Figure 1.1).

The event of a particular disease in the family may give rise to considerable anxiety if the patient feels that he may have inherited the disease and will inevitably manifest it. A patient presenting with chest pain and found to have no cardiac disease admitted to being

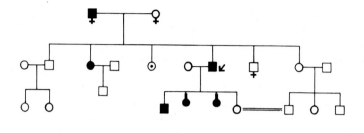

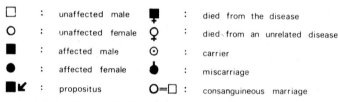

Figure 1.1. *Documentation of a family tree.*

anxious about himself because his father died of a myocardial infarct; a patient with recent onset of headaches had lost a brother as a result of a cerebral tumour.

Much information can be obtained from previous medical records. Many clinicians find it advantageous to familiarise themselves with the patient's previous history before interviewing the patient. Care must be taken, however, not to be unduly biased by the previous medical record and the clinician should be as critical of the information and diagnosis recorded in the medical notes as he would be of the patient's own interpretation of his symptoms.

Difficulties with the Examination

There are a number of circumstances which hinder the taking of an adequate history. The patient may have difficulty in communicating with doctors because of an unfortunate previous experience with the medical profession; because of uncertainty regarding the role of the doctor, for example whether the doctor would be prepared to become involved in a difficult domestic situation; and, most importantly, because of a limited appreciation of the significance of his complaints. Patients do not always remember clearly, or in logical time sequence, and they frequently omit symptoms of major clinical significance. Symptoms may be offered in the belief that the doctor will find them important; the patient may avoid symptoms which are socially embarrassing or which arouse strong emotions. The clinician may have difficulty in understanding the patient. Words may be used by the patient which can be misinterpreted — 'sick', 'loose motions', 'heartburn', 'indigestion' — and it is essential that the doctor determines to his own satisfaction precisely what the patient means. The clinician should also appreciate that various 'inteference factors' can limit or disrupt his communication with the patient, for example impatience, irritation, fatigue and preoccupation with other matters. Patients who are depressed and withdrawn will not volunteer much information and the history will need to be extracted with patience and tolerance. At the other extreme is the loquacious hypermanic person who rambles. Occasionally an angry, aggressive patient is encountered and the clinician must respond calmly and with tolerance and attempt to determine the cause of the resentment.

It is impossible to obtain reliable information from a confused patient. Likewise no history is obtainable from the unconscious individual or the young child. Information from relatives, friends or bystanders is necessary and the source of such information, and the reason for it being obtained, must be recorded. If the patient should recover sufficiently to give a coherent history this is added to the case notes. Attempts should be made to interrogate by writing if the patient is deaf or aphasic.

When a patient is seen with a parent, spouse, or some other relation or friend, it is helpful to interrogate the patient with the help of his companion and then question each separately. This can be arranged easily while the patient is undressing. It may happen that the spouse or parent gives the history to the exclusion of the patient. This circumstance is noted and every effort should be made to question the patient on his own.

The clinician must be critical about accepting a patient's explanations and associations. Patients frequently seek an explanation for their symptoms and include this in their history as established facts. When difficulties are recounted about personal and particularly marital relationships it is necessary to be aware that only one side of the problem is being presented and it is helpful to hear the view of the other person involved before making a final judgement.

It may not be possible or prudent to undertake a comprehensive interview under all circumstances. It is unwise to spend much time in obtaining a detailed history when an ill patient with myocardial infarction is first seen; the details can be obtained later when the patient has recovered.

Doctors should beware of making comments like 'poor historian', 'unco-operative patient', or other such comments. While this may be a correct statement it is not uncommonly the case that an inexperienced clinician has been unable to establish rapport with his patient and that the fault lies as much with the doctor for not being tolerant and understanding as with the patient for being unhelpful.

Concluding the History

When it is clear that the patient has no further relevant information to impart he should be told that a physical examination will be undertaken. By this stage the clinician should have made some assessment of the patient's personality and anticipated his reactions to being examined: embarrassment, or fear. The patient is reassured as the case may be and instructed where to go and what clothes to remove.

THE PHYSICAL EXAMINATION

The physical examination is in some respect secondary to the history. Many diseases are diagnosed on the history alone and it is difficult to obtain the fullest information from a physical examination if no history has been obtained. This is partly because the history will indicate which body system is at fault and partly because after the history the clinician may have some idea of the diagnosis and therefore look for specific signs, for example, delayed relaxation of the reflexes in hypothyroidism or buccal pigmentation in Addison's disease.

Initial Impressions

Much information about the physical condition of the patient can be obtained while the patient is giving the medical history. An alert clinician will notice the gait of the patient as he enters the consulting room: spastic, ataxic, high-stepping or shuffling. While the patient talks it is possible to observe his manner, and actions. Speech defects should be apparent early on. Abnormalities of pigmentation, the presence of cyanosis, anaemia, and jaundice can be recognised. Such preliminary observations are particularly important in endocrine disorders because a more detailed examination of the body systems may not be obviously abnormal. A nervous, fidgeting, tremulous patient with prominent eyes will suggest hyperthyroidism; a dull, lethargic patient with a gruff voice should suggest hypothyroidism.

Physical Conditions of the Examination

The patient should be examined in a good light and under comfortable circumstances. The room should be warm, well ventilated and quiet. All patients are seen completely undressed except for a pair of briefs. Females should remove all their top garments; if they feel embarrassed they can wear their brassiere as long as this is removed to enable the breasts to be palpated and to permit an adequate examination of the chest and heart. The undressed patient is covered by a blanket. Patients may feel awkward on being asked to undress and the necessity for this will have to be explained. A polite, gentle and calm approach will be necessary to reassure the patient.

From the history the clinician will be aware of any physical disability of the patient who can then be placed in the most comfortable position. Although the ideal posture for the patient at the beginning of the examination is lying on the back at an angle of 45°, patients with dyspnoea may be more comfortable sitting upright, while pain in the hip may affect how the patient lies. During the examination a painful area must be anticipated and the examination made gently and with care. A clinician who unwittingly or unnecessarily hurts a patient may lose all chance of establishing a satisfactory relationship with that patient. Notwithstanding, every effort should be made to undertake a complete examination of an affected region.

Method of Examination

Despite the growing technology available to medical practitioners and the wealth of laboratory data to aid in the making of a diagnosis, the physical examination remains a fundamental technique for obtaining valuable data. The examination must be performed thoroughly and competently using correct techniques for examining systems and organs and eliciting physical signs. It is also necessary that the significance of a physical sign is appreciated; thus a palpable liver is not necessarily indicative of hepatomegaly, for it may be a normal liver displaced downwards by over-inflated lungs. The clinician must develop a method of examination which is both comprehensive and economical of time. His method should be applicable to all circumstances be it hospital or home. The approach and technique may differ from one clinician to another. The essential point is that by the end of the examination the patient has been examined adequately and no physical sign has been overlooked. As in the case of the history taking, so with the physical examination, circumstances may not permit a detailed examination, for example, the shocked patient who is admitted with a myocardial infarct. Under such circumstances the examination should be confined mainly to the system at fault and only vital functions of the other systems tested. These systems can and should be examined in greater detail once the patient has recovered. All clinicians should devise for themselves a form of examination which is rapid but not comprehensive and this usually means omitting a detailed examination of the respiratory and nervous systems. Chest radiographs are now universally obtainable. A neurological examination can be performed rapidly if attention is directed mainly to muscle power and reflexes but modalities of sensation and individual muscle function are evaluated only if the history indicates the need.

It is convenient to organise the technique of physical examination around systems: cardiovascular, respiratory, gastrointestinal, etc. Another way is to examine the patient by starting at the head and working down to the toes, disregarding the traditional body systems. Either method is reasonable, but there are advantages conceptually and diagnostically in examining according to systems. To make a physical examination by adhering strictly to a system approach can be time-consuming and it can be more economical of time and energy to adopt a compromise between the two extremes. The head and neck are examined, then the anterior chest, the posterior chest, the abdomen and then the nervous system and locomotor systems. Since it is important that the patient feels at ease it is helpful to commence the examination by examining the hands and pulse, the face and neck and the lymph glands. This can be done without the patient having to be uncovered.

The general technique for the examination of most systems, organs or lumps is by inspection, palpation, percussion and auscultation. The patient should always be viewed in a good light. Natural sunlight is preferable to artificial illumination particularly when trying to detect jaundice. It is frequently helpful to inspect an area from more than one position when, for example, a lump is being examined. Palpation is always as gentle as possible. In general it is preferable that all palpation is made with the tips or the pulps of the fingers or the palm of the hand, whether it be to feel for a mass, or to detect changes in skin temperature, or to feel for noises in the chest or a cardiac thrill. Percussion is undertaken by pressing the third (middle) finger of the left hand firmly against the skin. The finger is then struck either on the second phalanx or the terminal phalanx by the third (middle) finger of the right hand which is used as a hammer (Figure 1.2, a and b). The technique of effective percussion is to have the finger firmly pressed to skin and to use a free pendular action of the right wrist: the movement is not of the arm or of the finger. The examiner listens for the noise elicited by the percussion although much information can also be obtained from the vibrations transmitted to the percussed finger.

As a rule the physical examination is conducted most efficiently from the right-hand side of the couch. Left-handed clinicians occasionally find it more comfortable to examine from the left-hand side and certain modifications in examining technique become necessary, for example, palpating for the spleen. But the examiner should be prepared to examine the patient from more than one position. The chest movements are evaluated best by viewing the patient from the front; the neck can be examined from the front and back; the left ankle jerk is easier to elicit when standing on the left side of the patient than on the right.

In many situations, in either the hospital or surgery, it will be possible to have the patient's height, weight and temperature recorded and the urine examined before he is seen by the doctor. It is essential that the height, as well as the weight, of children is obtained. The body temperature can be obtained orally (from under the tongue), rectally or from the skin (axilla, groin or natal cleft). Rectal temperatures are the most reliable and are of particular value in hypothermic patients when special low reading thermometers are necessary. The rectal temperature is about 0.5°C higher than oral readings. Skin temperatures are about 0.5°C lower than oral ones, but unless taken carefully by leaving the thermometer in position for sufficient time they can be inaccurate. In most

situations the oral temperature is recorded. It is normally 37.0 ±
0.5°C. A diurnal range is present with the lower temperature
occurring in the morning.

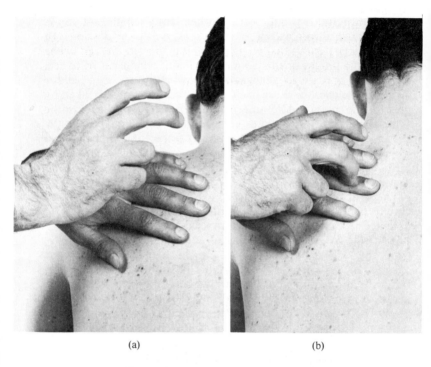

(a)   (b)

Figure 1.2, a and b. *Technique of percussion.*

General Assessment

The first step in the examination is to form an impression of how
acutely ill the patient is. This decision will determine the extent of
the initial examination. A decision may need to be taken at this
early stage regarding resuscitation and appropriate therapy. The
patient may be collapsed, shocked, weak and confused, pale in
appearance, sweating with cold cyanosed extremities. Dehydration
is recognised from a dry tongue, sunken eyes, and poor tissue

turgor. Postural hypotension, tachycardia and marked peripheral vasoconstriction are features of severe sodium depletion. These are relatively crude signs of salt or water depletion and usually become apparent after the loss of about four to six litres of body fluid and a sodium deficit of 650 to 1300 mmol. A general survey of the patient is made including the hands, arms, face, neck, limbs and trunk. Body habitus, nutrition, rashes, lumps and abnormal pulsations are noted. The general demeanour of the patient is observed and at this stage it is helpful to make a mental note whether the patient appears thyrotoxic, myxoedematous or parkinsonian.

Head and face

During the history there will have been the opportunity to observe various cranial and facial features. A large head is seen in hydrocephalus and in Paget's disease (Figure 1.3); frontal bossing is a feature of rickets. The colour of the face depends on many factors

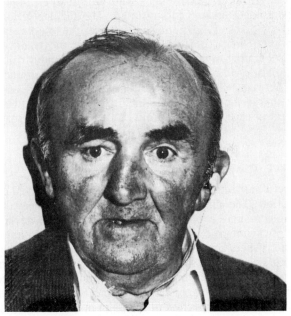

Figure 1.3. *Paget's disease of the skull.*

including racial pigment, ultraviolet tanning, capillary tone and haemoglobin level. Facial pallor should be distinguished clearly from anaemia which is detected best by looking at the conjunctiva. Conjunctival pallor is seen when the haemoglobin is reduced below 9 g per 100 ml. The colour also depends upon whether the haemoglobin is oxygenated or reduced. Normally arterial oxygen saturation is 97 per cent; when this falls below 80 per cent the blue colour of cyanosis may be apparent. An adequate haemoglobin concentration is necessary to recognise cyanosis which will not occur at haemoglobin levels below 5 g per 100 ml. Other factors which will influence skin colour include bilirubin (jaundice, yellow colour), carotinaemia (yellow discoloration), uraemia (light brown 'muddy' colour), carboxyhaemoglobin (bright pink colour) and methaemoglobin and sulphaemoglobin (blue colour).

An overall impression can be made of obesity. Tables are available as a guide to ideal weight judged according to sex, age and height; measurements of skin fold thickness can be made with calipers. For general purposes most clinicians rely on a visual impression of excess subcutaneous fat. Abnormal distribution of adipose tissue occurs in Cushing's syndrome or when large doses of corticosteroid drugs are administered. The fat deposition occurs particularly on the face ('moon face'), over the lower cervical and thoracic vertebrae ('buffalo hump') and on the trunk. Loss of weight is a feature of many disease states and probably results from a combination of poor diet, malabsorption, and altered metabolism. Diseases characteristically accompanied by weight loss include thyrotoxicosis, diabetes mellitus, pulmonary tuberculosis, malignant disease, and the various causes of fat malabsorption.

Hands and feet

The careful inspection of the hands provides a great deal of useful information. The shape is altered in acromegaly where the hands broaden to assume a 'spade-like' appearance; ulnar deviation is a feature of rheumatoid arthritis; arachnodactyly is seen in Marfan's syndrome. There may be swellings on the fingers from gout or Heberden's nodes. The small muscles of the hand may be wasted as part of a generalised wasting state, but when the wasting is confined to the hands alone it suggests a neurological or myopathic disorder or disuse atrophy. Inspection of the palm may reveal a contracture of the palmar fascia with flexion deformity of the fourth and fifth fingers known as Dupuytren's contracture. Palmar erythema is a mottled red discoloration of the thenar and hypothenar eminence occurring in liver disease, rheumatoid arthritis, thyrotoxicosis and pregnancy. The appearance must be distinguished from the normal pink homogeneous palmar flush often seen in states of vasodilatation.

The nails are inspected for general shape, contour and condition. There is marked variation in the shape of the nails. The nails may be misshapen from biting or breaking. They may be discoloured from dirt or from cigarette smoke. Fungal infection results in thickened, discoloured nails; psoriasis affecting the nails is recognised by pitting and pigmented dystrophy. Fine white streaks or blotches on the nail are a common finding in normal people and thought to indicate previous trauma to the nail. In iron deficiency the nail may show longitudinal ridging and increased brittleness while in severe deficiency the nail assumes a spoon shape: koilonychia.

White nails (leuconychia) are a feature of chronic liver disease and are related to hypoalbuminaemia. White bands across the nail are a consequence of severe acute illness. Small, linear, 'splinter' haemorrhages under the nails occur in infective endocarditis although they may occur in normal people, probably as a result of minor trauma.

Clubbing of the fingers and toes is an important index of disease. The nail bed becomes thickened and boggy which is appreciated by palpating the nail bed to elicit fluctuation. The finger to be tested is held between the thumb and the third finger while the index finger is used to palpate the skin over the base of the nail (Figure 1.4). Normally only slight fluctuation is present; a tendency for the tissue to feel springy, boggy or fluctuant is the feature of clubbing. Not all the fingers may show clubbing initially. The other characteristic of clubbing is filling-in and obliteration of the angle between the nail and the nail bone. The overlying skin appears shiny and red. The curvature of the nail along both the longitudinal and lateral axis is more marked, producing a beaked or clubbed appearance. In gross cases the fingers are thickened and the finger pulp hypertrophied; the appearance resembles that of a drum-stick (Figure 1.5).

A tremor of the outstretched hands is a feature of many neurological and metabolic disorders: flapping tremor in portasystemic encephalopathy, fine tremor in thyrotoxicosis, coarse tremor in chronic alcoholism and in the elderly.

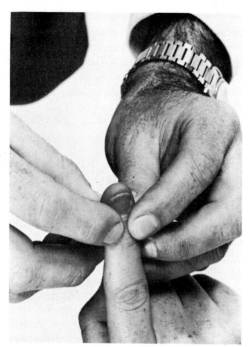

Figure 1.4. *Examination of clubbing of fingers.*

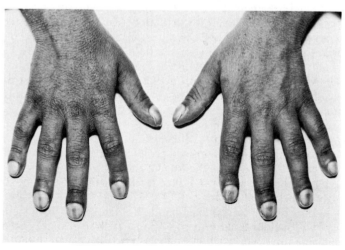

Figure 1.5. *Appearance of clubbing.*

Examination of a lump

Most lumps in the body can be examined according to a general scheme. The procedures of inspection, palpation, percussion and auscultation are used, but in addition one or two other techniques are employed. The information should be recorded according to the following scheme.

Site. The exact position is described with reference to adjacent structures. Any attachment to skin, muscle, bone or other structures is recorded. A comment is made as to whether the mass is fixed or mobile.

Size. The dimensions of the lump are measured and recorded in centimetres, the measurement being along the horizontal and vertical axis. If it is not possible to make a precise measurement, for example if the mass is intra-abdominal or in the pelvis, either an approximate measurement is given or the lump is described in terms of common objects: the size of a grape, walnut, golf ball, orange, tennis ball, melon, football. Such descriptions, while being vivid, are no substitute for accurate measurements.

Shape. The mass is described as being round, oval or irregular.

Surface. The surface may be smooth or irregular. The lump may be nodular, and the nodules are small or large. The surface characteristics of intra-abdominal masses may be difficult to determine depending upon the thickness and granularity of the adipose tissue on the anterior abdominal wall.

Sensitivity. A lump may be tender or non-tender. Many benign tumours are non-tender whereas most inflammatory masses are tender.

Temperature. A mass may feel warm, which suggests an inflammatory cause, although rapidly growing malignant lumps can also cause an increase in the skin temperature because of new vessel formation, increased blood supply and vasodilatation. The overlying skin may look reddened. Vascular anomalies may feel warm.

Margins. Benign tumours generally have well-defined margins separating the mass from the surrounding tissue. This is often not the case with inflammatory and malignant lumps.

Consistency. A swelling may be hard or soft and there are varying degrees of firmness. The commonly used descriptions are: bony, hard, firm, rubbery, soft and fluctuant. Fluctuation is elicited by placing both forefingers on the mass and pressing with one finger. If the lump is fluctuant an impulse will be felt by the other finger. Alternatively the mass is felt between finger and thumb and indented by the forefinger. Fluctuation should be detected in two places before it is considered to be present. While fluctuation is usually indicative of fluid, some very soft tumours such as fibromas or even neurofibromas may be fluctuant.

Pulsation. Some tumours pulsate. If the mass pulsates in all directions it is regarded as demonstrating direct or expansile pulsation which is indicative of a mass involving blood vessels, for example, an aneurysm. Pulsation in one plane only is evidence of transmitted pulsation and suggests that the mass is abutting upon a large blood vessel, for example, a retroperitoneal mass. However, an aneurysm may be filled with blood clot and may not show direct pulsation.

Percussion. This is generally of limited value. A resonant note indicates an air-filled mass, for example a distended stomach or loop of bowel.

Auscultation. A variety of sounds may be heard when listening over a lump.
Murmurs. A systolic murmur may be detected over vascular benign or malignant tumours. Another vascular noise to be detected is a venous hum which is a soft continuous low-pitched humming noise. Despite an increased blood supply it is unusual for inflammatory masses to be accompanied by a bruit. Characteristically a venous hum or a systolic murmur can be heard over large vascular thyroid glands. Primary and secondary tumours of the liver may be associated with either a systolic murmur or a venous hum.
Friction. Intra-abdominal masses may incite a peritoneal inflammatory reaction which results in the production of a friction sound, or rub. A coarse, rough, grating sound is heard over the area on deep breathing. A friction rub may be heard over a very large spleen when it indicates splenic infarction, and occasionally over an enlarged liver. A rub may be heard in plastic peritonitis.

Other sounds to be heard include bowel sounds in hernias and the fetal heart beat in a gravid uterus.

Transillumination. By placing a torch against the mass and shining the light it is possible to detect whether the mass transluminates. Transillumination is a characteristic of fluid-containing lumps, although milky fluid transluminates poorly and blood-filled masses not at all; some lipomas may show transillumination. The sign is helpful in scrotal swellings: a hydrocele transluminates but not a testicular tumour. But a testicular tumour may be present in association with a hydrocele.

The documentation of a swelling is aided by an appropriate diagram (Figure 1.6).

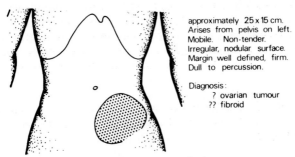

approximately 25 x 15 cm.
Arises from pelvis on left.
Mobile.   Non-tender.
Irregular, nodular surface.
Margin well defined, firm.
Dull to percussion.

Diagnosis :
       ? ovarian tumour
      ?? fibroid

Figure 1.6. *Description of a lump.*

CONCLUDING THE INTERVIEW

Once the examination has been completed the patient is instructed to dress and the interview is ended by the clinician explaining the outcome of the examination and what further steps are required. This is a very important stage of the interview. The patient will be anxious or curious and failure to explain the nature of the illness, or the procedures planned or the treatment required, can lead to much misunderstanding and even ill-feeling in the future. The patient is given the opportunity to ask questions and the replies should be as frank and explicit as possible. The continued co-operation of the patient is essential, particularly when the management of the illness is tedious or trying. It is at this initial stage of the doctor—patient contact that a healthy rapport is established which will support the relationship during difficult periods in the future.

TECHNIQUE OF RECORDING THE INTERVIEW

The interview may be recorded in a variety of ways. The most commonly used method is to write down an abstract of what the patient has said and what has been found on physical examination. To do this properly requires training. Handwriting must be legible and sufficient detail must be included to describe the symptoms and signs clearly and provide an indication for subsequent decisions. One of the difficulties with this time-honoured technique is that the clinician is only half-concentrating on the patient, frequently glancing away from the patient to his notes. Patients find this disconcerting and it can have the effect of disturbing the free flow of thought and words. However, with experience it is possible to record the essential features of the history without disturbing the patient or inhibiting the development of rapport.

Another technique is to make only brief notes during the history taking and at a later stage rewrite these in a more detailed form. This ensures a comprehensive history but is excessively time-consuming. The method may be used to advantage by those learning the technique of recording the interview. The use of tape recorders ensures a verbatim record of the interview but is not generally applicable to clinical medicine.

Although the student may find it helpful to record the physical findings during the examination, with a little experience it is possible to complete the examination and then write the record. Since the physical examination is on more formal lines than the history it is generally easier to remember and record the findings after the examination. Many institutions use detailed structured case sheets and these have the advantage that they can serve as a guide to what must be examined.

THE RELIABILITY OF CLINICAL METHODS

It must be recognised that the clinical examination is a relatively unreliable method of obtaining data. Agreement between physicians over the ability to elicit physical signs has not been subjected to intensive study but it appears that there is a greater agreement rate between physicians the more normal the subjects are. Agreement over what is normal is usually easier than agreement over abnormality. Of even greater importance is the necessity to establish the reliability of many of the accepted signs in clinical medicine. There can be dispute over the character of a systolic murmur; studies have shown that considerable errors are made in the clinical assessment of prostatic size. Such information that is available gives little cause for complacency. Ways of increasing the reliability of the clinical data include a clearer definition of terminology, careful attention to examination techniques and methods of recording data, and avoidance of patient and physician fatigue.

MAKING THE DIAGNOSIS

It is essential that once the clinical examination has been completed a diagnosis or differential diagnosis (when a choice of two or more diseases is offered) is formulated as a basis for therapeutic decisions and to offer some prediction of the outcome of the illness. There are two stages, first the initial differential diagnosis, selected according to the clinical presentation, which serves as the basis for ordering various radiological and laboratory tests and for initiating therapy; and second the final diagnosis (which may include more than one disease), which takes into account the history, physical examination, laboratory data and clinical course. The importance of the medical history has been emphasised. A critical evaluation must be made of the data base and this requires learning, training and intelligence.

The diagnostic process can be represented in the following way:

Acquisition of data → Analysis of data → Therapeutic decisions
↓
are the data accurate?
↓
what is the problem?
↓
what is the cause?

Reliability of data implies reliability of the observations and not how they may be interpreted. For example:

History   : crushing retrosternal
                 pain   reliable
              dyspnoea   reliable

Examination	: tachycardia	reliable
	cardiomegaly	unreliable — observer error
	gallop rhythm	unreliable — observer error
	basal crackles	reliable
Radiology	: pulmonary oedema	reliable
Cardiograph	: S-T elevation over anterior chest leads	reliable
Laboratory	: Normal aspartate transaminase	unreliable — timing of blood sample

What is the problem? : chest pain
left-sided heart failure
pulmonary oedema

What is the cause? : acute anterior myocardial infarction

The experienced clinician will not be satisfied with this as the endpoint in the diagnostic exercise but will ask the further question 'Why should this particular patient sustain an infarct?', thereby setting in train a further diagnostic exercise.

The human mind analyses large amounts of data with difficulty and is not always impartial in selecting and evaluating information, being readily influenced by the most recent or outstanding clinical experience. The doctor sets about making a differential diagnosis by selecting from those diseases about which he has learnt. The less skilled clinician will compile a long list of diseases, many of which will not relate closely to the individual patient or his environment. The more useful and meaningful approach is to use the Bayesian or probabilistic method, in which an estimate is made of the probabilities of any one disease being responsible and on this basis a list is drawn up. This requires a thorough knowledge of disease and an appreciation of the incidence of different diseases in a particular community or environment. For example the differential diagnosis of bloody diarrhoea presenting in a native Scot who has not lived abroad would be ulcerative colitis, Crohn's disease and cancer of the colon, whereas a similar complaint in a patient residing in southern Africa would have *Shigella* dysentery or amoebiasis as likely causes.

The final diagnosis should include a statement about the physical illness, an appraisal of the emotional state and the patient's reaction to his illness, and an evaluation of the patient's social circumstances.

Problem-Orientated Medical Records

Weed (1970) has emphasised the advantages of compiling a list of problems on the basis of the clinical examination. The data in the record are organised not in terms of a diagnosis but rather around the various problems to which they pertain. In this way it is suggested that clinical notes can become structured, dynamic and comprehensive; they serve not only to aid medical care but also as a method of teaching. Furthermore such carefully structured notes should facilitate independent observations being made on how decision-making was achieved during the management of a patient. Thus problem-orientated medical records facilitate the introduction of some form of medical review or audit in the training of doctors.

Four basic elements in the medical record are recognised and the notes are organised around these.

1. The data base. Present, past and social history, physical examination and laboratory reports.

2. The problem list. By problems are meant medical or social difficulties as appreciated by the doctor or the patient. The list is not one of diagnoses. The problems are grouped as active and inactive or resolved.

3. The initial plan. This is a list of diagnostic procedures and therapeutic steps to be undertaken.

4. Progress notes. The progress notes should be related to the active problems and should contain the following elements:
  (i) subjective data
  (ii) objective data
  (iii) interpretation
  (iv) treatment
  (v) immediate plans.

5. Flow sheets. The use of a flow sheet enables data, particularly from the laboratory, to be maintained in an orderly and readily retrievable form.

6. Discharge summary. This is organised around the problem list.

This system has many advantages. It is not dependent on or restricted by a system of disease taxonomy; it lends itself to teaching and medical audit and if properly used should facilitate recall of information. On the other hand if care is not taken the notes can become lengthy, requiring much desk-time from the doctor and reducing the potential for information retrieval.

The traditional system of formulating a diagnosis or differential diagnosis and basing investigations and treatment accordingly has much to recommend it. There are advantages in thinking in terms of morbid anatomical or psychiatric diagnosis. The clinician in making the diagnosis and arranging patient care knowingly or unknowingly goes through the many steps which are clearly designated under the problem-orientated system. The many discussions and publications relating to the problem-orientated system have been to the benefit of those who wish to retain the traditional diagnostic approach, for they have emphasised the various aspects which should be covered when arriving at a diagnosis and planning subsequent management.

Whichever system is used, the traditional or the problem-orientated, the fundamentals of a good medical record depend upon the accuracy of the information which it contains, the clarity with which the information is expressed, the orderly organisation of the record around the symptoms, or diseases, or problems which are being treated and the careful recording of progress involving each facet of the clinical picture.

Once decisions are taken about management these are recorded in the notes. It may be that a series of blood tests and radiological investigations are required; these are listed in the notes. All treatment ordered is recorded together with what explanation and advice have been offered to the patient.

CASE RECORDS

The regular, accurate and tidy documentation of medical decisions and patient progress is essential to proper medical care. Adequate case records must be maintained for all patients whether they be seen in the ward, the outpatient clinic or the doctor's consulting room. The follow-up notes should give an account of the evolution of the patient's illness, new problems which have developed, management decisions taken and what information has been given to the patient.

A summary of the patient's illness is made at the time of discharge from hospital. This is a useful occasion to scrutinise the illness and the management in a critical way and can serve as an important learning experience.

Medical records are confidential documents. They may contain statements which could be embarrassing or alarming to the patient. An adequate history, and particularly a psychiatric interview, will inevitably contain confidences of the patient. Such information is relevant, valuable and should be recorded. It is essential that this information is respected, the privacy of the patient guaranteed and the confidentiality of the interview upheld.

SCHEME FOR THE RECORDING OF THE CLINICAL EXAMINATION

Name	Age	Record number
	Sex	Marital status
Address		Telephone number
Name of family doctor		Next of kin
Date of admission		Date of discharge

Present History

A chronological account of all the major symptoms.

Systemic enquiry

Cardiovascular system: pain, dyspnoea, orthopnoea, syncope, fatigue, oedema, palpitations, cramps, paraesthesia and changes in colour of legs and feet.

Respiratory system: cough, sputum, haemoptysis, dyspnoea, pain, wheeze.

Abdomen and renal: sore mouth, tongue, dysphagia, appetite, weight loss, bowel habit, stools, vomiting, pain, jaundice, pattern of micturition day/night, dribbling, retention, dysuria, appearance of urine, haematuria, loin pain.

Metabolic and endocrine: weight, hair distribution, growth and development.

Menstrual history: age of menarche, number of days and estimate of amount of bleeding, length of cycle, last menstrual period, intermittent bleeding, dysmenorrhoea, premenstrual tension, age of menopause, postmenopausal bleeding, vaginal discharge.

Locomotor system: pain, stiffness, swelling, locking of a joint.

Skin: rashes, pigmentation, pruritus, lumps.

Blood: colour, bleeding, bruising.

Nervous system: headache, vision, diplopia, hearing, tinnitus, vertigo, taste, smell, speech, alterations in consciousness, faints, fits, involuntary movements, weakness, paraesthesia, sphincter control.

Psychiatric: preoccupation and worries, altered mood state, insomnia, memory disturbance, recent life-changes, stresses.

Past History

Childhood illnesses, immunisations, accidents, allergies, medical, surgical and obstetric events.

Drug History

Current and previous drug therapy response, adverse reactions.

Personal and Social History

Diet, smoking and alcohol habits, occupation, previous occupation, recreation, housing, financial state, relationship within the family and at work, social support. Visits to other countries.

Family History

Account of health, illnesses and deaths of the spouse, children, parents, siblings and other relevant family members.

History about an infant or child

Antenatal information: health of mother during pregnancy.

Natal: character of labour.

Neonatal: cry, colour, flaccidity, gestational age, birth weight, jaundice, transfusions.

Later life: feeding, infection, immunisation, development.

Physical Examination

General assessment

How ill is the patient, shock, dehydration, presence of pain.

Height, weight, temperature.

Nutritional status, skeletal deformities.

Appearance of head, face, mouth, ears.

Appearance of eyes: exophthalmos, squint, pallor, redness, jaundice.
Examination of neck: thyroid, trachea, neck veins.
Examination of skin, hands, nails.
Lymph nodes: cervical, supraclavicular, axillary, epitrochlear, inguinal, femoral, abdominal.
Examination of breasts.
Examination of any specific lumps.
Presence of oedema.

Cardiovascular system

Pulse: feel bilaterally for temporal, carotid, radial, brachial, femoral, popliteal, dorsalis pedis and posterior tibial. At the radial record rate, rhythm, volume, character and condition of vessel wall.
Blood pressure: lying, standing.
Venous pressure: height, character of waves.
Praecordium: Inspection: deformities, dilated vessels, impulses.
　　　　　　　Palpation: site and character of apex beat, other impulses, thrills.
　　　　　　　Percussion: cardiac dullness, other dullness.
　　　　　　　Auscultation: at mitral, tricuspid, pulmonary, aortic and other areas. Record heart sounds, other sounds, murmurs, friction sound.

Respiratory system

Presence of clubbing, cyanosis, nature of breathing.
Appearance of sputum.
Inspection: shape and movements of chest.
Palpation: position of trachea, apex beat, chest movements, vocal, fremitus.
Percussion: character of note, area of cardiac dullness, upper border of liver dullness, other dullness.
Auscultation: breath sounds, voice sounds, adventitious sounds.

Abdomen

Inspection: teeth, tongue, gums, scars, distension, veins, hernias, discoloration, masses, movements, faeces.
Palpation }liver, spleen, kidney, stomach, bowel, bladder, other masses.
Percussion
Rectal examination: inspection of anus, digital examination.

Metabolic and endocrine

Appearance of body habitus.
Relative proportions of limbs and trunk.
Pigmentation, distribution of hair.
Examination of eyes.
Chvostek's sign, Trousseau's sign.
Secondary sexual characteristics.
Scrotum: penis, testis, spermatic cord.
Vaginal examination: inspection of vulva, digital examination of vagina, cervix, uterus and ovaries.

Locomotor system

Ears, feet and hands for gouty tophi.
Movements, tenderness, swelling involving: shoulder, elbow, wrist, hands, fingers, hip, knee, ankle, feet.
Test for active and passive movements.
Spine.

Nervous system

Mental state: orientation, emotional state, personality, intellectual functions.
Speech: dysphasia, dysarthria.
Agnosia and apraxia: tactile, visual and auditory agnosia.
Neck stiffness

Cranial nerves:		
I	:	sense of smell.
II	:	visual acuity, visual fields; examination of optic fundus.
III IV VI }	:	external and internal muscles of the eye.
V	:	sensation on face, masseter muscles.
VII	:	facial movements.
VIII	:	hearing, vestibular function. Weber and Rinne tests.
IX X }	:	palate, gag reflex, swallowing.
XI	:	trapezius and sternomastoid.
XII	:	movements of tongue.

Motor functions: gait, muscle tone, coordination, power.

Reflexes: *Tendon reflexes:* biceps, supinator, triceps, finger flexion, knee, ankle.

Superficial reflexes: abdominal, cremasteric, gluteal, anal, plantar.

Primitive reflexes: sucking, Moro, grasp, tonic neck reflex.

Involuntary movements: tics and habit spasms, myoclonus, tremor, chorea, athetosis.

Sensation: pain, touch, temperature, position, vibration, cortical sensation.

Psychiatric aspects of mental state

Behaviour and demeanour
Form of speech
Mood state
Preoccupations and content of thought
Abnormal perceptions and sensations
Cognitive functions
Insight and attitudes to illness

Blood

Bruising, petechiae, bleeding, haemarthrosis, soft tissue haematomas, lymph nodes. Haemoglobin, haematocrit, white blood count, differential count, blood smear, erythrocyte sedimentation rate.

Urinalysis

Appearance of urine.
Chemical analysis: protein, sugar, ketones, bilirubin, urobilin, porphyrins, blood.
Microscopy: white cells, red cells, casts, crystals.

Summary of Findings

Diagnosis or Differential Diagnosis (or Problem List)

Physical
Psychological/psychiatric
Social

Investigations Ordered

Therapy

Patient Information

Progress Notes

Final Diagnosis and Discharge Summary

FURTHER READING

Engel, G. L. & Morgan, W. L. Jr (1973) *Interviewing the Patient.* London: W. B. Saunders.

Feinstein, A. R. (1973) The problems of the problem-oriented medical record. *Annals of Internal Medicine,* **78,** 751-762.

Koran, L. M. (1975) The reliability of clinical methods, data and judgments. *New England Journal of Medicine,* **293,** 642-646, 695-701.

Weed, L. L. (1969) *Medical Records, Medical Education and Patient Care.* Chicago: Chicago Year Book Medical Publishers.

Wright, H. J. & Macadam, D. B. (1979) *Clinical Thinking and Practice.* Edinburgh: Churchill Livingstone.

Wulff, H. R. (1976) *Rational Diagnosis and Treatment.* London: Blackwell Scientific Publications.

2 The Cardiovascular System
D. Emslie-Smith

THE HEART

A patient can have severe cardiovascular disease, for example, aortic valve disease, malignant hypertension or even myocardial infarction, and yet have no symptoms until a late stage. The four most significant symptoms of heart disease are *dyspnoea, chest pain, palpitations* and *syncope.* Some symptoms are interpreted wrongly by the patient as being due to heart disease and it is essential that he should be asked very carefully about the details of his symptoms, using direct questions, and often demanding in answer a straight 'yes' or 'no'. Direct questions should not be confused with leading questions, which are couched in a form that suggests to the patient that he should answer in a particular way.

HISTORY

Dyspnoea

Shortness of breath is the commonest symptom of heart disease. However, many patients with no heart disease complain of dyspnoea because of pulmonary disease, or because they are describing as 'breathlessness' some other abnormality of respiration. When a patient complains of breathlessness it is very helpful to ask him to demonstrate how he breathes when he feels breathless. The demonstration may show at once whether the breathing suggests cardiac dyspnoea, which resembles the physiological hyper-ventilation after exercise, or the shallow hyperventilation or occasional deep sigh of anxiety. This deep sighing respiration is sometimes described by patients in curiously stereotyped terms such as 'I can't seem to get a satisfactory breath', or 'I don't seem to get to the bottom of it'.

Cardiac dyspnoea is associated with an increased amount of blood in the lungs as a result of failure of the left side of the heart, usually of the left ventricle but sometimes, as in mitral stenosis, of the left atrium. It is thought that the increased volume of blood in the lungs reduces its compliance and that the sensation of breath-lessness is related to the increased effort needed to expand abnormally rigid lungs. Because cardiac dyspnoea is a symptom of left-sided cardiac failure it is more severe during increased cardiac work, for example physical exercise.

It is possible to grade dyspnoea, and a four-point scale of severity has been introduced. This commonly used method of grading dyspnoea has some drawbacks: for example, some patients with mitral stenosis may have no breathlessness on exertion but may have acute pulmonary oedema, precipitated perhaps by the onset of atrial fibrillation or of tachycardia during pregnancy. Such patients do not easily fit into the grading system and it is probably more realistic to grade a patient's dyspnoea by recording just what he can or cannot do without becoming breathless. The question 'What have you had to give up doing?' is often useful. If the physician is unable to decide clearly by talking to the patient whether he has exertional dyspnoea he should go with him for a short walk, preferably upstairs. Many hospitals have flights of stairs whose use as the basis of readily available exercise tolerance tests is often neglected.

When a patient is breathless at rest the dyspnoea is often worse on lying down, possibly because the descent of the diaphragm is impeded. It is important therefore to ask patients how many pillows they use at night. If a patient has to be propped up to be comfortable the dyspnoea is described as *orthopnoea*. The patient should be asked directly whether he ever wakes up breathless during the night. If so, he should be asked about all the circum-stances, for in *paroxysmal nocturnal dyspnoea* the patient is wakened with the intense breathlessness of *pulmonary oedema*, often accompanied by wheezing *(cardiac asthma)*. He is usually forced to sit up and often gets out of bed and walks about. He may even go to a window and throw it open for fresh air. This behaviour tends to shift blood from the lungs to the legs and feet and so relieves the pulmonary oedema and the dyspnoea.

The patient should also be asked whether he has a *cough* because pulmonary oedema insufficient to cause obvious dyspnoea is sometimes responsible for a short dry irritating cough, especially on exertion. If the patient admits to a cough he should be asked whether he coughs up *sputum* and if so what it is like. Purulent sputum can occur in the chronic bronchitis associated with anoxic pulmonary heart disease but also with the winter bronchitis of mitral stenosis. Four kinds of *haemoptysis* are associated with heart disease, and all four can be present at different stages of mitral stenosis.

1. When pulmonary oedema is unrelieved the alveoli and airways fill with a pale pink frothy exudate, which may well spill out from the nose and mouth. This is usually a terminal event.

2. A few red streaks in a purulent or mucopurulent sputum are common in winter bronchitis, which occurs particularly in mitral stenosis.

3. Occasionally, rather early in the natural history of mitral stenosis, patients can have quite a large haemoptysis of fresh blood ('pulmonary apoplexy'). This may be the result of rupture of bronchopulmonary anastomoses in the lung and it resembles the brisk haemoptysis of cavitating pulmonary tuberculosis.

4. Patients confined to bed may develop phlebothromboses in the legs or pelvis. Thromboembolism may then cause pulmonary infarction with the production of the characteristic sputum, at first red homogeneous clots which later darken to a brownish colour.

Chest Pain

There are many causes of *retrosternal pain*; it is therefore most important to decide whether pain is the result of cardiac ischaemia. *Cardiac ischaemic pain* is felt either as *angina pectoris* or else as the similar, but longer lasting pain of *myocardial infarction*.

There are four aspects of cardiac ischaemic pain that help to characterise it: the site, the quality and the duration of the pain, and its relation to cardiac work.

Site. Cardiac ischaemic pain is most often felt behind the midsternum in a diffuse area that may be covered by a fist. It also occurs across the whole of the front of the chest. It may radiate to one or other shoulder, more often the left, and down the inner border of one or other, or both arms, more usually the left, as far as the elbow or even to the wrist or finger tips. It may also radiate up either one or both sides of the neck and into the lower jaw, sometimes being felt in the gums. It radiates less frequently to the back and down into the epigastrium. The pain may not present in all these sites simultaneously; for example it most commonly starts behind the sternum and only later spreads to other sites. Again, when these other sites are involved the pain may be felt there as distinct from that behind the sternum; thus a patient may feel retrosternal pain and a separate pain in the left shoulder radiating a little down the inside of the left arm. Sometimes the pain begins in a peripheral site such as the arm and then spreads up the arm to the shoulder, only later to be felt substernally ('reversed angina').

The diffuse distribution of the pain is important in diagnosis. A patient should be asked to point to the pain. If he can localise it with a finger tip it is not cardiac ischaemic pain. When asked to indicate its site patients very often place a clenched fist in front of the sternum or grip their chest with both hands. These characteristic gestures give information not only about the localisation of the pain but also about its character.

Duration. Unless the patient has had a cardiac infarction the duration of cardiac ischaemic pain (angina) is minutes, not moments or seconds. The patient should be asked the direct question 'If you stop when you get the pain, how long does it take to go away?'. If he answers in terms of minutes he should then be asked whether this refers to 'minutes by his watch' or whether he really means 'moments'. If the answer is, for example, 'Just two or three seconds, I suppose', the pain is most unlikely to be angina, which lasts two to three minutes.

Quality. It is extraordinarily difficult to describe the character of pain, and the more articulate and introspective the patient the more difficult this seems to be. The patient should be asked 'What sort of pain is it?' or 'What does the pain feel like?' It is surprising, and most useful for the clinician, that the character of cardiac ischaemic pain is so frequently described in terms such as 'gripping', 'crushing', 'squeezing' or 'tight'. Occasionally, of course, the pain is described in other ways, such as 'burning'. Intelligent and articulate patients may sometimes deny it is actually pain but describe it as intolerably severe discomfort, but the 'discomfort' is still described by the adjectives mentioned.

Relation to cardiac work. Cardiac ischaemic pain comes *during* increased cardiac work and not after it; thus angina is felt during exercise and not after the exercise has been completed. While a common cause of increased cardiac work is physical exertion, another common cause is tachycardia, caused by strong emotion or dysrhythmia. The term 'cardiac ischaemic pain on effort' for angina tends to make the student forget tachycardia as an important cause. Common conditions in which emotion can lead to angina occur while watching an exciting football match or other sporting event, either on the spot or while sitting quietly at home watching the event on television. Such cardiac work reduces filling of the ventricles during shortened diastole, causing an impaired cardiac output and reducing coronary blood flow.

It is, however, during exercise that angina is usually felt. First of all it may only be felt on fairly severe exercise but as the coronary blood flow becomes increasingly restricted the angina occurs after less exertion. Thus at the start it may often be felt only on climbing stairs or walking up a steep hill against the wind, but later may occur even when the patient is walking quite quietly along the flat. Cold weather and a full stomach bring it on more readily. Often a patient who walks to work knows exactly how far he can go before the pain appears, and as time goes on he may find that this distance diminishes. The patient cannot 'walk off' the pain. He is forced to stop because of its increasing and intolerable severity. This enforced stop may be embarrassing for him and he may disguise it, for example by looking into a shop window. Often, of course, the pain is accompanied by dyspnoea; sometimes the dyspnoea comes before the pain, sometimes the pain begins before the breathlessness.

Angina may occur with the first exertion of the day, and when the patient recovers after resting, it does not return again unless much more exercise is taken ('second-wind angina'). For example a golfer may feel it on the first green, but then be able to complete 18 holes without another attack ('first-hole angina').

For some reason cardiac ischaemic pain is sometimes relieved by belching and by the ingestion of alkalis. This encourages the patient's hope that he has indigestion. Rapid relief from angina is often produced by a trinitrin tablet allowed to dissolve under the tongue. The effect of trinitrin is rapid and the pain disappears earlier than it would otherwise do. If a patient says that trinitrin tablets help his pain but that it takes about ten minutes, either the pain is not angina or that particular trinitrin tablet is not effective.

Cardiac ischaemic pain does not always have the characteristic four features, but if three of them are present the diagnosis is highly probable, even in the rare 'variant angina' that comes during rest. It cannot be stressed too strongly that the diagnosis of cardiac ischaemic pain is made by taking a careful history. A patient may have angina without any physical signs, and with a normal electro-cardiogram and a normal cardiac silhouette on x-ray.

The pain of cardiac ischaemia arises in the same way as the pain of an ischaemic skeletal muscle exercised beyond the point where metabolites are removed by perfusion of blood (see section on intermittent claudication). The typical sites of radiation are still quite unexplained.

Myocardial infarction

The pain of *myocardial infarction* is typical cardiac ischaemic pain but the duration is much longer than two or three minutes and it may occur at rest. It can last for hours or several days. It is often accompanied by other symptoms about which specific enquiries should be made. They are dyspnoea, sweating, faintness, vomiting, and a feeling of fear — perhaps even fear of death. Patients rarely complain spontaneously of fear but will readily answer 'Yes' when asked 'Were you frightened?'.

Other forms of cardiovascular pain

The pain of a *dissecting aneurysm of the aorta* can be very similar to that of cardiac infarction. It is usually very severe and sometimes radiates to the back, loins or other sites unusual in myocardial infarction. It may be accompanied by transient obliteration or inequality of peripheral pulses or by changing neurological signs from involvement of vasa nervorum. When the dissection proceeds backwards towards the aortic sinuses the coronary ostia themselves may become occluded and genuine myocardial infarction can complicate the clinical picture. The pain of *pericarditis* is often a dull ache in the retrosternal region that may sometimes be influenced by respiration. It is sometimes accompanied by referred pain at the tip of the left shoulder, although, compared with angina, the pain is sharp and feels rather superficial. An *aneurysm of the thoracic aorta* may erode the bone of the vertebrae or sternum, causing severe pain, sometimes described as 'boring', and said to be worse during the night.

Chest-wall pain

Many patients who may think they have heart disease have pain in the chest that is quite different from cardiac ischaemic pain. It is often localised to a very small area and the patient may be able to point to it with one finger. It is frequently felt as a stab or a series of jabs 'like a knife'. In between stabs there may be a long-continued dull ache in the region or more diffusely round about it. Careful palpation of the muscles in the intercostal spaces and more superficially in the chest wall may identify points of extreme tenderness accurately localised at or near the site of the pain. Sometimes, when the examiner 'springs' the xiphoid cartilage, the patient experiences acute pain resembling the one he experiences spontaneously. Similarly, pressure on a single costosternal joint may be found to cause the pain. These types of 'chest-wall pain' are very common and naturally cause much anxiety. However, cardiac neurosis itself seems to be associated with jabbing pain, localised to one spot very often near the apex beat, where the patient thinks his heart lies. It has none of the characteristics of cardiac ischaemic pain and the patient's complaint of breathlessness, when analysed by careful questioning, is often shown to consist of the deep sighs of anxiety.

Other causes of retrosternal pain

Retrosternal pain that may mimic that of a cardiac infarction can be produced by oesophageal disease, and spondylosis of the lowest cervical and upper thoracic spine. A massive pulmonary embolism may cause severe retrosternal pain associated with collapse, dyspnoea and intense cyanosis. The pain from sternal erosion by an aneurysm of the ascending aorta is chronic and unlikely to be confused. There are many other causes of pain in the anterior chest, but enquiry about their site, character and duration usually rapidly excludes a cardiac cause.

Palpitation

When a patient becomes aware of the beating of his heart in his chest the experience is 'palpitation'. It is perhaps surprising that so few people are aware of their heart's action except, for example, after severe exercise when it is accepted as a normal phenomenon. Sometimes people find that they cannot settle down to sleep lying on their left side because they feel their heart beating; they usually accept this and go to sleep lying on their right side, but sometimes the discovery alarms them, as does palpitation arising in other circumstances.

Palpitation is only occasionally a symptom of heart disease but its nature must always be exactly elicited by careful questioning. It is necessary to find out the speed and regularity of the heart beats, whether there have been preceding attacks, whether there is any precipitating factor recognised by the patient and whether the patient has been suspected of having heart disease or is receiving tablets such as digitalis. The answers may suggest a paroxysmal tachycardia of some kind.

The heart beat may be felt as regular or irregular, fast and fluttering or slow and thudding. When a patient complains of palpitation he should be asked to represent it by tapping on the table. This quickly allows the physician to determine the approximate rate and whether or not it is regular. Palpitation may be associated with sinus tachycardia, perhaps from emotion, or with almost any dysrhythmia except possibly the bradycardia of complete heart block. One of the commonest causes is *ectopic beats* ('extrasystoles', 'premature contractions'). These are sometimes felt as a thump, sometimes as if the heart had 'missed a beat', sometimes 'like something turning over'. Such feelings may occur as a single event, or they may be grouped to cause a vague intermittent fluttering feeling. The palpitation of ectopic beats is most commonly associated with states of anxiety, fatigue and lack of physical fitness but they are alarming and immediately direct the patient's attention to his heart, thus forming a basis for the development of a cardiac neurosis.

Syncope

While sudden transient loss of consciousness caused by heart disease *(cardiac syncope)* is rather uncommon, vasomotor syncope is a common symptom. Consciousness is lost in syncope because cerebral perfusion is inadequate for a short time.

Cardiac syncope

When the cardiac output becomes inadequate because of an intrinsic fault in the heart syncope may result. Ventricular fibrillation or standstill (asystole) following a cardiac infarction may last only a few moments but may cause syncope; if the dysrhythmia lasts longer twitching and convulsions develop and death usually occurs after about two minutes. Severe stenosis of the aortic or pulmonary valves so restricts the stroke volume that on exercise the cardiac output may not be great enough to sustain the cerebral blood flow; *'effort syncope'* may then occur. A special type of cardiac syncope is the *Adams—Stokes attack*. Although loss of consciousness is a feature of a typical attack, minor failures of cerebral perfusion may cause only transient dizziness. In the full syncopal form the patient suddenly loses consciousness without warning. He falls, and lies as if he were dead, limp, pale and pulseless, with fixed dilated pupils, but still breathing. If an attack lasts long enough he may twitch or have a convulsion. When the cardiac output increases full consciousness suddenly returns and a striking facial flush (reactive hyperaemia) is seen. The cardinal signs that differentiate Adams—Stokes attacks from other causes of syncope or convulsions are the absent pulse and the characteristic flush. Adams—Stokes attacks are usually caused by ventricular standstill or a fast ventricular dysrhythmia in a patient with complete heart block, but they can be caused by any change of cardiac rhythm and heart block need not be present between attacks.

Rarely a left atrial myxoma causes syncope by the pedunculated tumour temporarily obstructing the mitral valve and reducing the cardiac output.

Vasomotor syncope

This term embraces all syncopal attacks caused by a fall in cerebral perfusion as a result of sudden lowering of the peripheral resistance. It includes, for example, the syncope of orthostatic hypotension either from prolonged standing or produced by too large a dose of a potent antihypertensive drug. The commonest example is the simple 'faint', often provoked in susceptible individuals by strong and conflicting emotions and preceded by symptoms and signs of autonomic activity, such as lightheadedness, yawning, sweating and pallor.

Pressure on the carotid sinus can cause syncope from hypotension secondary to the bradycardia induced by the baroreceptor reflex, but this form of syncope only rarely occurs spontaneously, usually in older patients while turning their heads or suddenly looking up or down. The danger of using carotid sinus pressure in an attempt to slow a fast heart rate, either in the diagnosis or in attempted treatment, should be realised.

Fatigue

Feelings of fatigue and lassitude occur in patients with heart disease. Fatigue occurs in low cardiac output states particularly after exertion and certainly this is true, for example, of patients who have mitral incompetence. Lassitude is common in chronic infections, and infective endocarditis is no exception. However, when a patient complains of lassitude expressed in terms such as 'It's that awful tired feeling, doctor!' the commonest cause is usually found to be an anxiety state, the feeling of lassitude being associated with other typical features, such as lack of concentration, difficulty in getting to sleep and occasional deep sighs.

Ankle Oedema

Swelling of the ankles is usually found on clinical examination but is sometimes a presenting complaint. Most patients with oedema of the ankles do not have cardiac failure, for there are many other causes, including chronic venous insufficiency from varicose veins, venous obstruction and hepatic or renal disease. Sometimes the ankles are swollen, not because they are oedematous, but because they are simply 'thick' in configuration. When oedema of the ankles is the result of heart disease it is accompanied by other signs of congestive cardiac failure, including a raised jugular venous pressure. If the patient has recently been treated with diuretics or digitalis, however, the venous pressure may fall before all the oedema has had time to disappear. Simple questioning about medication can resolve this problem.

Headache

Headache is only very rarely a symptom in cardiovascular disease, but a characteristic headache present on waking in the morning seems to be reasonably common in hypertensive patients. It disappears when the hypertension is adequately treated.

Previous History

The patient should always be asked directly whether at any time a doctor has suggested that there might have been anything wrong with his heart, or has commented on the presence of a murmur. The significance of the answers must be assessed by the physician after he has examined the patient; for example, it often emerges that the mention of a murmur many years previously has been the cause of a severe cardiac neurosis.

The patient should also be asked directly whether at any time he has suffered from rheumatic fever or 'St Vitus' dance' (Sydenham's chorea). If he answers 'Yes', he should then be asked whether he was in bed with it, and if so for how long, and whether anyone made any comment about heart murmurs at the time. Women who have borne children should be asked about their pregnancies and whether they were complicated by any sign of heart disease or by pre-eclamptic toxaemia. It is common for mitral stenosis to be detected for the first time in the antenatal clinic, and the hyperkinetic circulatory state of the first few months of pregnancy can often precipitate pulmonary oedema in a patient with critical mitral stenosis who was previously unaware of dyspnoea on effort.

Social History

The patient should be asked about the amount of physical exertion involved in his daily work, and whether there are stairs at home or at work. The assessment of how handicapped a patient is, for example by breathlessness, can only be made by bearing these important factors in mind. As always, the patient should be asked about his smoking habits and his consumption of alcohol, for ischaemic heart disease is much commoner in patients who smoke many cigarettes and an excessive consumption of alcohol causes a cardiomyopathy.

Family History

The taking of the family history should include questions about the incidence of heart disease, especially congenital and ischaemic heart disease, hypertension and strokes. Tact is needed, of course, to avoid alarming the patient unduly.

PHYSICAL EXAMINATION

The physical examination should be made systematically. The inexperienced are always in too much of a hurry to auscultate. The normal circulation changes from moment to moment under emotional, nervous and humoral influences; for example, the cardiac output may double with excitement. There are also anatomical and functional variations at different ages. This great variability must always be remembered and allowed for.

Although it is generally convenient to examine patients lying in bed or on a couch, propped up at an angle of about 30 to 45°, some physical signs are better elicited with the patient standing up. Signs of anxiety should be noted, for example the excessive axillary sweating so commonly seen in adolescents or the characteristic deep sighing respirations of the anxious. The patient's complexion is observed for any abnormalities such as pallor, pigmentation and the 'café au lait' complexion sometimes seen in infective endocarditis. An unusual distribution of body hair occurs in myxoedema, panhypopituitarism, haemochromatosis and Cushing's syndrome. The characteristic features of the many diseases in which the cardiovascular system is involved may be apparent. Paget's disease, thyrotoxicosis, myxoedema, acromegaly, myopathies, Down's syndrome, Marfan's syndrome, Hurler's syndrome, Turner's syndrome and the Holt—Oram syndrome should be borne in mind. In the elderly the cardiovascular effects of thyrotoxicosis may occur in the absence of the usual clinical evidence of an overactive thyroid.

Thorax

Particular attention should be paid to the shape of the thorax, noting any sternal deformity, either protrusion (pigeon breast) or depression (funnel chest); the former is sometimes the result of long-standing right-ventricular hypertrophy, particularly in congenital heart disease in children; the latter produces physical signs that may falsely suggest heart disease. The thoracic spine should be inspected, for scoliosis can displace the heart from its normal position and give a spurious impression of its size. An unduly straight thoracic spine can also cause misleading appearances in the cardiac silhouette on chest x-ray. Skeletal abnormalities such as these may be associated with innocent bruits, late-systolic murmurs and 'clicks' on auscultation. Dilated veins under the skin of the thorax may suggest caval obstruction while pulsating arteries in the intercostal spaces, especially interscapular, suggests coarctation of the aorta. An aneurysm of the ascending aorta may produce a swelling on one or other side of the sternum, or in the suprasternal notch, which may pulsate, and over which a systolic bruit is heard and sometimes a thrill felt.

Head

Much information may be obtained from a careful inspection of the head. In acute rheumatic fever nodules may be felt in the occipital aponeurosis. Careful examination of both retinae with an ophthalmoscope gives the only opportunity of looking at arterioles and venules, and allows an appreciation of changes in them, for example in hypertensive retinopathy. Inspection of the conjunctivae often gives a better clinical indication of whether a patient is anaemic than inspection of the palms. Pupillary reflexes should be tested if there is a suggestion of aortic incompetence: an Argyll Robertson pupil suggests syphilis. The characteristic shimmering iris caused by the lens dislocation of Marfan's syndrome is unmistakable. Scleral vessels may be congested in polycythaemia and the sclera may be icteric. The cornea should be inspected for an arcus.

The cheeks should be examined. Their complexion is muddy in haemochromatosis, brick red in polycythaemia and some patients with longstanding mitral stenosis and pulmonary hypertension have a characteristic 'malar flush' consisting of dilated venules in the cyanosed skin of the cheeks. Some patients with severe aortic valve disease have a very pink-and-white complexion. The skin of patients with scleroderma is often shiny and firmly attached to the underlying tissues of the nose and brow. The characteristic rash of systemic lupus, with its butterfly distribution across the nose and cheeks, is sometimes seen. The head is unduly large in Paget's disease, and, rarely, may nod with every heartbeat when there is severe aortic incompetence (de Musset's sign).

The inside of the mouth should be carefully inspected for *central cyanosis*. Cyanosis of the lips may often be peripheral cyanosis, as commonly seen in children who have stayed too long in cold water. It is not satisfactory to inspect the tongue, because the dorsum of the tongue is often coated and the large veins on the under surface give a false impression of blueness to the tissues there. It is best to inspect the mucous membrane inside the mouth opposite the molar teeth and if this is cyanosed the cyanosis is central in origin. Minor degrees of central cyanosis are hard to detect without experience. The condition is not clinically detectable until the arterial P_{O_2} is about 50 mm Hg (arterial oxygen saturation less than 85 per cent), and about one-third of the cardiac output bypasses the lungs by a shunt that may be anatomical (cyanotic congenital heart disease) or physiological (ventilation/perfusion abnormality). These figures are based on a normal haemoglobin level of 15 g/dl, because cyanosis occurs only when there is more than 5 g/dl of reduced haemoglobin. When there is polycythaemia, therefore, as is common in cyanotic congenital heart disease, or severe anoxic pulmonary heart disease, cyanosis is deeper. The high-arched palate of Marfan's syndrome is obvious if looked for.

Neck

In the neck the thyroid should be palpated for enlargement and the examiner should auscultate for systolic bruits, not only over the thyroid but also in areas related to the carotid and vertebral arteries on each side (Figure 2.1). In elderly women the right common

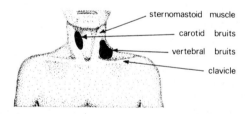

Figure 2.1. *Sites in the neck for auscultation of arterial bruits.*

carotid artery is sometimes kinked and pulsating; it is important not to confuse this with an aneurysm. Sometimes when there is a coarctation of the aorta there is an obvious, slowly swelling pulsation of the carotid arteries, and even of the subclavian arteries, visible above the clavicles. The carotid pulses should be palpated for the abnormalities of wave form characteristic of various valve lesions (see below). Occasionally in peripheral arterial disease or dissecting aneurysm of the aorta one or other carotid artery is less easily palpable, or even impalpable. In the arteritis of Takayasu's disease the carotid arteries may be impalpable.

The neck should also be inspected for the pulsations of the internal jugular vein (p. 67). When an aortic aneurysm presses on the left bronchus the trachea is pulled downward with each systole. This may be detected by eliciting the *tracheal tug*. The examiner should stand behind the seated patient and apply steady upward pressure with the tip of a forefinger on the patient's cricoid cartilage.

Hands

Inspection of the hands may show the characteristic changes of rheumatoid arthritis which are sometimes associated with aortic valve disease, or arachnodactyly, commonly associated with Marfan's syndrome. The palms may be pale when the patient is anaemic or have a blotchy erythema of the hypothenar and thenar eminences when there is liver failure or hypercapnia. There may be erythematous patches (Janeway lesions) in infective endocarditis or pigmented creases in Addison's disease. The fingers may be cold and pale and exhibit Raynaud's phenomenon in some cases of peripheral arterial disease. The skin of the fingers may be tightly bound down to the subcutaneous tissues in scleroderma. The pulps of all ten digits should be systematically squeezed to exclude the tender Osler's nodes of infective endocarditis. The nails should be carefully inspected for the presence of subungual splinter haemorrhages; although these are most commonly the result of trauma they can also be associated with infective endocarditis. Severe iron deficiency anaemia is suspected if there is koilonychia. Capillary pulsation of the nail bed can be elicited in the normal finger, especially when vasodilated, by pressing down the free border of the nail and inspecting the junction between the proximal pink area and the distal pale area produced by the pressure. When the pressure is critical the capillary pulsation can be seen as a rhythmical movement of the junction between the pale and pink regions. Capillary pulsation is often obvious in aortic incompetence. It may be demonstrated in the nail bed, or by pressing a glass slide against the mucous membrane of the everted lower lip. Capillary pulsation has no useful place in the actual diagnosis of aortic incompetence. In acute rheumatic fever nodules may be demonstrated in the tendon sheaths of the dorsum of the hand by making the patient clench his fist. Clubbing of the fingers is found in cyanotic congenital heart disease, and in some patients with pulmonary heart disease or infective endocarditis.

Elbows

Nodules are found on the back of the elbows in acute rheumatic fever, rheumatoid arthritis and gout. In the antecubital fossa the brachial artery can normally be palpated and used for sphygmomanometry; if arteriosclerotic, it may be seen as a kinked vessel, contracting with each pulsation *('locomotor brachialis')*. The antecubital veins are the most convenient for venepuncture.

The Arterial Pulse

The pulse wave is not the result of the passage of blood along the arteries at 0.5 m/sec but is a pressure wave that travels at about 7 m/sec and is propagated by the incompressible blood both forward and laterally; the lateral movement distends the arterial wall and gives rise to the pulse wave. The propulsive force conveys the pulse wave down the arterial system from the aortic root.

Careful examination of the pulsation of eight accessible arteries is essential. They are the temporal, carotid, brachial, radial, femoral, popliteal, posterior tibial, and dorsalis pedis arteries. Palpation of each of these arteries has its own particular usefulness in the assessment either of heart disease or of peripheral vascular disease. Thus the *temporal artery* may be tender or obliterated in temporal arteritis, and the palpation by the examiner of his own temporal artery may be useful, as explained later, to check on the pulsations of his own digital pulps. The *carotid artery* is the accessible artery nearest the arch of the aorta and so gives the best indication of the arterial wave-form. Careful palpation of the *brachial artery* by firm pressure from the examiner's thumb gives a fair idea of the wave-form if for some reason the external carotid artery is difficult to feel; the arterial blood pressure is measured during sphygmomanometry (see below) by auscultation over the brachial artery which should always be palpated before measuring the blood pressure. The *radial artery* is, of course, the most conventional artery to choose for palpation of the pulse and it is very convenient because it is always accessible with a patient fully clothed. The *arterial pulses in the legs* are reduced or absent when there is obliterative arterial disease (see below) and absent or delayed in coarctation of the aorta; that is, the *femoral pulse*, if present, is transmitted later than the brachial in contrast to the normal state in which pulsations of the brachial and femoral pulses are felt as simultaneous. During the progression of a dissecting aneurysm of the aorta one or more of these arteries may disappear either temporarily or permanently.

An appropriate artery, usually the radial or carotid, is conventionally palpated to assess five aspects of the pulsation: the rate, the rhythm, the pulse pressure, the shape of the pulse wave, and the 'state of the arterial wall'. It is important that the pulses are always felt on both sides. When there is difficulty in deciding upon the character of the arterial pulse it is helpful to palpate the carotid artery.

Rate

The radial pulse is best felt by the examiner placing the tips of the first three fingers in the groove that lies just proximal to the radial styloid and between the radius and the flexor tendons. The patient's hand should be passively supported. Sometimes the radial artery does not lie in the groove, in which case it usually runs an aberrant course over the radial styloid where it can be easily seen pulsating under the skin.

Usually the pulse rate indicates the rate of cardiac contraction. It should be timed with a watch, preferably over one minute and certainly over not less than one-quarter of a minute. With experience, the normal unhurried pulse rate of about 65 to 75 beats per minute can be recognised, but for faster or slower heart rates careful timing is essential. The heart rate of infants cannot be accurately counted by palpation; cardiac auscultation is needed. The heart rate is increased *(tachycardia)* normally in infants and young children and at any age during and after exercise, excitement or anxiety. Tachycardia accompanies fever and other conditions associated with an increased metabolic rate, for example thyrotoxicosis, or conditions involving a hyperkinetic circulatory state (Table 2.1). In some types of 'circulatory shock' there is also tachycardia.

A slow heart rate *(bradycardia)* is common in fit young people, but can also be abnormal. Sinus bradycardia, caused by depression of the activity of the sinoatrial node, is sometimes seen after a cardiac infarction and also sometimes accompanies acute virus illnesses and typhoid fever; a raised intracranial pressure sometimes causes a slow pulse rate by a reflex mechanism. High-grade atrio-ventricular (AV) block (complete heart block or for example 3:1 AV block) can cause a slow pulse rate.

Table 2.1. *Hyperkinetic circulatory states.*

Physiological
  Exercise
  Emotion (excitement, anxiety)
  Pregnancy

Pathological
  Pyrexia
  Anaemia
  Hypoxia and hypercapnia
  Thyrotoxicosis
  Arterio-venous fistulae
    (including Paget's disease of bone)
  Hepatic failure

Some dysrhythmias (see below) produce a regular pulse rate which may be fast or slow, and auscultation may greatly help their correct interpretation. Thus, coupled ectopic beats may not eject enough blood into the aortic root to promote a pulse wave that reaches the radial artery. The dysrhythmia may then be mis-diagnosed as sinus bradycardia unless the premature and abnormal heart sounds are listened for. Pulse rates lower than about 50 may be associated with complete heart block.

Paroxysmal tachycardias, both atrial and ventricular, are usually much faster than sinus tachycardia — so fast in infants, in fact, that it may be difficult to count the rate even on auscultation. The correct diagnosis of all dysrhythmias can only be made by the electrocardiogram (see below). Atrial flutter with 2:1 AV block often gives a regular heart rate of about 160 and with 4:1 AV block the rate may seem normal.

Rhythm

Careful attention to the normal rhythm of the pulse shows that it is hardly ever absolutely regular. *Sinus arrhythmia* is a normal feature at almost any age but perhaps more noticeable in younger patients. It is most obvious when the patient is told to breathe more slowly and much more deeply than usual. The pulse rate speeds towards the end of inspiration and then slows during early expiration. During expiration the filling of the left ventricle is increased, with an accompanying increase in stroke volume and blood pressure which stimulates baroreceptors and the vagus to cause reflex slowing of the heart. If the rhythm of the pulse seems to be more irregular than can be explained by sinus arrhythmia, the examiner must ask himself whether the irregularity is a *regular irregularity* that follows a repetitive pattern, or an *irregular irregularity*, in which the pulsations seem to be totally chaotic with no discernible pattern at all. A regularly irregular pulse is usually the result of ectopic beats (premature contractions, extrasystoles) but can also be associated with Wenckebach periods (see below). When a premature contraction follows every normal ventricular contraction (coupled ectopic beat) the pulse has a characteristic double rhythm called *pulsus bigeminus* or 'coupling' which is the result of the normal beat followed by the ectopic beat which is succeeded by a compensatory pause (Figure 2.2).

An irregularly irregular pulse is most commonly caused by atrial fibrillation in which the AV node only irregularly transmits some of the innumerable stimuli it receives. Occasionally when there are very frequent ectopic beats the pulse is also irregularly irregular. The rapid and irregular ventricular contractions are associated with varying lengths of diastole and consequently with different amounts of diastolic ventricular filling. The stroke volumes therefore vary and the smaller stroke volumes fail to produce a pulse wave that reaches the wrist, so the pulse rate felt there is slower than the heart rate which can only be appreciated by auscultation *(pulse deficit)*.

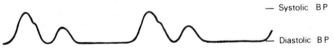

— Systolic BP

— Diastolic BP

Figure 2.2. *Pulsus bigeminus caused by coupled ventricular ectopic beats.*

Pulse pressure

The pulse pressure is the difference between the systolic and the diastolic blood pressures, that is, the amplitude of the arterial pulse wave. It is, of course, only measured accurately by sphygmomanometry but unusually high and unusually low pulse pressures can be identified, particularly by palpation of the brachial artery. The pulse pressure of an artery roughly determined by palpation is traditionally referred to by the misleading term 'volume'. The pulse pressure at the site of palpation of any artery bears no relation to the volume of blood flowing under the finger. The traditional usage of the term depends on an indirect relationship between the pulse pressure and the left ventricular stroke volume that initiates the pulse wave. This relationship is so unreliable that the term should probably be dropped. The pulse pressure is raised, and the pulse described as 'bounding' in hyperkinetic circulatory states (Table 2.1). The pulse pressure is increased, and the wave-form altered, when there is an increased run-off from the large arteries in late systole or early diastole, either backward because of incompetence of the aortic valve or a left-to-right shunt, or forward because of peripheral vasodilatation.

A pulse with a low pulse pressure *(pulsus parvus)* may be the result of a low stroke volume due to left ventricular failure or tachycardia with impaired ventricular filling as a result of shortened diastole. On the other hand it may be caused by an obstruction to left ventricular outflow, such as stenosis of the aortic valve, or thickening of the arterial wall in the elderly. Peripheral pulses may be impalpable when there is peripheral vasoconstriction caused by cold or shock.

If the arterial pulse is recorded by an indwelling cannula and an accurate recorder, with respiration recorded simultaneously, it can be shown that during inspiration the systolic, diastolic and mean pressures and the pulse pressure are all reduced. During inspiration the intrathoracic pressure becomes more negative and the lung expands; blood then pools in the pulmonary vessels and filling of the left side of the heart is reduced. This reduction has a greater effect on the left ventricular stroke volume than the increased venous return has on the function of the right side of the heart. The variation in pulse pressure is not normally detectable by palpation, or by indirect arterial pressure measurement (sphygmomanometry). However, when it is exaggerated it is readily detectable by palpation, and is then rather misleadingly called *pulsus paradoxus.* Pulsus paradoxus is most commonly felt during acute attacks of asthma when the great increase in ventilatory effort produces correspondingly great haemodynamic changes in the lungs and ventricles. It is also present when filling of the ventricles is restricted, for example by constrictive pericarditis or by a peri-cardial effusion. The mechanism in this case is not certain; it is possible that the descent of the diaphragm during inspiration may increase the pericardial restriction.

When the left ventricle fails it may contract regularly, but alternate contractions are less powerful. As a result alternate stroke volumes, and hence pulse pressures, are regularly higher and lower *(pulsus alternans)* (Figure 2.3).

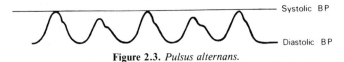

Figure 2.3. *Pulsus alternans.*

Shape of arterial wave-form

The normal arterial wave-form (pressure pulse) varies in different parts of the arterial tree. Its purest form is recorded from the root of the aorta (Figure 2.4) where, during the ejection phase of left ventricular systole, the ascending limb of the aortic pressure pulse is steep and interrupted before its summit by a flattening or notch, called the *anacrotic* notch. During the phase of reduced ejection the falling part of the tracing is less steep and when the aortic valve shuts there is a momentary increase in pressure in the aortic root producing the *dicrotic* notch before the aortic pressure sinks gradually during the rest of diastole. The farther away from the aortic root the arterial wave-form is recorded the more it is distorted, the ascending limb becoming steeper, the systolic pressure higher and the diastolic pressure lower because of the reflection of the pressure waves from, for example, branching parts of the arterial tree. Normally no anacrotic notch is present in peripheral arteries and although the dicrotic notch can easily be recorded by indirect pressure measurements, such as by a pressure capsule held firmly over the artery, it is not usually palpable as a notch by the fingers. The normal arterial wave-form is easily appreciated by the examiner's thumb pressed firmly on the

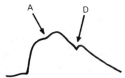

Figure 2.4. *Form of pressure pulse directly recorded from the root of aorta. Arrows indicate the anacrotic (A) and dicrotic (D) notches.*

patient's brachial artery, the elbow being held fully extended. The examiner can feel and see his thumb rising sharply during the upstroke of the pulse, or percussion wave, and then falling sharply for a short distance. For the rest of diastole the thumb sinks much more slowly to its diastolic position.

The shape of the arterial wave-form is most accurately detected at the bedside by careful palpation of the carotid artery (Figure 2.5, A and B). The examiner should feel for the artery with the first two or three fingers of his right hand in the anterior triangle of the neck just medial to the medial edge of the sternomastoid muscle. The arterial impulse is usually fairly easily felt but palpation is sometimes difficult, and is almost always uncomfortable for the patient.

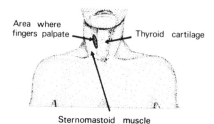

Area where
fingers palpate ⟶   ⟵ Thyroid cartilage

Sternomastoid muscle

Figure 2.5A. *Site for palpation of the carotid artery.*

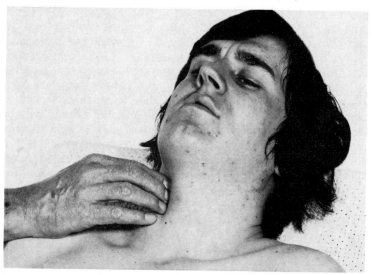

Figure 2.5B. *Palpation of the carotid artery.*

The examiner should remember, too, that the carotid sinus lies in this region and that stimulation of it can lead to syncope; the carotid arteries should never be palpated simultaneously on both sides. Attention should be paid to the speed of both the rise and the fall of the pressure pulse and to the presence or absence of obvious notches. An abnormally slow rising pulse with a delayed peak is characteristic of aortic valve stenosis (Figure 2.6A). The narrowed valve slows ventricular ejection and a plateau, or even an anacrotic notch, may be felt before the delayed peak (*plateau*, or *anacrotic pulse*). If the stenosis is severe the pulse pressure is often low and such a pulse is sometimes described as *pulsus parvus et tardus*.

Rapid ventricular ejection causes a rapid upstroke and if this is transmitted to the periphery it imparts to the palpating finger an abrupt, almost flicking, sensation. This sensation is similar to that said to be experienced when playing with a Victorian toy called a *waterhammer*. When the systolic percussion wave is short and the fall of the pulse wave is rapid the pulse is said to be *collapsing*. Such a pulse wave occurs when there is a rapid run-off of blood from the aorta, either backward into the left ventricle through an incompetent aortic valve or forward into a dilated peripheral circulation. Almost always a fast-rising pulse is also a collapsing one, so the terms 'collapsing' and 'waterhammer' have come to be used as though they were synonymous. The most important cause of such a pulse is aortic incompetence. Because the left ventricle must eject an increased volume of blood in the normal time in order to maintain a normal stroke volume the systolic pressure is raised. There is usually a compensatory peripheral vasodilatation that reduces the volume of regurgitant blood and encourages a forward flow in diastole. A large quantity of blood is therefore rapidly ejected in early systole into dilated arteries that empty rapidly in diastole. The diastolic pressure is therefore unusually low. This wave-form, with low diastolic and high systolic pressures, and

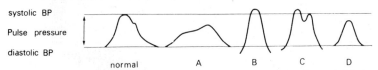

systolic BP

Pulse pressure

diastolic BP

normal   A   B   C   D

Figure 2.6. *Diagrammatic representations of normal and abnormal arterial wave-forms and pulse pressures. A, anacrotic (plateau) from aortic stenosis; B, Corrigan's (water hammer and collapsing) pulse in aortic incompetence; C, pulsus bisferiens from combined aortic stenosis and incompetence; D, 'small collapsing' ('jerky') pulse in mitral incompetence.*

waterhammer and collapsing qualities, is called *Corrigan's pulse* (Figure 2.6B). Such a pulse is exaggerated if gravity is made to assist the retrograde run-off of blood, thereby increasing the pulse pressure further. This is traditionally done at the bedside by palpating the radial artery in a special way. Instead of feeling the artery in the usual manner with the finger tips in the groove just medial to the radius, the whole arm is held above the patient's head by the examiner's hand so that his first three fingers lie flat across the palmar aspect of the patient's wrist (Figure 2.7).

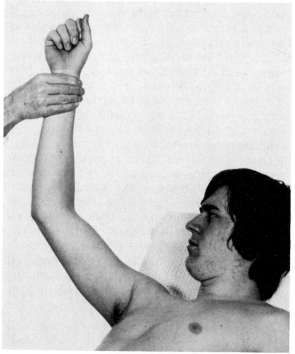

Figure 2.7. *Method for palpation of Corrigan's pulse in the radial artery.*

Some of the highest pulse pressures recorded occur with aortic incompetence and are often associated with capillary pulsation visible in mucous membranes if looked for by special methods (see above). Any conditions that cause a high pulse pressure can cause a collapsing pulse. Similarly, in complete heart block the long ventricular diastole allows increased ventricular filling, so a large stroke volume is ejected into an arterial system that has become relatively empty and causes a collapsing pulse. Occasionally the pulse pressure is not high but the rise and fall of the pulse wave is rapid. The pulse then has a characteristic jerky quality, as is sometimes felt in patients with mitral incompetence or obstructive cardiomyopathy (Figure 2.6D).

Corrigan's sign is not the same as Corrigan's *pulse*. The sign consists of a strikingly jerky, *visible* pulsation of the carotid arteries, and is usually the result of severe aortic incompetence.

When the aortic valve is both stenosed and incompetent the pulse may be neither anacrotic nor a Corrigan's pulse, but a mixture of the two. The palpating finger on the carotid artery may feel rapid oscillations referred to as *carotid shudder* and, rather rarely, over either the carotid or the brachial artery a true double beat can be felt, known as *pulsus bisferiens* (Figure 2.6C). Obstructive cardiomyopathy also sometimes produces this type of pulse.

A second form of double-peaked pulse wave is the result of a palpable dicrotic wave. This is felt when the blood pressure is normal or low, the arteries elastic and the peripheral resistance low, as in the young; the classical association usually mentioned is with typhoid fever, perhaps because in the early stages the pulse rate is unusually low, despite the fever.

Pulsus alternans is often more easily detected from the brachial than from the radial artery, but it is best demonstrated — and indeed sometimes spontaneously noticed — while the blood pressure is being recorded by sphygmomanometry. The beats with the higher systolic pressure cause Korotkoff sounds first but after the pressure in the cuff has dropped a few mm Hg the lower pressure beats produce sounds and the rate of the sounds therefore exactly doubles. Alternation can often be seen in the oscillation of the head of the column of mercury in the sphygmomanometer.

'State of the arterial wall'

Before the routine use of the sphygmomanometer crude estimations of the blood pressure were made by gauging roughly how much pressure was needed to obliterate the pulse. This technique has rightly been rejected. The traditional crude estimation of the 'state of the vessel wall', made by a rolling palpation of the radial artery by the finger tips, should be rejected also. It is true that in older people the artery is more easily palpable than in the young but the condition in which it is most obviously abnormal, Mönckeberg's sclerosis, where the artery feels like corrugated gas piping, is associated neither with an increased peripheral resistance and hypertension nor with obliterative arterial disease. The ritual yields no valuable information.

The Arterial Blood Pressure

The arterial blood pressure can only be measured accurately by a direct intra-arterial recording using a cannula with an adequate lumen. In clinical practice, of course, it is measured by sphygmo-manometry. The mercury manometer is the simplest and most reliable apparatus though it is heavy, bulky and less convenient, especially for domiciliary practice, than aneroid instruments. Even with the mercury instrument, however, it is necessary to make sure that the glass manometer tube is clean, that there are no air bubbles in the mercury column, no air leaks in the valve or rubber bulb and that the cuff is not only wide enough and long enough to encompass the arm adequately, but also that the stitching round the inflatable rubber pad is intact so that when the pressure is raised the pad does not herniate from below the cloth.

The basic principle underlying the technique is that the cuff when inflated exerts a pressure cone throughout the soft tissues of the limb sufficiently deep to occlude the artery whose blood pressure is being measured. The size of the cuff relative to the size of the arm is therefore important. A very fat arm needs a cuff wider than the standard one, while a narrower cuff is necessary for a child. Fallaciously high pressures are recorded from fat people if this fact is not recognised.

The brachial artery is usually chosen and the cuff is applied to the arm well above the antecubital fossa. The inflatable pad should be arranged so that it lies over the artery with the tubes leaving it from the upper edge, and the rest of the cuff should then be wrapped carefully round it so that there are no creases and the whole of the pad is firmly bound to the arm (Figure 2.8). The arm should be arranged so that the cuff is at the level of the heart and the brachial artery in the antecubital fossa should be identified by palpation. The examiner should then prepare to listen for the Korotkoff sounds by placing the diaphragm part of his stethoscope over the brachial artery. He then inflates the cuff until either the mercury column rises to the top of the manometer or the radial pulse on the same arm is no longer felt by his palpating finger. Only by one of these techniques will he avoid occasionally reading a systolic pressure that is falsely low, caused by the 'auscultatory gap.' By releasing the valve slightly he should allow the mercury column to fall slowly, listening carefully while he does so. The Korotkoff sounds begin as soft muffled thuds and the manometric level at which they are first heard is taken as the *systolic blood pressure.* As the pressure falls they usually become steadily louder and more clearly tapping until they suddenly become muffled. This point of sudden muffling is taken as the *diastolic blood pressure.* As the pressure then continues to fall the sounds become softer and eventually disappear. Occasionally they are heard until the mercury column falls to zero. Occasionally, too, they disappear for a few mm Hg fairly soon after the systolic pressure has been identified, only to reappear again well above the diastolic pressure. This is the *auscultatory gap.*

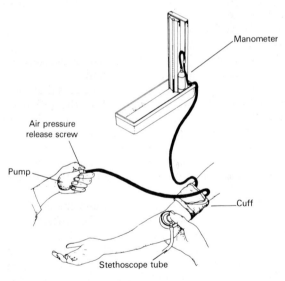

Figure 2.8. *Sphygmomanometry.*

It is very difficult indeed to record a 'basal' blood pressure. Patients are frequently excited and tachycardia raises the blood pressure. Verbal reassurance seldom helps. Indifference to the procedure through familiarity, though most helpful, is very time-consuming. For this reason the pulse rate should always be counted and recorded when the blood pressure is measured. Continuous intra-arterial recording of the blood pressures of healthy and hypertensive patients throughout the 24 hours of a normal day has shown how variable the pressure is, and how tiny emotional stimuli can immediately produce considerable changes that may last quite a long time. It is therefore fatuous to delude oneself that by sphygmomanometry one can record a blood pressure to an accuracy of 2 mm Hg, as was once suggested. Probably it is unrealistic to attempt anything more accurate than a measurement to the nearest 5 mm Hg.

The blood pressure may not be the same in each arm, differing in normal people by perhaps 10 mm Hg systolic and 5 mm Hg diastolic. When a normal person stands the systolic pressure often rises and it certainly should not fall more than about 20 mm Hg. The diastolic pressure also rises, by up to about 10 mm Hg. Hypertensive patients who are being treated with drugs to lower the blood pressure frequently have postural (orthostatic) hypotension and on standing the blood pressure may fall considerably. If the blood pressure is taken with the patient standing, after exercise, the pressure may be even lower. Postural hypotension also occurs in patients with abnormal autonomic nervous function, for example in diabetes mellitus or old age.

The point at which the sounds suddenly become muffled ('phase four') has long been accepted in the United Kingdom as the best index of the diastolic pressure but for many years physicians in the United States were encouraged to regard the point at which the sounds disappeared completely ('phase five') as the diastolic pressure. Recently, phase five has been recommended for international use, probably because it is easier for semi-trained personnel to identify. The point of sudden muffling correlates well with intra-arterial recordings, and avoids the anomaly of a patient with a zero diastolic pressure. Although insurance companies sometimes ask for a record of the point at which the sounds disappear clinicians are generally encouraged to adopt the British criterion. The best practice is to record the systolic pressure, and both phase-four and phase-five diastolic pressures when they differ.

Occasionally it is desirable to record the blood pressure in the legs. This is conveniently done with the patient lying prone, with inflatable cuffs on the thighs, and the examiner auscultating the popliteal artery. Because the thighs are much thicker than the arms, specially wide cuffs have to be used. If they are not available a sphygmomanometer pad can be placed appropriately and held tight against the thigh by crepe bandages; this expedient is not nearly so satisfactory. The blood pressure in the legs is normally higher than that in the arms, even when the patient is lying down. In the presence of coarctation of the aorta, when the femoral pulse may be delayed or impalpable, the blood pressure in the legs may be lower than that in the arms, or unrecordable.

The Venous Pulse

From a careful inspection of the jugular venous pulse the examiner can obtain two important pieces of information: an estimate of the *venous pressure*, which is approximately the filling pressure of the right atrium, and the *form of the venous pulse waves*, which gives information about haemodynamic events in the right atrium and ventricle and the function of the tricuspid valve. Unfortunately, there is no other part of the examination of the cardiovascular system, apart perhaps from auscultation, which is performed less competently, and apparently with less appreciation of the purpose, than the inspection of the jugular venous pulse.

Veins are the great capacitance vessels of the circulation and unlike arteries they are not circular in cross section until they are fairly full. As the volume of blood in a section of vein increases, it changes the shape of the vessel from an ellipse to a circle. Only then does the circle increase in diameter, that is, distend. Depending upon the volume of blood in a section of vein the vein will be collapsed (elliptical) or full (circular) or distended. There is a good relation, though not a linear one, between the volume and the pressure of blood flowing in a large vein, but visible venous pulsation is much more the result of volume changes within the vein than of changes in pressure. This is easily demonstrated at cardiac catheterisation when the pressure changes in the superior vena cava are disappointingly small, although the visible pulsation of the internal jugular vein may be striking.

The *form of the pulse waves* in the jugular vein is a function, then, of cyclical changes in volume that distend the fully filled vein. It gives information about intracardiac events. On the other hand, the clinical estimation of the *venous pressure* does indeed depend on the pressure of blood in the vein, because the vein will not be filled, that is, it will not have a circular cross section but will be 'collapsed' and invisible in the neck whenever the atmospheric pressure is greater than the pressure of blood in the vein. When the pressure inside the vein exceeds the atmospheric pressure the vein will be full, and will pulsate because of the cyclical changes in the volume of blood it contains.

Because the wall of a vein is very distensible compared with that of an artery, increases in the volume of blood within it increase its diameter, so the pulsation sought by careful inspection will not be along the long axis of the vein but directed radially. In the case of the jugular vein it will therefore appear not as an up-and-down movement, like that of mercury in a sphygmomanometer which rises and falls with each arterial pulse between the systolic and diastolic pressures, but rather an inward and outward pulsation of the skin and soft tissues overlying the vein. This pulsation is the important thing to look for at the outset, for the highest point at which it can be identified, and above which the vein is collapsed, identifies the venous pressure so long as the pulsation does not reach the ear lobes.

The pencil-thin external jugular vein should be ignored completely, even when it is easily visible and obviously pulsating, because it can produce both falsely high and falsely low impressions of the venous pressure. The student should train himself rather to identify the less obvious pulsations of the much larger internal jugular vein which lies more deeply, below the sternomastoid muscle and in the anterior part of the posterior triangle in the lower part of the neck, just lateral to the clavicular insertion of the sternomastoid (Figure 2.9). Its pulsations will not be seen unless the patient is first placed in a position in which the venous pressure is able to fill the vein against the effects of gravity, atmospheric pressure and the intrathoracic negative pressure, all of which tend to make the vein collapse.

The patient should be propped up comfortably at an angle of about 45° to the horizontal with his head resting so that the sterno-mastoid muscles are relaxed; if they are taut they prevent the transmission of internal jugular venous pulsation. If necessary, the chin should be gently lifted by the examiner so that wrinkles of skin in the anterior and posterior triangles are smoothed out. It is sometimes helpful to turn the head slightly away from the side of the neck that is being inspected. The patient will often try to help, but should be discouraged if the sternomastoid or platysma contracts. The examiner should then look carefully at the lower part of the sternomastoid and the surrounding skin and soft tissues for the double outward pulsation of the normal venous pulse.

Inexperienced examiners may find it hard to distinguish between arterial and venous pulsation in the neck. In fact only rarely is there any real difficulty. The venous pulsation is usually double and, even if not, it is usually of comparatively low amplitude, slowly swelling and subsiding and involving the soft tissues at the root of the neck in the area already described. On the other hand the visible pulsation of the normal carotid artery is much more abrupt, always single and most easily seen and felt in the anterior triangle of the neck medial to the medial border of the sternomastoid. It is easy in cases of doubt to palpate the carotid arterial pulsation on one side of the neck while looking at the venous pulsation on the other.

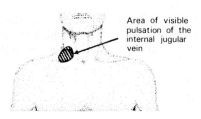

Area of visible pulsation of the internal jugular vein

Figure 2.9. *Area of visible pulsation of the internal jugular vein.*

It is sometimes said that venous pulsation is not palpable, but this is a misleading half-truth; pulsation of a vein with a normal venous pressure cannot be felt, but when the vein is distended and the venous pressure is really high the pulsation is often palpable.

When the venous pressure is normal its pulsations should just be apparent above the clavicle when the patient lies at an angle of 45°. If they cannot be seen the patient should be lowered to, say, 30° and the examiner should look again. The pulsations are diffuse, and of low amplitude as a rule, and their identification is often helped by the careful use of lighting and shadows cast over the area of inspection either by a careful arrangement of the collar of the patient's shirt or pyjamas, or by his chin or the sternomastoid itself. Either daylight or artificial light may be used and the pulsations of the internal jugular vein, especially on the right, can often be clearly seen as the edge of the shadow seems to move with them (Figure 2.10). Since the pulsations are outward ones, and not up and down, they can often be seen on either side of the root of the neck by the examiner looking at the patient full face rather than from one side; in this case the patient's head should be in the midline, with the chin not turned to either side. If the patient lies flat, or almost flat, venous pulsation is rarely observed, probably because the jugular veins are then fully distended. When a patient with a normal venous pressure sits bolt upright no venous pulsation will be seen in the neck because the internal jugular vein will be collapsed down to a level below the clavicles.

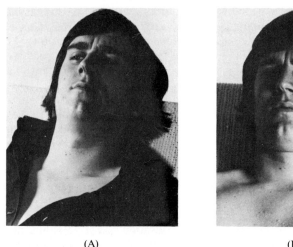

(A)   (B)

Figure 2.10. *The use of light and shade in observing pulsation of the right internal jugular vein. A, light source from patient's right side, shadow of collar thrown on area; B, light source from patient's left side, sternomastoid throws shadow.*

Jugular venous pressure

There are no valves between the right atrium and the superior vena cava nor between the superior vena cava and the internal jugular vein. The level to which the internal jugular vein is not collapsed but is distended and pulsating is for practical purposes the right atrial pressure and can be expressed in centimetres of blood. The upper level of pulsation should then rationally be related to the level of the right atrium, and the venous pressure measured directly. The surface markings of the right atrium with the patient lying at different angles to the horizontal are not known by many. By a time-honoured clinical convention, therefore, the venous pressure is measured as the vertical distance between a horizontal plane passing through the highest point of visible venous pulsation and another horizontal plane passing through the *sternal angle* (manubriosternal joint), with the patient in any position. This expedient convention is justified by the convenient fact that, within the general errors of clinical method, the distance between the mid-right atrium and the sternal angle is almost the same despite the position of the patient (Figure 2.11).

Once the upper level of pulsation of the internal jugular vein has been identified it is easy to measure with a centimetre scale the distance between the horizontal plane that intersects it and that which intersects the sternal angle. This measurement should be recorded as the jugular venous pressure. When the patient is lying at an angle of about 45° the normal venous pressure thus measured is about three centimetres. Theoretically it should fall on inspiration and rise on expiration because of the effect of the lowered intra-thoracic pressure during inspiration, but in practice this fall on inspiration is often not apparent in quite normal young individuals; there may, however, be an obvious change in the amplitude of pulsation during the different phases of respiration.

When the right atrial pressure is raised the pressure and volume in the superior vena cava and the internal jugular vein are also increased, and the point in the neck at which the upper level of pulsation is visible is higher than normal. With the patient at 45° the high right atrial pressure of right heart failure may produce internal jugular venous pulsation that is visible as high up as the lobe of the ear, which may be moved by the pulsation. When this is so it is not possible to measure the height of the venous pulse accurately with the patient at 45°. Sitting the patient upright may then allow the upper border of pulsation to become visible, but if not, the head of the venous pressure is, in a sense, intracranial, and the pressure cannot be measured by this method. Rhythmic displacement of the ear lobes by an underlying pulsation is almost always caused by *venous* pulsation, except occasionally when it is associated with Corrigan's sign, the striking visible carotid pulsation of severe aortic incompetence.

The form of the venous pulse

Pressure tracings from the right atrium recorded during cardiac catheterisation show two main waves named *a* (atrial) and *v* (ventricular) and a less obvious and more transient wave called the *c* (closure) wave. The upstroke of the *a* wave is associated with

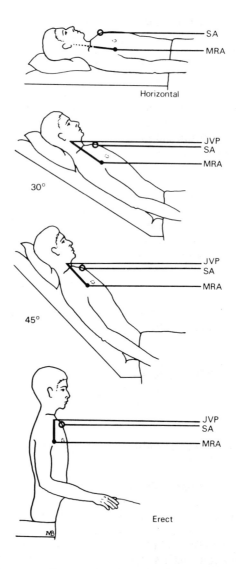

Figure 2.11. *Diagrams to illustrate the relationship of the normal internal jugular venous pressure (JVP) to the sternal angle (SA) (manubriosternal joint) and the clavicle with the subject in four different positions. The vertical distance between the sternal angle and the mid right atrium (MRA) remains relatively constant. When the patient lies at 45° to the horizontal, venous pulsation is just above the clavicle.*

atrial systole, its downslope with atrial diastole. This downslope is continued into a fall in pressure known as the 'x descent' probably associated with the 'descent of the base' of the heart when the AV ring moves towards the apex during isometric contraction of the ventricles. This x descent is interrupted by the c wave caused by the closure of the tricuspid valve. As blood continues to fill the right atrium against a closed tricuspid valve during ventricular systole the v wave rises, but when the tricuspid valve opens again very early in diastole the atrium empties, and the v wave subsides as the 'y descent'. These variations of atrial pressure are transmitted back a short way into the great veins and are accompanied by considerable changes of volume in the veins.

The normal pulsation of the internal jugular vein also has three components, a, c and v, that occur about 80 msec after the pressure waves in the right atrium. In the jugular pulse, however, the c wave is not caused by the closure of the tricuspid valve, but by the transmitted pulsation of the neighbouring carotid artery. It is, however, of little importance, because although the c wave of the jugular pulse can be mechanically recorded from skin of the neck in the jugular phlebogram, it is not visible and the normal venous pulse appears therefore as a double pulsation consisting of the a and v waves (Figure 2.12).

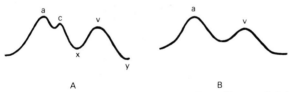

Figure 2.12. *A, normal jugular phlebogram as mechanically recorded; B, jugular venous pulse as usually seen.*

Disturbances of haemodynamics in the right side of the heart are reflected in the venous pulse (Figure 2.13). In atrial fibrillation the right atrium does not contract, so there is no a wave. Usually only the v wave is visible and because there is only a single pulsation it may be mistaken for that of the carotid artery. The single v wave of atrial fibrillation occurs appreciably later than the palpable pulsation of the carotid artery. Rarely a double venous pulsation is seen in atrial fibrillation but here the first pulsation is the c wave transmitted from the carotid artery. This again can be identified by simultaneous palpation of the carotid artery.

When the strength of atrial systole is abnormally increased, because of chronic resistance to atrial outflow, for example with pulmonary arterial hypertension, tricuspid stenosis or pulmonary stenosis, or else when, because of a dysrhythmia, the atrium contracts against a closed tricuspid valve, the *a* wave is larger than normal. In the neck it often appears as an obvious characteristically flicking wave, appreciably earlier than the carotid arterial pulse. When the cause is pulmonary arterial hypertension, pulmonary stenosis or tricuspid stenosis, every *a* wave is a 'giant' one. When, however, the atrium contracts against a closed tricuspid valve because of a dysrhythmia, it need not do so regularly; for example with atrial extrasystoles, and in complete heart block, there will only occasionally be a giant *a* wave. Such *a* waves, by a quite illogical confusion of ideas, are traditionally called *'cannon waves'* (see pp. 109—110).

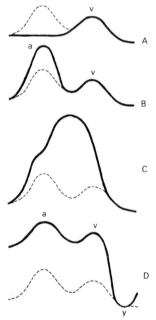

Figure 2.13. *Abnormal jugular venous wave-forms. A, atrial fibrillation; B, pulmonary arterial hypertension (giant a wave); C, tricuspid incompetence; D, pericardial restriction. The broken line represents the normal jugular venous pulse.*

It is often taught that with tricuspid stenosis the slow blood flow across the valve produces a slow *y* descent, but in practice a slowly falling *v* wave is hardly ever apparent on inspection of the jugular pulse, though the giant *a* wave is.

When the tricuspid valve is incompetent, most commonly in right heart failure because of ventricular dilatation without corresponding lengthening of the chordae tendineae, the atrial pressure rises during ventricular systole. In the right atrial pulse the *x* descent is obliterated and replaced by a positive systolic wave. The same change occurs in the venous pulse and the characteristic pulsation of tricuspid incompetence is of a slowly swelling, single wave. On its upstroke a slight hesitation may sometimes be seen, corresponding to the *a* wave, which, with the *v* wave, has been engulfed by what is virtually 'ventricularisation' of the superior vena cava and the internal jugular vein. With tricuspid incompetence the inferior vena cava is also similarly distended and the whole liver becomes pulsatile.

When the filling of the right ventricle is prematurely arrested, for example by the stiff pericardium of constrictive pericarditis or by a large pericardial effusion, the venous pressure is usually raised and if there is sinus rhythm the *a* and *v* waves are discernible. The most conspicuous wave, however, is the *y* descent, caused by the opening of the tricuspid valve and the consequent sudden reduction in intra-atrial pressure.

Pressure on the anterior abdominal wall raises the intrathoracic pressure and hence the pressure in the vena cava and jugular veins. The consequent rise in jugular venous pressure *(hepatojugular reflux)* may help to identify the venous pulse, and is particularly conspicuous in patients with tricuspid incompetence. Partial obstruction of the retrograde flow down the inferior vena cava increases that up the superior vena cava and into the jugular veins.

Hepatic Pulsation

Systolic pulsation of the liver can be detected in cases of severe tricuspid incompetence more often than is usually thought so long as the right technique is employed. With the patient propped up at about 45° the examiner should stand on the patient's right side with his wrist held rigid so that the dorsum of his hand and the dorsal aspect of his forearm are in the same plane. He should clench his fist so that the metacarpophalangeal joints are flexed at right angles and the four fingers held together. He should then place the first phalanges of the fingers so that they fit snugly into the patient's lower right intercostal spaces about the mid-axillary line over the area beneath which the enlarged liver lies (Figure 2.14). Keeping his hand and wrist in this position, and varying the pressure applied to the patient's intercostal spaces, he will soon detect the 'lever' of his forearm moving outward and inward with the patient's respiration. Closer observation and finer adjustment of the pressure will allow

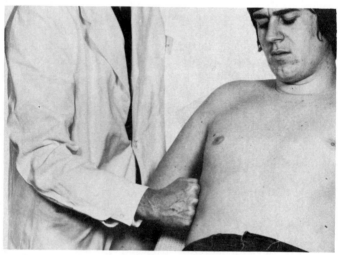

Figure 2.14. *Method of palpation for hepatic pulsation (see text).*

him to feel and see pulsations superimposed on the respiratory movements; these pulsations are systolic, and coincident with the typical single pulsations of tricuspid incompetence visible in the internal jugular vein. The examiner should then move his hand and lay it flat on the right hypochondrium. If the liver is enlarged below the costal margin he will then be able to feel, and often to see, the same systolic pulsations, this time directed anteriorly. Pulsation in two directions at right angles to one another is, of course, characteristic of intrinsic, rather than transmitted, pulsation.

Praecordial Pulsations

The *apex beat* or *apical impulse* is defined as the point farthest down and farthest out in the intercostal spaces of the praecordium at which the palpating finger clearly feels the outward movement of the cardiac impulse. The cardiac impulse is a systolic event but its cause is uncertain since the apex of the heart retracts from the chest wall during systole. In systole, however, the shape of the heart changes, the ventricles become plumper and the distance between the AV ring and the apex shortens, the base of the heart moving downward and forward. It is assumed that these movements are responsible for the localised pulsation of the apex beat. X-rays show that the actual apex of the heart is about one inch lower down than the palpable apex beat.

In thin normal subjects the apex beat can usually be felt, and often seen, as a slight single pulsation narrowly localised in the fifth left intercostal space about the *mid-clavicular line*, that is, a line parallel with the mid-sternal line, running downward from a point halfway between the sternoclavicular and the acromioclavicular joints. The position of this line has to be determined for each individual because of the varying sizes and shapes of the thorax. The position of the apex beat is recorded with reference to this line or, if it is displaced to the left, with reference to the *anterior axillary line*, a line also parallel to the mid-sternal line but running down from the point where the edge of the pectoralis muscle meets the chest wall; or the *mid-axillary line.* The use of the nipple as a reference point is unsatisfactory and measurement from the mid-sternal line, though perfectly accurate, is not commonly used. The determination of the apex beat must be made with the patient lying either flat on his back or propped up a little and tilted neither to one side nor the other. It is not unusual for the apex beat in perfectly normal subjects to be imperceptible by either sight or palpation. The thicker the subcutaneous fat the more difficult it is to locate the apex beat accurately, or even to feel it at all. When the heart is enlarged the apex beat is displaced downward and outward, and may even be felt in the seventh intercostal space in the mid-axillary line.

The pulsations of the apex beat can be more critically analysed if they are graphically recorded by apex cardiography (Figure 2.15). The main outward pulsation is caused by ventricular systole but this is preceded by a smaller pulsation associated with the atrial contraction and followed by an inward pulsation that marks the opening of the AV valves. When there is atrial hypertrophy, or unusually forceful atrial contraction, the *atrial impulse* may be palpable as a bifid apex beat. It is best felt with the patient lying a little to the left side and the examiner's hand placed flat on the chest wall so that the extended fingers lie over the area of the apex beat.

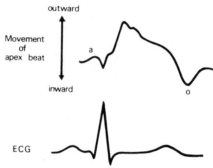

Figure 2.15. *Normal apexcardiogram and ECG showing the small atrial contribution* (a) *and the retraction at* o, *the time of opening of the AV valves.*

A strikingly 'tapping' single apex beat is caused by the vibrations associated with a loud first heart sound, as in mitral stenosis, and is not a sign of right ventricular hypertrophy as was once wrongly taught.

The powerful and prolonged systolic contraction of a hypertrophied left ventricle transmits a systolic pulsation to the ribs and other structures of the chest wall overlying it. This pulsation is best felt by the examiner's hand, placed firmly on the left praecordium with the thumb pointing upwards just medial to the nipple, the palm and metacarpophalangeal joints lying below the nipple and the extended fingers curving round the chest wall to the anterior axilla. The sustained heave can be felt and seen. The direction of the systolic impulse is downward and outward (Figure 2.16).

When there is gross left ventricular hypertrophy systolic retraction may be noticed in the intercostal spaces near the lower left sternal border.

The right ventricle lies not only to the right of the left ventricle, but also above it and anterior to it, below the sternum and the left sternal edge. When the right ventricle is hypertrophied its prolonged and more powerful pulsation lifts the sternum and the left

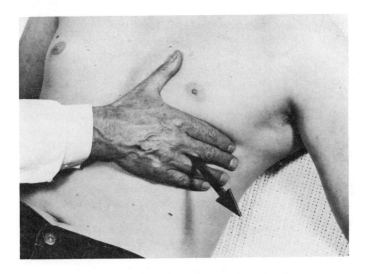

Figure 2.16. *Palpation for the heaving impulse of left ventricular hypertrophy. The pointer indicates the direction of the impulse.*

sternocostal joints. If the examiner places the palm of his hand, with the extended fingers pointing upward and parallel to the midsternal line, over the left sternal edge he will be able to feel and see the bony structures lift during systole, and his hand move with them. The direction of this impulse is anterior (Figure 2.17). This pulsation can also be seen if the examiner looks tangentially across the sternum, though he may have to stoop to do so. These two sustained systolic 'heaves' with their characteristic sites and directions are almost always valid clinical evidence of right and left ventricular hypertrophy. Sometimes, however, a left parasternal lift is felt over a tense pericardial effusion. These sustained heaving impulses should not be confused with the much jerkier cardiac pulsations sometimes felt in thin patients, and especially in children, with tachycardia and increased cardiac activity, but no heart disease.

Rarely, when the pulmonary artery is greatly enlarged, for example by long-standing pulmonary arterial hypertension, its pulsation may be detected by two fingers pressed firmly into the second or third left intercostal space to the left of the sternum.

Other pulsations are sometimes visible in the praecordium and

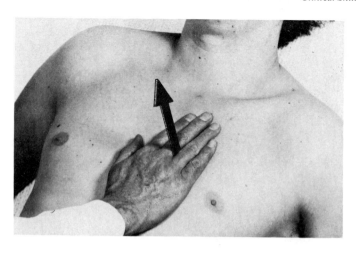

Figure 2.17. *Palpation for the left parasternal lift of right ventricular hypertrophy. The pointer indicates the direction of the impulse.*

xiphisternal region. In patients with aortic coarctation a large collateral flow often develops through tortuous and dilated internal mammary arteries. These can sometimes be seen pulsating at either edge of the sternum in the intercostal spaces. In thin patients a curious ripple is sometimes seen in intercostal spaces to the right of the sternum; it is perhaps particularly common in patients with atrial septal defects and Ebstein's anomaly, and is probably associated with atrial contraction. Pulsations are often seen in the xiphisternal region. These are usually either transmitted from the heart which lies just above the diaphragm, or else from the underlying aorta. They have no diagnostic value.

An aneurysm of the ascending aorta may cause pulsation that may be visible or palpable in the suprasternal notch or on either side of the sternum. On palpation a thrill may be felt. After a large myocardial infarction there may be abnormal systolic movements of the left ventricle that cause unusual systolic pulsations to become visible on the left praecordium; they may be transient, due to ventricular dyskinesis or, rarely, permanent, from a ventricular aneurysm. Hypertrophic obstructive cardiomyopathy sometimes gives rise to a double impulse at the apex. This double impulse is usually associated with a fourth heart sound but is occasionally due to a double ventricular thrust.

Percussion

Percussion for the borders of the heart is valueless, except in one condition. When a pericardial effusion is large enough to distend the pericardium to the right of the sternal edge, careful percussion from the region of the right nipple towards the edge of the sternum may demonstrate stony dullness. Even this sign, by itself, is insufficient for the diagnosis of a pericardial effusion, and other evidence, such as raised venous pressure with a characteristic pulsation, should be sought.

Auscultation

Stethoscopes

To most laymen the stethoscope is much more symbolic of medicine than the caduceus and certainly the livelihood of a practising clinician, and sometimes the life of a patient, depends upon its efficient use. The cliché that the stethoscope does not matter so much as what happens between its ear-pieces is only a half-truth: the whole truth is that competent auscultation, that is *directed listening* as opposed to just *hearing*, demands not only careful and prolonged ear training but also an adequate instrument.

Many studies have been made of the physical properties of stethoscopes and their different components. There is general agreement among physicists and practising cardiologists that a stethoscope should have two types of chest-piece, a diaphragm and a bell. When firmly applied to the praecordium the diaphragm chest-piece transmits high-pitched sound more efficiently than the bell, whereas the bell, lightly applied, turns the underlying skin into a diaphragm and transmits low-pitched sounds better than the diaphragm chest-piece. All modern stethoscopes have both bell and diaphragm incorporated in one chest-piece, allowing the auscultator to use one or the other by a simple movement. There are many varieties of both diaphragm and bell chest-pieces and it is well known that some are less efficient than others. The chest-piece is connected to the metal tubing of the head-piece by rubber or plastic tubing preferably with a lumen of one-eighth inch diameter. Ideally the tubes should not be longer than 10 inches and should have thick walls to exclude extraneous sound. The ear-pieces must fit the external auditory meatuses so that they completely exclude all sound except that coming from the chest-piece. Even the slightest leak of external sound not only distracts the auscultator but actually impairs auditory acuity. This implies not only that the ear-pieces must be exactly the right size to fit the auscultator's ears — and the shape and size of external auditory meatuses vary greatly — but also that the metal head-piece arms must be adjustable to allow the ear-piece to lie in the external meatus at exactly the correct angle to suit the individual ear. The spring between the arms of the head-piece must of course be strong enough to hold the ear-pieces firmly in position.

Some of these ideal properties are difficult to combine satisfactorily in practice; for example short lengths of thick tubing are not very flexible and make the stethoscope difficult to fit into a pocket. Some of the most efficient chest-pieces are bulky. Some of the voguish, lightweight 'slimline' stethoscopes have bells so inefficient that they have led practitioners grown accustomed only to their use to conclude that a diaphragm chest-piece is as efficient as any bell in conveying low-pitched sounds. Moreover, the human audiogram varies from person to person and changes over the years, for example when high-frequency deafness starts in middle age. It follows, therefore, that there can be no universally recommended stethoscope. Each clinician must find by trial and error the model that serves him best, and many experienced auscultators use hybrid specimens, perhaps even with chest-piece, tubing and ear-pieces derived from three different original instruments.

Cardiovascular sound

Doctors, professional musicians and wireless telegraphists are among the few groups of workers whose livelihood depends on their ability to listen critically. Nowadays we are surrounded by such constant noise that we subconsciously put up a barrier to hearing. It is all the more difficult, therefore, to learn not only to hear but to listen, and not only to listen but to listen in a positively directed manner.

Cardiovascular sounds are, in physical terms, merely vibrations whose frequencies lie within the range of human hearing. These vibrations are caused by turbulent flow, or sudden accelerations or decelerations in the flow, of blood in the semi-fluid heart and large vessels. For example, sudden changes of velocity produced by the opening and closing of cardiac valves produce only momentary turbulence that causes transient sharp sounds, whereas more prolonged turbulence produces sounds of longer duration known as *'murmurs'* or *'bruits'*. Most of the vibrations lie below the threshold of human hearing. The human audiogram shows that the normal threshold is lowest for frequencies about those of human speech. For sounds that have a much lower or higher pitch the ear is comparatively deaf: in these frequency ranges lie many important heart sounds and murmurs. In addition, heart sounds and murmurs may be so faint that they can hardly be heard even after prolonged auscultation. For these two reasons auscultation demands intense mental concentration using a faculty that most people normally have learned to neglect. The student must realise clearly that it is no use putting the ear-pieces of a stethoscope into his ears and the chest-piece on a patient's chest and then letting his mind be a neutral though receptive blank. He must deliberately and systematically listen with all his powers of concentration for what he expects he may hear, and also to detect the absence of what he would normally expect. To do this he must, of course, have a clear idea of what he is listening *for*, both in health and in disease.

The musical term 'pitch' refers to the frequency of vibration. A high-pitched sound such as is made by a violin or piccolo is associated with a high-frequency vibration. A low-pitched sound such as is made by a double bass or bassoon is associated with relatively low-frequency vibrations. The musical term 'timbre' is associated with the purity of the wave-form of the vibration, for example the number of harmonics included, and corresponds to the difference in quality between a note of the same pitch played, for example, by a violin and by an oboe.

Areas of auscultation

Surface markings of the four heart valves are often as shown on Figure 2.18A. It must be remembered, however, that the two ventricles lie not vertically in the chest but almost horizontally on the diaphragm, with the interventricular septum at an angle of about 45° to the anteroposterior axis of the thorax. The atria lie behind rather than above the ventricles, so the mitral and tricuspid valves lie side by side. Because the right ventricle is not only to the right of the left ventricle but also above and anterior to it, the tricuspid valve has identical relations to the mitral valve, and the inflow tracts of both ventricles are only separated by the interventricular septum.

Turbulence and eddy formation occur in a tube when the velocity of flow exceeds a critical value, determined, among other things, by the diameter of the tube. The energy involved in turbulent flow and eddy formation produces the vibrations associated with heart sounds and murmurs. The turbulence occurs downstream from the site of obstruction or dilatation or cusp movements and intra-cardiac phonocardiography has shown that heart sounds and murmurs are loudest downstream from their site of origin, that is, downstream from the heart valves in the case of the heart sounds, and downstream from stenoses or dilatations in the case of murmurs. This downstream projection of sounds from the site of their production explains the traditional 'areas of auscultation' of the four heart valves. Sounds arising from the aortic valve are projected to the second right intercostal space at the sternal edge and down the left sternal edge over the ascending and first part of the descending aorta. Sounds arising from the pulmonary valve are heard around the second left intercostal space. Because the mitral and tricuspid valves with their corresponding ventricular inflow tracts lie side by side, sounds arising at the AV valves are projected to areas of the chest wall very near to one another; those from the mitral valve are best heard at or just internal to the apex beat, while

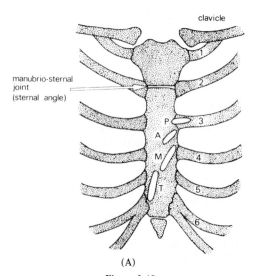

(A)

Figure 2.18.

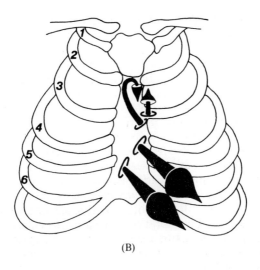

(B)

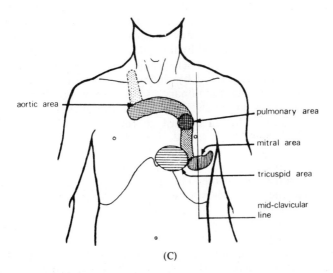

aortic area

pulmonary area

mitral area

tricuspid area

mid-clavicular line

(C)

Figure 2.18. *Surface markings of heart valves, auscultatory areas and the propagation of murmurs: A, surface markings of heart valves; B, direction of blood flow, and therefore of propagation of turbulence from the valves; C, areas on chest where sounds and murmurs arising at the four valves are usually best heard.*

those from the tricuspid valve are best heard over a slightly less localised area at the lower left sternal border or the bottom end of the sternum.

Auscultation of the xiphoid region is often rewarding, especially when heart sounds are difficult to hear elsewhere because of pulmonary disease.

Heart sounds

Before Laennec invented the stethoscope auscultation was performed with the examiner's ear held firmly against the chest. Anyone who does this can easily hear two heart sounds with every cardiac cycle. The *first heart sound* is the longer and louder of the normal heart sounds. It is associated with the start of ventricular systole and is caused by vibrations set up by the closure of the AV valves. Often there are two main groups of vibrations within the first heart sound and on auscultation with the stethoscope the first sound can be heard to be 'split'. This splitting is the result of the closure of first the mitral, and later the tricuspid, valve. The vibrations are most intense downstream from the AV valves, where the turbulent flow arises, so the first heart sound is best heard at an area of the chest wall near the apex beat. Because of its length and the comparatively low frequency (musical pitch) of its components it is traditionally represented by the syllable 'lub'. The *second heart sound* consists of two shorter groups of vibrations of higher frequency. They are caused by the sudden closure of, first, the aortic, and then the pulmonary, valve. They are best heard downstream from these valves in an area on the chest wall about the second intercostal space just to the right and left of the sternum. The second heart sound, being shorter and of higher pitch than the first heart sound, is traditionally represented by the syllable 'dupp'. The interval between the first and second heart sounds is ventricular systole. The interval between the second heart sound and the first heart sound of the next cardiac cycle is ventricular diastole.

The untrained ear may not appreciate the split between the aortic and pulmonary valve components of the second heart sound. Careful auscultation, however, during slow continued respiration confirms that the second heart sound is only single during the phase of full expiration. During the inspiratory phase the increase in the negative intrathoracic pressure increases the volume of blood in the right ventricle and this significantly delays the closure of the pulmonary valve, and hence the pulmonary component of the second heart sound. The second heart sound then sounds more like 'trupp'. At the height of inspiration the delay in the closure of the pulmonary valve is maximal, the split between the aortic and pulmonary components is widest and the sound may be represented as 'tu-rupp'. During expiration the split narrows again. This 'movement' of the splitting of the second heart sound is most easily heard in young people in the erect position. The appreciation of the splitting of the second heart sound forms a useful first test of a beginner's ability to use his stethoscope. When only the first and second sounds are audible the rhythm is normal duple rhythm and the sounds can be represented as 'lub-dupp' (Figure 2.19).

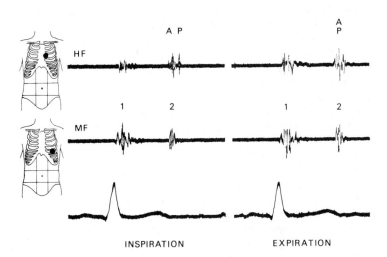

Figure 2.19. *Phonocardiogram of a normal young adult. One microphone at the left sternal edge provides a high frequency (HF) record, the other at the region of the cardiac apex provides a medium frequency (MF) record. 1 and 2, first and second heart sounds; A and P, vibrations associated with closure of the aortic and pulmonary valves. Lead II ECG at bottom. On inspiration the increased negative intrathoracic pressure increases the filling of the right ventricle in diastole. The increased right ventricular volume delays closure of the pulmonary valve; the pulmonary valve closure sound (P) is delayed causing audible splitting of the second heart sound (40 msec, in this record). On expiration pulmonary valve closure occurs so soon after aortic valve closure that the second heart sound seems single on auscultation. From Bell, Emslie-Smith and Paterson (1980) in* Textbook of Physiology *with kind permission of the publishers (Edinburgh: Churchill-Livingstone).*

In children and young adults a short muffled low-pitched sound is often heard in early diastole; this is the *third heart sound*, which has been shown to occur towards the end of the phase of rapid ventricular filling. The vibrations responsible for it are probably set up in the blood at a time when the left ventricular wall is changing from a state of active relaxation to one of passive distension and when the mitral valve system reaches a certain tension. A third heart sound gives a *triple rhythm* to the cardiac cadence and the sounds can be represented as 'lub-dupp-um'. An audible *fourth heart sound* (atrial sound) is abnormal though it can sometimes be demonstrated in normal people by phonocardiography. It resembles the third heart sound in duration and pitch but occurs just before the first heart sound and is associated with the contraction of the atria and the flow of blood through the AV valves. The triple rhythm of an atrial sound has a cadence that can be represented as 'tu-lub-dupp'. If the heart rate is fast and there is a triple rhythm the cadence is described as a *'gallop rhythm'*. When both the atrial sound and the third heart sound are audible the rhythm is *quadruple* ('tu-lub-dupp-um'); when the heart rate is fast the third heart sound of one cardiac cycle may coincide with the atrial sound of the next, the rhythm will then again be a triple one and is referred to as *'summation gallop'* (Figure 2.20). Triple rhythms are often best heard at the apex or near the xiphoid.

How to auscultate

The student should realise that it is impossible to listen critically for more than one thing at a time. For example, he should not attempt to assess the cadence of heart sounds at the same time as listening for murmurs; he should train himself to listen separately for high-pitched and low-pitched sounds. When he is deliberately listening — 'tuned-in' — for low-pitched sounds he will not be able to hear high-pitched sounds unless they are very loud; when he is 'tuned-in' for high-pitched sounds he will not hear low-pitched ones. This principle is particularly important when there are loud easily heard sounds whose frequency is well above the threshold of human hearing. Such sounds 'capture the ear' and it needs intense concentration to disregard the obvious and concentrate on other parts of the cardiac cycle for faint sounds that are difficult to hear. Of course experienced clinicians can frequently identify, for example, the auscultatory sounds of severe mitral stenosis almost at once, but the student would be well advised to adopt the policy of trained cardiologists and use the technique of non-simultaneous identification, only subsequently assembling the various components of the auditory pattern into a whole. It is probably lack of appreciation of this technique that leads some to believe that even the most skilled cardiologist is incapable of distinguishing four separate sounds that may occur within about 200 msec: for example, two components of the second sound, the opening snap of the mitral valve and a third heart sound.

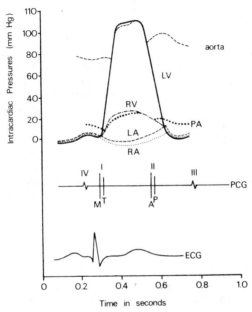

Figure 2.20. *Relationships between haemodynamic events in the cardiac cycle and the four 'normal' heart sounds recorded on a phonocardiogram (PCG). I, first heart sound; II, second heart sound; III, third heart sound; IV, fourth heart sound (atrial sound). M, T, A and P represent closure of the mitral, tricuspid, aortic and pulmonary valves respectively.*

The student should adopt a systematic approach to auscultation. He should start by putting the diaphragm part of his chest-piece at the pulmonary area and listen for the second heart sound. When he hears it split and unsplit on normal respiration he can feel that he has begun to be 'tuned-in'. The first sound is then readily identified, occurring simultaneously with the upstroke of the carotid arterial pulse. The basic cadence of the heart sounds should be given time to imprint itself on the mind before the stethoscope is moved inch by inch to other areas of the praecordium where extra sounds are commoner. Individual practice will vary, but from the pulmonary area the auscultator might move to the aortic area, then 'inch' down the left sternal border, finishing up at the mitral area, at or internal to the cardiac apex. At each site he must listen with the diaphragm for high-pitched sounds and with the bell for low-pitched sounds with a pause between each spell of concentrated listening.

After each spell he should ask himself the questions of the following catechism.

1. Do I hear the first heart sound? If so, is it loud, as in mitral stenosis, or soft, or even variable in intensity as in complete heart block; is it split or unsplit?

2. Do I hear the second heart sound? If so, is it loud or soft, split, or unsplit? If split, do its components move in a normal manner with respiration or not? 'Reversed splitting' with the two components widening on expiration occurs in left bundle-branch block and left ventricular failure.

3. Do I hear any other heart sound? If so, is it in early diastole, that is, a third heart sound, or is it in presystole, that is, an atrial or fourth heart sound?

4. Do I hear any short sound that is not one of these heart sounds, for example a short, high-pitched clicking sound? If so, is it in systole or in diastole? At what phase of systole or diastole is it heard; for example, early or mid-systolic or early diastolic? (Figure 2.21).

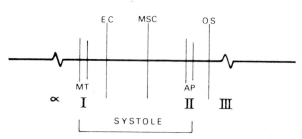

Figure 2.21. *The normal heart sounds (as in Figure 20) with three other short sharp sounds: EC, early systolic ejection click; MSC, mid systolic click; OS, opening snap of mitral (or tricuspid valve); α, atrial sound (fourth heart sound).*

5. Is there any other sound? It so, is it a murmur or pericardial friction?

6. If it is a *murmur*, where is it loudest? Does it radiate in any direction? Is it systolic or diastolic or both? (Figure 2.22). If the murmur is systolic, what is its type, for example ejection or regurgitant? (see below). If it is diastolic, at what stage of diastole does it start; for example, does it follow the second heart sound immediately *(early diastolic murmur)* or is there a clear gap between the second heart sound and the onset of the murmur *(mid-diastolic murmur)*?

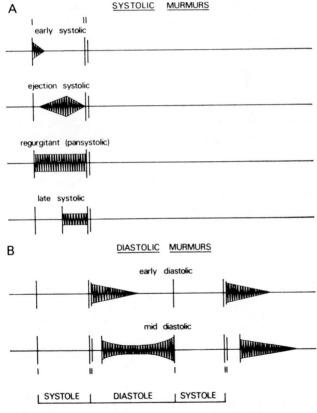

Figure 2.22. *Diagram of common systolic (A) and diastolic (B) murmurs. I and II indicate first and second heart sounds.*

7. If there is both a systolic and a diastolic murmur are they separate murmurs *(to-and-fro murmur)* or is there a single murmur that waxes and wanes in intensity throughout the whole cardiac cycle *(continuous murmur)*? (Figure 2.23).

The answering of this catechism takes time and much concentration but its use provides the very best training in auscultation for the student and for the experienced practitioner the best means of missing no clue of diagnostic help.

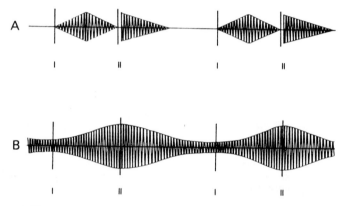

Figure 2.23. *(A) 'To-and-fro murmurs' consisting of an ejection systolic murmur and a separate early diastolic murmur; (B) continuous murmur.*

This systematic auscultation is reinforced by a systematic method of recording what has been heard. A good way is to record diagrammatically what the auscultator would expect a phono-cardiogram (page 116) to show. Figure 2.24 shows a series of such diagrams. Transient sounds such as heart sounds and clicking sounds are represented by simple vertical lines above and below the baseline, murmurs as zig-zag lines. The length and loudness of murmurs can also be indicated by numbers representing clinical gradings. It is convenient to represent the gradings of length below the line and the gradings of loudness above the line. Additional information such as directions of radiation of murmurs and points of clarification can easily be added.

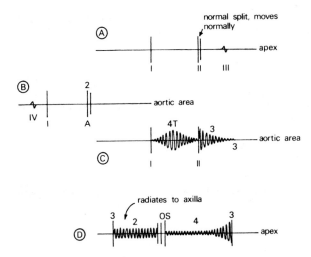

Figure 2.24. *Method of recording heart sounds and murmurs. Heart sounds are labelled with Roman numerals, loudness as grades (out of 4) above the line, length similarly but below the line. A, normal sounds, young adult; B, atrial sound and loud aortic closure sound at aortic area as in hypertensive heart disease; C, loud ejection systolic murmur with thrill (T) and early diastolic murmur as in aortic stenosis and incompetence; D, loud first heart sound, pansystolic murmur, mitral opening snap and mid-diastolic murmur with presystolic accentuation, all at the apex, as in dominant mitral stenosis with some incompetence.*

Murmurs

It is only necessary to watch a river to realise that turbulent flow occurs in certain well-defined conditions, for example where there is a sudden narrowing of the stream, where some obstruction projects into the stream or where the stream suddenly widens. Murmurs that arise from turbulent flow are propagated in the direction of flow from the site of their production and are heard in the areas of auscultation described earlier. Mitral valve murmurs are heard around the apical impulse, tricuspid valve murmurs more medially. Only rarely, when there is gross right ventricular hypertrophy, are murmurs that originate in the tricuspid valve heard best to the right of the sternum. Murmurs arising at the aortic valve are projected in the direction of flow and therefore follow the course of the ascending and descending aorta in the thorax. Consequently, they are best heard about the second right intercostal space, across the sternum at about this level and down the left sternal border; they may even be heard a little internal to the apex beat. Murmurs arising in the pulmonary valve are projected in the direction of flow along the course of the main pulmonary artery and are best heard to the left of the sternum about the level of the second intercostal space (see Figure 2.18).

If the velocity of blood flow across the comparatively narrow aortic and pulmonary valves is high, for example with excitement, exercise or fever, and in almost all children, turbulent flow is common during the ejection phase of ventricular systole even when there is absolutely no abnormality of the valves. An *innocent flow murmur* is the result. When turbulence is great enough the intensity of vibrations produces not only a very loud murmur but also a palpable vibration called a *thrill*.

Systolic murmurs

Murmurs heard between the first and second heart sounds are systolic, those heard between the second heart sound and the first heart sound of the next cardiac cycle are diastolic. Systolic murmurs are associated with movement of blood during ventricular systole either *forward* during *ejection* through the aortic or pulmonary valve, or *backward*, from ventricle to atrium, by *regurgitation* through an incompetent mitral or tricuspid valve. A third cause is ejection of blood from a high-pressure left-sided chamber through a septal defect into a right-sided chamber with a lower pressure, for example the left-to-right shunt through a ventricular septal defect. Four types of systolic murmur are usually described, depending on their timing during systole (Figure 2.22A).

Early systolic murmurs. These murmurs are short diminuendo murmurs immediately after the first heart sound. Although they are often seen on phonocardiograms they are seldom discernible on auscultation, merely sounding like a rather indistinct first heart sound; indeed, the vibrations may represent rather slow damping of the vibrations involved in the production of the first heart sound. They have no pathological significance.

Ejection murmurs. These murmurs are caused by the turbulence arising from the ejection of blood across abnormal aortic or pulmonary valves, or by the ejection of blood with increased velocity across normal valves. They can therefore be of either physiological or pathological significance. On the phonocardiogram they have a characteristic appearance. Immediately after the first heart sound there is a short silent gap. The murmur then starts and is diamond shaped, the vibrations rapidly increasing in amplitude and then diminishing again. The point of highest amplitude of the diamond corresponds with the time of maximum velocity of ejection across the valve (Figure 2.25). This diamond shape gives to the murmur a characteristic short, brusque, crescendo—diminuendo property. When the murmur arises at the aortic valve the vibrations end before aortic valve closure and the aortic component of the second sound may be clearly heard. When the murmur arises at the pulmonary valve, however, the turbulent blood flow may not have subsided at the time the aortic valve shuts, so the vibrations on the phonocardiogram can be seen to pass through the aortic closure sound to end before the pulmonary closure sound; the aortic component of the second sound is not heard because it is hidden in the end of the ejection murmur but the pulmonary component is usually audible. The commonest causes of ejection systolic murmurs are listed in Table 2.2.

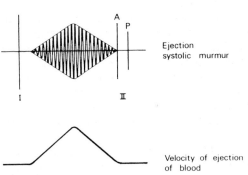

Figure 2.25. *Turbulence from ejection of blood across the aortic valve causes a diamond-shaped ejection murmur that starts after the first heart sound and ends at the aortic closure sound.*

Regurgitant murmurs. When the mitral or tricuspid valve is incompetent blood flows during ventricular systole not only forward through the semilunar valves but also backward through the incompetent valve from the high-pressure ventricle into the low-pressure atrium. Unlike the ejection systolic murmur, which is caused by turbulent forward flow against a relatively high and

Table 2.2. *Commoner causes of ejection systolic murmurs.*

Physiological

  Rapid flow through normal semilunar valves
      Childhood and adolescence
      Hyperkinetic circulatory states (Table 2.1)

Pathological

  Rapid flow through normal pulmonary valve
      Atrial septal defect (see text)

  Flow through abnormal semilunar valves
    (a) With pressure gradient across valve
      Aortic valve stenosis (rheumatic or congenital)
      Pulmonary valve stenosis (congenital)
    (b) Without pressure gradient
      Aortic valve sclerosis (in elderly)
      Bicuspid aortic valve (congenital)
      Aortic valve incompetence (see text)

  Left ventricular outflow tract obstruction
      Hypertrophic obstructive cardiomyopathy (HOCM, IHSS)
      Subaortic stenosis

  Ventricular septal defect (see text)

changing aortic or pulmonary artery resistance, the regurgitant blood flow across an atrioventricular valve sets up turbulence that is more or less uniform throughout the whole of systole. The shape of the murmur is determined by the pressure gradient responsible for the turbulent flow that causes it. Figure 2.26 shows the gradient and murmur in mitral incompetence. Since the pressure gradient between the ventricle and the atrium does not end with the closure of either the aortic or pulmonary valves a phonocardiogram often shows that the murmur actually continues for a short time after the second sound. This is not, however, audible on auscultation but the murmur does sound as if it occupies the whole of systole from the first heart sound to the second heart sound, even obliterating the second heart sound. It is therefore called a *pansystolic* (or holosystolic) murmur. Pansystolic murmurs vary greatly in loudness. When they are soft they are appropriately described as 'blowing' but when they are loud they can have a rough quality almost resembling that of an ejection murmur; when the vibrations are unusually regular they may have a musical quality. The pansystolic murmur of mitral incompetence from papillary muscle dysfunction, ruptured chordae tendineae or prolapsing mitral valve cusp often sounds louder or more musical towards the end. When the heart beats with normal sinus rhythm the pansystolic murmur of tricuspid incompetence is louder during inspiration because there is then an increased volume in the right ventricle as a result of the increased venous return. When the cardiac rhythm is irregular, as in atrial fibrillation, respiration has no effect on the loudness of the murmur.

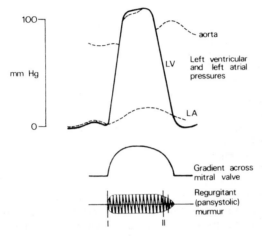

Figure 2.26. *When the mitral valve is incompetent there is regurgitation of blood during systole from the left ventricle to the left atrium and the left atrial pressure is abnormally raised. Turbulent flow is related to the ventriculo-atrial gradient and causes a pansystolic murmur.*

Late systolic murmur. This murmur starts about mid-systole and continues up to the second sound. Phonocardiograms sometimes show that it is immediately preceded by a sharp, high-pitched mid-systolic click, and occasionally the click is audible (see Figure 2.22A). Because there is such a long pause between the first heart sound and the onset of the murmur late systolic murmurs are frequently misdiagnosed as early diastolic murmurs. The fact that their timbre is quite different from any early diastolic murmur merely adds to the confusion. They are often quite loud, of medium frequency and only their timing gives rise to difficulty. For many years these late systolic murmurs were regarded as 'innocent' murmurs, but it is now appreciated that they occur in three conditions. Most commonly they are associated with 'subvalvar' mitral incompetence where, because of an abnormality of the chordae tendineae or the papillary muscle one cusp of the mitral valve fails to close during systole. They are also heard in left ventricular obstructive cardiomyopathy when the hypertrophied muscle of the outflow tract contracts abnormally late in systole giving rise to a special kind of delayed ejection murmur; they also arise from a coarctation of the aorta.

Not all murmurs can be forced precisely into one or other of these categories: for example, the murmur of tricuspid incompetence is not always absolutely pansystolic, sometimes falling silent before the second sound, and the murmur of a ventricular septal defect is often a 'long ejection' murmur starting earlier and seeming to last longer than a 'typical' short ejection systolic murmur arising from one of the semilunar valves.

Ejection systolic murmurs are often best heard at the aortic and pulmonary areas. The pansystolic murmur of mitral incompetence is best heard at the apex and may radiate out to the axilla while that of tricuspid incompetence is best heard internal to the apex at the left sternal edge and may radiate to the mid-sternal area. Late systolic murmurs are usually loudest near the apex, while the characteristic murmur of ventricular septal defect is usually loudest about the middle of the sternum at the level of the third or fourth intercostal space, or near the right sternal edge. The ejection murmurs of aortic and pulmonary stenosis may radiate to the carotid regions above the clavicle.

Diastolic murmurs

There are three types of diastolic murmur, named according to the point in diastole at which each begins (Figure 2.22B). The commoner causes of diastolic murmurs are listed in Table 2.3.

Table 2.3. *Commoner causes of diastolic murmurs.*

Early diastolic murmurs (EDM)
Aortic incompetence
(Pulmonary incompetence, see text)
Mid-diastolic murmurs (MDM)
Mitral stenosis
(Tricuspid flow murmur from large ASD, see text)
(Mitral flow murmur from large VSD, see text)
(Short MDM in mitral incompetence, see text)

Early diastolic murmurs. Early diastolic murmurs are associated with turbulence arising from regurgitation of blood backward into the ventricle across an incompetent aortic or pulmonary valve. Phonocardiograms sometimes show a very short gap between the appropriate valve closure sound and the onset of the murmur but this gap is never appreciated by the ear. The murmur sounds as though it immediately follows the second heart sound. It is relatively high-pitched, and frequently resembles a breath sound both in pitch and timbre. This is the main reason why an early diastolic murmur can best be heard when the patient has emptied his lungs and stopped breathing ('expiratory apnoea'). Its quality is often described as 'blowing' but a much better term would be 'breathing'. Occasionally it is rougher or even musical. The phonocardiogram shows that the vibrations have greatest amplitude at their start and then diminish progressively. The murmur is therefore a diminuendo one. It can be loud or soft, short or long. Soft early diastolic murmurs are often difficult to hear even by trained auscultators and when high-frequency deafness begins in middle age they are the first murmurs to be missed.

Figure 2.27 shows the pressure gradient responsible for the turbulent flow in aortic regurgitation and the way in which it is

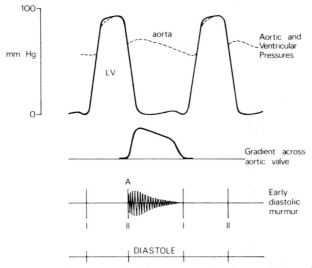

Figure 2.27. *When the aortic valve is incompetent there is regurgitation of blood during diastole from the aorta to the left ventricle. Turbulence is related to the aorto-ventricular gradient and causes a diminuendo early diastolic murmur.*

related to the murmur. Because early diastolic murmurs are high-pitched they are best heard with the diaphragm of the stethoscope firmly applied to a site downstream from the aortic or pulmonary valve, for example the aortic area or the second left interspace or down the left sternal border. They are best heard with the patient leaning slightly forward, holding his breath after full expiration (Figure 2.28). Most early diastolic murmurs are caused by aortic incompetence. The murmur of pulmonary incompetence is rare, even when there is evidence of pulmonary arterial hypertension.

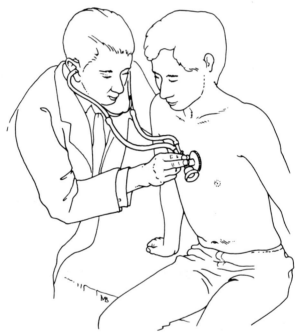

Figure 2.28. *Optimal conditions for hearing early diastolic murmurs. The examiner uses the diaphragm of his stethoscope firmly applied to the aortic area or left sternal edge. The patient is leaning slightly forward with his breath held in full expiration.*

Mid-diastolic murmurs. The term 'mid-diastolic' suggests that this murmur starts in mid-diastole, which is not strictly true. The phonocardiogram shows that it begins early in diastole but well after the second heart sounds. On auscultation this silent gap is so obvious that the murmur sounds as though it starts about mid-diastole. Mid-diastolic murmurs are caused by the turbulent flow of blood through a narrowed mitral or tricuspid valve. Figure 2.29 shows the pressure gradient between the atrium and the ventricle and its relationship to the 'shape' and duration of the murmur of mitral stenosis. Mid-diastolic murmurs are of very low frequency indeed, and most beginners fail to hear the murmurs even when they are quite loud because of failure to realise that is is necessary to listen 'tuned in' to such low pitches; thinking about the rumble of distant thunder or the sound of double basses in an orchestra may help the beginner to 'tune in' low enough. These murmurs are

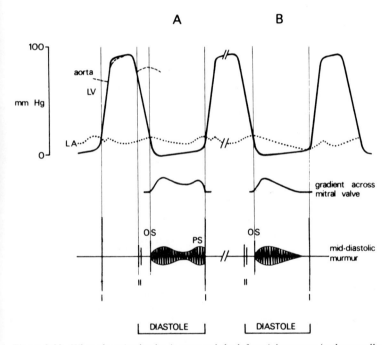

Figure 2.29. *When the mitral valve is stenosed the left atrial pressure is abnormally raised and the narrowed valve causes turbulent flow during ventricular filling in diastole. The turbulence is related to the AV gradient. In A there is sinus rhythm and atrial contraction increases the gradient before the mitral valve closes. The turbulence causes a mid-diastolic murmur with a presystolic accentuation (PS). In B there is atrial fibrillation so there is no presystolic murmur. Despite the rhythm the high AV gradient causes a loud first heart sound when the valve shuts and a mitral 'opening snap' (OS) when it opens.*

therefore often described as 'rumbling'. When they are short they can easily be confused with a third heart sound for they have much the same frequency. When they are long and the patient has sinus rhythm they end in a presystolic accentuation or presystolic murmur (Figure 2.29A). Because of their low pitch, mid-diastolic murmurs are best heard with the bell of the stethoscope lightly applied to the skin. The mid-diastolic murmur of mitral stenosis is best heard at or internal to the apex, and especially when the heart is slowing after a little exercise and the patient is lying flat and turned at about 30 to 45° towards his left side (Figure 2.30). The

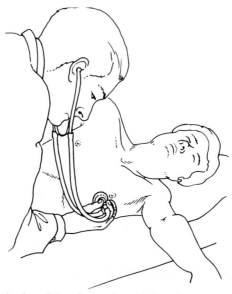

Figure 2.30. *Optimal conditions for hearing mid-diastolic murmurs. The patient has been exercised and then lies down, turned approximately 45° to his left side. The examiner uses the bell of his stethoscope lightly applied at or medial to the apical impulse. He listens especially carefully when the heart rate begins to slow.*

murmur of tricuspid stenosis is heard only slightly more medially. As with the murmur of tricuspid incompetence, so long as the patient has sinus rhythm the murmur of tricuspid stenosis becomes louder on inspiration because of the increased blood flow caused by the increased volume of the right ventricle during inspiration. This respiratory effect is abolished in the presence of atrial fibrillation.

Presystolic murmurs. When the mitral or tricuspid valves are stenosed atrial contraction with sinus rhythm increases the gradient across the valve and the turbulent flow through the narrowed valve causes a presystolic murmur (Figure 2.29A). With mitral stenosis this produces the presystolic accentuation; occasionally in tricuspid stenosis it is the only murmur heard and becomes louder during inspiration.

The two common diastolic murmurs, which are always abnormal, and therefore important, can often be difficult to hear but they should not be difficult to distinguish. Apart from the fact that they are both diastolic they do not have a single other feature in common; they are different in timing, pitch, timbre and site and are made easier to hear by different manoeuvres and different postures of the patient and by using different chest-pieces of the stethoscope.

The diagnostic value of murmurs

As soon as one can identify a murmur as systolic or diastolic one has already taken a large diagnostic step. The trained auscultator can tell one from the other at once, because just as he can distinguish a dog's bark from a sheep's bleat, he knows, for example, that no diastolic murmur sounds like the systolic murmur to which he is listening. The student often has difficulty, however, and must make use of as much help as he can find. When listening over the apex, if the chest-piece lifts, it does so during systole. Palpation of the carotid pulse helps some students. The best guide however remains the first and second heart sound; when 'lost' the student should return to the pulmonary area, or wherever the two sounds are clearest, and then 'inch' towards the site where the murmur is loudest. The next step is to identify the systolic murmur as ejection (diamond shaped) or regurgitant (pansystolic). Ejection murmurs usually arise either at the aortic or pulmonary valves while regurgitant murmurs arise at the mitral or tricuspid valves. Similarly early diastolic murmurs arise at the aortic or pulmonary valves while mid-diastolic and pre-systolic murmurs arise at the mitral and tricuspid valves. Abnormal cardiac valves and congenital cardiac defects give rise to auscultatory abnormalities apart from murmurs and the auscultatory syndromes of various common cardiac lesions are often very characteristic.

Mitral stenosis

When the mitral valve is narrowed the left atrial pressure is abnormally high and the atrioventricular pressure gradient in diastole is greater than normal. When the abnormal valve shuts it causes a larger vibration than usual which can be heard as an abnormally loud first heart sound and often felt at the apex as a 'palpable' first heart sound or 'tapping apex beat'. In the absence of mitral incompetence systole is silent and the pulmonary and aortic components of the second heart sound are usually separable, though if there is pulmonary arterial hypertension the pulmonary component may be so loud that the second heart sound seems single. If the anterior cusp of the mitral valve is pliant, when the stenosed valve opens the anterior cusp sets up transient vibrations that are seen on the phonocardiogram and heard through the diaphragm of the stethoscope as a high-pitched sharp snapping sound, the *'opening snap'* of the mitral valve. The opening snap has been likened to the sound caused when a spinnaker fills but the mechanical analogy is not very accurate. It is usually best heard at the lower left sternal edge and internal to the apex beat. It is sometimes louder during inspiration and usually causes no confusion with the much lower pitched third heart sound. The mid-diastolic rumble starts with the opening snap and, if the patient has sinus rhythm, it becomes louder with the presystolic accentuation up to the first heart sound of the next cardiac cycle. The 19th century French cardiologist Duroziez attempted to imitate the characteristic cadence in his mnemonic 'ffout-ta-ta-rrrou', in which 'ffou' represents the presystolic murmur, the terminal 't' of ffout the loud first heart sound, 'ta-ta' the second heart sound and opening snap and 'rrrou' the mid-diastolic rumbling murmur. Many now find the sounds 'rroo-upp, ta-ta' represent that cadence better, starting with the mid-diastolic rumble ('rroo'), including the presystolic accentuation to the loud first sound ('upp'), the systolic pause (comma) and the second sound and opening snap ('ta-ta').

Mitral incompetence

In mitral incompetence the first heart sound is not abnormally loud and the second heart sound may not be heard at the apex because of the pansystolic murmur, which may radiate out towards the axilla. Unless there is accompanying mitral stenosis there is no opening snap but there is often a low pitched third heart sound and sometimes a short mid-diastolic rumble. Not all rumbles in diastole are caused by mitral stenosis, even when the mitral valve is diseased (see pages 106, 107 and Table 2.3).

Aortic incompetence

The only evidence of aortic incompetence may be a very soft, short, high-pitched early diastolic murmur, but it may, of course, be long and loud. When there is free aortic regurgitation the increased velocity of ejection of the larger stroke volume causes an ejection systolic murmur that need not imply any stenosis of the valve. The very rare murmur of pulmonary incompetence is indistinguishable on auscultation and the lesion can only be reliably established by pulmonary angiography.

Aortic and pulmonary stenosis

Stenosis of either the aortic or the pulmonary valve causes a loud ejection systolic murmur at the appropriate area. The exact timing of the murmurs varies as described above. If there is poststenotic dilatation of either the aorta or the pulmonary artery there may be in early systole a sharp high-pitched clicking sound (aortic or pulmonary *ejection click*) (Figure 2.21). Unlike the opening snap of mitral stenosis a pulmonary ejection click is often best heard in expiration. With severe aortic stenosis the aortic closure sound may be soft or impossible to hear.

Atrial septal defect

The increased flow of blood through the right ventricle and across the pulmonary valve causes an ejection systolic murmur in the pulmonary area. Sometimes the two components of the second sound are widely split at all phases of respiration *(fixed splitting)*, because the large left-to-right shunt across the atrial septum keeps blood flow across the pulmonary valve maximal irrespective of the respiratory cycle. This increased blood flow sometimes produces turbulence at the tricuspid valve which causes a rumbling mid-diastolic murmur audible in the tricuspid area.

Ventricular septal defect

The characteristic long ejection murmur heard over, or to the right of, the sternum about the third intercostal space is often loudest with comparatively small defects and may be associated with a very easily felt thrill. If the pulmonary vascular resistance is high, however, the murmur may be shorter, softer and of pure ejection type, with no thrill. A loud third heart sound caused by rapid left ventricular filling is fairly common. To maintain a normal stroke volume in the presence of a left-to-right shunt the filling of the left ventricle is increased and the increased flow across the mitral valve may produce a rumbling mid-diastolic murmur at the apex *(diastolic 'flow murmur')*. It is present in about half the patients, and in most of those in whom the pulmonary blood flow is over 2.5 times the systemic blood flow.

Patent ductus arteriosus

Because the pressure in the aorta is above that in the pulmonary artery throughout both systole and diastole, patency of the ductus arteriosus causes a continuous left-to-right shunt from aorta to pulmonary artery. The blood flow and turbulence are greatest about the time that the semilunar valves close and give rise to a characteristic *continuous murmur* which waxes and wanes. At the time when the murmur is loudest, a loud second heart sound can often be recognised. This murmur has a rough quality and is sometimes therefore referred to as a *'machinery murmur'* (see Figure 2.23B). It is heard in the pulmonary area and below the left clavicle, and can only be confused with the softer continuous murmur that is the result of increased blood flow through the great veins in the neck *(venous hum)*. The venous hum is louder above the clavicle than below, and can be stopped completely by obliterating the venous return in the neck by a firmly applied finger, and often altered or abolished by turning the head and bending the neck from side to side.

Eponymous murmurs

Students are often confused by the eponyms that have been attached to murmurs by some of their teachers. The Gibson murmur is that of patent ductus arteriosus. The Austin Flint murmur is a mid-diastolic murmur heard at the apex in cases of gross aortic incompetence without mitral stenosis. Its exact cause is uncertain. The Graham Steell murmur is the rare early diastolic murmur of pulmonary incompetence. The name of Carey Coombs is sometimes attached to a short mid-diastolic rumbling murmur heard at the apex in children with active rheumatic carditis; its cause is uncertain but it does not signify established mitral stenosis. Duroziez's murmur is a 'clinical toy'. In severe aortic incompetence the backward and forward movement of blood in the aorta is exaggerated; if a stethoscope is placed over a large artery such as the brachial or femoral, and the artery is partially occluded by a finger, proximal to the stethoscope, at a certain critical pressure the blood flowing to and fro under the stethoscope gives rise to a to-and-fro murmur that can easily be heard.

The grading of cardiac murmurs

The loudness of cardiac murmurs may be graded in different ways. Six grades of loudness are often used, particularly in the United States and by cardiologists in the United Kingdom. In this six-grade scale a Grade 1 murmur is only just audible by a skilled auscultator in very favourable conditions; a Grade 2 murmur can be heard as 'soft' by ordinary auscultation; a Grade 3 murmur is louder and easily heard; a Grade 4 murmur is loud; a Grade 5 murmur is the loudest murmur inaudible without the aid of a stethoscope and a Grade 6 murmur is so loud that it can be heard without a stethoscope.

It will be appreciated that there is little practical difference between a Grade 1 and a Grade 2 murmur, the difference depending mainly on the skill of the auscultator. Similarly there is little practical difference between a Grade 5 and a Grade 6 murmur. In the United Kingdom therefore, the loudness of cardiac murmurs, like the severity of any physical sign, is commonly graded out of four, corresponding to the time-honoured clinical adjectives of degree, 'mild', 'moderate', 'considerable' and 'gross'. With the four-grade system a Grade 1 murmur can be heard after a short period of determined auscultation, a Grade 4 murmur is the loudest murmur possible, and Grades 2 and 3 are intermediate. There is much to recommend this simpler form of grading; the loudness of murmurs is a very subjective matter and even with phonocardiography satisfactory methods of estimating loudness are lacking. Whichever system is adopted, it should be clearly indicated in any records; for example a murmur might be described as 3/6 or 2/4.

Pericardial Friction

Normally the small amount of serous fluid between the visceral and parietal pericardium allows the heart to move freely within the pericardial sac. With pericarditis, however, the fibrinous exudate produces *friction sounds* as the heart moves. These sounds can occur during systole or diastole or both, but are not confused with murmurs because their timbre is quite different. They are scratchy or crunching sounds, like pleural rubs. Although they arise in the pericardium their intensity may be influenced by respiration. Occasionally, when there is pleurisy of the surface of the lung near the heart, pleural friction sounds are linked to the cardiac cycle and are called pleuro-pericardial friction, but the lesion responsible is a pulmonary, not a cardiac one. Another type of pulmonary sound linked to the cardiac cycle, but not directly attributable to the heart, is the clicking sound heard in the region of the cardiac apex in some cases of left-sided pneumothorax.

Carotid Sinus Pressure

This important manoeuvre can be used in the clinical diagnosis of arrhythmias and, for some, in the treatment. The exact technique is important. With the patient lying propped up the right carotid artery is palpated at the level of the upper border of the thyroid cartilage while the clinician listens to the patient's heart with his stethoscope and continues to do so throughout the manoeuvre. With his thumb the clinician presses the artery firmly against the bodies of the cervical vertebrae for several seconds, massaging it gently as the pressure is maintained. The moment the cardiac rhythm is heard to alter the pressure must be stopped. If the rhythm does not change the left carotid sinus should be stimulated but on no account should both carotid sinuses be pressed simultaneously.

Cardiac Dysrhythmias

The accurate diagnosis of dysrhythmias can only be made with an electrocardiograph (Figures 2.36—2.43). Sometimes, however, an instrument is not available and the patient's condition is such that urgent treatment must be given. In these circumstances only the diagnosis may be attempted on clinical grounds alone. *Sinus tachycardia* must be distinguished clinically from atrial flutter or supraventricular tachycardia. It usually varies in rate, especially when the patient is told to hold his breath, and is seldom faster than about 140 beats per minute. Carotid sinus pressure causes gradual slowing. During a *supraventricular paroxysm of tachycardia* the loudness of the first heart sound is constant because of the fixed relation between atrial and ventricular systole. In some AV nodal tachycardias (high junctional tachycardias) the right atrium contracts against a closed tricuspid valve and obvious rapid and regular *a* waves can be seen in the jugular pulse. Pressure on the carotid sinus either has no effect, or ends the paroxysm abruptly. *Atrial flutter* may be suspected clinically when a regular tachycardia has a ventricular rate of about 160 beats per minute (flutter with 2-1 AV block) or when the rate changes frequently (flutter with changing AV block). Occasionally flutter waves may be seen in the jugular venous pulse as rapid small *a* waves, and very rarely indeed, when there is a high degree of AV block, 'flutter sounds' can be heard on auscultation. Carotid sinus pressure increases AV block while pressure lasts, so the ventricular rate slows appropriately and may then increase in a stepwise manner.

The key to the clinical diagnosis of *atrial fibrillation* is the chaotic rhythm: the pulse is irregularly irregular and on auscultation no pattern can be recognised in successive cardiac cycles. No *a* wave is present in the venous pulse. Sometimes, when the ventricular rate is slower than usual, it may be hard to distinguish atrial fibrillation from frequent ectopic beats or from atrial flutter with changing block.

In *ventricular paroxysmal tachycardia* the ventricular rate is high, usually over 180 beats per minute, often over 200. The first sound can sometimes be heard to vary in intensity because of the varying relationship between atrial and ventricular systole. Occasional 'cannon waves' may be seen in the neck for the same reason. Multiple low-pitched extra heart sounds are very occasionally heard. Carotid sinus pressure has no effect whatever on the rhythm.

In *complete heart block* the ventricular rate is often as slow as 30 beats per minute, but it may be as fast as 60 when the pacemaker is high in the junctional conducting tissue. The rate varies little with exercise. The bradycardia is associated with a collapsing pulse. Because of the varying times between atrial and ventricular contraction there is a varying intensity of the first heart sound, the occasional very loud ones being called 'cannon sounds'. Occasional giant *a* waves are seen in the jugular venous pulse; the cannon sounds are heard when the interval between atrial and ventricular contraction is minimal, so that the AV valves close on a partly filled ventricle, whereas giant *a* waves are the result of atrial systole against a closed tricuspid valve: cannon sounds and cannon waves do not always occur simultaneously, and the term 'cannon wave' is therefore doubly unintelligible. There is often evidence of cardiac enlargement. Sometimes separate atrial sounds can be heard, usually at the lower left sternal border, and occasionally a third heart sound or a short mid-diastolic murmur follows some beats. The patient may give a characteristic history of Adams—Stokes attacks.

Examination of the Rest of the Thorax

If coarctation of the aorta is present striking arterial pulsation can often be seen in the enlarged and tortuous collateral vessls in inter-costal spaces, as well as in the internal mammary arteries on either side of the sternum. The best way to look for this arterial pulsation is to have the patient, stripped to the waist, bend over the back of a chair and hold the front of the seat with his hands. The lighting should be arranged so that it falls tangentially across his back between the scapulae, which are held far apart by the position of the arms. The tortuous pulsatile vessels are thrown into relief by the contrast of light and shade. Pulsating vessels may also be palpated.

Auscultation of the lung bases during deep respiration may detect fine crackles that do not clear on coughing, suggesting pulmonary oedema. With severe pulmonary oedema, of course, the fine crackles are not confined to the bases but are heard more widely over the lungs. Pleural effusions caused by congestive cardiac failure produce the appropriate physical signs.

Abdomen

The liver should be percussed and palpated to decide if it is enlarged and whether it has intrinsic pulsation caused by tricuspid incompetence (see above). The spleen should also be palpated; it may be enlarged in congestive cardiac failure and sometimes in bacterial endocarditis when it may be tender. The abdominal aorta runs only a short distance below the anterior abdominal wall, lying on the top of the vertebral bodies. Its pulsation is often visible and normally always palpable. In elderly people it is often kinked and sometimes it is dilated by an aneurysm. In congestive cardiac failure and constrictive pericarditis ascites may be a prominent feature. Auscultation of the abdomen may lead to the discovery of arterial bruits. These usually arise in the aorta but occasionally are the result of a unilateral renal artery stenosis and are audible to one or other side of the umbilicus and often slightly above it.

Oedema

Cardiac oedema accumulates in the most dependent parts of the soft tissues. When the patient is ambulant it is therefore most obvious in the ankles and may well become more obvious as the day goes on. When patients are confined to bed, however, the oedema may be present in the sacral area or the backs of the thighs where pitting can be elicited by firm and fairly long sustained pressure. Sometimes a pillow against the sacrum prevents the fluid accumulating there and the pad of pitting oedema is displaced upwards towards the lower lumbar region. When oedema is gross it also involves the genitalia.

Legs

The legs should be examined for oedema, for evidence of peripheral arterial disease and for varicose veins (see p. 137). In Marfan's syndrome there is a tendency to dislocation of the patellae, with a long patellar ligament. The feet should be examined for pes cavus, for clubbing of the toes — less easy to identify than clubbing of the fingers — and for splinter haemorrhages. The ankle jerks may be affected in neurosyphilis which may be accompanied by aortic valve disease.

Urine

The urine must always be examined for the presence of protein or sugar and microscopically for the presence of a deposit including red cells and casts.

FURTHER INVESTIGATIONS

Non-Invasive Investigations

Two simple investigations are essential to complete a reasonable examination of the cardiovascular system: they should be as much part of the routine as the history and the clinical examination. They are a chest x-ray and an electrocardiogram.

Chest x-ray

A good quality posteroanterior (PA) x-ray of the chest gives much useful information not only about the heart but also about the pulmonary vasculature. The position of the heart in the thorax varies according to the shape of the thorax. Patients with long narrow chests tend to have narrow vertical cardiac silhouettes, while patients of broad stocky build have high diaphragms and more horizontal hearts. Cardiac screening, by fluoroscopy (see below), shows the heart's chambers pulsating, the diaphragms moving on respiration and the cardiac silhouette altering its shape and position with respiration. It is therefore very important that a single x-ray should be a six-foot film taken on full inspiration with exposure factors that produce appropriate penetration to show the

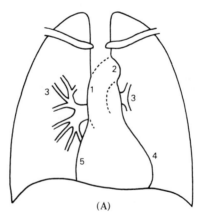

(A)

Figure 2.31A. *The cardiac silhouette in a PA chest x-ray. 1, the ascending aorta; 2, aortic arch (knuckle); 3, left and right pulmonary arteries radiating outwards from the hila; 4, left ventricle; 5, right atrium.*

pulmonary vasculature. The cardiac silhouette in the PA view normally appears as shown in Figure 2.31B. The left atrium and the right ventricle cannot be identified individually in this view but can be seen by special oblique views of the heart (see below). The size of the heart as a whole can be reasonably assessed by the 'cardiothoracic index', the ratio of the maximum width of the cardiac silhouette to the maximum width of the thorax measured from rib to rib; normally it is not greater than 50 per cent. Enlargement of the left ventricle and right atrium are readily identified and widening of the aortic arch and left pulmonary artery are often obvious. Enlargement of the left atrium can often be seen as an

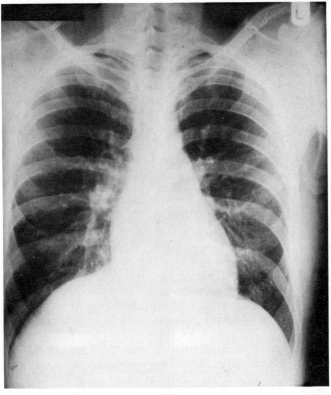

(B)

Figure 2.31B. *The cardiac silhouette: normal PA x-ray.*

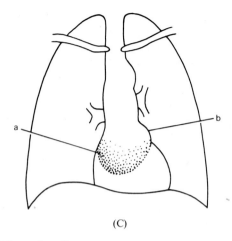

(C)

Figure 2.31C. *The cardiac silhouette: a large left atrium shows as a denser shadow (a) and the left atrial appendage as (b).*

area of extra density within the cardiac silhouette (Figure 2.31C) while enlargement of the left atrial appendage sometimes causes an extra bulge on the left border of the cardiac silhouette between that of the pulmonary artery and the left ventricle. From about the apex of the left ventricle to the surface of the diaphragm there is often a less dense triangular opacity caused by a pad of fat in the pericardium.

The PA x-ray of chest also shows both main pulmonary arteries and many of their smaller branches (Figure 2.31, A and B). The pulmonary veins are normally invisible but when they contain an abnormal volume of blood, as for example when there is pulmonary venous hypertension, they become visible as vertical vessels in an area below the clavicles as shown in Figure 2.32. There are no physical signs of pulmonary venous hypertension, which frequently precedes pulmonary oedema, and evidence for it, in the form of congested upper pulmonary veins, must be sought on the chest x-ray.

Pulmonary oedema is seen, even when there may be no audible crepitations on auscultation, as a diffuse opacity at both hila with a characteristic 'bat's wing' distribution (Figure 2.33). Chronic interstitial oedema, with thickening of the interlobular septa of the lung, can be suspected by the appearance of septal lines (Kerley's B lines), short, thin horizontal lines extending inwards for a centimetre or two from the periphery of each lung field for a few centimetres above the diaphragm (Figure 2.34).

Long-standing severe pulmonary arterial hypertension some-times results in peripheral oligaemia of the lung fields, the outer thirds of which look abnormally radiolucent; this is the result of peripheral vasoconstriction of the pulmonary arteries ('pruning' of the pulmonary arterial tree).

The enlargement of certain cardiac chambers may be best demonstrated by films taken in the right or left anterior oblique projections while the oesophagus contains a barium suspension. The right anterior oblique view normally shows the oesophagus to be only slightly curved, but left atrial enlargement displaces it obviously backward. The left anterior oblique view shows enlarge-ment of the left ventricle. The left lateral view shows both ventricles and the left atrium almost as well as the left anterior oblique projection (Figure 2.35).

Cardiac 'screening'

Fluoroscopy of the heart is useful in detecting abnormal pulsation of individual chambers, as for example when a ventricular aneurysm is suspected, and for the identification of calcification of the valves. Although calcified valves may be noticed in a single x-ray film in one or other projections as dense opacities within the cardiac silhouette, the actual valve involved can usually only be identified by watching the direction of movement of the opacity during systole and diastole.

Electrocardiogram

The standard, 12-lead, scalar (surface) ECG is the second essential addition to the cardiological examination. It can give important evidence about the cardiac rhythm, hypertrophy of the atria and ventricles, disturbances of electrical conduction within the heart, for example bundle-branch block and AV dissociation, as well as indications of myocardial abnormalities such as hypoxia, injury and infarction. Electrocardiography is the only sure way of accurately diagnosing a dysrhythmia or of identifying the site of an infarction during life. Figures 2.36 to 2.50 give some examples of characteristic abnormal ECGs. In skilled hands the more complicated vectorcardiogram (VCG) occasionally gives extra information, for example by sometimes confirming the presence of an infarction when there is left bundle-branch block.

Phonocardiography

By the use of microphones, suitable frequency-filters and oscilloscopic recording, graphical records can be made of heart sounds and murmurs. It is important to understand that the trained human ear is a far finer instrument than the best phonocardiogram (PCG) and can hear, for example, soft high-pitched early diastolic murmurs that cannot be recorded. 'Routine phonocardiography', performed by a technician from microphones applied at the four conventional areas of auscultation through high, medium and low frequency filters, is valueless. A phonocardiographic record is only as good as the auscultator who supervises the recording, carefully selecting the sound he wants to record and the site at which it is best heard. The ordinary phonocardiogram cannot distinguish between different timbres, for example the PCG of pericardial friction may be indistinguishable from murmurs. The main use of the phonocardiogram is for the accurate timing of sounds and murmurs and the clear demonstration of certain very transient sounds such as the systolic click at the start of a late systolic murmur. In this situation the murmur captures the ear but the click may not be heard on auscultation though it is quite obvious on a PCG.

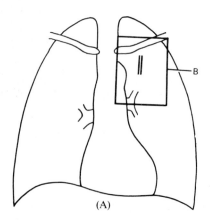

(A)

Figure 2.32. *B shows part of a PA chest x-ray from the position indicated in A, showing the upper pulmonary veins which may be visible as vertical vessels when dilated by blood (pulmonary venous hypertension).*

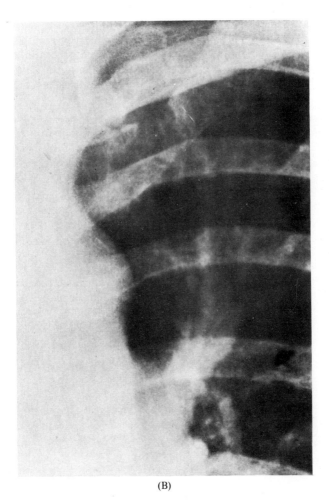

(B)

Figure 2.32.

Indirect recording of pulsations

By applying a pressure capsule to the skin above the pulsation of the heart, an artery, the internal jugular vein or a distended liver, a graphical record can be obtained. Indirect carotid arteriograms and jugular phlebograms may be useful to time events in the

phonocardiogram, or for demonstration purposes, but the wave-
forms are not identical with those recorded directly from inside the
vessel and are very readily distorted by variations in pressure,
obliquity of application of the capsule and other variations of
technique. The indirect recording of the apical impulse (apex cardiography is also sometimes useful in the same way (Figure 2.15).

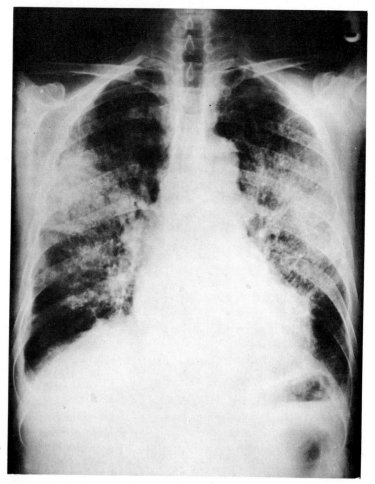

Figure 2.33. *PA chest x-ray showing the characteristic distribution of the diffuse opacity of pulmonary oedema.*

Echocardiography

In echocardiography sound waves are reflected from various parts of the heart and recorded throughout successive cardiac cycles against time on the base line. In skilled hands it can give valuable information about pericardial effusions, enlargement of chambers and movements of individual valve cusps. Here again it is possible to produce fallacious records, for the exact angle of the exploring sound wave is absolutely critical.

Invasive Investigations

Haematological investigation

The hyperkinetic circulatory state that results from any severe anaemia may mimic heart disease, and when anaemia accompanies heart disease the patient is more easily breathless and the clinical picture is confused. The presence of bacterial endocarditis or other infection may be suspected by the unexpected finding of anaemia, leucocytosis or a high ESR.

Valsalva's manoeuvre

A great deal is sometimes made about the diagnostic help afforded by the haemodynamic changes that occur during and after Valsalva's manoeuvre (forced expiration against a closed glottis). Although the changes in heart rate and blood pressure involved are interesting in physiological terms, and may be abnormal, either in heart failure or when there is defective autonomic circulatory control, they are only identified accurately by direct recording of the arterial pulse through an indwelling cannula. It is much easier to diagnose heart failure by hearing fine crackles at the bases of the lungs, by seeing pulmonary oedema on a chest x-ray or by observing a raised jugular venous pressure. Valsalva's manoeuvre is an interesting 'clinical toy', like the demonstration of capillary pulsation, the production of Duroziez's murmur or the 'pistol shot' sound over peripheral arteries demonstrable in cases of severe aortic incompetence. No cardiologist actually diagnoses aortic incompetence by finding these physical signs; he does so by hearing the characteristic murmur.

Cardiac catheterisation

Under fluoroscopic control, usually with an image intensifier, cardiac catheters can be introduced into peripheral veins and arteries and pushed towards the heart to explore the great veins, the aorta or the four cardiac chambers. They can be used as probes to pass through abnormal communications between cardiac chambers and vessels, for example atrial and ventricular septal defects, or a patent ductus arteriosus. They can be attached to manometers to record intravascular pressures and demonstrate pressure gradients by withdrawal of the catheter tip across heart valves. Through them samples of blood can be obtained from any site in the heart or central circulation. Analysis of the oxygen content of mixed venous blood from the pulmonary artery can be used to calculate the cardiac output by the Fick principle. Blood samples from other sites allow the calculation of blood flows across shunts between cardiac chambers. Through a catheter in the pulmonary artery dye may be injected to measure cardiac output by the dye-dilution technique.

Special catheters with electrodes at the tip are used to record the intracardiac electrocardiogram and direct recordings can be made

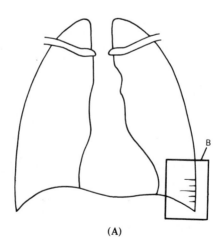

(A)

Figure 2.34.

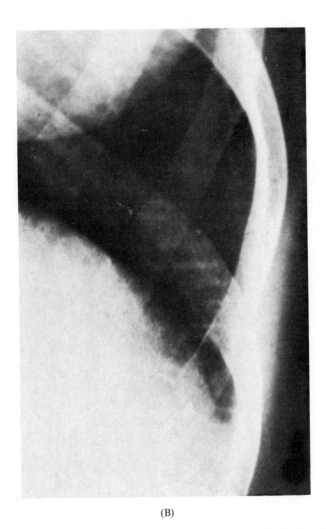

(B)

Figure 2.34. *B shows part of a PA chest x-ray from the position indicated in A, showing septal lines (Kerley's B lines).*

of the electrical impulse travelling through the AV nodal tissue, the bundle of His and the right and left bundle branches of the special conducting system of the heart. Other cardiac catheters have at the tip a special platinum electrode capable of producing an electric potential in the presence of hydrogen: when such a hydrogen electrode is sited in a cardiac chamber a lung-to-electrode circulation time can easily be made by allowing the subject to inhale a breath of pure hydrogen gas; intracardiac left-to-right shunts can thus be readily confirmed. Minute microphones at the tips of cardiac catheters have been used to identify the sources of normal and abnormal heart sounds.

A radio-opaque fluid ('contrast medium') can be injected into any chamber of the heart or into the great vessels (angiocardiography). The passage of this opaque medium through the heart can be recorded by rapid still or ciné x-ray photography and gives useful information about the anatomy of the chambers and the

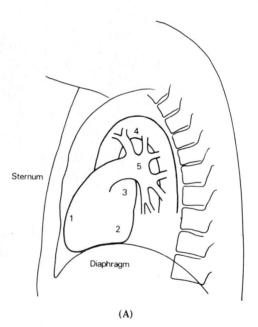

(A)

Figure 2.35.

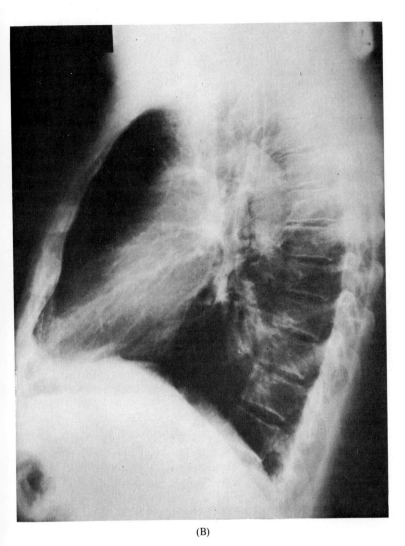

(B)

Figure 2.35. *Left lateral chest x-ray (B) with diagram (A) indicating the sites of various structures. 1 = right ventricle; 2 = left ventricle; 3 = left atrium; 4 = aorta; 5 = pulmonary artery.*

flow of blood between them. Both coronary arteries can be selectively catheterised and the coronary arteriograms thus obtained demonstrate the coronary arterial circulation. In skilled hands cardiac catheterisation is an invaluable part of the investigation of many patients with heart disease, providing information obtainable by no other method.

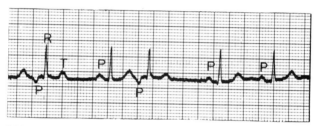

Figure 2.36 *Electrocardiogram, lead II, showing two supraventricular extrasystoles. The ectopic focus is low in the atrium or in the AV junctional tissue. Atrial excitation occurs in a direction the reverse of normal. The first and third P waves are therefore inverted. Ventricular conduction is normal so the abnormal premature P waves are followed by normal premature QRST complexes. (Figures 2.36 to 2.43 come from G. H. Bell, D. Emslie-Smith and C. R. Paterson,* Textbook of Physiology, *10th edition (1980) with kind permission of the authors and Churchill-Livingstone, Edinburgh).*

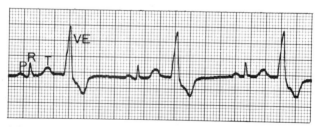

Figure 2.37. *ECG, lead II, showing ventricular extrasystoles (VE) following each normal complex. The abnormal spread of excitation from the ectopic pacemaker below the divisions of the conducting tissue causes wide and abnormally shaped QRST complexes.*

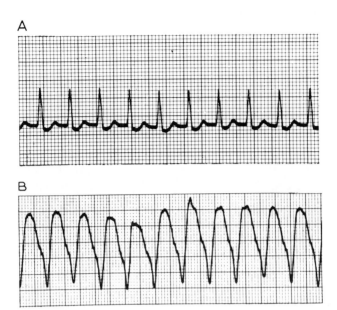

Figure 2.38. *Paroxysms of tachycardia. A. Supraventricular (atrial) tachycardia; because the ectopic pacemaker discharges above the division of the AV conducting system the QRST complexes have a normal shape. B. Ventricular tachycardia; the ectopic pacemaker lies below the division of the AV conducting tissue, so the complexes are bizarre, like ventricular extrasystoles.*

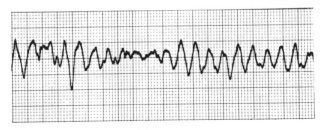

Figure 2.39. *Ventricular fibrillation. There are no recognisable P waves or QRS complexes. The chaotic cardiac electrical activity gives rise to random oscillations only.*

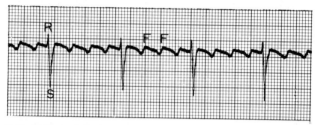

Figure 2.40. *ECG, lead II, showing atrial flutter. A regular succession of characteristically abnormal P waves (F or flutter waves) indicates the abnormal excitation of the atria but the ventricles respond only to every fourth beat. There is therefore '4:1 AV block'.*

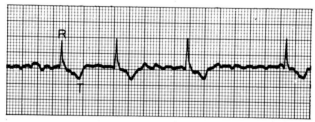

Figure 2.41. *ECG, lead II, showing atrial fibrillation. Low voltage irregular oscillations of the base line represent the atrial arrhythmia. The QRS complexes occur irregularly because the AV node can transmit only some of the impulses it receives. In this record the T wave is inverted because of an abnormality of repolarisation.*

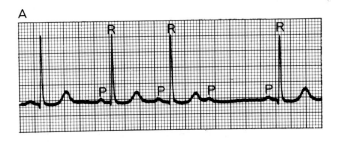

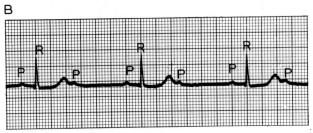

Figure 2.42. *Two forms of incomplete heart block. A. The PR interval increases from complex to complex because the impulse takes an increasingly long time to traverse the AV node; eventually the impulse is not conducted to the ventricles and no QRS complex follows the P wave. The cycle then begins again ('Wenckebach periods'). B. There is no QRS complex after every second P wave because of failure of AV conduction ('fixed' 2:1 AV block, 'dropped beats').*

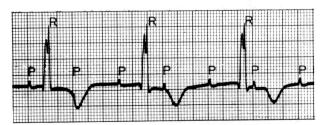

Figure 2.43. *Complete heart block. The P waves occur regularly at a rate of 100 per minute and represent atrial systole at this rate. The wide and abnormal QRS complexes also occur regularly, but at a much slower rate (45 per minute) and represent the discharge of an independent ventricular pacemaker. Atrial and ventricular activities are entirely dissociated.*

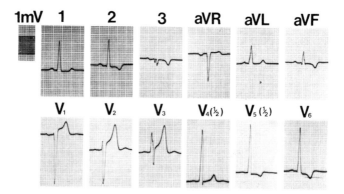

Figure 2.44. *Left ventricular hypertrophy. Note the high-voltage QRS complexes and inverted T waves in left chest leads (V5 and V6). '(½)' indicates that the record was taken with the sensitivity of the instrument set at half the normal value shown under '1 mV' at the top left hand corner of the figure.*

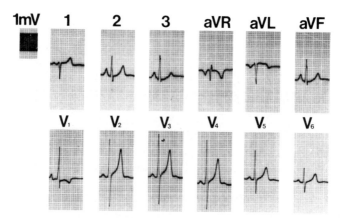

Figure 2.45. *Right ventricular hypertrophy. Note the right axis deviation in leads 1 and 3 and the high R waves in right chest leads with an inverted T wave in lead V1. In addition the P wave in lead 2 is high and spiked, suggesting right atrial hypertrophy ('P pulmonale').*

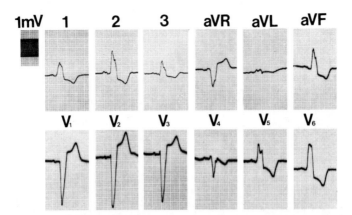

Figure 2.46. *Left bundle-branch block. Note the wide slurred QRS complexes with inverted T waves in leads related to the left ventricle. In addition, the P wave is wide and bifid in lead 2, suggesting left atrial hypertrophy ('P mitrale').*

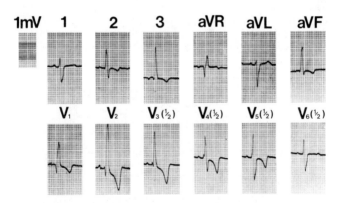

Figure 2.47. *Right bundle-branch block. Note the wide, polyphasic QRS complexes with inverted T waves in right chest leads, and the wide, slurred S wave in leads 1 and V5 and V6.*

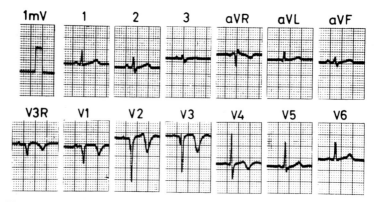

Figure 2.48. *Antero-septal cardiac infarction. Note the wide deep Q waves with steeply inverted T waves in right chest leads.*

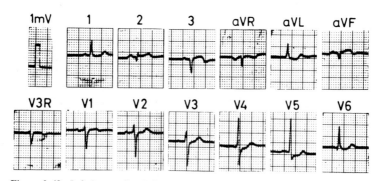

Figure 2.49. *Inferior cardiac infarction. Note the abnormal Q waves in leads 2, 3 and aVF, whose axes run toward the diaphragmatic surface of the heart.*

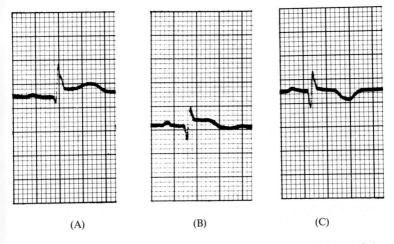

(A)   (B)   (C)

Figure 2.50. *Typical sequential changes in lead aVF of a patient with an inferior myocardial infarction. A: Day of infarction; elevation of ST segment. B: Next day; q is deeper and wider, and there is still ST elevation. C: 12 days later; no ST elevation, but pathological Q and inverted T.*

ARTERIES

A number of disorders affect the arteries. The clinical features vary with the acuteness of onset of the condition and the way in which the arterial disease affects the tissues of the body. The two commonest conditions that serve to illustrate these principles are atheroma (or arteriosclerosis) and the vasospastic condition typified by Raynaud's syndrome.

Atheroma (Arteriosclerosis)

The principal effect of atheroma is narrowing of the arteries (stenosis) which may eventually cause complete block; the tissues then depend on the enlargement of collateral vessels ('obliterative arterial disease'). The other effect is weakening of the wall of the vessel, producing an aneurysm or rupture of the vessel with haemorrhage.

History

The taking of the family history should include questions about the occurrence of cardiovascular disease including hypertension, cardiac infarction and diabetes mellitus. Enquiries should be made about the patient's past history including hypertension, angina, diabetes mellitus or hypothyroidism, and smoking.

Pain. Three types of pain occur in obliterative arterial disease: the sudden agonising pain of an acute arterial occlusion, pain in the muscles on exercise, and rest pain in the feet.
Intermittent claudication. The patient will complain of dull cramp-like pain on walking a certain distance. The pain increases in severity until he stops; it then goes away. Often this pain is accompanied by a feeling of coldness in the foot and some loss of feeling or a 'pins and needles' sensation. The commonest site is in the calf when the block is in the superficial femoral artery between groin and knee. Claudication may also affect the buttocks when the site of arterial blockage is the distal aorta or common iliac vessel *(Leriche syndrome).* Pain in the foot is less common and indicates small vessel disease.

The claudication distance is fairly constant for the patient on the flat, but is shorter when walking uphill or upstairs or against a stiff wind, all of which demand more muscular activity. It may diminish spontaneously if an adequate collateral circulation develops. If not, and if the disease progresses, the distance diminishes and a new pain (rest pain) is experienced.
Rest pain. This is the burning pain felt in the forefoot especially during the night when the foot warms up under the bedclothes but the blood supply is insufficient to sustain the increased metabolic demand. Although the foot feels hot to the patient, it will be cold to the touch. Characteristically relief is obtained by pulling the foot out of the bed and especially by placing it on a cold surface. When rest pain is severe the patient may sit up all night with the foot on cold linoleum.
Coldness. This is usually noted by the patient in the ischaemic limb as is paraesthesia. Ulceration of the skin may be present over the pressure areas.

Physical examination

It is important to remember that arterial disease affects many of the arteries in the body although it may be clinically more evident in one area. The whole of the cardiovascular system must therefore be examined. It is necessary always to compare the affected limb with the apparently normal one.

Colour. This varies from pale skin through normal to a dusky red or cyanotic appearance when poor perfusion has resulted in stagnation of blood in dilated arterioles. Eventually gangrene may appear.

Temperature. The difference in temperature in the two limbs can easily be appreciated by passing the fingers of the hand down the limbs. In the affected limb a gradation of temperature change may be evident near the ankle.

Trophic changes. The poor blood supply to the skin, hair, nails and digital pulps produces changes in these tissues. The skin becomes puffy and dry and later, thin, taut and shiny. The hair becomes sparse or absent, the pulps of the tips of the fingers and toes flatten and the nails become thick, curved and ridged.

Ulcers and gangrene. Ulcers in the skin that result from occlusion of small arteries are rounder, more clearly demarcated and are surrounded by less inflammation than the ulcers associated with venous insuffiency. Gangrenous extremities are obvious, but incipient gangrene may appear as unduly pale or cyanosed digits or areas on the heel. Sometimes a line of demarcation can be seen between the gangrenous and normal tissue.

Paraesthesia. Altered sensation with hypoaesthesia of glove or stocking distribution may be present.

Arterial pulses. In the lower limb the femoral pulse is felt below the mid-inguinal point; the popliteal by palpating the artery against the upper end of tibia with the knee bent; the posterior tibial is felt as it passes in the groove behind and below the medial malleolus; and the dorsalis pedis is felt just lateral to the extensor hallucis tendon. The popliteal pulse is the most difficult to feel. The arteries in both limbs should be compared. Where there is a difference in pressures in the femoral artery or a thrill is felt in one, the arteries are auscultated. A thrill or murmur indicates proximal arterial narrowing.

Much information on the degree of ischaemia can be gained from observation of the lower limb on elevation and dependency.

With the patient on his back both legs are raised by the observer to at least 45°. If ischaemia is marked, pallor will be noted in the pulps of the toes and the sole of the affected forefoot. Pallor can also be produced by asking the patient to flex and extend the ankle as if he were walking — a paddling motion. When he has 'walked' his claudication distance, calf pain will occur and the foot may become pale.

Following elevation the legs should be allowed to hang down over the edge of the couch and the foot observed for reactive hyperaemia and the time of venous filling which is normally 5 to 30 sec. Pallor on elevation and rubor on dependency with delayed venous filling indicate severe ischaemia.

Obliterative Arterial Disease of the Upper Limb

This is not exactly similar to that in the lower limb. It usually presents with patchy gangrene of the skin of fingers caused by emboli thrown off from proximal atheroma. Sometimes claudication of the forearm muscles may be present. The blood pressure should be measured in both arms and a difference of more than 20 mm Hg suggests proximal narrowing.

An interesting syndrome — *subclavian steal syndrome* — is sometimes seen when the subclavian artery is severely narrowed or blocked at its origin. On exercising the arm muscles the patient experiences dizziness, faintness and possibly diplopia as blood flows reversely down the vertebral artery to supply the limb, thus reducing the flow in the basilar system ('stealing' blood).

The patency of the radial and ulnar arteries can be tested by making the patient clench his fist while the examiner obliterates both arteries with his thumbs. When the patient unclenches his fist the palmar skin is pale. The patency of each artery is tested by removing the thumb from it and watching the palmar hyperaemia.

Vasospastic Conditions

The patient suffers from attacks in which the hands especially, and sometimes the feet, become pale, then blue, and then red, because of spasm of the arteries. In its primary form with no known cause it is known as Raynaud's disease and when there is a definite aetiological cause it is called Raynaud's syndrome.

There is often a family history, especially on the female side, of sensitivity to cold. Patients with Raynaud's disease are usually young women aged 15 to 40 years with a long history of ischaemic attacks in both hands. When the condition occurs in an older group and is unilateral one should exclude a collagen disease, a disorder of immunoglobulins, atheroma, vibrating tool injury and cervical rib.

In Raynaud's disease there is little to note except cold hands. Changes in skin pigmentation, telangiectasis, oedema, ulceration, calcification and digital atrophy suggest scleroderma.

Further investigations for Raynaud's disease

The fingers are x-rayed to exclude rheumatoid disease and digital calcification. An x-ray of the neck will exclude a cervical rib. Blood is examined for haemoglobin, ESR, cold agglutinins and the RA latex test.

Further Investigations of Arterial Disease

Arteriography. Injection of contrast material into an artery outlines the vascular anatomy and demonstrates the site and degree of disease. It is performed when there is a hope that surgery may be possible. It is senseless and dangerous to perform arteriography on patients with severe cardiac or cerebral vascular disease in whom improvement of claudication distance by surgery may result in an earlier heart attack.

Thermography. The thermoscan measures the infra-red radiation emitted from the limbs. These radiations are a measure of the temperature of the skin and are thus related to the blood flow through the skin. It is not yet in general use largely because of the expense of the machine.

Other techniques. These include oscillometry, now replaced by Doppler or ultrasound blood flow detectors, venous occlusion plethysmography, estimation of skin blood flow using radio-isotopic clearance and skin blood pressure. These methods are still being evaluated.

VEINS

In the investigation of disorders of veins, enquiries should be made about previous pregnancies, periods of prolonged bed rest, surgical operations or long journeys by air or sea, any previous venous thrombosis, contraceptive pills and oestrogen therapy.

History

Pain

Three sorts of pain are associated with common venous disorders: the diffuse throbbing 'bursting' pain of severe phlebothrombosis, the more localised pain associated with superficial thrombophlebitis and the generalised ache of chronic venous insufficiency from varicose veins.

Tiredness

Patients with chronic venous insufficiency often complain of 'heaviness' or 'tired' feelings in the legs, particularly after much standing or walking. These feelings worsen during the day, and are relieved by lying down, or elevating the legs.

Signs

Deep phlebothrombosis

Pulmonary thromboembolism is a regrettably common cause of death both inside and outside hospital. Often patients who are found at autopsy to have pulmonary infarctions from this cause, or deep venous thromboses in the legs, have no symptoms, so the physician must be constantly vigilant and seek for the physical signs that suggest the presence of phlebothrombosis in the calf muscles. Slight swelling of the calf, with increased turgor of the flaccid muscles may be the only abnormality, and the circumference of the calf on the abnormal side may be greater than that on the other side when measured with a tape measure. Superficial veins on the dorsum of the foot and over the anterior aspect of the tibia may be more distended on the affected side, and the skin on that side may be warmer. There may be tenderness on palpation of the calf, in the popliteal space, or over the saphenous opening of the femoral vein. The skin may be slightly cyanosed and there may even be slight oedema of the foot or ankle, particularly of the tissues behind the medial malleolus. If the patient's foot is passively dorsiflexed by the examiner with the knee held straight there may be pain in the calf *(Homans' sign)* but this manoeuvre carries some risk of causing thromboembolism, so it is rarely used.

Superficial thrombophlebitis

Evidence of thrombophlebitis may consist of palpable hardening of the affected superficial vein, with accompanying signs of inflammation — tenderness and redness of the overlying skin.

Varicose veins

The dilated tortuous varices of the large superficial saphenous veins are usually obvious, especially when the patient stands. Other evidence of incompetence of the communicating veins between the superficial saphenous system and the deep femoral veins are rather localised bluish protrusions in the skin overlying the communicating veins — the so-called 'blow-out areas'. Another common form of varicose veins consists of microvarices, a fan-like arrangement of small tortuous veins radiating in the drainage area of incompetent communicating veins. Varicose veins, and the incompetence of communicating veins that causes them, lead to chronic venous insufficiency of the legs with a tendency to ankle oedema and chronic gravitational (nutritional) changes in the skin: eczema, brownish pigmentation and ultimately ulceration, commonly over the lower medial aspect of the tibia above the ankle.

Trendelenburg's Test

This commonly used clinical test is aimed at deciding whether the valves in the communicating veins are incompetent. With the patient lying, the veins in the legs should be emptied by passively raising the leg. Pressure should then be applied at the saphenous opening either by a thumb or a tourniquet with a pad. The patient should then stand up. Rapid filling of the varicose veins from below means that the valves in the communicating veins between the superficial and deep venous systems are incompetent. If there is little filling of the veins within half a minute pressure should be removed. Immediate filling from above then suggests incompetence at the junction of the saphenous and femoral veins.

Further Investigations

Further investigations of venous insufficiency or obstruction include the use of ultrasound and phlebography, either by the injection of radio-opaque contrast medium and subsequent x-ray photography, or by radioisotope techniques, for example the injection and tracing of fibrinogen labelled with ^{125}I.

MICROCIRCULATION

Retinal Vessels

The retinal vessels seen with an opthalmoscope are described in the section on opthalmoscopy.

Other Microcirculatory Lesions

In various forms of vasculitis, for example polyarteritis and the vasculitis associated with some collagen disorders such as rheumatoid arthritis, microinfarcts may be seen in the skin. These may appear around the nail beds or at the tips of the fingers as small dark necrotic lesions. Livido reticularis that is not induced by heat, as in erythema ab igne, may also be associated with vasculitis. The tender Osler's nodes of infective endocarditis (page 53) may not be embolic but have an immune basis.

FURTHER READING

Birnstingl, M. (Ed.) (1973) *Peripheral Vascular Surgery.* London: Heinemann.
Dubin, D. (1974) *Rapid Interpretation of EKGs: a Programmed Course,* 3rd edition. Tampa, Florida: Cover Publishing Co.
Finlayson, J. K., Kenmure, A. C. F. & Short, D. S. (1978) Cardiac signs for students: the wheat and the chaff. *British Medical Journal,* **i,** 1471-1473.
Keele, K. D. (1963) *The Evolution of Clinical Methods in Medicine.* London: Pitman.

Leatham, A. (1977) *Introduction to Examination of the Cardiovascular System.* London: Oxford University Press.

Oram, S. (1971) Clinical examination. In *Clinical Heart Disease,* Chapter 2, pp. 43-64. London: Heinemann.

Parkinson, J. (1951a) Patient and physician. *Annals of Internal Medicine,* **35,** 307.

Parkinson, J. (1951b) Cardiac symptoms. *Annals of Internal Medicine,* **35,** 499.

Tavel, M. E. (1974) *Clinical Phonocardiography and External Pulse Recording,* 2nd edition. Chicago: Year Book Medical Publishers Inc.

Wood, P. (1968) *Diseases of the Heart and Circulation,* 3rd edition, Chapters 1 to 5. London: Eyre and Spottiswoode.

3 The Respiratory System
S. Clarke

Assessment of the respiratory system starts with a careful history followed by physical examination and chest x-ray which is of integral importance. Depending on the findings pulmonary function tests or other tests may then be required.

HISTORY

No respiratory history is complete without information about the six cardinal symptoms of respiratory disease, namely cough, sputum, haemoptysis, chest pain, dyspnoea and wheeze.

The importance of careful history taking cannot be over-stressed. It has long been known and recently been confirmed that a firm diagnosis can be made in a high proportion of patients based on the history alone and confirmed by physical examination and then special investigations (Hampton et al, 1975).

The previous medical history is important in respiratory conditions. For instance recurrent infections are seen in the winter in the chronic bronchitic, and attacks of dyspnoea and wheezing in the pollen season in the allergic asthmatic. The family history is equally important; for instance patients with unexplained dyspnoea may have a strong family history of allergy suggesting asthma. Similarly a history of pulmonary tuberculosis is highly relevant. The social history is important particularly with respect to industrial exposure at work, as for instance in the diagnosis of pulmonary asbestosis or pleural mesothelioma; similarly the history of cigarette smoking is of paramount importance in the diagnosis of chronic bronchitis and carcinoma of the lung.

Cough

The act of coughing may be involuntary or voluntary and is designed to clear secretions from the bronchial tree with an expiratory blast of air. At the start of coughing the subject takes in a maximum inspiration, the glottis closes transiently, the intercostal muscles and diaphragm then contract forcibly, generating a high intrathoracic pressure. The glottis opens and an explosive blast of air is expelled. The initial high intrathoracic pressure serves to initiate a high air flow and to narrow central airways thereby ensuring a high linear velocity along the bronchial walls and enabling secretions and debris to be expectorated forcibly. Often there are spasms of coughing but it should be remembered that only the first two or three, given when the lungs are fully inflated, are efficient while the remainder are inefficient and tiring. Further smaller airways, those distal to the subsegmental levels, tend to close during coughing and clearance of these is poor. At these sites and at the periphery the main clearance mechanism is the mucociliary escalator. Indeed in healthy subjects coughing is seldom required and is regarded essentially as a reserve mechanism for bronchial clearance. In these normal subjects a small volume of bronchial mucus is cleared and swallowed imperceptibly; the clearance of this into the stomach overnight explains the rationale for early morning gastric aspiration for Ziehl—Neelsen examination in suspected pulmonary tuberculosis when the patient is sputum-free.

The tracheobronchial tree is richly supplied with mucosal cough receptors, fibres from which are carried in the vagus nerve. Irritation of these receptors anywhere from the pharynx to the periphery of the lung may initiate coughing.

Chronic and therefore significant cough may be defined as one that lasts for more than two to four weeks. Cough with upper respiratory infections is common and insignificant. The causes of a chronic cough are many and depend on such factors as smoking habits and industrial chest exposure. In practice the commonest causes are:

Chronic bronchitis. This is defined by the clinical history alone (Medical Research Council, 1965) as a chronic or recurrent increase above normal in the volume of mucus secretion sufficient to cause expectoration — which is not caused by localised broncho-pulmonary disease (such as bronchiectasis). In practice the diagnosis is made when a patient has a chronic or recurrent cough with sputum on most days for at least three months of the year for at least two consecutive years.

By contrast emphysema is an anatomical diagnosis made when there is an increase beyond the normal in the size of the air spaces distal to the terminal bronchioles and accompanied by destruction of the alveolar walls. As such, although emphysema may be present in the lungs of chronic bronchitics it is impossible to define it precisely in life, though certain radiographic features and a low gas transfer may suggest its presence.

Pneumonia of various types, or *lung collapse* due to bronchial obstruction.

Asthma, particularly when dry nocturnal cough is a feature, with or without wheezing. Occasionally these features may be confused with paroxysmal nocturnal dyspnoea, and cardiac asthma with left ventricular failure.

Bronchial carcinoma, frequently associated with haemoptysis.

Pulmonary tuberculosis.

Bronchiectasis, where sputum may be copious.

Parenchymal lung disease such as fibrosing alveolitis or pulmonary oedema.

Foreign bodies.

The cough may have specific features depending on the site of irritation or nature of the background disease. In chronic bronchitis early morning cough may be severe but remit following expectoration of sputum while the attendant wheezing and dyspnoea may then improve for the rest of the day. In these patients coughing may also be troublesome when they lie down at night; this may be due to redistribution of secretions, narrowing of dependent airways or elevation of the diaphragm.

Cough may be a feature of laryngitis or tracheitis which may cause retrosternal pain mimicking angina. With recurrent laryngeal palsy cough becomes bovine in type due to incompetence of the cords. A post-nasal drip at night may cause cough and the association of sinusitis and bronchiectasis is well known. In the latter sputum is usually copious. Finally, being under voluntary control, cough may be nervous in origin and a feature of anxiety.

Sputum

Though on many occasions cough may be dry, equally so the presence of bronchial secretions is a potent causative factor and hence sputum is often expectorated. The volume, colour, consistency and odour may vary widely. It is important to inspect the sputum as this gives some information about the underlying cause. In chronic bronchitis the sputum is usually clear, white or grey, and this usually turns green or yellow in the presence of infection. In bronchiectasis the sputum may be copious, infected and layered (pus and mucus). In lung abcess the sputum may be foetid, particularly when anaerobic organisms are present.

In bronchial asthma the sputum may be thick, sticky and clear and may contain plugs and microscopic particles called Charcot—Leyden crystals and Curschmann's spirals; perhaps of greater importance is the presence of eosinophils which indicate an allergic reaction and on some occasions serve to distinguish between patients with asthma and chronic bronchitis. On occasion a profusion of eosinophils will colour the asthmatic's sputum, suggesting infection.

In lobar pneumonia the sputum is classically viscid and rusty though nowadays this is a rarity, and often the sputum may have no clear characteristics. The sputum may be pink and frothy in acute pulmonary oedema and occasionally in the rare alveolar-cell carcinoma.

Haemoptysis

Haemoptysis may be defined as the expectoration of blood or blood-stained mucus not due to bleeding from the upper respiratory (e.g. nose, gums) or gastrointestinal tract (e.g. haematemesis with aspiration). A 'single haemoptysis' usually lasts one to two days, being fresh initially and becoming progressively more stale. 'Repeated haemoptysis' continues longer than seven days or with a clear break; 'frank haemoptysis' indicates expectoration of pure blood without sputum. The patient should be questioned about the type, volume and duration of haemoptysis, and possible location (some patients indicate the site of origin), the presence of upper respiratory infection, any other bleeding tendency and smoking or industrial exposure.

Clinical examination should ascertain the presence or otherwise of nasal or oral bleeding, upper or lower respiratory tract infection and hypertension or heart disease and include chest x-ray, sputum culture and cytology. Limited information as to the cause may be drawn from the type of haemoptysis. That of active pulmonary tuberculosis and bronchiectasis is said to be brief and brisk while that of carcinoma is longer and may include clots. That of chronic bronchitis is nondescript but usually follows infection or severe coughing. That of medium-sized pulmonary embolism with infarction is frank, bright, profuse and frothy, initially indicating a site of origin deep in the lung. Finally it is often said that haemoptysis is rarely profuse or exsanguinating; this is not always the case and pulmonary mycetomas in old tuberculous cavities seem to have a particular tendency to bleed freely.

In a series of 324 patients presenting with haemoptysis, Johnston et al (1960) made the following diagnoses (Table 3.1) and these are of practical interest.

Table 3.1. *Diagnosis of 324 patients presenting with haemoptysis.*

Upper respiratory infection		24%
Normal		21%
Bronchitis		17%
Bronchiectasis		13%
Pulmonary tuberculosis	{ active	5%
	quiescent	6%
Pneumonia		6%
Cardiovascular disease	{ hypertension	2%
	mitral valve disease	2%
Carcinoma		2%
Others		2%

In assessing these figures it should be noted that in 45 per cent of patients no serious respiratory cause was found (24 per cent upper respiratory infection, 21 per cent normal). Equally bronchitis and bronchiectasis remain high on the list with a 30 per cent incidence. The inflamed bronchial mucosa is particularly susceptible to cough trauma in these conditions. Though the incidence of carcinoma in these figures is low, nevertheless it is an important cause to be ruled out by sputum cytology and bronchoscopy, particularly in male smokers over the age of 40 years. Pulmonary embolism presenting with haemoptysis and pleurisy, perhaps misdiagnosed as pneumonia, should be borne in mind as should rarer entities such as bronchial adenoma and systemic blood disorders.

Chest Pain

Chest pain should be considered in terms of type, site, radiation, precipitation, duration and relief. Some common respiratory causes are discussed below.

Tracheal pain is a raw retrosternal pain occasionally confused with angina and frequently noted in patients with upper respiratory virus infections which may track down the trachea. Influenza is a common cause. When the cough becomes loose and productive the pain goes. Pain may be particularly marked if there are prolonged spasms of coughing during which the trachea collapses allowing the inflamed mucosal surfaces to appose with each cough.

The *lung* itself is not well supplied with pain fibres but tumours and other space-occupying lesions either at the hilar regions or more peripherally may cause dull aching pain; also retrosternal pain may be caused by mediastinal lesions such as tumours and mediastinal emphysema.

The commonest type of pain related to the lungs is *pleural* pain reflecting the rich nerve supply of the parietal pleura. Pleural pain is usually localised and stabbing in type being made worse by any manoeuvre which apposes the pleural surfaces such as deep breathing, coughing or sneezing. Occasionally radiation may occur, particularly with diaphragmatic pleurisy to the shoulder, reflecting the common innervation of the diaphragm and dermatomes of the shoulder (C4—C5), and to the abdomen. The pain of dry pleurisy may be eased when an effusion develops separating the inflamed pleural surfaces.

Similar pain may be present with fractured ribs as with cough fractures in the bronchitic and there may be initial brief pleural pain in spontaneous pneumothorax. Chest pain may arise from the heart (angina, pericarditis), aorta, oesophagus or other mediastinal structures, from the posterior nerve roots (herpes zoster), and rib erosions (Pancoast tumour). Finally chest pain may be a reflection of anxiety. However before that diagnosis is accepted other possibilities must be firmly ruled out.

Dyspnoea

Dyspnoea (or breathlessness) may be described as difficult, laboured, uncomfortable breathing of which the patient is manifestly aware. However to understand the origin of this complex symptom it is necessary to know something of the factors controlling respiration.

Breathing is initiated and regulated by the rhythmic discharge of neurones located in the respiratory centre of the brain stem (pons and medulla). The activity of this centre is controlled by three sets of factors.

1. Local factors such as the general state of cerebral stimulation, the local P_{CO_2} and pH and the hypothalamic temperature. Increases in each of these stimulate the respiratory centre and respiration thereby.

2. Indirect stimuli, hypoxia or hypercapnia acting via the receptors of the carotid body.

3. Indirect stimuli via lung stretch (Hering—Breuer), irritant and J (juxta-capillary) receptors (via the vagus nerves) and others in the diaphragm and chest wall. The information which reaches the respiratory centre from the lung is used to maintain an appropriate level of alveolar ventilation.

Dyspnoea occurs when there is inequality between the forces applied and the resistance to breathing, the concept of 'length—tension—inappropriateness'. This imbalance may occur with alterations in the resistance (e.g. increased airways resistance in patients with airways obstruction) or compliance of the lungs and thorax (e.g. restrictive — 'stiff lung' in diffuse fibrosis), or increase in the frequency of breathing. Hypoxaemia, hypercapnia and acidaemia lead to hyperventilation and may be associated with the complaint of dyspnoea.

In other words dyspnoea may be a feature whenever the ventilatory capacity is reduced, whether by:

1. An obstructive defect — asthma, chronic bronchitis, or emphysema.

2. A restrictive defect — fibrosis, collapse, congestion, pleural effusion, pneumothorax, kyphoscoliosis or ankylosing spondylitis.

3. Weakness of the respiratory muscles as in myopathy or neuropathy; here the changes resemble those with restriction but the mechanics are quite different.

While concentrating on pure respiratory causes of dyspnoea other common clinical causes must be borne in mind. A useful clinical list would include:

1. Respiratory disease
2. Cardiac disease (by pulmonary congestion or oedema)
3. Anaemia (by unknown factors)

4. Obesity (by increasing the work of breathing and restricting the chest)
5. Thyrotoxicosis (by direct stimulation of the respiratory centre and increased O_2 consumption)
6. Anxiety.

At this point mention should be made of hyperventilation which leads to blowing off of CO_2 and consequent alkalosis with tingling in the lips and limbs, tetany and occasionally fits. This may occur with an organic cause (e.g. salicylate overdose where the acid pH drives respiration). It is most commonly of psychogenic origin, however, and often seen in the anxious person.

Dyspnoea may be further divided into acute, paroxysmal and progressive:

Acute dyspnoea may be a feature of spontaneous pneumothorax (particularly with tension), massive pulmonary embolism, lung collapse, massive pleural effusion or sputum retention.

Paroxysmal dyspnoea may be a feature of bronchial asthma with wheezing and airways obstruction. Equally so early left ventricular failure may present in a similar way (cardiac asthma) though often the patient will complain of paroxysmal nocturnal dyspnoea too. The latter is a reflection of increased (gravity-dependent) pulmonary blood flow and interstitial fluid accumulation as the patient gradually slides flat off high pillows.

Progressive dyspnoea is commonly a feature of respiratory disease such as chronic obstructive bronchitis, emphysema, chronic bronchial asthma, fibrosing or allergic alveolitis or pulmonary vascular disease (pulmonary emboli), as well as cardiac or other causes listed above.

An attempt should be made to assess the exercise tolerance in terms of distance walked on the flat, the number of flights of stairs climbed at a normal pace or other simple everyday activities such as household tasks or gardening. A system of grading may be used:

Grade 1. Normal

Grade 2. Dyspnoea only on hills or stairs

Grade 3. Dyspnoea on walking fast on the flat

Grade 4. Dyspnoea on walking further than 100 yards on the flat

Grade 5. Dyspnoea on washing, dressing or walking a few yards.

A '12-minute walking test', in which the distance covered is measured, has been introduced by McGavin, Gupta and McHardy (1976) for assessing disability in chronic bronchitis and other respiratory diseases. This test, being reproducible and objective, merits further use.

Wheeze

Wheezing is a musical noise produced not only by the human chest but by church organs and mouth organs, indicating a common mode of origin. Wheezing can be produced by the normal subject forcibly exhaling to residual volume when airways narrow critically. The student is urged to appreciate this for himself. Wheezing is of course a common complaint in patients with diffuse airways obstruction whether it be due to chronic bronchitis, emphysema or asthma. Patients vary widely in their appreciation of wheezing and in mild cases they may accept it as normal. Occasionally complaint may be voiced by an aggrieved spouse whose sleep is disturbed by nocturnal wheezing.

In asthmatics attacks of wheezing may be induced by exposure to the usual inhaled allergens (house dust, the house dust mite, pollens, etc.), by upper respiratory viral infections, by exercise and rarely by emotional upset. On occasion the nocturnal wheezing of asthma may be confused with that of cardiac asthma and early pulmonary oedema. In chronic bronchitics the wheezing and degree of airways obstruction may be made worse by intercurrent infections. Finally and less commonly wheeze may be unilateral due to local bronchial narrowing by tumour or foreign body. Further discussion on wheezing is included later in the section on physical signs.

PHYSICAL EXAMINATION

On appraisal the patient may look ill or well, and may be coughing, wheezing, breathless or blue. It is logical to start by examining the upper airways and neck, and then the chest, by inspection, palpation, percussion and auscultation. The patient should be reclining at about 45°, unclad and well illuminated. It saves time and movement if the front of the chest is examined and then the back.

Cyanosis is a blue coloration seen either in the central warm mucous membranes such as the buccal mucosa (central cyanosis), or in the cold periphery, hands or feet (peripheral cyanosis). To judge central cyanosis accurately is often difficult but when arterial oxygen saturation falls below 75 to 80 per cent (less than 6.0 to 7.3 kPa or 45 to 55 mm Hg partial pressure) then central cyanosis is invariably visible. Its presence, however, depends upon at least

5 g per cent of circulating haemoglobin being desaturated; as a consequence in severe anaemia cyanosis will not be seen, although the coincidence of disease enough to give anaemia and cyanosis is not particularly frequent and both may be associated with dyspnoea. Conversely patients with excess haemoglobin (polycythaemia) may readily have at least 5 g per cent haemoglobin unsaturated and appear plethoric and cyanosed.

Central cyanosis may be due to (1) asphyxia, (2) hypoventilation (e.g. respiratory depression or severe airways obstruction), (3) impaired oxygen transfer in the lungs, (4) venous—arterial shunts, either in the heart (e.g. Fallot's tetralogy) or lungs (Table 3.2).

Table 3.2. *Causes of central cyanosis.*

Respiratory	Cardiac (shunt)	Others
Chronic obstructive bronchitis	Fallot's tetralogy	Methaemoglobinaemia
Severe asthma	Transposition of aorta and pulmonary artery	Sulphaemoglobinaemia
Fibrosing alveolitis	Atrial septal defect[a]	
Pulmonary embolism	Ventricular septal defect[a]	
Hypoventilation (primary or acquired)	Patent ductus arteriosus[a]	
All the above conditions lead to ventilation perfusion ($\dot{V}/\dot{Q}$) abnormalities in the lung and cyanosis.		
Arteriovenous aneurysm ⎫ Lobar pneumonia ⎬ shunt		

[a] With reversed shunt.

Peripheral cyanosis is often seen in perfectly normal subjects exposed to cold as well as in those who have peripheral circulatory failure due to shock or other causes of low cardiac output such as mitral stenosis. Both types of cyanosis may of course coincide, for instance, in the patient with cardiogenic shock.

Dyspnoea may be obvious as the patient walks in or undresses and some idea of the cause of the shortness of breath may be clear from observation. For instance patients with chronic airways obstruction due to chronic bronchitis may show pursed-lips breathing (an attempt to reduce expiratory airways collapse and reduce the work of breathing) and they may be using their accessory muscles of respiration of which the sternomastoids are particularly prominent.

The facies may be revealing. The 'blue-bloater' type of chronic bronchitic aptly describes the face; the face may also be bloated by superior vena caval obstruction or Cushing's syndrome, often following corticosteroid therapy. By contrast in the 'pink-puffer' type of emphysematous patient the face is thin and pink though the patient may be very tachypnoeic.

Patients with severe chronic obstructive bronchitis may develop respiratory failure with CO_2 retention characterised by drowsiness, sweating, hot extremities with bounding pulse and dilated veins, and flapping tremor. CO_2 is a potent cerebral vasodilator and these patients may complain of headache, while examination of the optic fundi may show papilloedema due to congestion.

Inspection of the hands may reveal finger clubbing first described by Hippocrates and often associated with intrathoracic disease and less frequently with liver or gut disease (Table 3.3). With finger clubbing there is increased longitudinal and lateral curvature of the nail but the key feature with this sign is the loss of the normal angle (about 140°) between the nail and the cuticle. This is best observed by holding the fingers horizontal, level with the eyes and observing them from the side. Fluctuation or rocking of the nail bed may also be present and can be tested for. Where

Table 3.3. *Causes of finger clubbing.*

1. Thoracic tumours:	carcinoma of lung, mesothelioma of pleura, thymoma, lymphoma, neurofibroma, etc.
2. Diffuse pulmonary fibrosis:	fibrosing alveolitis (rarely in allergic alveolitis), asbestosis.
3. Chronic pulmonary infection:	bronchiectasis, abscess, empyema, cystic fibrosis.
4. Cardiac:	cyanotic heart disease—Fallot's tetralogy, transposition, atrial or ventricular septal defect or patent ductus arteriosus with reversed (R—L) shunt. infective endocarditis. arteriovenous aneurysm of lung.
5. Hepatic cirrhosis.	
6. Chronic bowel disease:	ulcerative colitis, Crohn's disease, coeliac disease.
7. Familial.	

clubbing is gross the terminal phalanges may assume the configuration of drum-sticks.

In finger clubbing there is a proliferation of subungual tissue. However, the precise aetiology remains unknown. Arterial hypoxaemia is a common but not invariable accompaniment, as may be seen from Table 3.3, and in certain cases correction of this will lead to regression of the clubbing (e.g. in Fallot's tetralogy). Increased blood flow to the terminal phalanges is often present and hypertrophy of the numerous arteriovenous anastomoses in the region of the nail bed may account for their change in shape. Where clubbing is due to tumour, removal of the tumour may lead to regression and indeed this may occur even after thoracotomy and sectioning of the vagus nerve in the thorax, suggesting neurogenic factors in its aetiology. Finger clubbing may be either an early or late sign of thoracic disease and of course it may be absent even in the presence of advanced disease. It has no particular predictive role. In practice it is seen most commonly with carcinoma of lung, cryptogenic fibrosing alveolitis, bronchiectasis, industrial lung disease such as asbestosis and in the various cyanotic heart disorders listed. In some instances finger clubbing is associated with hypertrophic pulmonary osteoarthropathy which may present with pain in the wrists and ankles suggesting a common aetiology.

The hands should also be inspected for cyanosis, abnormal pigmentation of the skin creases and for flapping hypercapnic tremor.

Examination of the neck is important since lymph glands in the neck may be associated with intrathoracic disease due to carcinoma, tuberculosis or reticulosis. Goitre may be associated with wheezing and inspiratory stridor when retrosternal, compressing the trachea.

In patients with chronic airways obstruction the accessory muscles visible in the neck may be constantly in use, the shoulders may be elevated and the hands fixed on the chair or bed rails. The jugular veins may be distended particularly during expiration when intrathoracic pressure is high in an attempt to overcome the expiratory airways obstruction. In cor pulmonale (right ventricular failure due to lung disease) the neck veins may be distended with a giant atrial wave visible; a right ventricular heave and peripheral signs of congestion with a large liver and oedema may be present. The jugular veins may be distended and fixed with superior vena caval obstruction, and venous anastomoses appear below the breasts.

Inspection

It is useful to view the thorax from both the front and the side. The configuration of the thorax is usually fairly symmetrical, moving relatively little during tidal breathing. Full expansion usually amounts to about 5 cm or so but this measurement is rarely made nowadays. Respiratory movement in men is chiefly abdominal and in women thoracic. There may be various deformities of the sternum such as pigeon chest and funnel chest (pectus excavatum) which are largely developmental in origin. Similarly kyphoscoliosis may be present and if severe compromise respiration. Deep sulci known as Harrison's sulci with indrawing of the ribs below the nipples used to be a feature of childhood rickets but may also be seen in patients who have had severe childhood asthma and in whom increased diaphragmatic activity has led to traction and indrawing of the lower ribs. Hyperinflation of the chest may be visible in patients with chronic airways obstruction and this is characterised by prominence of the sternum and a barrel-shaped configuration of the chest which appears to be held in a state of full inspiration. In this case expansion may be virtually negligible and the only movement is an upward and forward lifting of the thoracic cage as a whole like a bucket-handle.

In patients with restrictive defects of the lung, as opposed to airways obstruction, breathing may be rapid and shallow and the so-called 'door-stop' sign may be seen, where inspiration is stopped abruptly by restriction. This is probably best seen in patients with fibrosing alveolitis for instance. Again overall chest movement in this situation may be little though the thorax may appear quite normal in configuration.

Where there are local underlying abnormalities of the lung such as fibrosis, consolidation, collapse, pleural effusion or fibrosis, movement of the chest wall at that site may be visibly reduced and this should be carefully sought. A 'frozen' chest may reflect fibrosis after trauma or pleural effusion for instance. Often the apex beat can be visualised and its site confirmed by palpation.

The patient may be obviously tachypnoeic (breathing rapidly), the normal rate of respiration averaging between 12 and 16 per minute; the commonly recorded 20 per minute so often seen on the medical records reflects the sad fact that this measurement is rarely accurate. Tachypnoea itself may be due to anxiety, chest disease or cardiac disease and its origin usually becomes clearer as examination proceeds. Orthopnoea is said to be present when the patient can breathe normally sitting upright but becomes short of breath on lying flat. The commonest cause of this symptom is cardiac disease and incipient left ventricular or atrial failure leading to an increase in interstitial lung water, chiefly at the bases in the upright posture. On lying flat the pulmonary blood volume increases and is redistributed as is the interstitial fluid, accounting for the onset of dyspnoea, possibly via stretch or irritant receptors. Less often orthopnoea may be a feature of chronic obstructive bronchitis, where redistribution of bronchial secretions and postural changes in the airways on lying flat may account for bronchial irritability, coughing and dyspnoea. Additionally the diaphragms rise and the accessory muscles of respiration are less efficient.

Hyperpnoea or hyperventilation is usually due to anxiety though it may be induced by metabolic acidosis (e.g. uraemia, ketoacidosis or salicylate overdose). Where it is voluntary the patient complains of tingling, paraesthesiae, tetany and, rarely, fits due to the blowing off of CO_2.

Cheyne—Stokes respiration is seen in patients with cerebral and respiratory depression after strokes, with heart failure and in uraemia. The patient stops breathing for a matter of seconds, CO_2 builds up and initiates hyperventilation; CO_2 is blown off, the respiratory drive falls and apnoea follows. The cycle may be repeated at length. Occasionally this pattern is seen during sleep in the aged.

Palpation

The first step is to ascertain the position of the mediastinum by palpating the trachea and apex beat. There are two methods of palpating the trachea; the first is to slide the middle finger of the examining hand through the suprasternal notch directly backwards onto the trachea which if displaced will allow the finger to deviate to the opposite side. Alternatively finger and thumb may be used to lightly grip the trachea and examine its position. In different situations both techniques may be useful. Deviation of the trachea may be caused by goitre, by traction from upper lobe fibrosis, by pneumothorax or by displacement from a large pleural effusion.

The position of the apex beat, which usually lies in the fifth intercostal space within the mid-clavicular line and is the point furthest down and out where a distinct cardiac impulse can be felt, will give some indication of the position of the heart and therefore the mediastinum, assuming the heart is normal. If there is no other evidence of cardiac disease then fibrosis may pull the apex beat to the fibrotic side, whereas a space-occupying pleural effusion will push it in the opposite direction. Collapse of various lung lobes may have an effect while consolidation does not usually alter the mediastinal position. A thick chest wall or hyperinflated lungs may render the apex beat impalpable.

The next step is to confirm abnormalities of configuration or movement first noticed at inspection. Measurement of chest movement can be made by applying the flat of the hands to the chest wall with the thumbs placed centrally and the fingers lightly spread and gripping laterally; full inspiration then will shift the thumbs and give an indication of general and local expansion. This can be done over the upper and lower zones both anteriorly and posteriorly as well as the apices. By and large it is unusual to find anything that has not already been spotted by the keen observer on inspection.

Occasionally the crackles of a pleural friction rub or the vibrations of deeply pitched wheezes can be palpated. During palpation the axillae are examined for nodes and the breasts for lumps in the female. Naturally any obvious chest wall abnormalities seen at inspection should be palpated in the usual manner. Palpation of the voice sounds, tactile vocal fremitus, will be discussed below.

Percussion

The technique of percussion should be mastered by constant practice. It is usual to lay the left palm flat on the patient's chest with the fingers spread along the lines of the ribs and then percuss the middle phalanx of the middle finger. This should be done two to three times, care being taken not to leave the percussing finger applied to the motionless hand since this damps the vibrations and the quality of the percussion note. Examination should start by direct percussion of the clavicles and then continue down the front of the chest comparing both sides, the right upper zone with the left upper zone and so on. A similar plan should apply to examining the back of the chest and for this the patient should lean forward with the arms forward and crossed so that the scapulae are shifted laterally. Again the apices and the bases should be percussed carefully and the level of the diaphragm ascertained. Anteriorly dullness is found at about the level of the sixth rib, whereas posteriorly it is at the level of the tenth rib during quiet respiration.

The normal chest is resonant throughout. The diaphragm on the right is slightly higher ($\simeq$ 2 cm) than on the left due to the presence of the liver and indeed the liver can be percussed. Likewise the area of cardiac dullness can be percussed and both areas may be resonant when the lungs are hyperinflated. Naturally the percussion note depends upon the thickness of the chest wall and in very muscular or obese patients this may make the note less resonant. With hyperinflation or pneumothorax the percussion note may be hyper-resonant throughout.

The percussion note may be impaired wherever there are abnormal interfaces which damp out the vibrations. Thus dullness may be a feature of pleural or pulmonary fibrosis, collapse or consolidation. It is not really possible to discern between these by percussion alone though other physical signs may help. When fluid is present in the pleural cavity the percussion note sounds and feels stony dull. Stony dullness to percussion is probably the best sign of fluid in the pleural cavity. When learning it can best be appreciated by percussing beer in a barrel, wine in a cask or more likely rainwater in a water-butt. Once stony dullness has been appreciated it is not easily forgotten though of course its appreciation in the patient with a thick chest wall may be somewhat blunted.

Palpable Voice Sounds: Tactile Vocal Fremitus

After percussion it is useful to palpate for voice sounds over the upper middle and lower zones of the chest. This is tactile vocal fremitus and it is best appreciated by placing the ulnar border or the flat of the hand on the chest wall. Normally one can just appreciate the spoken words whether 99 or 1,1,1. However this sensation may be increased where there is underlying consolidation which amplifies the transmission of voice sounds. Conversely where there is fluid interposed such as pleural effusion, fremitus is absent and reduced where the lung is collapsed. In the presence of equivocal stony dullness absent vocal fremitus may indicate pleural effusion.

Auscultation

This is best done with the diaphragm of the stethoscope, which gathers more sounds of higher pitch. The chest should be examined in a logical sequence of upper, middle and lower zones, front, sides and back.

Normal vesicular breath sounds are soft, low-pitched and rustling in type. They are produced by turbulence in the air stream as it passes through the narrow larynx, and are transmitted back into the lungs to be modified by high-frequency attenuation by the branching sequence of the bronchial tree and by the lung parenchyma. The inspiratory phase is audible throughout and appears longer than the expiratory phase which follows without pause and fades into silence. This probably reflects the better transmission of breath sounds in the direction of flow towards the periphery on inspiration.

Bronchial breath sounds are louder, higher in pitch and blowing. They can best be appreciated by the student listening over the trachea. Again they reflect turbulent flow in the larynx just as with vesicular breathing. However transmission to the lung periphery is less modified by pneumonic consolidation or cavitation, and occasionally by pleural effusion and underlying collapse. The expiratory sound follows inspiration after a pause and is as long as or longer than the inspiratory sound with which it merges imperceptibly. The blowing quality of these sounds provides the clue to their origin and may be low, medium or high-pitched (tubular).

Nowadays this latter subdivision is somewhat academic. The main diagnostic value of bronchial breath sounds is in distinguishing pneumonic consolidation from collapse due to a mucus plug, bronchial carcinoma or foreign body.

Audible voice sounds: vocal resonance

This is the audible counterpart of tactile vocal fremitus and has a similar meaning; the patient says 99 or 1,1,1 and normally a buzzing noise is heard. With consolidation or cavitation louder bronchophony or whispering pectoriloquy may be heard, or bleating aegophony above a pleural effusion.

Added Sounds

There are three principal sounds added to the breath sounds, namely (1) crackles, synonymous with crepitations or râles, (2) wheezes, synonymous with rhonchi, and (3) pleural rub.

Crackles

Crackles may be simulated by rubbing hair between one's fingers or by a hairy chest. A few basal crackles may be heard in the normal upright subject breathing quietly and this probably indicates that airways are closing in the dependent lung bases during shallow breathing, an effect of gravity. Characteristically these crackles clear when the patient takes a deep breath or coughs and they are of no consequence, though to the beginner they may be misleading. The crackle is in effect a miniature explosion and is caused by the opening of airways on inspiration with equalisation of pressure along their lengths. It is no longer held that crackles represent the popping of bubbles in secretions in small airways during inspiration (though Laennec's original description of râle was the death rattle heard with sputum retention in dying patients). When crackles are numerous, widespread and persistent they are indicative of parenchymal and small airways disease. These explanations are insufficient to explain all the facts. Nevertheless *fine crackles* are heard in early pneumonic consolidation, *medium crackles* in pulmonary oedema and *coarse crackles* in bronchiectasis, lung abscess and allergic or fibrosing alveolitis. Crackles are not a common feature of chronic obstructive bronchitis, emphysema or asthma unless airways obstruction is severe, when they are early in inspiration and may be audible at the mouth. By contrast in restrictive lung defects such as fibrosing alveolitis, asbestosis and sarcoidosis, crackles are late in inspiration and rarely audible at the mouth.

Wheezes

Laennec suggested that musical wheezing was generated in the lungs in the same way as in a musical instrument. There are three types of instrument which possibly produce such noise: the organ pipe in which air oscillates after striking a sharp edge, a reed instrument such as an oboe or clarinet which depends on vibration of the natural reed, and a toy trumpet where sound is generated by a metal reed and its quality determined by the reed's mechanical properties alone. It seems likely that the toy trumpet provides the closest analogy to wheezing in the human lung rather than the more classical instruments. The bronchus is narrowed to the point of closure by expiratory pressure and when the linear velocity of air flow reaches a critical level, wheezing is generated. The linear velocity of air flowing through the stenosis plays a dominant part in determining the pitch; bronchial compliance plays a lesser part.

This may account for the occasional finding of a relatively silent chest in severe bronchial asthma where the gas flow is insufficient to generate wheezing. This is a pitfall for the unwary. The pitch of the wheeze is not therefore determined by the diameter and length of the airways involved as was originally thought.

The positive pressure exerted by effort plus the elastic recoil of the lungs and thorax during expiration tends to narrow intra-pulmonary airways so that wheezing is usually expiratory in phase. However narrowing of the trachea and central airways by virtue of retrosternal goitre or central carcinoma may be more fixed and lead to *inspiratory stridor.*

Wheezes are the hallmarks of airways obstruction, a charac-teristic feature of chronic bronchitis, emphysema and bronchial asthma. In chronic bronchitis with excessive secretions lining the bronchial tree, there are usually scattered lower-pitched sonorous wheezes, while in asthma where there is a combination of wide-spread smooth muscle spasm, mucosal oedema and secretions in the airways, there may be high-pitched musical wheezing. The airways obstruction may be completely reversible by broncho-dilators in asthmatics but only partially so (10 to 20 per cent) in bronchitics. The combination of wheezes and crackles may indicate bronchopneumonia, bronchiectasis or severe airways obstruction. Unilateral wheezing suggests discrete bronchial narrowing by mucus plug, tumour or foreign body (dentures or peanuts) and as such it may be inspiratory too.

Pleural rub

Friction between the parietal and visceral pleura can generate a creaky, crackling sound, resembling a window leather being rubbed. The sounds are usually loud, localised and often expiratory as well as inspiratory. These facts usually distinguish them from lung crackles but not always.

A pleural rub is heard where the pleural layers are roughened or inflamed with pneumonia, carcinoma or pulmonary infarct for example. With the development of an effusion the rub may vanish as the pleural layers are parted.

Other sounds

Finally with an air—fluid level in the chest, whether due to lung abscess or hydropneumothorax, a succussion splash may be heard on gently rocking the patient. This should not be confused with a splash sometimes audible over the full stomach or in pyloric stenosis. In pneumothorax the coin sign (bruit d'airain) may be elicited when a coin is placed on the chest wall and tapped with another coin, giving a typical ringing sound; however this is rarely needed to make the diagnosis and an expiratory postero-anterior chest x-ray is of infinitely greater value.

The physical signs of lung disease are summarised in Table 3.4.

FURTHER INVESTIGATIONS

Chest X-ray

The chest x-ray is an integral part of the examination of any patient with persisting chest symptoms. There is general agreement on how one should read a chest x-ray. Each component of a chest x-ray (Figure 3.1) should be scrutinised in turn and any abnormalities or discrepancies noted. On occasion however this leads to the student concentrating on normal features such as the ribs at the expense of missing obvious pulmonary shadows. It seems preferable to focus attention on obvious abnormalities first and then to proceed to the systematic scrutiny. Naturally if no obvious abnormalities are seen in initial appraisal the routine should be adhered to.

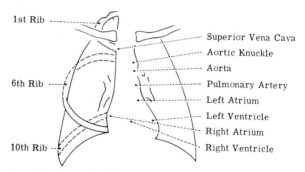

Figure 3.1. *Anatomical landmarks on the normal chest radiograph.*

The points to bear in mind when examining the chest x-ray are as follows:
1. The density of the film; the routine 2 m (6 ft) postero-anterior (PA) chest x-ray should be of such density that the vertebral bodies can be distinguished down to the mid-thoracic region; if

Table 3.4. Physical signs of lung disease.

Disease	Chest movement	Mediastinal shift	Percussion note	Breath sounds	Voice sounds	Added sounds
Chronic bronchitis Emphysema	Reduced, barrel-shaped, bucket-handle in type	0	Hyper-resonant	Vesicular, reduced, prolonged expiration	Reduced	Wheezes
Asthma	Variable depending on severity	0	,, ,,	,, ,,	,,	Wheezes
Pneumonic consolidation	Reduced locally	0	Dull	Bronchial	Increased, whispering pectoriloquy, aegophony	Crackles
Collapse	Reduced locally	Towards site	Dull	Vesicular, reduced or absent	Reduced	0
Pleural effusion	Reduced locally	Towards opposite side	Stony dull	Vesicular, reduced, bronchial at upper level	Reduced or absent, ? aegophony above	None; or pleural rub
Fibrosis	Reduced	Towards site	Dull	Bronchial	Increased	Crackles
Pneumothorax	Reduced locally	Towards opposite side	Hyper-resonant	Vesicular, reduced or absent	Reduced	0

they can be seen along its whole length the film is too hard, and if they cannot be seen at all the film is too soft.

2. The centering of the film can be noted by looking at the sterno-clavicular joints. Rotation may lead to spurious tracheal deviation or cardiac or hilar shadowing.

3. The trachea should be checked to see whether it is central and the mediastinum examined as well as the cardiac shadow for abnormalities in configuration and size; the normal cardio-thoracic ratio is less than 50 per cent.

4. The lung fields should be divided into three zones (Figure 3.2). The upper zones extend from the apex to the lower edge of the second rib anteriorly; the middle zones extend from there to the lower edge of the fourth rib anteriorly, including the hilar regions; the lower zones extend down to the diaphragm, and include the cardio- and costophrenic angles which should be sharp and clear.

5. The bony skeleton should be examined, particularly ribs and vertebrae, for fractures, porotic or sclerotic areas.

6. Finally general features such as the presence or absence of breast and other extraneous soft tissue shadows should be noted.

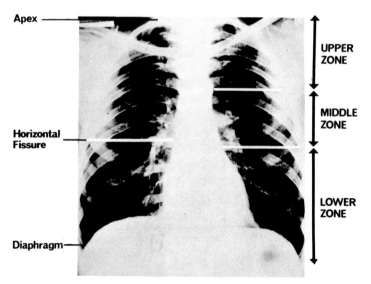

Figure 3.2. *Lung zones.*

The shadows within the lung fields are mainly caused by the pulmonary vessels and not the bronchi. Peripheral vessels may be pruned or lost in emphysema, pulmonary hypertension or multiple pulmonary embolism. Crowding of vessels is a feature of lobar collapse. The bronchi are only visible when their walls are thickened and expanded by bronchiectasis for instance, producing parallel or 'tramline' shadows.

The main or oblique fissure is visible only on the lateral x-ray, running from the fourth vertebral body across the hilum to the anterior third of the diaphragm. The horizontal fissure is seen only in the right lung, extending along the top of the fourth rib anteriorly, laterally to the sixth rib in the mid-axillary line and separating the right upper and middle lobes (Figure 3.3). These fissures change position with lung collapse, fibrosis or hyper-inflation.

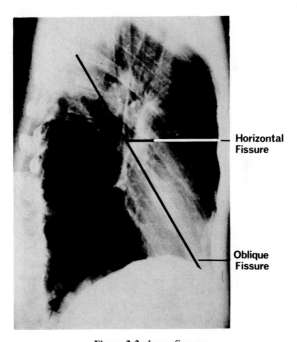

Figure 3.3. *Lung fissures.*

Pulmonary shadows

Collapse (Figure 3.4) leads to shrinkage of the lobe and shift of the fissures. Consolidation leads to no loss of volume (Figure 3.5), and an air bronchogram may be seen. Abnormal hilar shadows or peripheral 'coin' lesions are often due to carcinoma (Figure 3.6), though occasionally loculated fluid, infarction and inflammatory lesions may give a similar picture.

Diffuse pulmonary mottling may be caused by a wide range of diseases including miliary tuberculosis, sarcoidosis, pneumoconiosis and cryptogenic fibrosing or allergic alveolitis.

Pleural effusion is usually basal (with patient erect) filling in the costophrenic angles, and on occasion massive (Figure 3.7), with a curved, meniscus-like upper edge; a horizontal edge indicates an air—fluid interface. Bullae may be defined by fine linear shadows and cavities as apparent holes in shadows, when tuberculous or otherwise. Apical views and tomography may be needed to define them.

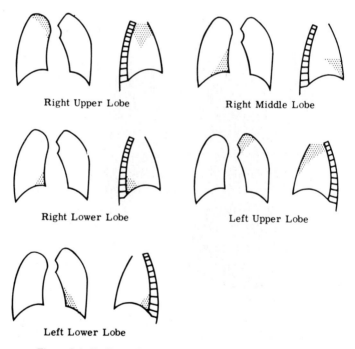

Figure 3.4. *Radiographic appearance of collapsed lung lobes.*

In clinical practice the changes seen on the x-ray usually concur with those suspected on clinical examination with some important exceptions. These include the asymptomatic apical infiltrate of early adult pulmonary tuberculosis, the asymptomatic hilar mass or coin lesion in the periphery of the lungs with bronchial carcinoma, and occasionally such entities as the bilateral hilar lymphadenopathy of sarcoidosis and mediastinal masses. Collapse or consolidation of various lobes of the lung give shadows as illustrated in Figure 3.4. In bronchiectasis there may be ring shadows indicating bronchial wall thickening. In pneumothorax the lung edge can be

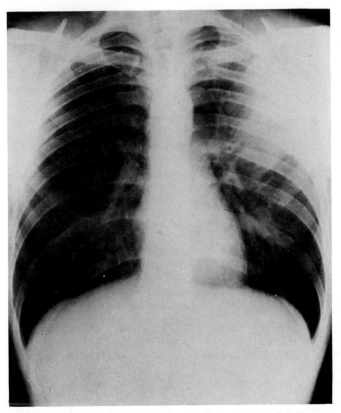

Figure 3.5. *Pneumococcal pneumonia in left upper lobe.*

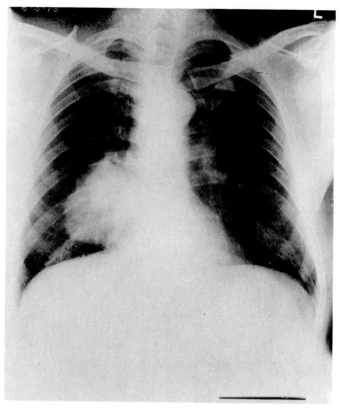

Figure 3.6. *Squamous cell carcinoma of bronchus in right lower lobe.*

seen displaced from the thoracic wall and this may be exaggerated if an expiratory film is taken (Figure 3.8). The diaphragm may be elevated (the right is 1 to 2 cm higher than the left due to the underlying liver) because of phrenic paralysis or overlying lung collapse or fibrosis.

In the diseases characterised by diffuse air-flow obstruction, namely chronic obstructive bronchitis, emphysema and asthma, the characteristic features seen are those of hyperinflation with horizontal ribs, hyperlucent lung fields and flat diaphragm; counting down, the anterior ends of more than six ribs may be seen above the diaphragm. In pulmonary hypertension the transhilar distance may be increased and the periphery of the vessels may be pruned.

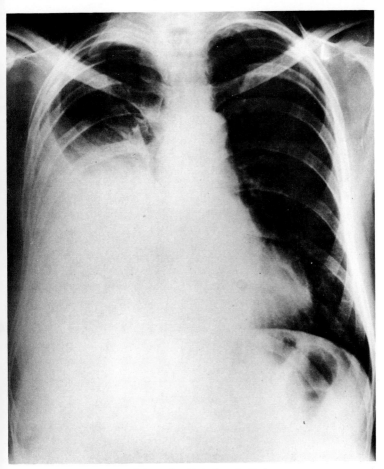

Figure 3.7. *Right-sided pleural effusion.*

A lateral chest x-ray should be requested if there is any doubt about the hilar regions. This will show whether the shadow is vascular or not, and pick up retrocardiac or posterior lesions. The costophrenic angles should be inspected carefully for fluid.

Special *apical views* may avoid overlying bony structures and show details of tuberculous infiltrates. *Tomography*, in which the x-rays are focused on various depths of the lung, is useful for demonstrating the nature of upper zone lesions whether infiltrates, cavities or 'coin' in type. Similarly hilar nodes and tumour may be confirmed.

Bronchography with iodised oil (e.g. Dionysil) instilled into the bronchial tree is useful to confirm bronchiectasis. It is not often required.

Fluoroscopy (screening) may be useful to check for diaphragmatic paralysis, where the high diaphragm moves upwards paradoxically on sniffing; or for abnormal cardiac pulsation.

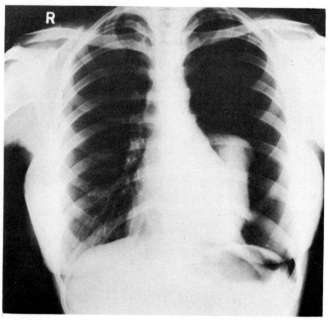

Figure 3.8. *Left pneumothorax with extensive collapse of the underlying lung.*

Sputum Examination

Sputum should be collected carefully, and an adequate fresh sample, uncontaminated by saliva, sent to the laboratory. Often an early morning sample is best. In suspected pulmonary tuberculosis where there is little sputum, early morning gastric aspiration is indicated on three consecutive days. Tuberculous cultures and sensitivities take from 8 to 12 weeks.

The next step is inspection of its characteristics by eye. Thereafter smear, culture and test for antibiotic sensitivities are indicated. An immediate smear and gram stain by the house physician may be rewarding and is frequently neglected. Usually the result should be confirmed by the microbiological laboratory, though urgent treatment may be necessary in the interim. Often nowadays the bacterial content of sputum in patients with acute respiratory infections has been significantly altered by antibiotics before testing takes place.

The sputum may show asbestos bodies in asbestosis and eosinophilia in asthma.

Sputum cytology is an important technique for diagnosing lung cancer. At least three specimens of sputum should be examined. This gives a positive result in over 50 per cent of cases.

Pulmonary Function Tests

Pulmonary function tests are an important part of the overall clinical assessment of the chest and lungs. They provide information on ventilation, perfusion and gas exchange (O_2 and CO_2) with objective numerical data which may support and clarify the clinical diagnosis. Their limitations should be (and frequently are not) appreciated. They may confirm a suspected diagnosis (e.g. asthma with reversible airways obstruction) but in many chest diseases the ultimate diagnosis is obtained by histology and lung biopsy. In this respect these tests are akin to renal or pancreatic function tests and should be accepted in like vein.

Depending on the nature of the clinical problem adequate information may be given by simple screening tests, which can be augmented as clinically indicated.

The usual screening tests can best be seen by reference to the report form shown in Figure 3.9. They can be divided into *lung volumes*, both *static* (VC), and *dynamic* (FVC, FEV_1, FEV% and PFR). These can be measured simply with a dry spirometer such as a Vitalograph and the PFR with a Wright peak flow meter or gauge. The VC is defined as the volume of a maximum expiration (from TLC to RV) after a maximum inspiration; the FVC, FEV_1 and PFR are measured on maximum forced expiration. The best of three readings is usually taken in each case. The lung volumes are shown in Figure 3.10. The static volumes give information about *restriction*, the dynamic volumes about air flow *obstruction*. The

PULMONARY FUNCTION REPORT

Diagnosis

Ht. cm. Wt. Kg. Smoking:

Hospital No.
Surname M/F
First Names M/S/W

D. of B.

Ward/Dept. Branch
Consultant
Doctor's Signature Date

LUNG VOLUMES			Predicted	Observed	% Predicted	After Broncho-Dilators
Vital capacity	VC	L				
Forced vital capacity	FVC	L				
☐ Forced expiratory volume, 1 sec.	FEV_1	L				
FEV_1/FVC		%				
Peak flow rate	PFR	L/min				
Expiratory reserve volume	ERV	L				
Residual volume	RV	L				
☐ Functional residual capacity	FRC	L				
Total lung capacity	TLC	L				
RV/TLC		%				

GAS TRANSFER		Predicted	Observed
Lung transfer T_LCO	$mmol.min^{-1}.kPa^{-1}$		
Rebreathing $P\bar{v}CO_2$	kPa		
☐ Arterial PO2	kPa		
,, PCO2	kPa		
,, pH	units		
,, base	mmol/l		

OTHER TESTS:

COMMENTS:

PULMONARY FUNCTION REPORT

Figure 3.9. *Pulmonary function report.*

complex static lung volumes include residual volume (RV) measured by either an inert gas dilution or plethysmographic method; TLC can then be calculated (RV + VC). *Gas transfer* is tested by measuring the uptake of a soluble test gas, carbon monoxide (0.3%), from a single vital capacity breath (transfer factor, $T_L CO$) and the PCO_2 is measured by a re-breathing method.

SI units are now used for the tests listed under Gas Transfer. For conversion, the following factors can be used:
$T_L CO$ (SI units) × 3 = $T_L CO$ in traditional units (ml/min/mm Hg)
$P\bar{v}CO_2$, PO_2 and PCO_2 (SI units) × 7.5 = value in mm Hg.

All these tests are non-invasive and take about half an hour to complete. Arterial blood gases can be estimated should the clinical situation warrant it (e.g. suspected respiratory failure).

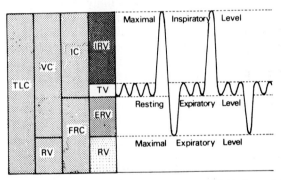

Figure 3.10. *Lung volumes. From Comroe et al (1962) with kind permission of the authors and the publisher (Chicago: Year Book Medical Publishers).*

Indications for pulmonary function tests are as follows:

1. Diagnosis. Pulmonary function tests may be valuable in the diagnosis of unexplained dyspnoea, respiratory failure, cyanosis or polycythaemia for instance. If pulmonary function tests are completely normal, then a respiratory cause of dyspnoea and the other abnormalities is unlikely.

Polycythaemia may be secondary to chronic hypoxic lung disease such as chronic bronchitis even when the patient is not overtly cyanosed. The level of hypoxaemia required varies and occasionally nocturnal hypoventilation may be sufficient provocation.

2. The assessment and management of patients with airways obstruction due to asthma, chronic bronchitis and emphysema. It is

imperative to make objective measurement of the degree of airways obstruction and its reversibility in all these conditions.

3. The preoperative assessment of patients requiring thoracotomy and lung resection for bronchial carcinoma or, less frequently, bronchiectasis, adenoma or other conditions.

4. The assessment of functional disability in patients with industrial lung disease for disability claims, where exercise testing may also be indicated.

Patterns of change in pulmonary function tests (Table 3.5)

Obstructive defects. These result in a low FEV_1 and $FEV\%$, reflecting airflow obstruction, and a high RV and RV/TLC ratio, reflecting hyperinflation. The latter reduces VC though TLC is normal and not restricted. The reversibility of airways obstruction is reflected by improvement in these measurements after inhaling a bronchodilator aerosol (e.g. isoprenaline or salbutamol), and gives a clue to the diagnosis; complete reversibility may be seen in the labile asthmatic patient, though often in the more severe asthmatic further treatment (e.g. a course of prednisone) may be necessary to judge this. Occasionally mild hyperinflation and high T_LCO may suggest background asthma even when flow rates are normal; positive skin-prick tests and sputum eosinophilia may support this

Table 3.5. *Lung defects.*

Pulmonary function test		Obstructive	Restrictive
Lung volumes	TLC	Normal	Reduced
	RV	Increased	Normal
	RV/TLC	Increased (hyperinflation)	Normal
	VC	Reduced	Reduced
Maximal flow	FEV₁	Reduced	Reduced[a]
	FEV%	Reduced	Normal
	PFR	Reduced	Reduced[a]
Gas transfer	T_LCO	Normal or reduced[b]	Reduced or normal
	P_O₂	Normal or reduced	Reduced, particularly on exercise, or normal
	P_CO₂	Normal or increased[c]	Reduced — by tachypnoea

[a] Reduced by loss of lung volume and not airflow obstruction.
[b] Occasionally raised in asthmatics.
[c] Occasionally reduced in asthmatics.

diagnosis. In chronic bronchitis the degree of airways obstruction is variable and reversibility ranges from 10 to 20 per cent; T_LCO may be either normal or low. In emphysema the same degree of airways obstruction and reversibility may be seen, but T_LCO is usually low. The airways obstruction in asthma and bronchitis is 'intrinsic' and confined largely to the bronchi themselves; in emphysema it is 'extrinsic' and a function of the diminished lung elastic recoil. In practice this does not appear to influence the degree of reversibility seen in chronic bronchitis or emphysema.

Restrictive defects. The TLC (and usually VC) are low; where restriction is due to abnormal chest wall for instance, transfer factor may be normal. With parenchymal lung disease such as fibrosing or allergic alveolitis, diffuse sarcoidosis or asbestosis, T_LCO is low and repeat measurements may be useful to monitor progression and the effects of treatment.

Gas transfer defects. A low T_LCO may suggest pulmonary vascular disease such as multiple pulmonary emboli or pulmonary hypertension. Often a low T_LCO is associated with arterial hypoxaemia (low PO_2) and respiratory failure. Scadding (1966) defined respiratory failure as:
1. Ventilatory defects
    i. obstructive (airways obstruction)
    ii. non-obstructive (restrictive or hypodynamic)
2. Gas transfer (or exchange) defects.

    In cyanosed patients or those with suspected respiratory failure in which, on occasion, clinical features may not be clear-cut, arterial blood gas measurement is imperative. A high PCO_2 (>6.7 kPa or 50 mm Hg) and low PO_2 (<8.0 kPa or 60 mm Hg) indicate hypoventilation and respiratory failure, whether central (primary or secondary to sedatives, trauma or meningitis), or peripheral (chronic obstructive bronchitis). A low or normal PCO_2 and low PO_2 indicate a gas transfer defect, seen in fibrosing alveolitis or pulmonary embolism and wherever there are ventilation perfusion ($\dot{V}/\dot{Q}$) inequalities in the lung or limited alveolo-capillary diffusion.

    The administration of 100 per cent O_2 (for about 25 min) may serve to distinguish whether hypoxaemia and cyanosis are cardiac or pulmonary in origin. With a right to left cardiac shunt or intrapulmonary shunt the PO_2 does not rise, or scarcely so, while with a $\dot{V}/\dot{Q}$ or diffusion abnormality it rises to reasonable levels (>26.6 kPa or 200 mm Hg).

Bronchoscopy

Bronchoscopy is indicated for bronchial carcinoma presenting with unresolved pneumonia, haemoptysis, hilar or peripheral 'coin' shadows, and for other unexplained bronchial and lung diseases. Mucus plugs and retained sputum can be aspirated and foreign bodies removed.

The recent advent of the flexible, fibreoptic bronchoscope has extended the range of vision to the upper lobes and periphery and has increased the usefulness of this technique for the investigation of a wide variety of lung diseases.

Pleural Aspiration

This is routinely used in the diagnosis and management of pleural effusion. It is normal to limit the volume of aspirate to 500 to 1000 ml, otherwise occasionally pulmonary oedema, heralded by coughing, may occur. Some characteristic features of pleural fluid are shown in Table 3.6.

Pleural Biopsy

Pleural biopsy should be done routinely at the time of pleural aspiration in almost every case. The Abrams needle is used as a 'crochet-hook' to biopsy the parietal pleura. Biopsy increases the diagnostic yield from the fluid alone by 30 per cent.

Lung Biopsy

This can be done by one of several methods:
1. Aspiration needle biopsy of solid masses, usually tumours.
2. Drill biopsy for diffuse lung disease.
3. Transbronchial biopsy for local or diffuse disease.
   All these techniques may be complicated by mild pneumothorax (20 per cent) and occasionally haemorrhage.
4. If all else fails then open lung biopsy is occasionally indicated.

Table 3.6. Pleural fluid characteristics.

Disease	Colour	Blood	Cells	Bacteria	Others
Congestive cardiac failure	Straw	—	—	—	—
Postpneumonic	,,	—	Neutrophils	±	—
Carcinoma	,,	+ +	Carcinoma	—	Pleural biopsy positive 40—60% Rapid recurrence
Tuberculosis	,,	—	Lymphocytes	+	Pleural biopsy positive 70—80%
Pulmonary infarction	,,	+ +	Eosinophils, Mesothelial	—	—
Trauma	—	+ +	Eosinophils	—	—
Emphysema	Cloudy	—	Neutrophils	+	—
Chylothorax	,,	—	—	—	High fats and cholesterol
Rheumatoid	Straw	—	Lymphocytes	—	Low sugar (<20 mg%, 1.11 mmol/l), high cholesterol and LDH, positive rheumatoid factor.
Pancreatitis	,,	—	—	—	High amylase

Diseases such as congestive cardiac failure or hypoproteinaemia (nephrosis and cirrhosis) lead to formation of a transudate (protein <30 g/l), the majority to an exudate (protein >30 g/l). Many effusions give intermediate levels and this is not of great value.

Skin Tests

Skin-prick tests to common allergens such as house dust and the mite, pets and pollens are useful in the diagnosis and management of asthma.

In the Mantoux test 0.1 ml of purified protein derivative (PPD) 1 to 5 tuberculin units (TU) is injected intradermally. It is read at 48 to 72 hours. The reaction when positive consists of induration and erythema. A diameter above 10 mm indicates previous tuberculous infection. In general the more florid the reaction, the more likely there is to be recent infection. This is used as a screening and diagnostic test.

Radioactive Lung Scan

Macro-aggregated ^{99m}technetium-labelled human albumin may be injected to give an index of lung perfusion. Retention and scanning is normally uniform, but may show single or multiple defects in embolic disease.

Ventilation scans may also be indicated in bullous disease.

FURTHER READING

Comroe, J. H., Forster, R. E., Dubois, A. B., Briscoe, W. A. & Carlsen, E. (1962) *The Lung,* 2nd edition. Chicago: Year Book Medical Publishers.

Cotes, J. E. (1979) *Lung Function,* 4th edition. Oxford: Blackwell.

Forgacs, P. (1967) Crackles and wheezes. *Lancet,* **ii,** 203.

Hampton, J. R., Harrison, M. J. C., Mitchell, J. R. A., Prichard, J. S. & Seymour, C. (1975) Relative contributions of history-taking, physical examination and laboratory investigations to diagnosis and management of medical outpatients. *British Medical Journal,* **ii,** 486.

Johnston, R. N., Lockhart, W., Ritchie, R. T. & Smith, D. H. (1960) Haemoptysis. *British Medical Journal,* **i,** 592.

McGavin, C. R., Gupta, S. P. & McHardy, G. J. R. (1976) Twelve-minute walking test for assessing disability in chronic bronchitis. *British Medical Journal,* **i,** 822.

Medical Research Council (1965) Definition and classification of chronic bronchitis for clinical and epidemiological purposes. *Lancet,* **i,** 448.

Scadding, J. G. (1966) Patterns of respiratory insufficiency. *Lancet,* **i,** 701.

4 The Abdomen

J. S. Morris and W. K. Stewart

The broad outlines of clinical history taking and examination have been presented in the opening chapter of this book, and the principles discussed apply to the clinical detection of renal and intestinal disease in similar manner to disease states in other systems. With respect to gastrointestinal disease, clinical history taking and examination have a particular relevance. Clinical assessment is used to decide whether symptoms require further investigation. If all patients with dyspepsia were to have a barium meal, for example, the resulting economic burden would be immense. In some diseases the diagnosis may be confidently made from the history, and this is particularly true of conditions such as carcinoma of the oesophagus and achalasia of the cardia.

A close doctor—patient relationship is particularly important in gastrointestinal disease because many of the symptoms and disorders have no effective treatment. Understandably, reassurance and education of the patient is often the only form of management available.

HISTORY: GASTROINTESTINAL DISEASE

Dysguaesia

Many people complain of a bad taste in the mouth. The most common cause is poor oral hygiene, but quite often no cause is

177

found and the complaint is dismissed as being of psychological origin. The symptom can occur in patients with chronic sinusitis and tonsillar infection. Dysguaesia has been described as a manifestation of cerebrovascular disease in the elderly, and a bad taste in the mouth is an extremely distressing complaint of those with inoperable stomach cancers and in patients with carcinoma of the oesophagus who have a Mousseau—Barbin or similar tube inserted to relieve the obstruction to swallowing.

Anorexia

In physiological terms there are two sensations which control the intake of food. The first of these is *hunger*, which is an unpleasant sensation, relieved by the intake of food. It can be regarded teleologically as a means of ensuring an adequate intake of calories. The second sensation is *appetite*, which is a pleasurable experience aroused by the thought, sight or smell of specific kinds of food. As such, appetite depends on the eating habits of a person's social or ethnic group. Feeding is controlled by two centres in the hypothalamus and brain stem. The laterally placed nuclei constitute the feeding centre, and the anteromedial nuclei act as a satiety centre. The stimuli which affect these centres are ill understood. It has been suggested that a low arteriovenous glucose difference stimulates the feeding centre, whereas a high glucose difference stimulates the satiety centre. Equally, the centres may be responsive to the changes in body temperature which occur after a meal.

With this poor understanding of the factors which control food intake, it is fortunate that loss of appetite seldom occurs as the sole manifestation of disease and when loss of appetite is organic there are other symptoms or physical signs which help to determine the cause. It has been claimed that loss of appetite for meat is an early symptom of carcinoma of the stomach, although there are no studies which support this hypothesis. Psychological factors play a large part in appetite disorders. Excessive appetite is discussed in Chapter 9.

Loss of Weight

Maintenance of body weight is dependent upon a whole range of factors, including appetite, energy expenditure and disease states.

In practical terms it is useful to remember that the six commonest causes of weight loss in clinical medicine are diabetes, thyrotoxicosis, neoplasms, malabsorption states, psychological disorders and tuberculosis.

Dyspepsia

This is a term which is used in a variety of ways. It generally implies epigastric discomfort, short of actual pain, experienced during or following a meal. There may be associated flatulence. *Flatulence* implies excessive gas in the abdomen. The patient may complain of either excessive belching, or abdominal distension (meteorism), or the passage of large volumes of flatus. Rarely, there is slight nausea. The lay term indigestion should be avoided because it may be used to indicate dyspepsia as well as actual epigastric pain or heartburn. Dyspepsia may accompany peptic ulcer disease, gastric cancer, gastritis, gallbladder disease or colonic disease. Not infrequently it is impossible to ascribe a cause.

Heartburn

This is the symptom of a burning retrosternal sensation which originates in the epigastric or lower sternal region and which radiates to the chest, deep to the sternum. The pain or discomfort may extend up to the throat. There may be associated regurgitation of gastric contents. The mechanism of heartburn is uncertain; it is a symptom of oesophageal dysfunction and indicates either oesophageal spasm or inflammation in response to an irritating fluid which may be acid or bile.

The symptom occurs with hiatus hernia, peptic ulceration, gastritis and gallbladder disease. It is common in pregnancy where it may be related to the combination of raised intra-abdominal pressure, those hormonal changes affecting the competency of the gastro-oesophageal sphincter mechanism, and the development of hiatus hernia. Severe heartburn must be distinguished from other causes of retrosternal pain such as oesophageal spasm (associated with tertiary contractions of the oesophagus), pericardial pain, angina pectoris and a myocardial infarct.

Waterbrash

This is an uncommon symptom in which there is a sudden rush of clear tasteless fluid into the mouth. Occasionally the fluid has a salty flavour. The term is not used if the fluid, either acid or bile, has obviously been regurgitated. The origin of the fluid is uncertain but may be from the salivary glands. Waterbrash is claimed to be a specific manifestation of a duodenal ulcer.

Dysphagia

Swallowing is a mainly reflex act which is controlled by a swallowing centre situated in the medulla. Food coming into contact with the fauces, the hypopharynx and the upper third of the oesophagus stimulates afferent impulses which travel along the superior branch of the vagus and the glossopharyngeal nerve to the medulla. Efferent impulses travel from the medulla through the nuclei of the fifth, seventh, tenth, eleventh and twelfth cranial nerves and the nucleus ambiguus. As a result of the reflex a series of peristaltic waves carries the bolus of food down the oesophagus and the arrival of the peristaltic waves at the gastro-oesophageal junction is preceded by relaxation of the physiological sphincter at the oesophagogastric junction. The control of sphincter relaxation is not clear, but it is influenced by a centre within the brain via the vagus nerve and by local humoral factors such as gastrin. The competence of the oesophagogastric junction probably depends mainly upon the sphincter; anatomical factors such as the diaphragm and the angle at which the oesophagus enters the stomach are probably not as important.

Dysphagia is the sensation of food sticking in the oesophagus *during the act of swallowing.* A similar symptom occurring at times other than during swallowing is referred to as *globus hystericus* and is of no organic significance. True dysphagia, however, always implies an organic disorder. Important causes include oesophageal cancer, peptic oesophagitis and stricture, and achalasia of the cardia. The patient is not always able to locate correctly the precise level of obstruction. Lower oesophageal causes of dysphagia for example, can give rise to symptoms in the suprasternal notch.

Pain and dysphagia

Dysphagia is not of itself a painful sensation, although pain is experienced by about 75 per cent of patients with achalasia. It may simulate that of a myocardial infarction and have a similar radiation. The frequency and duration of attacks of oesophageal pain in achalasia vary from patient to patient and even in the same patient. It is sometimes eased by drinking a glass of cold water. The cause of the pain is not understood.

Oesophageal pain also occurs in association with dysphagia due to a swallowed foreign body such as a fish bone. Here it is due to an associated oesophagitis and possible reflux of gastric contents. Bolus obstruction of an oesophageal carcinoma also causes pain.

Helpful clinical features in diagnosing the cause of dysphagia
(Figure 4.1)

Of all gastrointestinal symptoms, dysphagia is the one in which a clinical history is of greatest diagnostic help and it has been claimed that the cause of dysphagia can be deduced from the clinical history alone in over 80 per cent of patients. An organic obstruction of the oesophagus produces difficulty in swallowing solid foods in the initial stages and difficulty in swallowing liquids occurs much later in its course. Motor disorders, on the other hand, cause difficulty in swallowing both solids and liquids from the outset, particularly if these are very hot or very cold. Patients in whom dysphagia is due to motor abnormalities such as achalasia learn that swallowing is facilitated in the standing position or when a glass of water is drunk with the meal. They often adopt trick manoeuvres. Regurgitation of food is often associated with dysphagia, but the pattern of the dysphagia, i.e. the interval between swallowing and regurgitation, is seldom of diagnostic value.

Mucosal webs or rings of the lower oesophagus occasionally cause dysphagia. In these patients the history is often of help for they complain of intermittent dysphagia over many years. This occurs because the obstruction is completed by a bolus of food above a certain diameter and regurgitation of this bolus leads to complete remission of the symptom. Furthermore an oesophageal ring is not always constant. The patient then learns to avoid swallowing lumps of food without adequate chewing, although the possibility of developing dysphagia remains.

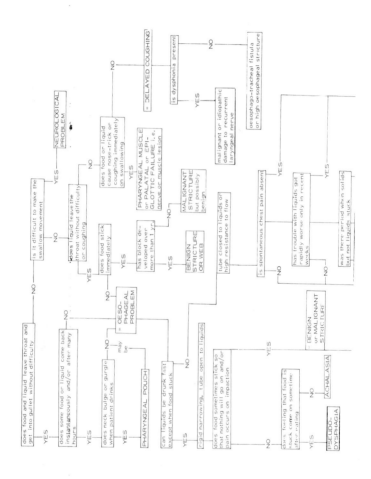

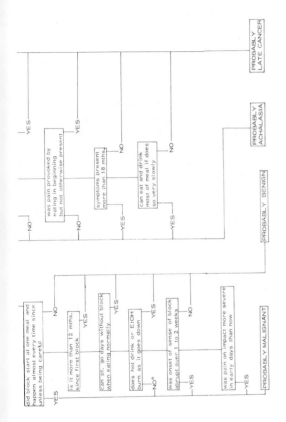

° If the other answers suggest a benign lesion,
the answer "NO" here indicates a ring stricture.

Figure 4.1. *Flow chart of questions for the diagnosis of the common causes of dysphagia. The doctor should ask himself these questions; they are not designed to be addressed to the patient. From Edwards (1976) with kind permission of the author.*

Vomiting

The act of vomiting occurs as the result of stimulation of two centres situated in the brain. The first, the vomiting centre in the lateral reticular formation, is stimulated by afferent impulses which arise within the gastrointestinal tract and in other organs such as the heart and mesentery.

The second centre is the chemoreceptor trigger zone in the floor of the fourth ventricle, and this is stimulated by drugs such as the cardiac glycosides and by metabolic abnormalities such as acidosis and uraemia. The efferent impulses arise only in the vomiting centre and stimulation of the chemoreceptor trigger zone leads in turn to stimulation of the vomiting centre.

Vomiting is usually preceded by nausea, although this may be absent when vomiting occurs as a manifestation of psychological disorders. Nausea is associated with a reduced gastric and an increased duodenal tone. Retching, which represents deep inspiratory movements against a closed glottis, follows the sensation of nausea. The final act of vomiting results from the sustained contractions of the muscles of the abdominal wall. It is important to distinguish between vomiting, which is the return of gastric contents, and regurgitation, which is a symptom of oesophageal disease. Regurgitation is unaccompanied by nausea, retching or straining.

Vomiting is usually associated with a number of other phenomena. Tachycardia is common, and hypersalivation or diarrhoea may occur. The hypersalivation and diarrhoea occur possibly because of the close anatomical relationships in the medulla of the control centres.

Certain characteristics of vomiting are helpful in suggesting its cause. Vomiting of *psychogenic* origin occurs most often just after a meal has started, and it is characteristic that the patient always manages to avoid vomiting in a public place. Early morning vomiting is a feature of *anxiety states*, but is also seen in *pregnancy* and *alcoholism. Intestinal obstruction* induces copious vomiting, and sometimes the vomitus has a faecal odour. The vomiting of food which has been eaten several hours or perhaps even a day earlier suggests *delayed gastric emptying.* The delay in gastric emptying is not necessarily the result of a mechanical obstruction to gastric outflow but may also result from motor disturbance of the stomach such as occurs in diabetes, scleroderma and hypokalaemia.

In the initial stages of pyloric obstruction, tone in the stomach wall is good, and vomiting of small amounts of fluid occurs. In the later stages of pyloric obstruction the stomach wall becomes atonic, and the vomitus is copious and less frequent, occurring only once every two or three days.

The character of the vomitus is sometimes useful. In obstructive vomiting the presence of bile indicates that the obstruction is distal to the pylorus. Blood in the vomit occurs only in oesophageal, gastric or duodenal disease.

Prolonged vomiting of any cause may produce a tear in the lower part of the oesophageal or gastric fundal mucosa which may bleed profusely (Mallory—Weiss syndrome). The recent development of endoscopy has shown that this sequence of events is more common than was formerly thought and the bleeding may follow only a brief bout of vomiting.

Abdominal Pain

Abdominal pain is the commonest presenting symptom of gastro-intestinal disease and may be the cause of considerable diagnostic difficulty. It has been estimated that almost one-half of those patients who present with the symptom elude precise diagnosis. Many of the diagnostic problems engendered by abdominal pain arise from our incomplete understanding of its mechanism. Normally the gastrointestinal mucosa is insensitive to noxious stimuli such as burning, pinching or cutting, although these stimuli may be painful when the mucosa is inflamed and if the pain threshold is lowered. The only stimulus which produces pain in the normal gastrointestinal tract, under experimental conditions, is distension. Within the intestinal mucosa are naked nerve endings which act as sensory receptors and stimulation of these nerve fibres leads to afferent stimuli which reach the central nervous sytem by a series of visceral nerves in anatomical proximity to the sympathetic nervous system. Within the spinal cord the afferent visceral pathway is probably identical with the fibres which carry painful stimuli from somatic areas. This accounts for the poor localisation of visceral pain.

Types of abdominal pain

Patients often find it very difficult to describe abdominal pain. Descriptive terms such as gnawing, burning, shooting or cutting are often used but they seldom have any diagnostic relevance. Colic is a severe form of abdominal pain which waxes and wanes in intensity and suggests the presence of an obstructing lesion within a hollow muscular structure or tension in its muscle wall.

Pain arising from disease within the abdomen is classified as visceral, somatic (or peritoneal) and referred pain which is located in structures outside the abdominal cavity.

Visceral (deep) pain arises in the hollow structures within the abdomen including its embryonic extensions, the bile and pancreatic ducts. Disease within these organs gives rise to deep-seated pain referred to the midline structure. The paucity of sensory receptors and the anatomical proximity of the afferent nervous pathway to the somatic pathway leads to poor localisation of the source of the pain. By and large pain originating from the stomach, duodenum and biliary and pancreatic ducts occurs in the mid-epigastrium, that from the small intestine around the umbilicus, and pain from the colon in the hypogastrium.

Somatic (peritoneal) pain. As disease within hollow intra-abdominal structures spreads to involve the surrounding peritoneum and the adjacent mesentery the pain develops a sharp, superficial quality and is easily localised by the patient. The peritoneum is richly endowed with nerve endings of cerebrospinal nerves derived from the 6th thoracic to the 1st lumbar segment, which provide the afferent pain pathway. Appendicitis illustrates both visceral and somatic pain. Initially the condition is associated with obstruction of the appendix; the pain is visceral, i.e. it is in the midline around the umbilicus. Since congestion of the appendix develops as a result of the obstruction, the surrounding peritoneum becomes inflamed and somatic pain develops which is felt in the lower right quadrant of the abdomen.

Peritoneal irritation gives rise to associated muscle spasm (guarding) and hyperaesthesia, probably as the result of stimulation of specific peritoneocutaneous and peritoneovisceral reflexes, although the precise neurological pathways are ill-understood.

Referred pain from the abdomen occurs by reflex stimulation of the sensory branches of the phrenic nerve. During fetal development the diaphragm is formed in the neck and migrates caudally. The diaphragm, with the phrenic nerve, is derived from the fourth spinal embryonic segment so that the central portion of the diaphragm and an area of skin over the clavicle, the supraclavicular fossa, the acromiom and the suprascapular fossa share a common innervation. Stimulation of the central region of the abdominal surface of the diaphragm thus gives rise to shoulder tip pain. Shoulder tip pain does not seem to occur when the thoracic surface of the diaphragm is stimulated, since this area of the diaphragm is less dependent on the phrenic nerve for its sensory innervation.

Peptic ulcer disease. The major symptom of peptic ulcer disease is epigastric pain or discomfort. The cause of the pain is not settled, although it is closely related to the presence of gastric acid for it has been shown that the pain of a peptic ulcer disappears when the gastric contents are removed and recurs when they are replaced. If the gastric contents are neutralised prior to replacement, however, the pain does not recur. Although acid in the stomach does not normally cause pain the presence of a peptic ulcer, and possibly the surrounding inflammation, lowers the pain threshold. It is extremely difficult to distinguish the pain of gastric and duodenal ulcer on clinical grounds. The time interval between eating and the onset of pain has little discriminating value, although nocturnal pain (that is, pain which wakens the patient, often at one to two a.m.) is slightly more common in patients with duodenal ulcer. The pain of peptic ulcer disease is usually relieved by antacids or by vomiting. It tends to be periodic and long periods of remission, up to many months, occur. A change in the severity or frequency of the symptoms suggests the development of a complication such as penetration or gastric outflow obstruction.

Reflux oesophagitis. The symptoms of oesophagitis include 'burning' retrosternal chest pain and reflux (acid regurgitation into the mouth) particularly on stooping. The important physiological abnormality which leads to reflex oesophagitis is incompetence of the lower oesophageal sphincter, which may accompany a hiatus hernia. Smoking, eating fats, glucagon and cholecystokinin all lower the sphincter pressure. A further abnormality seen in patients with reflux oesophagitis is a delay in the time in which acid is cleared from the oesophagus under basal conditions.

Gallstones. It is extremely difficult to prove a relationship between the existence of gallstones and abdominal symptoms. Many studies have shown that incompetence of the pyloric and lower oesophageal sphincter occurs in patients with cholelithiasis and it is possible that the accompanying regurgitation accounts for the dyspeptic symptoms which are sometimes described in gallstone disease. Surgical removal of gallstones for the symptoms of dyspepsia fails to produce relief in up to 50 per cent of patients. Gallstones which impact in the cystic duct, common bile duct or intestine give rise to severe abdominal pain.

Colonic disorders. The irritable bowel syndrome is increasingly recognised as a cause of colonic pain. The syndrome is associated with increased pressures within the lumen of the bowel. There are attacks of pain which. tend to occur after eating. The increased pressure possibly results from the colon being unduly sensitive to gut hormones such as cholecystokinin. Colonic pain occurs in the majority of patients with colonic carcinoma, although it is less frequent in patients with anorectal cancer.

Anal pain. Pain in and around the anus is unusual. Pain around the rectum sometimes occurs as a result of lesions of the lumbar spine or spinal cord. Proctalgia fugax is an extremely distressing symptom in which the victim is seized with spasms of severe rectal pain. The cause is unknown, although it has been shown that elevation of intracolonic pressure coincides with the pain. Rectal pain or discomfort associated with constipation is relieved by treatment of constipation. Lesions around the anus, such as a fissure-in-ano, are extremely painful and can interfere with normal bowel function with the development of constipation.

Pancreatic pain. Pain arising from disease of the pancreas may be felt in the anterior abdomen but it commonly radiates deep into the abdomen, 'through' to the back at a level of T8 to L1. Such pain may arise from primary pancreatic disease or be due to secondary involvement of the pancreas by a penetrating duodenal ulcer.

Food intolerance. Although patients often complain that abdominal pain is precipitated by food there is little objective evidence that specific foods cause pain. There is some evidence that the infusion of fat, but not protein, lowers the lower oesophageal sphincter pressure and this may account for the symptom of fat-induced dyspepsia. *Lactase deficiency* in the small intestinal mucosa may be associated with maldigestion of lactose. The fermentation of unabsorbed lactose to lactic acid by intestinal bacteria leads to abdominal pain, distension and diarrhoea in some patients.

Abdominal pain in childhood. Abdominal pain may occur in childhood for any of the reasons discussed above. Recurrent abdominal pain is, however, a particular problem. It occurs in up to 10 per cent of children but an organic cause is found in only five per cent of patients. When no organic cause for the pain can be discovered the pain is usually found to be periumbilical and it has been claimed the further away from the umbilicus the pain occurs the more likely it is to be organic in origin. Recurrent abdominal pain in childhood is occasionally a manifestation of depression and in a small number of children abdominal pain may be a symptom of epilepsy. The pain occurs in the absence of major convulsions but electroencephalographic changes occur and the pain may be alleviated by anticonvulsant drugs. In some children recurrent abdominal pain is a form of the irritable bowel syndrome. The long-term prognosis is unpredictable and the patient may continue to have bouts of pain into adult life.

Acute abdominal pain. A recent survey of patients with acute abdominal pain showed that the main causes for this complaint were appendicitis, diverticulitis, perforated ulcer, non-specific abdominal pain, obstruction, pancreatitis and cholecystitis. In reviewing the symptoms of which these patients complained it was found that the pain of acute appendicitis had usually localised in the right lower quadrant by the time the patient arrived at hospital and was seldom generalised. Generalised abdominal pain occurred commonly in patients with perforated peptic ulcer and localised pain confined to the upper abdomen was seen in less than half. Pain associated with diverticulitis most commmonly occurred in the left lower quadrant but it was occasionally generalised or umbilical. The pain of intestinal obstruction was around the umbilicus and the pain of cholecystitis and pancreatitis in the upper abdomen. Colic associated with impaction of a gallstone in the bile duct does not wax and wane as does renal colic but remains at a constant level of intensity. Rupture of an aneurysm of the abdominal aorta is another cause of severe, acute abdominal pain, which is frequently preceded for a period of two to three weeks by mild backache. The pain is usually periumbilical or in the lower abdomen. Occasionally the pain occurs in the back or in the legs and sometimes simulates renal colic.

Pelvic inflammatory disease gives rise to abdominal pain which may lead to diagnostic confusion. Salpingitis is usually insidious in onset and is only rarely unilateral. Unilateral abdominal pain occurs in salpingitis when the salpingitis coincides with ovulation. Rupture of an ectopic pregnancy causes severe pelvic and lower abdominal pain and about one-fifth of patients also have pain in the shoulder tip. The diagnosis is suggested by preceding amenorrhoea and slight vaginal bleeding coincident with the pain which occurs in about four-fifths of the patients. Large ovarian cysts sometimes twist on their pedicle. The tumour becomes congested and acute abdominal pain results.

Medical causes of the acute abdomen. Many medical conditions cause symptoms which suggest an 'acute surgical abdomen'. A *myocardial infarction* may give rise to pain which is felt only in the epigastrium and this occurs particularly in the elderly. *Lower lobe pneumonia* and *pulmonary infarction* may be confused with an acute abdomen, because the lower six intercostal nerves supply both the lower thoracic area and the abdominal wall. Lower lobe pneumonia is an important differential diagnosis of acute appendicitis in children. Gastric crises occur in *tabes dorsalis*, although this is less frequent as a manifestation of syphilis since the introduction of penicillin. Severe abdominal pain is a feature of *acute intermittent porphyria.* This condition is associated with a peripheral neuropathy and occasionally coma and epilepsy occur. Abdominal colic is a symptom of *lead poisoning. Ketoacidotic diabetes mellitus* is an infrequent cause of abdominal pain but should always be considered in difficult cases. Clinically, however, there appears to be a great danger of missing a surgical cause for abdominal pain in a patient with diabetic ketosis and caution should be exercised when a diagnosis of 'abdominal pain due to diabetes' is made. *Hypercalcaemia* is another cause of acute abdominal pain. In some patients hypercalcaemia leads to pancreatitis and in others there is an associated peptic ulcer, but in many the pains occur in the absence of these two conditions. Abdominal pain also occurs in Type I hyperlipidaemia, abdominal migraine, abdominal epilepsy, allergic purpura, haemochromatosis, and spinal cord and nerve root lesions.

Diarrhoea

Diarrhoea may be defined as the frequent passage of loose, unformed stools which have an increased water content.

Acute diarrhoea

Acute diarrhoea suggests an infective cause. Many organisms induce diarrhoea, and the manner in which they produce diarrhoea varies. The cholera vibrio produces an enterotoxin which reduces the net absorption of salt and water because there is an increased secretion of anions by the small intestinal mucosa. The increased anion secretion is mediated by adenyl cyclase and cyclic AMP. *Escherichia coli* may induce diarrhoea either by direct invasion of the intestinal mucosa or by the production of an enterotoxin which may have a similar action to the cholera toxin. Diarrhoea also results from invasion of the intestinal mucosa (mainly the colon) by organisms from the *Shigella* group, which are able to invade because of their ability to produce an endotoxin. The manner by which such organisms induce diarrhoea in pathophysiological terms is not known.

Chronic diarrhoea

Chronic diarrhoea results from a variety of changes in the physiology of the normal intestinal tract. Total bowel transit time is important, and when this is reduced, as in *thyrotoxicosis*, diarrhoea occurs. Diarrhoea also occurs when osmotic pressures within the gut lumen exceed the serosal osmotic pressure. *Disaccharidase deficiency* such as occurs in alactasia produces this type of diarrhoea because the unabsorbed sugars exert a profound osmotic effect. There are other mechanisms for the diarrhoea in lactase deficiency including lactic acid formation which possibly acts as a colonic irritant. *Steatorrhoea* leads to the accumulation of unabsorbed fatty acids within the bowel which are acted upon by colonic bacteria to form irritant hydroxy fatty acids. These hydroxy fatty acids have a structure which is similar to ricinoleic acid, an active constituent of castor oil. Recent work suggests that the hydroxy fatty acids interfere with the absorption of salt and water by the colon, thereby causing diarrhoea. Colonic absorption of salt and water is also impaired by bile acids which escape absorption when there is *disease or resection of the terminal small intestine.* Increased permeability of the small intestine occurs in the coeliac syndrome and this leads to the net exsorption of salt and water.

The appearance of the stool

The appearance of the stool of the patient with diarrhoea is often of diagnostic value. In cholera the stool is voluminous and watery with white flecks and it has been likened to rice-water. In malabsorption the stool is pale and bulky and floats on the toilet water, not because of the contained fat but because of the air trapped within the stool.

The colour of the stool is also important. In cholestasis the stool is pale and colourless but the faeces may be very pale in any type of fat malabsorption. Black tarry stools, melaena, occur as the result of gastrointestinal bleeding particularly from the upper intestine. Melaena should be distinguished from the grey-black stool of a patient taking oral iron. Bright red blood and/or mucopus in the stool infers inflammation or neoplastic change of the colonic mucosa. A small amount of mucus on the surface of the stool is a normal phenomenon. Excess mucus occasionally occurs in the stools of patients with an irritable bowel syndrome and in these patients the shape of the stool sometimes becomes ribbon-like or the stool is passed in pellets.

Constipation

It is difficult to define constipation in precise clinical terms. The word is used by some to indicate a reduced frequency of bowel actions. The majority of people in the United Kingdom have one or more bowel actions each day, but the range is wide, and perhaps the important consideration in terms of bowel frequency is a recent change from the normal habit. Most individuals passing a stool less than once every three days may be regarded as constipated. Others define constipation with respect to stool consistency and imply a hard stool which may cause discomfort or pain on defaecation.

The best objective measurement of constipation is to define it in terms of total bowel transit. This can be estimated radiologically by administering to the patient 20 radio-opaque markers and estimating the time in which the markers are excreted. In Western countries 75 per cent of the markers are expelled within 92 hours.

The act of defaecation can be considered as having two components, namely rectal filling and rectal emptying. The former depends on two factors, faecal bulk and the motor activity of the colon. If the faecal bulk is small the stool becomes dehydrated and bowel transit is slowed. Faecal bulk depends on the amount of non-absorbable residue and it is known that when the non-absorbable bulk of the diet is increased bowel transit is speeded.

Not a great deal is understood about the influence of the motor activity of the colon in producing constipation, although disturbed bowel motility with consequent increases in intraluminal pressures has been implicated as a cause of the abdominal pain and constipation which occur in patients with the irritable bowel syndrome (see p. 188).

Rectal emptying occurs as a result of a defaecation reflex, the centre for which is in the sacral segments of the spinal cord. The reflex is stimulated by rectal filling and efferent impulses travel along the sympathetic nerves to relax the upper anal sphincter. The lower anal sphincter is under voluntary control. The diaphragm and abdominal muscles are also important in the act of defaecation for their contraction increases the intra-abdominal pressure. Any neurological disease which involves the sacral spinal cord interrupts the defaecation reflex and leads to faecal retention. Because the lower anal sphincter is under voluntary control painful lesions around the anus such as a fissure may cause constipation.

Patients with constipation often complain of other symptoms which include headache, abdominal discomfort and distension, and sometimes poor appetite. The physiological explanation for these epiphenomena is not clear. It may be that they are psychological in orgin, perhaps resulting from the anxiety engendered by constipation.

Constipation of recent onset is of more serious import than is long-standing constipation. Pain, either before or during defaecation, suggests a motility disturbance as in the irritable bowel syndrome or an obstructing lesion.

Rectal Bleeding

Blood mixed in with the stool occurs when there is a bleeding lesion such as a carcinoma of the rectum or ulcerative colitis. Bleeding at the end of defaecation or which is only noticed on toilet paper after defaecation occurs in haemorrhoids. In the majority of situations the passage of fresh blood per rectum indicates anal, rectal or colonic bleeding but massive bleeding from the upper gastrointestinal tract sometimes produces bright red blood in the stool. Such patients usually show the clinical features of shock which is uncommonly present in patients with lower colonic bleeding.

Jaundice

Bilirubin is the pigment which is produced mainly by the breakdown of red blood cells in the reticuloendothelial system, although some bilirubin is formed during the de novo synthesis of red cells in the bone marrow and from the breakdown of other haems such as myoglobin. The bilirubin thus formed is insoluble in water and is transported in the plasma bound to albumin. Hence it cannot be excreted in the urine. Within the liver bilirubin is converted into a water-soluble substance by conjugation with glucuronide, a reaction which is mediated by the enzyme glucuronyl transferase. The mechanism of entry of the fat soluble form of bilirubin into the liver cell is a matter of some uncertainty although the recent discovery of the intracellular transport protein, ligandin, which has the ability to bind insoluble bilirubin, represents an important advance. The water soluble conjugated bilirubin is excreted through the bile canaliculus.

Cholestasis

Cholestatic jaundice infers that the elevated bilirubin is mostly conjugated, and that the alkaline phosphatase and other bile duct enzymes are elevated. The serum cholesterol concentration is raised. Liver cell enzymes (aspartate transaminase) are normal, or only slightly raised. There is bilirubinuria. Cholestatic jaundice may arise from either extrahepatic or intrahepatic causes.

One of the earliest symptoms of cholestasis is *pruritus* which is often most severe at night. The cause of the pruritus is not fully understood but may be related to the elevated serum levels of bile acids which occur in this condition. There is no evidence at present, however, which proves the relationship between either total bile acids or individual bile acids and pruritus. Pruritus may occur in cholestatic syndromes even when the degree of jaundice is not marked. Pruritus may also occur in diabetes mellitus, Hodgkin's disease, renal failure, polycythaemia rubra vera, hyperthyroidism and many skin disorders.

Jaundice associated with right upper quadrant pain suggests that a gallstone within the common duct is the cause. Painless obstructive jaundice is said to be a feature of carcinoma of the head of the pancreas, but in about 70 per cent of patients some degree of anterior abdominal or back pain is present. Cholestasis of either intra- or extrahepatic origin leads to darkening of the urine and light-coloured stools. The light-coloured stools are due to the failure of bile pigments to enter the intestinal tract. Because liver cell function is usually intact, however, the bilirubin is conjugated and the water soluble pigment is excreted by the kidney to cause darkening of the urine. In pure cholestatic jaundice the urine has no urobilinogen.

Intrahepatic cholestasis is most commonly caused by viral hepatitis and drugs, particularly the phenothiazines. Sometimes recurring attacks of cholestatic jaundice occur — benign intra-hepatic cholestasis. Less commonly cholestasis occurs as the result of the Dubin—Johnson or Rotor syndrome in which the excretion of conjugated bilirubin from the liver cell is impaired.

Hepatocellular jaundice

Hepatocellular jaundice is due most commonly in the United Kingdom to viral hepatitis, drugs or cirrhosis. Liver function tests show raised transaminase levels, moderate elevation of the serum alkaline phosphatase and only slight change in the serum choles-terol. The diagnosis of hepatocellular jaundice depends on a careful history in which particular attention should be paid to jaundiced contacts, possible modes of transmission (for example, recent blood transfusion, injections, tattoos, homosexual contacts) and a careful drug history. Clinical examination may reveal extrahepatic signs of liver cell disease.

Unconjugated hyperbilirubinaemia

Haemolytic jaundice is rarely severe, and the serum level of bilirubin seldom exceeds 4 mg per cent. It rarely poses a diagnostic problem. Unconjugated hyperbilirubinaemia occurs in perhaps 10 per cent of the population who are otherwise normal (Gilbert's syndrome). It is associated with the deficiency of the conjugating enzymes in the liver cell — glucuronyl transferase. Very low levels or even absence of glucuronyl transferase occur in the Crigler—Najjar syndrome. Occasionally patients recovering from viral hepatitis may have a transient unconjugated hyperbilirubinaemia. Patients with unconjugated hyperbilirubinaemia do not itch and the urine contains urobilinogen but no bilirubin.

HISTORY: URINARY SYSTEM DISEASE

The cardinal symptoms comprise localised renal pain, ureteric colic, disordered micturition, alteration in the volume or appearance of the urine and urethral discharge.

Renal pain

Renal pain, like ureteric colic, is always lateralised and, in direct contrast with gastrointestinal pain, never affects the central abdominal area. The pain is usually felt in the loin or so-called posterior renal angle where there may also be tenderness to finger-tip pressure. On occasion renal pain is also felt anteriorly below the lateral costal margin. Although renal tissue itself is insensitive, renal pain as described can arise from stimuli such as increased tension applied to the renal capsule, pelvis or pedicle. Many disorders of the renal parenchyma such as glomerulonephritis are without local pain throughout their course.

Ureteric colic

Ureteric colic is a lateralised, often severe pain which is experienced in the loin, flank, groin and testicular—labial areas (Figure 4.2). This pain stems from adjacent smooth muscle reacting to an obstructive ureteric lesion. Characteristically the pain spreads sequentially from above downwards towards the testis or labium majus. The level of the pain — loin and flank, groin and testis — reflects in some measure the level of the causative obstructive lesion. Ureteric pain is phasic, waxing over 20 to 30 minutes and waning for longer periods in between. The exacerbations may be severe and are accompanied by cold sweats, nausea, vomiting and restlessness. While the causative obstruction is most commonly a radio-opaque calculus, identical colic may stem from a non-opaque uric acid stone or even from a blood clot. Concomitant slight haematuria is usual.

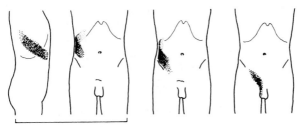

Figure 4.2. *Distribution and radiation of renal and ureteric pain.*

Bladder function disorders

The disorders of bladder function are diverse and include pre-cipitancy, dysuria, strangury, increased frequency, slowing of the stream and hesitancy, retention and incontinence of urine.

Precipitancy implies the urge to pass urine without the ability voluntarily to postpone the act of voiding. When present alone precipitancy suggests a bladder sphincter defect, including those that are neurological in basis, but accompanied by dysuria it is the result of bladder irritation, usually by cystitis.

Dysuria is the term for uncomfortable or painful micturition. Such pain accompanies and may well persist briefly after voiding. The pain of dysuria is felt mainly in the urethra especially at the external urinary meatus although the causative irritant usually lies within the bladder where the trigonal area is highly sensitive. When severe the pain persists after voiding accompanied by an urge to micturate which cannot be assuaged. Such dysuria is given the distinctive name *strangury*. Sometimes bladder irritation produces discomfort localised by the patient just above the pubis.

Frequency of micturition. While increased frequency of micturition may occur without any increase in the rate of formation of urine, an increased flow of urine or polyuria understandably is usually accompanied by an increase in the frequency of micturition as well as in the volume of urine expelled. Normal adults do not habitually need to waken from overnight sleep for micturition and a regular requirement to waken to void urine during the overnight hours is the special variant of increased frequency termed *nocturia*. By day or by night, increased frequency of micturition may occur despite a normal unchanged rate of formation (and output) of urine especially when the cause of the frequency affects the bladder control mechanism. When polyuria is also present, increased frequency is a simple consequence of diuresis at the renal level. Polyuria first made manifest by nocturia is a common early symptom of chronic renal failure.

Retention of urine. Gross disturbance of bladder function is made manifest by either, or both, urinary retention or incontinence. Normal micturition and continence of urine are the end result of the functions of the bladder sphincters including the vesico-ureteric mechanisms and the detrusor muscle coordinated by the related spinal reflex arcs, all of which are controlled from the cerebral level. In each patient it is necessary to identify the basis of defective micturition and bladder control in terms of obstruction, atony or muscle weakness, or neurogenic defect. Involuntary retention of urine within the bladder occurs in acute and chronic forms, the latter being alternatively termed 'retention with overflow'.

Acute retention of urine is the state of vesical overdistension by urine, developing within a matter of hours and due either to organic obstruction of outflow or to a defect in the expulsive mechanism. Most characteristic is the acute retention resulting from sudden urethral obstruction caused by prostatic enlargement, when the affected elderly male presents in distress with a painful, tensely distended bladder which, although tender, is easily palpable above the pubis. The patient in these circumstances is unable to void more than a few drops of urine at a time and cannot relieve himself of the intolerable urge to pass urine. Acute retention of urine is usually preceded over weeks or months by premonitory alterations in voiding which the patient has disregarded. Acute retention can also result from neurological lesions such as transverse myelitis or traumatic cord transection and, in some of these at least, the bladder distension is devoid of pain or other sensation. Post-operative urinary retention can occur in patients with prolapsed lumbar intervertebral disc lesions.

Female as well as male patients who are ill with unrelated severe illness such as pneumonia, meningitis or hemiplegia may develop urinary retention without any obvious lesion in the bladder or its nervous controls and without obvious pain. The routine care of such severely ill and all comatose patients includes a check on urine volume output rate and routine abdominal examination for the bladder state.

Chronic retention of urine develops insidiously in most patients and may first be brought to attention simply as slowness of micturition with a thin feeble stream. Other effects which may be present singly or in various combinations are nocturia, hesitancy, the need to strain down, dribbling after voiding, the need to void little and often and loss of voluntary control in greater or lesser degree. These patients, commonly males, have usually tolerated their urinary symptoms over periods of weeks or months and they are often quite unaware that their bladder is over-distended with urine. Accordingly, it is important when examining the abdomen deliberately to inspect and palpate for possible urinary bladder distension, especially in the presence of incontinence or any other progressive difficulty connected with micturition. The chronically distended bladder is usually painless, non-tender and may well reach up as a dome-shaped swelling from behind the pubis almost to the umbilicus. As with acute retention of urine, chronic retention may develop on the basis of organic obstruction, impaired detrusor contractility or be secondary to a neurological defect. The underlying cause must be identified. Most commonly, in elderly male patients with urine-soiled clothing and health impaired with azotaemia, a condition of urinary retention with overflow results from progressive organic urethral obstruction produced by benign hypertrophic or neoplastic prostatic enlargement.

Occasionally, as in diabetic autonomic neuropathy, the bladder may be partly denervated on the afferent side without any spinal cord lesion and vesical atony with retention and overflow results. Slowly developing lesions of the spinal cord at or above the sacral segments which govern sphincter and detrusor muscle control may produce disturbed micturition with an appreciable residual bladder volume even after attempted emptying of the bladder.

Incontinence of urine. Incontinence of urine, like retention, can result from a variety of pathological lesions. In children nocturnal incontinence or enuresis is commonly present in the absence of a demonstrable organic lesion but in individual patients such lesions must be considered. Similarly incontinence in the elderly, both by day and by night, may arise for no obvious lesion. Rectal impaction with accumulated faeces or vascular lesions in the neuraxis may contribute to such incontinence. Adult males are rarely troubled with incontinence of urine but, when it arises, a neurological lesion such as multiple sclerosis should be suspected. Incontinence of urine in multiparous women, which is troublesome only when the patient is ambulant, is usually due to a muscular pelvic floor defect (a uterine prolapse) but the possibility of a vesicovaginal fistula must be excluded by detailed examination.

Naturally, the average patient has difficulty in distinguishing between unduly frequent voidings of less than normal volumes of urine on the one hand and increased frequency of micturition combined with *polyuria* and large voidings on the other hand. Dysuria accompanying increased frequency of micturition suggests that the causal lesion is present at bladder level while increased frequency with increased thirst and polydipsia but without dysuria points to underlying polyuria. When uncertainty remains it is necessary to measure the volume of urine produced over a timed interval of adequate duration — conventionally 24 hours.

The 24 hour urine volume in normal individuals approximates to 1500 ml, within wide limits between about 500 and 2000 ml. A useful approximation is a normal production rate of 1 ml of urine per minute, that is, 1440 ml per 24 hours. The rate of production is not uniform, there being a physiological overnight cut-back in urine formation which is usually lost under conditions of polyuria, hence the occurrence of nocturia in chronic renal failure and other causes of diuresis. On average, adults void on four to seven occasions during each day, each bladder emptying being 300 to 400 ml in amount. Some habitually void smaller volumes and more often than others. Since there is a good deal of individual variation in these respects, the clinician places most diagnostic credence upon observed change in established habits rather than divergences from a rather arbitrary 'normal' value for frequency of bladder emptying, volume of voiding and urine production rates.

Change in the appearance of the urine encompasses a wide variety of alterations both physiological and pathological. Complaints by the patient that the urine is 'strong' or 'dark' may refer to physiological variations, psychoneurotic misinterpretations or real abnormalities of odour or pigmentary content, depending upon the patient. As the physicians of the 15th century found, it is always desirable for the clinician to inspect a fresh sample of urine in a clear glass container. *Turbidity* may reflect phosphate precipitate in alkaline urine, red blood cells or pyuria. Present in more than trace quantities in the urine, red blood cells produce the frank red coloration of overt *haematuria.* Because red discoloration of urine may occur due to diet-derived dyes (eosin or beet, etc.) it is always desirable to examine microscopically, under a cover slip, a wet film preparation of centrifuged urine, the so-called sediment. A specimen of the sediment obtained from 10 ml of freshly collected urine will often afford important diagnostic information. This examination cannot be delegated to the laboratory since, to be of most value, the specimen should be freshly collected — some would say 'still warm'.

In the case of haematuria the patient should be questioned about its relationship to the phases of the urine stream. Initial and terminal haematuria both suggest blood loss of vesical or posterior urethral origin. Renal bleeding usually produces a blood loss which is uniformly dispersed throughout the urine stream. Bleeding per urethram apart from micturition indicates a ureteric lesion.

Discharge of secretion or exudate from the urethra which may be purulent is usually noticed by the male between acts of micturition as 'dripping' and/or soiling of the undergarments. Urethral discharges from the short female urethra are usually slight in amount and are sometimes unobserved or even wrongly attributed to the vagina. Urethral discharge is relatively common in male patients and may indicate gonorrhoea or nonspecific urethritis. Occasionally a patient's complaint of discharge, with little or none being evident on examination, may be the result of a morbid preoccupation possibly stemming from fear, guilt or other psychogenic abnormalities. All such discharges require to be investigated both microscopically and bacteriologically. Every ulcerated lesion on the genitalia must be regarded potentially as a syphilitic chancre until cautious examination (using protective gloves) and appropriate laboratory tests show otherwise.

Family history

A family history is often of importance in gastrointestinal and renal disorders, many of which have a familial basis such as coeliac disease, ulcerative colitis and Crohn's disease, familial polyposis coli and polycystic kidneys. The knowledge of similar symptoms occurring in other members of the family, therefore, can be of diagnostic help. Wilson's disease (hepatolenticular degeneration), haemochromatosis and renal polycystic disease have a strong familial basis, and the diagnosis of either of these conditions should prompt the close investigation of other members of the family.

PHYSICAL EXAMINATION

General Examination

A careful general examination is of much value in patients with abdominal disease because gastrointestinal and renal diseases produce many systemic manifestations.

Hands

Examination of the hands often provides diagnostic clues in patients with gastrointestinal disease. *Finger clubbing* occurs in association with cirrhosis, coeliac disease, Crohn's disease and ulcerative conditions of the colon. The cause of the relationship is unknown. Fibrosis of palmar fascia occurs in alcoholic liver disease and a Dupuytren's contracture is produced.

In liver disease the skin of the palm is reddened (palmar erythema). This sign is not invariably present in chronic liver disease, and may also occur in rheumatoid arthritis, thyrotoxicosis and during pregnancy. In some families, the skin of the palms of the hands and the feet becomes excessively keratinised (tylosis) and members of these families have a high incidence of carcinoma of the oesophagus.

In iron deficiency anaemia the nail bed is pale and the nails may be brittle and spoon shaped (koilonychia). In chronic liver disease the nails are sometimes white (Terry's nails), although 'half-and-half nails', in which the proximal half of the nail is white and the distal half normal coloured, are also described. In chronic renal disease a brown nail bed is sometimes seen. Finally, the hands may show changes of progressive systemic sclerosis with narrowed tapered fingers and ischaemic changes which may be associated with dysphagia or intestinal malabsorption. The telangiectases of hereditary haemorrhagic telangiectasia classically are distributed around the edge of the nail.

Pigmentation

Pigmentation of the skin occurs in chronic renal disease, in liver disease, and as a result of intestinal malabsorption. Isolated pigmentation occurs in acanthosis nigricans, a rare velvety, brownish skin eruption, which, when it occurs in patients over the age of 40 years, is strongly suggestive of an intestinal malignancy.

In patients with jaundice, the presence of scratch marks suggests that the jaundice is cholestatic. In long-standing cholestatic jaundice, cholesterol deposits are seen around the eyes (xanthelasma) and also in skin elsewhere (xanthomas) particularly on the extensor surfaces. Unlike the xanthomas associated with other forms of hypercholesterolaemia, tendon involvement is rare. The earliest recognition of jaundice is in the conjunctivae and the yellow colour may be recognised when the serum bilirubin concentration is greater than 3.0 mg/100 ml (50 μmol/l). Good, natural light is essential.

Naevi

Among the other skin lesions which occur in liver disease, *spider naevi* are probably the commonest. A typical spider naevus consists of a central arteriole with branching vessels radiating from it. There is a surrounding zone of erythema, and pressure on the central point leads to blanching of the spider. In liver disease, the majority of spiders occur on the area of skin drained by the superior vena cava and only rarely elswhere. The reason is not known. The cause of spider naevi in liver disease has not been explained although it is possible that they result from imbalance of the sex hormones. Vascular spiders also occur during pregnancy, in rheumatoid arthritis and even in normal people. In healthy individuals the number of spider naevi seldom exceeds five. Spider naevi must be distinguished from Campbell-de-Morgan spots which are cherry red and elevated above the skin, and purpura which does not blanch on pressure.

Some patients with chronic liver disease have numerous small vessels randomly scattered through the skin in a similar distribution to spider naevi. This skin change has been called paper money skin because of the resemblance of the lesion to red silk threads coursing through the old American dollar note.

Vitiligo

Vitiligo occurs as areas of skin depigmentation and is known to have an autoimmune basis. It appears in both white and coloured people and in this latter group is particularly distressing. It occurs in autoimmune liver conditions. Necrotic skin lesions and acne may also be encountered in autoimmune liver conditions.

Other skin disorders

Apart from the relationships between the liver and the skin, there are other associations between the skin and the gastrointestinal tract. Various *vitamin deficiencies*, particularly of the B group, may accompany malabsorption and skin disorders such as pellagra may develop. Deficiency of vitamin C causing scurvy is very rarely seen as a result of malabsorption. The various lesions of scurvy, however, are important, for they occur in undernourished, elderly patients. The patient is generally unwell and the petechial haemorrhages occur in the skin and in the periosteum of long bones. Haemorrhagic gum lesions are classical. On the other hand various skin disorders may be associated with disordered gastrointestinal function. The most important of these is *psoriasis* which is associated with malabsorption (dermatogenic enteropathy). *Dermatitis herpetiformis* (Figure 4.3) is an irritating skin eruption which occurs particularly on extensor surfaces. It is associated with a gluten-induced enteropathy which is probably identical to coeliac disease. *Ulcerative colitis* may be accompanied by erythema nodosum — tender painful nodules on the extensor surfaces of the legs; rarely there may be a distressing skin condition called

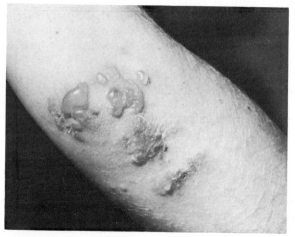

Figure 4.3. *Classical lesions of dermatitis herpetiformis on the elbow. From Alexander (1975)* Dermatitis Herpetiformis, *with kind permission of the author.*

pyoderma gangrenosum, in which there is indolent irregular cutaneous ulceration, with undermined blue margins. This occurs mainly on the legs and is not necessarily related to the activity or extent of the colitis. Pyoderma gangrenosum is not always associated with inflammatory bowel disease and approximately 50 per cent of those who have the condition have no known associated disorder. The skin and gut may be jointly affected by disorders such as scleroderma, polyarteritis nodosa, pseudoxanthoma elasticum and Ehlers—Danlos syndrome. Many skin changes occur in the uraemic state including purpura, itching, and a 'muddy' pigmentation. When the blood urea is very high secretion into the sweat can result in precipitation of urea crystals on the forehead — uraemic frost; purpura is present in many uraemic patients.

Other systemic manifestations of abdominal disease

The joint involvement accompanying gastrointestinal disorders is described in Chapter 7. Eye involvement, particularly an iritis or uveitis, is seen in ulcerative colitis. In Wilson's disease (hepato-lenticular degeneration) a characteristic brown copper deposit may be seen just internal to the limbus on the nasal and temporal margins of the cornea (Kayser—Fleischer ring). The deposition is in Descemet's membrane on the posterior surface of the cornea. The ring is more easily seen by slit lamp examination.

A variety of neurological disorders may occur after a surgical portacaval shunt, or as a result of large natural shunts in patients with chronic liver disease. The neurological picture includes deep coma, loss of intellectual ability and basal ganglion and extra-pyramidal syndromes. The most characteristic physical sign is the flapping tremor which is seen when the outstretched hand is extended (asterixis). Flapping tremor also occurs in chronic renal disease, congestive heart failure and chronic hypercapnia.

Examination of The Mouth

The mouth should be inspected in good light, and attention should be paid to the buccal mucosa, the tongue (including its under-surface) and the opening of the parotid ducts which are found opposite the upper molars on the buccal mucosa. The state of the gums and teeth should be noted.

Ulcerative and bullous lesions of the buccal mucosa

Aphthous ulcers (Figure 4.4) are most common on the inside of the upper or lower lips. Characteristically they are painful. Such ulcers are common in patients with coeliac disease and ulcerative colitis. They are often indistinguishable from the ulcers which are found in Behçet's syndrome. However, aphthous ulcers unrelated to major disease occur in about 20 per cent of the population. In early life, the sex incidence is equal, but in later life they tend to occur more frequently in females.

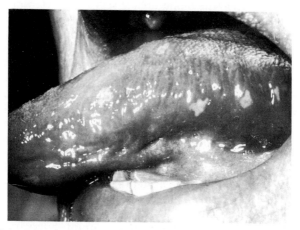

Figure 4.4. *Aphthous ulcers on lateral border of tongue. Courtesy of Professor D. K. Mason, Glasgow Dental Hospital and School.*

A variety of primarily dermatological diseases may also affect the mouth. These include erythema multiforme, lichen planus (Figure 4.5), pemphigus and pemphigoid. The lesions of erythema multiforme appear as large bullae which rapidly break down and are covered with a tenacious haemorrhagic exudate. Lichen planus commonly occurs on the inside of the cheeks opposite the occlusal lines and on the dorsal and posterolateral aspects of the tongue. The characteristic lesion is a fine meshwork of white lines at the intersections of which are white papules about two mm in diameter. In 50 per cent of patients with pemphigus the disease starts in the mouth. The lesions appear as blisters surrounded by a white cuff. There is splitting up of the interconnecting bridges between cells so that bullous lesions can be produced by gentle rubbing of the

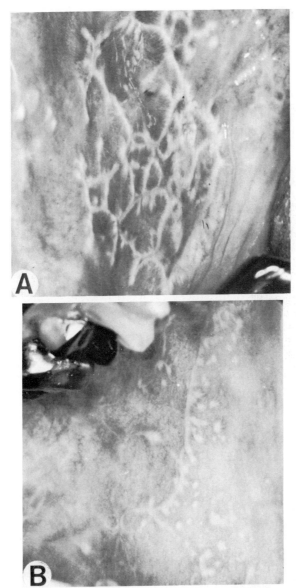

Figure 4.5. *Oral lichen planus. (A) Reticular type. (B) Papular type. From Pindborg, J. J. (1980) in Oral Manifestations of Systemic Disease (Ed.) Jones, J. H. & Mason, D. K., with kind permission of the author.*

mucosa (a positive Nikolsky's sign). Pemphigoid tends to occur in older patients (above 60 years) than does pemphigus and the lesions are found particularly on the hard palate and gums, this being an important differentiation from pemphigus.

Traumatic ulcers

These should be considered in the differential diagnosis of bullous or ulcerative lesions within the mouth. The trauma may be obvious, but on occasion these ulcers occur as the result of habit.

White patches within the mouth

Leukoplakia appears as a white membrane which is adherent to the buccal mucosa or tongue (Figure 4.6). The condition may result from trauma or be idiopathic. Not all cases are pre-malignant. Leukoedema is a thin, greyish, opalescent web on the mucosa resulting from trauma. It is not a precursor of leukoplakia. Oral moniliasis is a common cause of white lesions within the mouth. The lesions are not adherent, have a more diffuse distribution than

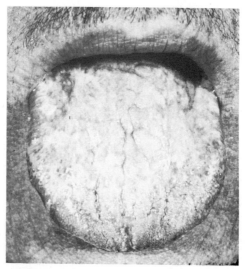

Figure 4.6. *Leukoplakia of tongue. Courtesy of Mr D. Downton, Royal Free Hospital, London.*

leukoplakia and are surrounded by a small margin of erythema. They are frequently painful. In infants they must be distinguished from milk curds which can be scraped off readily and there will be no erythema.

Pigmented lesions within the mouth

Peutz—Jegher's syndrome (Figure 4.7). The brown, blackish or bluish-grey pigmented spots of this condition occur typically on the lips, although they are also seen on the skin around the mouth and around the eyes and ears. Although a rare condition, it is important to recognise, for it may be associated with small intestinal polyps which may bleed or form the apex of an intussusception.

Other pigmented lesions. Pigmented lesions within the mouth are not uncommon in otherwise normal people, and may be frequent in coloured people. In adrenal insufficiency the pigment is found as a bluish discoloration on the inside of the cheeks opposite the molars. Similar pigmentation occurs rarely in malabsorption,

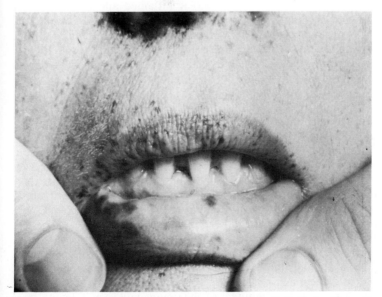

Figure 4.7. *Peutz—Jegher's syndrome. Courtesy of Mr D. B. E. Foster, University Hospital of Wales, Cardiff.*

thyrotoxicosis and haemochromatosis. Heavy metal poisoning from mercury, bismuth or lead produces a dark line just below the gingival margin. The line is reputed to occur because of the deposition of metallic sulphides produced by the action of bacteria from the gingival inflammation which is invariably present. Greenish-yellow discoloration of the teeth occurs in some children who survive kernicterus. The colour is due to the deposition of bilirubin. A similar discoloration results from the deposition of tetracycline in both the first and second dentitions of children. Such discoloration should be distinguished from the yellow plaques on the side of the teeth which occur in gingivitis.

Fordyce spots. These yellow spots, which are the size of pinheads, represent ectopic sebaceous glands, and are found on the lips and buccal mucosa. Although present before puberty they become more obvious in adult life. They may be seen in up to 80 per cent of patients.

Gingivitis

This lesion of the gingival mucosa occurs commonly in adults. The mucosa at the apex of the teeth is inflamed and friable so that bleeding occurs readily. Pockets of pus and debris are found and these produce a characteristic odour. In advanced stages of the disease the teeth become loose and are eventually lost. Gingival hypertrophy may be seen in association with scurvy, leukaemia and drugs such as phenytoin sodium (Figure 4.8).

The Tongue

The tongue is a neuromuscular structure covered by a mucous membrane. The surface area of the mucous membrane is increased by the formation of folds of epithelium or papillae. There are three main types of papillae. The circumvallate papillae number from 10 to 12 and are found on the dorsum of the tongue at the junction of the anterior two-thirds and the posterior third. They assume a V formation centred on the foramen caecum. The fungiform papillae are found at the apex and along the lateral aspects of the tongue. They are usually barely visible, but on occasion, even in the normal patient, they are red, large, round and smooth. The filiform papillae cover the remainder of the tongue and vary in length from one to three mm.

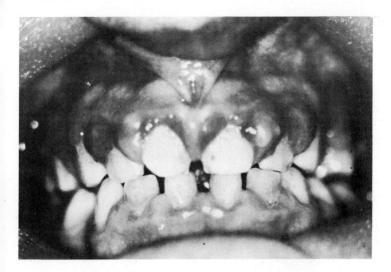

Figure 4.8. *Gingival hypertrophy following administration of phenytoin sodium. Courtesy of Dr C. Scully, Glasgow Dental Hospital and School.*

General abnormalities of the tongue

In states which produce dehydration the tongue is dry. In extreme dehydration there may be an associated parotitis. A dry mouth (xerostomia) also occurs in Sjögren's syndrome in which there is impaired secretion of saliva and also of tears. A dry tongue is also common in mouth breathers and tobacco smokers. In amyloid disease, myxoedema and acromegaly the tongue is large.

Variations in the appearance of the tongue

Fissured (scrotal) tongue (Figure 4.9). This is a common appearance in which clefts are found on the dorsum of the tongue. Occasionally the clefts are visible only when the tongue is viewed in profile.

Median rhomboid glossitis*. This is a developmental abnormality in which filiform papillae are absent from the dorsum of the tongue

---

*Medium rhomboid glossitis is possibly a fungal infection rather than a congenital abnormality.

so that a diamond-shaped area of denuded mucosa is seen in front of the foramen caecum. This area of the tongue represents the remains of the tuberculum impar which has been caught up between the two halves of the developing tongue.

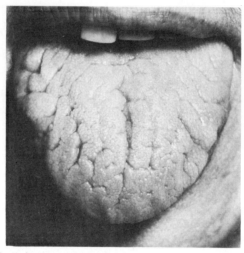

Figure 4.9. *Scrotal tongue. Courtesy of Mr D. Downton, Royal Free Hospital, London.*

Black hairy tongue (Figure 4.10). This is seen only rarely. The filiform papillae are overgrown — sometimes four times longer than their original length. Most cases have no identifiable cause but the condition may sometimes be caused by antibiotic therapy.

Furring of the tongue. Furring of the tongue occurs in smokers, mouth breathers and in any condition which causes dehydration. Furring of the tongue is not caused by constipation. There is heaping up of squamous epithelium on the filiform papillae resulting from inadequate cleansing of the tongue which ordinarily occurs during chewing.

Geographic tongue (Figure 4.11). An area of filiform papillae is lost from the dorsum of the tongue. The smooth pink mucosa contrasts sharply against the mucosa covered with normal papillae.

The characteristic feature is that the appearance of the tongue changes from day to day.

Marginal indentation of the tongue. This occurs when the lateral borders of the tongue are moulded to the contours ot the teeth. It occurs in normal people.

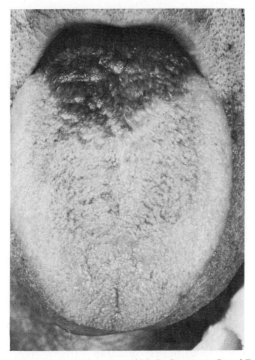

Figure 4.10. *Black hairy tongue. Courtesy of Mr D. Downton, Royal Free Hospital, London.*

Carcinoma of the tongue. Carcinoma of the tongue occurs most commonly on the lateral borders, but on occasion is found on the posterior third of the dorsum or on the under surface. The tumour is usually ulcerated with firm raised edges but sometimes there is no ulceration and the only physical sign is firm induration. For this reason palpation, in addition to inspection, is mandatory in the patient who complains of pain in the tongue. Palpation of the tongue is undertaken by placing a finger on the dorsum and underside of the tongue and also by feeling from the lateral aspects. It is courteous to wash the hands before and after the examination.

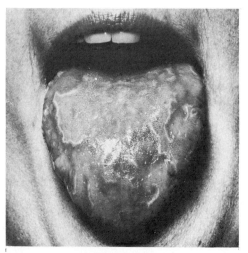

Figure 4.11. *Geographic tongue. Courtesy of Mr D. Downton, Royal Free Hospital, London.*

PHYSICAL EXAMINATION OF THE ABDOMEN

For the purpose of recording physical signs and also for placing the site of abdominal pain the abdomen is divided into nine areas (Figure 4.12): right upper quadrant (right hypochondrium), epigastrium, left upper quadrant (left hypochondrium), right lumbar, umbilical, left lumbar, right lower quadrant (right iliac fossa), suprapubic (hypogastrium), left lower quadrant (left iliac fossa).

Careful methodical inspection of the abdomen is always valuable because masses, enlarged viscera and peristalsis may be visible when they are not readily palpable. The abdomen is best viewed with light falling across it tangentially so that any swellings are thrown into relief and it may be more convenient for the clinician to be sitting. With the patient breathing quietly it may be possible to see an enlarged liver bulging in the right upper quadrant and descending with respiration, or a spleen descending in an oblique direction from the left upper quadrant. Other masses, particularly in the epigastrium, may also be seen.

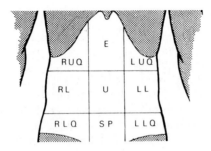

Figure 4.12. *Areas of the abdomen. See text for explanation of symbols.*

Generalised distension occurs when the intestine is distended by gas, when there is ascites, by an ovarian cyst or an enlarged uterus. The appearance of the umbilicus is sometimes of help in distinguishing between the various causes of abdominal distension. The umbilicus is unchanged in gaseous distension; with ascites it is everted; in the presence of an ovarian cyst it is drawn up and vertical. It is sometimes difficult to be sure that the abdomen of an obese patient is or is not distended by an intra-abdominal lesion.

Visible peristalsis is an extremely important physical sign. Occasionally peristalsis is visible in thin, otherwise normal, individuals. Most often however, peristalsis indicates obstruction to the forward passage of gastrointestinal contents. Peristalsis running from left to right in the upper part of the abdomen infers gastric outflow obstruction. Most commonly this is caused by pyloric stenosis, but occasionally occurs in the absence of a mechanical obstruction as a result of a disturbance of gastroduodenal motility. When visible peristalsis is present, it is often accompanied by a succussion splash (page 223).

Small bowel obstruction gives rise to a different pattern of peristalsis. Numerous segments of small bowel contract and relax in an irregular manner and the peristalsis has no recognisable pattern. The abdomen has been described as like a 'bag of worms' or a 'step ladder' in this condition. Visible peristalsis is not an inevitable sign of small bowel obstruction, and often the only sign is central abdominal distension. Peristalsis is also uncommon in patients with large bowel obstruction. Here, distension is found mainly in the flanks and peristalsis runs from right to left.

Operation scars

Scars of previous operations are important for they may be relevant to the patient's current illness. Surgeons nowadays perform many different operations through a paramedian incision, so that it is difficult to decide the precise operation solely from the location of the operation scar. A right lower quadrant 'grid iron' incision usually indicates a previous appendicectomy, and an oblique (Kocher) incision in the right upper quadrant usually denotes a previous cholecystectomy. An abdomen with many operation scars suggests a Munchausen syndrome, although many laparotomies may be done in patients with unrecognised porphyria.

Abdominal wall veins

Veins over the abdominal wall become more obvious when there is obstruction to the blood flow in the portal vein or inferior vena cava (Figure 4.13). The normal venous flow is from the umbilicus upwards to the thorax and from the umbilicus down to the groin. In portal hypertension the flow of blood is always away from the umbilicus. A dilated cluster of veins radiating from the umbilicus is known as a caput medusae. When such veins are seen an examination for a bruit should always be made over the area extending from the xiphisternum to umbilicus. A venous hum suggests patency of the main portal vein (page 233). In inferior vena caval blockage the flow of blood is always upwards from below the umbilicus. The veins are usually situated at the sides of the abdomen and represent the collateral channels between the inferior and superior vena cavae. Conversely in blocks of the superior vena cava the flow of blood is downwards to the umbilicus. There is seldom difficulty in deciding whether dilated veins over the abdomen are the result of liver disease (portal hypertension) for other signs of liver disease are usually present.

In *acute pancreatitis* or as a result of retroperitoneal haemorrhage blood tracks retroperitoneally and bruising may occur around the umbilicus (Cullen's sign) or in the flanks (Grey Turner's sign). The signs may be seen following acute haemorrhagic pancreatitis, ruptured tubal pregnancy and a leaking aneurysm of the abdominal aorta.

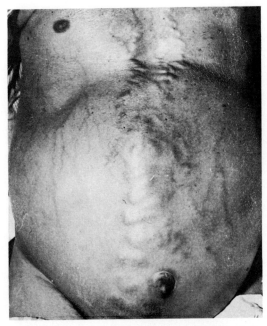

Figure 4.13. *Visible engorged veins in a patient with alcoholic cirrhosis. There is gross ascites in addition.*

The inspection of hernial orifices

Femoral herniae are seen below the inguinal ligament and are more laterally placed than are direct or oblique inguinal herniae. Sometimes a femoral hernia is not visible and it is then necessary to palpate the femoral canal. *Direct inguinal herniae* bulge forward through the inguinal triangle and lie close to the os pubis. Because the neck of the hernial sac is wide it may not be clearly seen but it rarely strangulates (Figure 4.14). *An oblique inguinal hernia* passes down the inguinal canal towards the scrotum. If it is not visible, an attempt should be made to provoke its descent by asking the patient to cough when he is standing. Sometimes such a hernia is only palpable when a finger is put into the external abdominal ring. A recent study indicates that clinical differentiation of direct and indirect hernias is far from accurate. It is essential to examine the hernial orifices in any patient with intestinal obstruction.

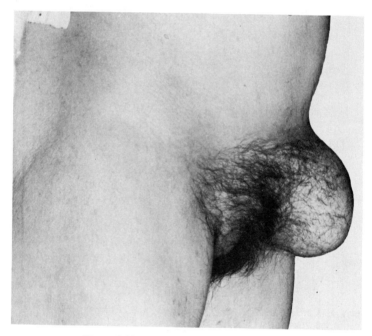

Figure 4.14. *Strangulated left inguinal hernia.*

Palpation of the abdomen

There are three aspects to abdominal palpation. Initially, the palpation should be superficial; this serves to define areas of tenderness and assures the patient that the doctor is making all possible attempts to avoid causing discomfort. Secondly, the abdomen should be palpated deeply and if tenderness is present attempts should be made to elicit rebound tenderness. Deep palpation also allows any palpable mass to be defined and characterised. Finally, the abdomen should be palpated in order to detect enlargement of any of the intra-abdominal organs.

In order for the abdomen to be examined properly the patient should be lying flat with one pillow under the head. This is not always possible if the patient is dyspnoeic. Successful examination of the abdomen is never possible when the patient is tense and attempts should be made to put the patient at his ease. Examination should be carried out in warm, pleasant surroundings, and it is always easier to examine a patient on an examination couch than on a soft, low hospital bed. When the muscles of the abdomen are tense, it is sometimes useful to get the patient to flex his knees. Palpation should always be done with sensitive pads of the fingers rather than the finger tips. The hands should be warm. It is just as important for the clinician to be relaxed and comfortable. He should adopt a position, depending upon the height of the couch or bed, which enables him to palpate freely and without inhibiting discomfort. Standing, sitting at the side of the bed or even kneeling may each be appropriate.

Superficial palpation. During superficial palpation it is important for the examiner to watch the patient's face. Often a wince is the only admission that a patient may make of tenderness. When an area of tenderness is defined an attempt should be made to elicit *rebound discomfort.* This is done by pressing sharply over the area of the tenderness and suddenly releasing the hand. As the abdominal wall muscles spring back into place the underlying peritoneum is stretched and pain is produced if the parietal peritoneum is inflamed. Rebound tenderness also occurs when a similar manoeuvre is performed on the side of the abdomen opposite to that where superficial tenderness was found. A similar physical sign occurs over an inflamed gallbladder. Here the patient is asked to take a deep breath and at the height of inspiration, when the gallbladder descends the palpating hand is sharply pressed. If the gallbladder is inflamed pain occurs (Murphy's sign). This sign is positive in most patients with acute cholecystitis.

When only the visceral peritoneum is inflamed the anterior abdominal muscles are not tensed until the inflamed area is palpated at which point there is voluntary contraction of the muscles — *voluntary guarding.* If the parietal peritoneum is also involved by inflammation there is reflex spasm of the anterior abdominal wall muscles and that part of the abdominal wall is tense and hard — *reflex rigidity.* Such physical signs indicate acute, localised peritonitis. When a hollow organ within the abdomen ruptures, the peritonitis is generalised and the abdominal wall contracts and splints the underlying peritoneum producing a 'rigid' abdomen. Areas of tenderness in the abdomen are often associated with cutaneous hyperaesthesia. These should be regarded as physiological phenomena, rather than useful physical signs.

Deep palpation. During deep palpation, an attempt is made to detect any abnormal masses within the abdomen. It should be remembered that the descending colon is palpable in over 90 per cent of normal individuals. It is usual to palpate the aorta in a thin person, particularly a female who has had multiple pregnancies and has a lax abdominal wall. The aorta is normally sensitive to pressure. A palpable aorta must be distinguished from aneurysmal dilatation or irregularity of the aorta. If an abnormal mass is found it should be defined anatomically and its characteristics and mobility noted (see page 25). Scars of previous operations often cause problems in deciding whether or not an abnormal mass is present because of the underlying fibrous tissue. Divarication of the rectus muscles which occurs after multiple pregnancies enables the examiner to palpate deeply into the abdomen.

Palpation of the liver

An adequate palpation of the liver cannot be made unless the patient is lying flat. The edge of the index finger is laid parallel to the liver edge which strikes the finger as the liver descends on inspiration (Figure 4.15). Alternatively the finger tips of one or both hands are placed parallel to the right costal margin and the patient is asked to take a deep breath through the open mouth (Figure 4.16). Firm but gentle pressure is required and normally the edge of the liver will be felt to move downwards as the patient breathes in. The liver edge is normally palpable in the epigastrium and in the right upper quadrant on deep inspiration. If the liver edge is more than one to two cm below the costal margin it can be considered enlarged. The best position at which to define hepatomegaly is opposite the edge of the ninth costal cartilage. The liver is more easily felt in women and children. However, before labelling a liver as being enlarged it is always necessary to define, by percussion, the upper border. This is normally at the level of the fifth to sixth intercostal space. Clearly a liver margin felt four cm below the costal margin does not indicate hepatomegaly if the upper border

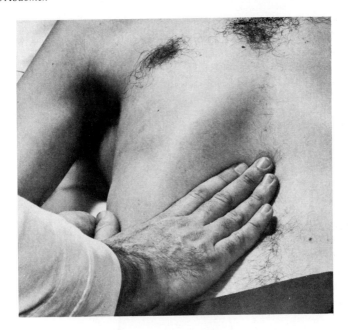

Figure 4.15. *Palpation of the liver.*

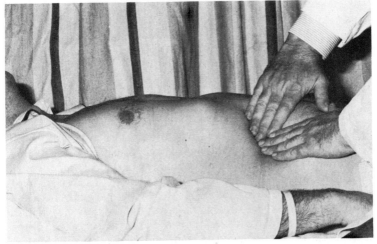

Figure 4.16. *Palpation of the liver.*

of the liver is percussed out at the seventh intercostal space. Failure to define the upper border of the liver is the commonest reason for making an erroneous diagnosis of liver enlargement.

Another reason for a false diagnosis of hepatomegaly is the Riedel's lobe (Figure 4.17). This is an abnormally prominent extension of the right lobe and may extend to the pelvic brim. It is long and narrow while the remainder of the liver is of normal size. Since the lobe is laterally placed it can be confused with the right kidney. Both may be felt by bimanual examination. A Riedel's lobe is commoner in females. If the liver margin cannot be felt with the fingertips an attempt can be made to define the lower margin by percussion, the resonance of the gut giving way to dullness over the liver. This is a much less accurate way of defining liver size than by

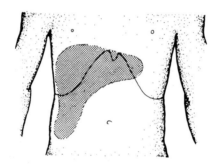

Figure 4.17. *Anatomical configuration of Riedel's lobe.*

palpation. A very large liver may be overlooked if palpation is commenced too close to the costal margin. It is always wise to begin palpating in the right lower quadrant, moving upwards towards the right upper quadrant with each breath.

When the liver is palpable, and particularly when enlarged, it is necessary to observe the following features: liver edge, is it sharp, or blunt, regular or irregular; liver surface, consistency, tenderness, pulsation. The edge is blunted, rounded and tender in congestive cardiac failure which is probably the commonest cause of hepatomegaly in the United Kingdom. Metastatic malignant disease is another common cause of hepatomegaly and the liver may be hard and irregular with palpable lumps; but a smooth firm hepatomegaly may also occur in secondary malignant involvement of the liver. It is rare to be able to palpate umbilicated nodules in the liver; such nodules are characteristic of necrotic malignant deposits. A cirrhotic liver may be large and irregular in shape and it is usually hard. Other causes of hepatomegaly include extrahepatic bile duct obstruction, infiltration with fat or amyloid, and congestion due to obstruction of the hepatic veins or venous radicles.

A small liver can only be detected by percussion when there is reduction in the upper level of dullness and there is resonance along the lower costal margin. Detection of reduced liver size is a more valuable sign than hepatomegaly since there are only two causes and each can be distinguished readily from the other on clinical grounds: acute liver failure and cirrhosis of the liver. Because a cirrhotic liver is often shrunken the nodules are not palpable.

It is necessary to auscultate for arterial bruits and friction sounds over an enlarged liver (p. 233).

Palpation of the stomach

The stomach is normally not palpable even if it is abnormally distended. Indeed the distension is often more easily seen than felt. If gastric outflow obstruction is suspected a *succussion splash* may be tested for: the patient is gently rocked from side-to-side while the examiner places his ear close to the abdomen and listens for a splashing sound. A splash is only of significance if the patient has had nothing to eat or drink within two to three hours of the examination. Tumours of the stomach may be felt as a hard mass in the left upper quadrant which moves on respiration. In congenital pyloric stenosis it is occasionally possible to feel the hypertrophic sphincter to the right of the midline in the epigastrium.

Palpation of the spleen

The spleen is never palpable in the healthy adult since its anterior pole lies in the mid-axillary line well behind the costal margin. The technique of palpating the spleen is important. The palpation is difficult and unless done properly an enlarged spleen may not be felt. The main reason for this is that the inexperienced tend to move the examining hand and 'search' for the palpable spleen rather than to let the spleen come down to strike the hand during respiration. The palpation of the spleen requires a bimanual technique in which the left hand is placed posteriorly over the lower costal margin and the front, right hand, is placed flat on the right hypochondrium with the fingers opposite the ninth to tenth rib, just below the rib margin (Figure 4.18). The patient takes a deep inspiration through the open mouth and at the same time the left hand gently rotates the rib cage forwards. The enlarged spleen is recognised by the tip hitting the right hand fingertips. Any attempt to 'dig' or palpate deeply by the right hand may result in the spleen riding over the fingers and thereby be overlooked. Palpation for the spleen should be anterior and lateral from the tenth rib. The spleen may be percussed as a dull area posteriorly in the ninth, tenth and eleventh

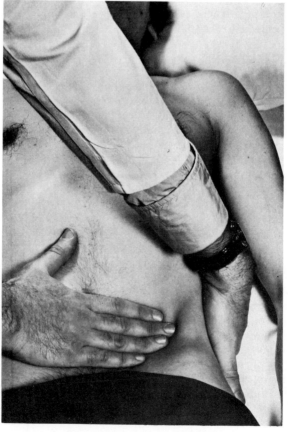

Figure 4.18. *Palpation of the spleen.*

costal spaces. This is a poor and inaccurate method of determining spleen size.

A spleen is distinguished from a left kidney and other masses in the left upper quadrant, such as colon, stomach and tail of pancreas, by the fact that the edge comes out from under the rib cage, it moves early in respiration, the edge has a well-recognised notch, it enlarges obliquely towards the right lower quadrant and it is dull to percussion. These features distinguish an enlarged spleen from a renal mass which enlarges downwards, is resonant and is felt bimanually with the posterior left hand palpating in the loin. However, occasionally massive spenomegaly can be felt by bimanual palpation.

A very large spleen may be overlooked if palpation is not begun in the right lower quadrant. The causes of massive splenomegaly include myelofibrosis, chronic myeloid leukaemia, Gaucher's disease, malaria and kala-azar. The spleen is also enlarged in portal hypertension, infective endocarditis, sarcoidosis, haemolytic states, polycythaemia rubra vera, and infections such as tuberculosis, viral hepatitis, infectious mononucleosis and typhoid fever.

The spleen, which is only just palpable, becomes more readily palpable if the patient lies on his right side with the left arm extended (Figure 4.19). This is useful in confirming a palpable mass in the left upper quadrant as a spleen, but is of no value as a technique for the routine detection of splenic enlargement.

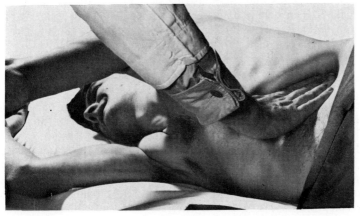

Figure 4.19. *Palpation of the spleen.*

Palpation of the pancreas

The normal pancreas is not palpable and it is only occasionally that a pancreatic tumour or pseudocyst can be felt in the upper abdomen. The mass is usually deep-seated unless it is very large. There may be resonant bowel overlying it. While a pancreatic mass does not move with respiration this is not invariably so and some slight downward movement may occur at the end of a deep inspiration.

Palpation of the gallbladder

In any jaundiced patient an attempt should be made to feel the gallbladder. The detection of an enlarged gallbladder is difficult and a gallbladder may be shown to be grossly distended at laparotomy and yet be undetected clinically by experienced clinicians. The gallbladder only becomes palpable when the bile duct is obstructed below the entry of the cystic duct. It is said that if the gallbladder is palpable in the presence of obstructive jaundice then the cause of the obstruction is other than a gallstone and is more likely to be neoplastic (Courvoisier's law). However this is often misleading since a distended gallbladder is so frequently missed on abdominal palpation. When the gallbladder is palpable it presents as a smooth cystic swelling in the right upper quadrant of the abdomen. The swelling occurs in the midline near the ninth costal cartilage, but may be lower if it is pushed down by an enlarged liver. The gallbladder may also be distended if the cystic duct is blocked when it may be distended with mucus (mucocele) or pus (empyema). Rarely, a hard nodular carcinomatous gallbladder may be palpated and such patients are usually icteric.

Palpation of the kidney

Examination of the kidney commences with a check for renal angle tenderness. In minimal degree this consists of pain produced by finger-tip pressure localised to the angle formed by the last rib and the lateral border of the sacrospinalis. Renal angle tenderness suggests that the renal capsule is distended or irritated, as in an obstructive nephropathy or active pyelonephritis. Marked renal angle tenderness occurs in the presence of a renal carbuncle or perinephric abscess and can interfere with subsequent bimanual palpations.

The examination of either kidney is made bimanually, the left hand in the loin below the last rib and lateral to the sacrospinalis with the right hand placed anteriorly (Figure 4.20). The patient is asked to breathe in deeply and during this the hands are approximated. A kidney will be felt as a smooth rounded structure moving downwards during inspiration. If the hands are brought together *before* inspiration the kidney cannot descend and it may not be palpated. In lean, well relaxed, normal individuals, the lower poles of both kidneys, especially the right, may be felt. In a few very thin patients, usually females, both lower poles or even an entire kidney can be held or moved between the hands. Such mobility was formerly regarded as abnormal, but it is simply the consequence of a paucity of perirenal fat.

The kidney is usually felt best by the posterior hand. By manipulating the kidney forward with this hand it may be possible to feel the organ indistinctly with the anterior hand. A kidney is recognised by the rounded lower pole (this is not as sharp as either a liver or a splenic edge), the organ moves late in respiration, it enlarges directly downwards, it lies deep in the abdomen, and is usually resonant to percussion because of overlying colon.

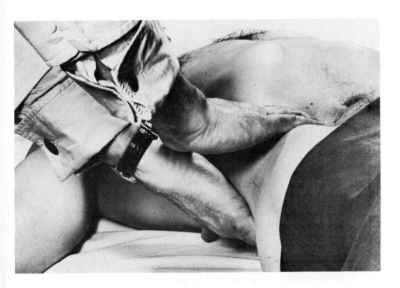

Figure 4.20a. *Palpation of the kidney.*

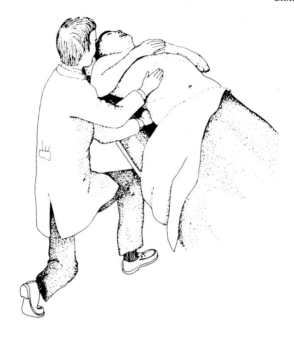

Figure 4.20b. *Palpation of the kidney.*

A normal kidney is slightly tender on palpation.

A renal mass may be due to a hydronephrosis, tumour or cyst formation. Massive enlargement of both kidneys is usually the result of polycystic disease. Some enlargement of one kidney with a non-functional or non-existent kidney contralaterally may simply represent compensatory hypertrophy of the remaining kidney. Occasionally a normal kidney may be more readily palpable than is usual because of its displacement by hepatic enlargement, or an adrenal or other retroperitoneal tumour.

Diminution in kidney size usually cannot be detected by bimanual examination. The small kidney of chronic glomerulonephritis and pyelonephritis therefore requires radiographic demonstration. A plain anteroposterior film of the abdomen is usually sufficient for the purpose, but occasionally tomography, possibly combined with the nephrogram phase of excretory urography, is required for measurement of size and appreciation of shape and cortical width.

Ascites

The presence of intraperitoneal fluid is suspected when there is abdominal distension with bulging flanks and possibly an everted umbilicus (Figure 4.13). The method of demonstrating ascites is by 'shifting dullness'. Percussion is started from the midline at the umbilicus and continued laterally. An initial resonant note will give way to dullness. The point of transition is noted on the skin and the patient turned over towards the side. After waiting a few seconds percussion is repeated and if fluid is present the upper level dullness will have shifted to be closer to the midline while the opposite flank will have become more resonant. Shifting dullness is the best clinical indication of ascites and preferable to attempting to detect a 'fluid thrill'. Unfortunately the detection of fluid in the abdomen is not easy. No movement of free fluid may be detected while a loaded colon can move as the patient turns thereby giving a positive sign of shifting dullness.

Ascites must be differentiated from an ovarian cyst where, in contrast to free fluid, there is dullness in the centre of the abdomen. A grossly distended stomach and distended small bowel in conditions associated with steatorrhoea may also be misleading.

The presence of ascites makes palpation of the intra-abdominal organs difficult. In this situation the technique of *ballottement* is used. The fingertips are dipped sharply into the abdomen and the displacement of the fluid above any organ such as an enlarged liver or spleen, or an abnormal mass, will give a tapping impression. By making a series of such movements it may be possible to map out an organ or mass.

When ascites is diagnosed it is always necessary to undertake a diagnostic tap. The fluid may be clear, purulent, blood stained or chylous. Causes for ascites include peritoneal inflammation, for example tuberculosis, metastatic malignant disease, cirrhosis of the liver, hypoalbuminaemic states such as nephrotic syndrome and protein—calorie malnutrition and congestive heart failure.

Examination of the bladder

This forms part of the routine assessment of the abdomen by palpation, Ideally, every patient will have voided urine before being examined, and in these circumstances, the normal bladder is empty, non-tender and placed retropubically within the true pelvis. Young children provide the exception, their bladders normally being substantially above the pelvis. A urine-distended bladder, as in acute retention, is palpable as a dome-shaped swelling which projects from the pelvis towards the umbilicus. A blader so distended is always dull to percussion. Chronic urinary retention ('retention with overflow incontinence') can be associated with a melon-shaped bladder swelling, the apex of which can reach the umbilicus even in adults. At best, even in chronic retention, the edges of the distended bladder are ill defined to palpation and through the abdominal wall at least there appear some similarities between a distended bladder and a moderately sized uterine enlargement. Except in the most chronic retention palpation over a distended bladder usually elicits tenderness and a desire to micturate. When doubt arises the nature of a supposed bladder swelling, especially in women, can often be clarified by passing a urethral catheter with full aseptic precautions and then re-examining the abdomen. The distended bladder must be distinguished from other masses arising from the pelvis including ovarian and uterine enlargements.

Examination of the hernial orifices

This should be undertaken routinely and the examination of the hernial orifices is of particular importance in patients with intestinal obstruction.

Indirect inguinal hernia. Normally the internal abdominal ring lies 1.25 cm above the inguinal ligament, and midway between the pubic symphysis and the anterior superior iliac spine. The external abdominal ring lies 1.25 cm above and 1.25 cm lateral to the pubic spine and will not admit the tip of the finger. An oblique, indirect inguinal hernia can be seen or felt as a bulge running obliquely above the inguinal canal. In males the external abdominal ring can be palpated by invaginating the little finger into the scrotum and in the presence of an indirect inguinal hernia the little finger will enter the ring and pass along the inguinal in an upward and lateral direction. In females the diagnosis is more difficult but an impulse on coughing and a swelling can be detected in the labium major.

Direct inguinal hernia. A direct inguinal hernia leaves the abdomen through Hesselbach's triangle, being bounded medially by the outer margin of the rectus abdominus muscle, laterally by the deep epigastric artery and below by the medial half of the inguinal ligament. The hernia lies above the inguinal ligament and does not descend into the scrotum.

In contrast to the indirect inguinal hernia, a direct hernia lies behind the spermatic cord and a finger inserted into the external abdominal ring passes directly into the abdomen. Pressure over the indirect inguinal ring will obliterate the cough impulse from an indirect inguinal hernia but not a direct inguinal hernia. In males an inguinal hernia must be distinguished from a hydrocele, a femoral hernia, maldescended testis and a lipoma of the cord. In females the differentiation includes a femoral hernia and a hydrocele of the canal of Nück.

Femoral hernia. A femoral hernia passes vertically down the femoral canal as far as the saphenous opening at which point it tends to curve upwards towards the inguinal ligament. The impulse or swelling is found below the inguinal ligament and lateral to the pubic tubercle. The differential diagnosis includes an inguinal hernia, a saphenous varix and a psoas abscess.

Umbilical hernia. In adults the herniation is through the linea alba usually above and occasionally below the umbilicus. As the hernia enlarges it assumes an oval shape and droops downwards. In infants the hernia passes directly through the umbilical ring.

Epigastric hernia. This is a protrusion of fat through the linea alba. It is situated in the midline usually midway between the umbilicus and the xiphisternum.

Incisional hernia. This occurs through the site of an abdominal incision.

Divarication of the recti

This is a common condition usually found in multiparous females. When the patient strains a gap is seen between the recti through which bulge the abdominal contents. The separated recti can be felt easily when the abdomen is relaxed.

Distinction between an intra-abdominal and extra-abdominal mass

Occasionally there may be uncertainty whether a mass lies within the abdominal cavity, or within or superficial to the anterior abdominal wall. The distinguishing feature is that intra-abdominal swellings cannot be felt when the abdominal wall is tensed whereas masses within the wall can still be felt or even become more prominent. In order to tense the abdominal muscles the patient is asked to press the forehead against the examiners's left hand while the right hand palpates over the mass.

Percussion of Other Organs or Masses

Percussion is of limited value in deciding whether solid intra-abdominal organs are enlarged. The technique is only of some assistance in the examination of the liver. Percussion is sometimes valuable in deciding the nature of a mass in the left upper quadrant of the abdomen. If the dullness to percussion over the mass is continuous with dullness over the ninth, tenth and eleventh intercostal spaces in the mid-axillary line then the mass is likely to be spleen.

Resonance over a mass is occasionally helpful. The kidneys bear a fairly constant relationship to the gas-filled colon. An enlarged kidney is, therefore, usually associated with a band of resonance across it. This physical sign is only confirmatory for a palpable mass and a band of resonance alone should never be taken as evidence of renal enlargement.

Auscultation of the Abdomen

This is an important part of the abdominal examination. Auscultation should always be carried out in quiet surroundings and in deep expiration, so that sounds are not obscured by breath sounds. The bell of the stethoscope should be used, and this should be lightly applied to the abdomen. Firm pressure of a stethoscope over a major vessel in a thin person can induce a vascular bruit.

Abdominal vascular sounds

The hearing of a bruit in the abdomen does not necessarily signify disease, for a bruit is commonly heard in normal people, particularly the young. These 'physiological' murmurs arise from the abdominal aorta (arterial) and from the inferior vena cava (venous). Pathological murmurs from the heart may also be heard in the abdomen, those arising from the aortic valve being most common. The location of abdominal bruits is shown in Figure 4.21.

Arterial murmurs are also heard in the abdomen when major blood vessels are constricted. The commonest cause of an arterial murmur is a renal artery stenosis, but arterial murmurs are heard in many patients with hypertension when there is no obstruction to blood flow in the renal artery. Arterial murmurs also arise in obstruction of the superior mesenteric artery, and in coeliac axis compression. Pancreatic tumours which compress the splenic artery can produce an abdominal bruit. A murmur over the liver

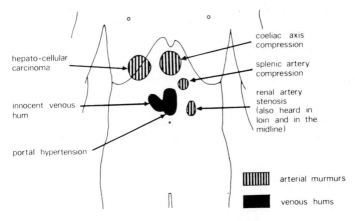

Figure 4.21. *Location of vascular sounds in the abdomen.*

occurs with primary and secondary tumours of the liver and alcoholic hepatitis; occasionally a murmur may be heard over an enlarged spleen. Arterial murmurs occur in small abdominal aortic aneurysms, but are seldom heard when the aneurysm is large. Abdominal arterial murmurs are more likely to be significant when they radiate out from the epigastrium or are heard in the loins or lower quadrants. A diastolic component to the murmur also makes it more likely that the murmur is significant.

Although less common than innocent arterial murmurs venous hums arising from the inferior vena cava are heard in normal individuals. A venous hum is heard in some cases of cirrhosis; the umbilical vein, which usually obliterates soon after birth, opens up as a result of portal hypertension and a venous hum develops. The hum may be intensified and easier to hear when the patient is standing. Hearing such a murmur infers patency of the main portal vein, because the umbilical vein drains into the left branch of the portal vein and is therefore of help in the differential diagnosis of portal hypertension.

Arteriovenous malformations within the abdomen give rise to continuous low-pitched murmurs which are diffuse.

Bowel sounds

Bowel sounds are of less diagnostic value than vascular sounds. The origin of the sounds is debatable although it is likely that they all derive from the small intestine. The rhythm and frequency of bowel sounds in the normal individual vary considerably. Up to 30 bowel sounds may be heard in one minute, but the lower limit of normal is undefined, and bowel sounds should not be considered absent until none has been heard over a period of at least four minutes. The frequency of bowel sounds tends to be reduced after a meal. It is difficult to assess the value of qualitative changes in bowel sounds, although it is a commonly held clinical impression that high pitched 'tingling' sounds signify mechanical intestinal obstruction or paralytic ileus.

Friction noises

Friction noises are occasionally heard over the spleen or the liver, particularly after splenic venography and following liver biopsy. They are also heard over an area of splenic infarction or over a neoplasm or abscess of the liver.

Rectal Examination

The rectal examination is an essential part of the clinical examination. The procedure should be explained to the patient who will require reassurance. At all times it is essential to be gentle and unhurried. The examination is most easily performed when the patient is in the left lateral position with both legs flexed. Alternatively, the patient can be in the knee-elbow position, although this is less comfortable, impossible in the aged or very ill and usually causes the patient some embarrassment. Before the finger is inserted into the anus, the perianal skin is carefully inspected. This area of the body is prone to a number of skin conditions including anal warts, fungal infections and psoriasis. Skin tags are occasionally seen around the anus and these may be the cause of perianal discomfort and pruritus. These may be the end stage of haemorrhoids or acute perianal haematomas or an indication of an anal fissure. Regional ileitis causes a bluish discoloration of the skin. Haemorrhoids can also be seen as bluish swellings, particularly when the patient bears down simulating a bowel action. They occur classically in the positions of 3, 7 and 11 o'clock when the midline of the body is in the 12 o'clock position. An acute perianal haematoma may be seen as a cherry-sized blue swelling at the anal margin.

When the external examination of the anus is complete, the gloved finger which is lubricated is placed into the anus. The finger is inserted from a posterior direction between the gluteal folds and gradually inserted with gentle rotation. If there is any suspicion of pain it may be helpful to lubricate using a local anaesthetic cream. Sphincteric tone is first assessed. The external and internal sphincter can be distinguished. A lax sphincter occurs in neurological disorders, particularly those in which the lower spinal cord is affected, and a tight sphincter is usually an indication that the patient has found it difficult to relax adequately or there is a fissure. If the introduction of the finger into the rectum causes pain then an anal fissure should be suspected. This appears as a linear 'tear' at the posterior or anterior anal verge. The cause of such fissures is not known, although they are thought to represent undue spasm of either the internal or external anal sphincter in response to rectal distension.

Normally the rectum should be empty but just prior to defaecation and in constipated subjects the rectum will contain faeces. The finger is inserted as deeply as possible and rotated in all directions. Posteriorly the coccyx and sacrum will be felt, laterally the pelvic wall and anteriorly the urethra and prostate in the male and cervix in the female. It may also be possible to feel the uterus and adnexa. Bimanual palpation using the left hand on the anterior abdominal wall may help to determine the site and size of any mass. Lesions high in the rectum are sometimes felt more readily when the patient bears down as if having a bowel action. Faecal matter within the rectum occasionally causes some confusion if felt through the mucous membrane and may be called polyps.

The normal prostate is smooth, firm and the lateral lobes can be felt separated by a median groove. An enlarged prostate can be detected but it is seldom that the cause of the enlargement can be determined with certainty by digital examination. An abnormally small prostate occurs with oestrogen therapy and hypopituitarism. The prostate will be very tender and 'boggy' if an abscess is present. Anal and rectal cancers can usually be recognised readily as craggy ulcers or proliferating tumours.

The cervix can be palpated and it may be possible to distinguish the small 'acorn' nulliparous cervix from the larger, more patulous cervix of the multiparous patient. The uterus, especially if retroverted, can be felt particularly if the bimanual techique is used. Ovaries may be felt laterally in thin patients or if the organs are enlarged by a cyst or tumour. The pouch of Douglas in the female and the rectovesical space in the male may be the site of tumour deposits. A 'boggy' swelling in this area suggests a pelvic abscess. If the inflamed appendix is in the pelvic position tenderness is elicited on rectal examination.

When the finger is withdrawn the finger is examined for blood and if desired any stool on the glove can be tested for blood. It is courteous to clean the anus once the examination is completed.

Proctoscopy

A variety of proctoscopes (anoscopes) is available. The instrument is lubricated and then carefully inserted using the same technique of gentle rotation as with the digital examination. The patient is in the same position as for digital examination. It is always wise to precede anal or rectal endoscopy with a digital examination and thereby avoid causing the patient unnecessary pain.

The mucous membrane is inspected. It should be pink and glistening with thin rectal valves. Any ulceration, inflammation, polyp or tumour mass is noted and a biopsy taken. Haemorrhoids are recognised by asking the patient to strain (reassuring him at the same time that he will not have an accident) and noting the presence of blue distended veins in the 3, 7 and 11 o'clock positions. Anal fissures may be visualised but frequently it is not possible to undertake endoscopic examination unless the patient is anaesthetised.

Sigmoidoscopy

Most gastroenterologists prefer to perform sigmoidoscopy before proctoscopy. Sigmoidoscopy is best performed in a special room in which there is a table which can be tilted and elevated but nonetheless sigmoidoscopies performed in the general outpatient department are often quite adequate.

Various forms of sigmoidoscopes are available. For general outpatient use a narrow-bore 25-cm instrument is useful for it is more easily manoeuvred and more comfortable than the wider bored instruments. With the patient in the left lateral position, the lubricated, warmed sigmoidoscope is gently introduced into the rectum. As soon as the rectum is entered the obturator is removed and the further passage of the instrument is carried out under direct vision following the lumen of the bowel. The sigmoidoscope is advanced up the rectum preferably without the insufflation of air. This is usually easily accomplished until the rectosigmoid junction is reached at a distance of between 13 and 15 cm from the anus. Here the lumen of the bowel passes anteriorly and to the left. Once the sigmoidoscope has been advanced to the fullest possible depth, it is withdrawn slowly and it is during withdrawal that insufflation of air is of value in distending the bowel. Any suspicious lesion within the bowel should be biopsied. Once a biopsy has been done the biopsy site should be carefully inspected and any undue bleeding is usually easily controlled by the pressure of a cotton swab on a long forceps. The appearance of the mucosa should be carefully assessed. The normal mucosa is salmon pink and the venous pattern is readily seen. When ulcerative proctitis or colitis is present the mucosa is inflamed, friable and bleeds easily when swabbed. Ulcers are only occasionally seen.

Against a background of proctitis the presence of obvious ulceration suggests granulomatous (Crohn's) colitis. Occasionally solitary ulcers are seen in the rectum. Biopsy of a rectal valve in the inflamed rectum should be undertaken with care, and is best performed on the posterior wall of the rectum below the peritoneal reflection.

Barium enema is best avoided in the 24 hours following a biopsy of the rectum, for it is during this period that the remote danger of bowel perforation is greatest.

Examination of the Child

An adequate abdominal examination cannot be made if the child is crying. Although the abdominal muscles may relax when the child stops crying to inspire, the period is too short for satisfactory palpation. The infant may be calmed by being offered a feed from a bottle; an older child requires gentle reassurance, and a relaxed patient approach. If the child refuses to lie flat the abdominal examination may be undertaken conveniently with the child held in the mother's arms, or sitting on her knee, or standing on her lap. The clinician attempts to palpate the abdomen by approaching from behind the child. It is essential that the examiner's hand is warm, that he is gentle and that areas of tenderness are palpated with extreme care.

The principles of the examination are the same as in adults. Because a child employs mainly diaphragmatic respiration there is much abdominal wall movement. Absence of this occurs in peritonitis. The hernial sites should always be examined particularly in a child with abdominal pain or vomiting. The lower border of the liver is normally palpable up to two cm below the costal margin and the spleen is palpable in 10 per cent of normal infants. The spleen readily enlarges in minor febrile illnesses of childhood and may be felt frequently in these children. It tends to enlarge vertically downwards rather than in the oblique direction in adults. A young child who is unable to cooperate fully when asked to 'take a deep breath' may be induced to do so if asked to 'give a hard blow' which will inevitably necessitate a deep breath. The kidneys are often felt in normal children and palpation of a full bladder is not uncommon.

It may be possible to feel the pyloric tumour of congenital hypertrophic stenosis in male infants. It should be sought during feeding by palpating just below the liver edge lateral to the right rectus muscle. Gentle pressure is used. An acorn-like mass will be felt to contract and relax intermittently over an interval of 10 to 15 minutes. Inspection of the abdomen in these infants may reveal gastric peristalsis situated in the epigastrium moving from left to right.

The mass of an intussusception may be felt as a sausage-shaped, soft tumour in the right upper quadrant. Other masses which might be encountered include a Wilm's tumour, neuroblastoma, and mesenteric and retroperitoneal lymph nodes. The rectal examination should be performed with particular gentleness using the little finger if necessary. The greatest care should be taken to avoid needless pain if an anal fissure is present and, indeed, it may not be possible to perform the examination. The nature of anal sphincter tone is noted and whether the rectum contains faeces. The narrow, empty rectal segment in Hirschprung's disease may be encountered.

Examination of Urine

Testing of urine is mandatory for all patients who are referred to hospital either as outpatients or for admission. It is a desirable part of every general medical examination, including those undertaken in general practice, since these inexpensive tests afford a relatively high yield of positive results with diagnostic significance. The minimum examination is an inspection of freshly passed urine and chemical tests for protein, glucose and, in all dark-coloured specimens, for bile pigments in addition.

Colour and transparence

In health urine presents varying shades of amber colour and is transparent when freshly voided. As personal experience will have shown, the intensity of the hue varies greatly with concomitant water output, the amount of the rather obscure pigments urochrome and uroerythrin being fairly constant from day to day. Dietary changes also have marginal effects on the basic amber colour.

Urine left to stand exposed to air may show one or more of three changes. The amber colour of urine gradually develops a darker orange tinge as colourless urobilinogen, present in normal amounts, is converted by oxidation to urobilin, which is a brown pigment. This feature is marked when larger quantities of urobilinogen are present as, for example, in haemolytic anaemia. Secondly, some of the mucin present in urine may appear as a hazy colourless cloud floating in the urine. Thirdly, the less soluble inorganic salts may precipitate out, forming finally a sediment at the bottom of the vessel. In general, precipitated mucin and amorphous and crystalline salts are clinically unimportant, representing the effect of cooling and concentration (urates) or alkalinity (inorganic phosphates). When bacterial decomposition occurs within the urinary tract the urine as voided may show turbidity due to precipitated phosphate, be alkaline and smell of ammonia.

Disease often alters the colour of urine by introducing an abnormal and recognisable extra pigment, for which reason it is well worth while inspecting freshly passed urine as a routine. Colour and/or transparency change in urine, as passed or apparent after standing, can suggest one or other underlying disease but each colour is not unique to one pigment (see Table 4.1) and a possibility based on inspection should be verified by a specific test.

Loss of transparence indicates the presence of suspended particulate material such as pus cells, erythrocytes, bacteria or amorphous crystals of phosphates or urates. These differ in the associated colour change.

Table 4.1. *Abnormal colours in urine*

Colour	Pigment	Causation
Brown-black	Methaemoglobin	Haemolysis or urinary bleeding
	Melaninogen melanin[a]	Disseminated melanoma
	Homogentisic acid[b]	Alkaptonuria
	Phenolic oxidation products	Lysol poisoning
Red-brown	Haemoglobin/methaemoglobin[a] admixture ± RBC	Haemolysis or urinary bleeding
	Myoglobin	Rhabdomyolysis
Pink-red	Porphyrins[a]	Porphyria
	Beet colourant	Beetroot ingestion; genetic predisposition
	Drug dyes	Pyridium, rifampicin or other drugs
Red	Haemoglobin ± RBC	Haemolysis or urinary bleeding
	Myoglobin	Rhabdomyolysis
	Porphyrins	Porphyria
Yellow-orange	Urobilin[a]	Excessive in haemolysis and certain stages of hepatitis
Yellow	Tetracycline	Antibiotic therapy
	Riboflavin	B vitamin medication
Yellow-brown or green	Bilirubin	Cholestatic jaundice
Green-blue	Methylene blue	Sweet colourants; de Witt's pills
Milky	Pus cells	Urinary infection; analgesic nephropathy
	Fat globules	Chyluria

[a] Intensified on standing by conversion from precursor chromogen.
[b] Oxidation on standing darkens colour.

Odour

The aromatic fragrance of urine is often complicated by unidentified excretory products derived from the diet. Infected urine can smell of stale fish or ammoniacal decomposition or be odourless. Acetone can impart a fruity smell to urine during ketosis with ketonuria. In general, while patients are quite often perplexed by the 'strong smell' of their urine, odour is rarely an important discriminating factor in diagnosis.

Urinary solute concentration

In the formation of urine from glomerular ultrafiltrate, renal tubular activity adjusts the relative proportions of water to total solute. The effect of this work, the state of 'concentration' or 'dilution' of the urine, can be judged crudely by the colour of the urine in the absence of abnormal pigments or estimated by specific gravity or osmolality methods. Because the daily output of the physiological pigment urochrome is fairly constant, the intensity of the amber colour of urine varies directly with the concentration of total urinary solute. Pale urine is generally dilute urine.

Specific gravity (SG) measurement by urinometer provides a less than perfect index of solute concentration in urine. The instrument, a simple hydrometer calibrated for use at room temperature (15°C), is inexpensive and convenient. The physiological range on ordinary diet is SG 1.007 to 1.022. Random samples taken over the course of a day vary greatly. After abstinence from fluids for 12 hours overnight the morning urine is usually at least SG 1.020. This concentration test is evidence against the presence of diffuse renal disease. Because a specific gravity measurement is the ratio of the mass of a unit volume of urine relative to the mass of a like volume of distilled water, the specific gravity of urine is influenced by the presence in urine of large heavy molecules such as glucose, radiological contrast media or protein without there being any proportionate change in the physiologically important total urinary solute concentration.

Since tubular work adjusts the relative numbers of water to solute molecules — numbers of particles being material and not mass — osmometry is the preferred measure of urine concentration/dilution. Unfortunately, unlike the urinometer for specific gravity, osmometers are expensive and laboratory based. When on an average diet, adult subjects excrete urine in the osmolal range

200 to 1200 mmol/kg water. During prolonged fluid deprivation healthy kidneys will conserve water by forming concentrated urine in the range 900 to 1200 mmol/kg water. Water loading, as by one litre of water ingested within twenty minutes, should result in a brisk diuresis with solute concentration falling below 100 mmol/kg water in one of the hourly urine collections secured during the four hours after ingestion. Plasma osmolality is about 290 mmol/kg water and the ratio of urine/plasma osmolalities represents accurately the extent of concentration or dilution work undertaken by the renal tubule.

Urine concentration (water conservation) and urine dilution (water excretion) tests are usually described in the context of discriminating between healthy and early diseased kidneys. The dilution test also forms the basis of some clinical investigations involving pituitary and adrenocortical functions as well as nephrons. Urine dilution is not impaired by renal disease before concentrating capacity is affected. Because rapid water ingestion is unpleasant and can induce water intoxication in the presence of renal disease, the dilution test is best avoided in these circumstances. Occasionally, as in medullary cystic disease of the kidneys or tubular injury during hypercalcaemia from a variety of causes, inability to conserve water at renal tubular level results in the constant production of dilute urine (pale, low SG and low osmolality) to which the patient responds by increased fluid intake (polydipsia). Water turnover is increased to avoid dehydration.

Reagent dip strips and tablets for urinalysis

Systems of diagnostic 'dip strip' tests have been formulated by the Ames Company and by the Boehringer Corporation. While convenient and reliable, these tests require detailed understanding. Like virtually all tests, they are liable to false positive or negative results in particular circumstances. Drugs and their metabolites in urine are important in this context. Comprehensive information in attractive ready-to-use form is available to medical students on application to Ames and Boehringer.*

A useful multireagent dip strip for general use is Labstix (Ames), which indicates pH and detects protein, glucose, ketones and blood in urine. Success with multireagent strips requires a strictly timed

---

*Ames Co., Division of Miles Laboratories Ltd, Stoke Poges, Slough SL2 4LY.
Boehringer Corporation (London) Ltd, Bell Lane, Lewes, East Sussex BN7 1LG.

routine with ordered sequence in reading. It is wise to commence with single agent strips before proceeding to multireagent strips since the latter are a little complicated to read.

Hydrogen ion concentration (pH), output rate (titratable acidity) and net acid output

On the usual meat and fish diet the urine produced in health is of acid reaction (pH 4.5 to 6.0). An exceptional diet (e.g. vegetarian) or disease with acid—base upset (e.g. pyloric stenosis) can induce reactive formation of alkaline urine. Most commonly, urine alkaline (ph $>$ 7) when voided is indicative of infection by a micro-organism capable of urea-splitting with release of ammonia. One renal tubular disorder, renal tubular acidosis, is characterised by the continued production of only slightly acid or even alkaline urine in the presence of systemic acidosis and stems from a failure of secretion of hydrogen ions by the tubules. Urine acidity is checked on fresh urine using pH-sensitive colorimetric dip strips. Analysis of acid—base status may require measurement of the amount of non-volatile acid being excreted in buffered form from the titratable acidity and ammonium outputs in terms of net millimoles of hydrogen ion per 24 hours (normal adult value 40 to 80 mmol/24 hours). Titratable acidity and pH measurements are not undertaken as a routine although there is some justification for noting pH more commonly. The common form of renal failure is not accompanied by the excretion of notably less acidic urine (hydrogen concentration or pH), although the output of buffered hydrogen ion (titratable acidity) and hydrogen ion as ammonium are both reduced and in consequence net hydrogen ion output (acid output) per unit of time is reduced.

Protein

Albumin, the commonest abnormal protein found in urine, is readily demonstrated with dip strips (e.g. Albustix, Ames) based upon the protein error of acid—base indicator reagents. The dip strips are semiquantitative. Buffered indicator in the test strip reacts with protein and, in doing so, the yellow indicator colour changes to a shade of green without there being any pH change within the dipstrip because of the buffer. False positive results can stem from the reagent buffer effect being overcome by alkaline urine or contaminating quaternary ammonium disinfectants. The sensitivity of Albustix is adjusted to give a 'trace' positive result with 200 mg albumin per litre urine. Normal individuals excrete less than 150 mg protein per 24 hours, mostly as globulins derived from the kidneys (Tamm—Horsfall protein) and urinary tract. When the water output rate (urine volume per 24 hours) happens to be low, 'trace' positive proteinuria to Albustix can occasionally be found in normal people, especially in concentrated 'first' morning urine specimens. Protein error-based dip strips are rather insensitive to non-albumin proteins such as globulins. Thus Albustix may give false negative results with haemoglobin, Bence Jones proteins and mucoprotein when traditional heat coagulation tests for protein in urine are positive.

There is still an occasional role for the older protein tests such as heat coagulation using boiled acidified urine or precipitation using drops of 25 per cent sulphosalicylic acid. Bence Jones proteins (kappa or alpha immunoglobulin light chains) precipitate out well before boiling temperature and re-dissolve on boiling. The detection of Bence Jones immunoglobulin in urine is uncommon but virtually pathognomonic of abnormal proliferation of plasma cells in bone marrow, that is, myelomatosis. Although these light chain globulins are readily excreted by glomerular filtration they may damage renal tubules and result in 'myeloma kidney'.

Except for 'trace' proteinuria, all instances of proteinuria should be graded by the rate of excretion in terms of grams of protein per 24 hours and not simply by the concentration in a single casual sample of urine. Proteinuria in excess of two grams per 24 hours can be taken as indicative of a glomerular lesion provided a para-protein such as Bence Jones globulin is excluded. Heavy persistent proteinurias (>5 grams/24 hours) eventually lead on to the nephrotic syndrome state, manifested by gross dependent oedema, hypoalbuminaemia and hyperlipaemia. Glomerular lesions, usually glomerulonephritis, less commonly amyloid disease, diabetic or hypertensive nephropathies and other processes, cause proteinuria by increasing the permeability of the glomerular structure to normal plasma proteins, especially albumin. In general, with certain exceptions, persistent proteinuria implies glomerular abnormality, commonly chronic glomerulonephritis.

Bence Jones globulin is tested for in the ward sideroom by adding a small amount of 50 per cent acetic acid and saturated aqueous sodium chloride solution to urine in a test tube. The globulin is recognised as a precipitate formed at room temperature which clears on boiling and reappears on subsequent cooling. In this test albumin is precipitated but does not dissolve on boiling. Unfortunately albumin and Bence Jones globulin may both be present when the characteristics of the former conceal the latter. Urine protein electrophoresis, the conclusive laboratory method for Bence Jones protein, should be resorted to when there is any doubt.

Proteinuria, with more than 150 mg per 24 hours excreted persistently, does occur in some healthy individuals below 30 years of age and is regarded as benign since renal disorder does not eventuate. This proteinuria has the feature that it is undetectable in urine collected over a period of time when the individual is supine. It appears when he or she is upright, hence the name orthostatic or postural proteinuria. The first morning urine, the one traditionally selected for testing, is characteristically protein-free in individuals with orthostatic proteinuria. Postural proteinuria is quite a common finding in young people being examined prior to military service, employment or for insurance purposes. It appears to wear off with increasing age. Other benign but evanescent proteinurias are associated with vigorous exercise such as marathon running or febrile illnesses.

Glucose

The specific test for glucose, as distinct from reducing substances in general, is glucose oxidase based. In the presence of atmospheric oxygen and glucose the oxidase produces hydrogen peroxide, which reacts with a suitable chromogen to give a diagnostic colour change. Several forms of glucose oxidase dip strip are available commercially. All are immersed momentarily in urine, tapped free of excess fluid and read in air. Clinistix (Ames) is read at 10 seconds, when a purple colour indicates $\geqslant 5.5$ mmol glucose per litre urine. The different chromogen system in Multistix (Ames) gives green-brown colours when positive but is of comparable sensitivity. Clinistix and Labstix (Ames) are qualitative. Diastix strips (Ames) are available for the semiquantitative estimation of glucose in blood plasma and are not to be confused with strips for tests on urine.

Benedict's alkaline copper sulphate solution, the traditional test for urine sugars, is reduced by several substances (galactose, lactose, fructose, pentose and ascorbic acid) other than glucose. Although non-specific, the alkaline copper reduction reaction provides a convenient semiquantitative test for glucose in urine.

Clinitest (Ames) is a kit form of this reagent, in which five drops of urine are diluted in a test tube with ten drops of water. Addition of the reagent tablet initiates an exothermic reaction which, with glucose (and/or reducing sugars) produces coloured precipitates, green through yellow to orange brown, indicating amounts of glucose in the urine under test between 14 and 110 mmol per litre (0.25 to 2 g/dl). It should be remembered that Clinistix is inherently more sensitive to glucose at the lower end of the concentration range and can be positive for glucose in low concentration when Clinitest is negative. Clinitest is not specific for glucose, and positive results with these tablets and a concomitant negative with Clinistix may reflect other reducing substances such as ascorbic acid, non-glucose sugars like lactose or fructose, or homogentisic acid as in alkaptonuria.

In routine testing it is usual to test with a specific qualitative agent such as Clinistix (or the glucose oxidase component of Labstix). Positive tests must be checked quantitatively. Anomalous results call for repetition and, if confirmed, necessitate a check on the details of these tests in the technical literature.

Glucose may be present in urine for a variety of reasons, of which diabetes mellitus is the most important but not necessarily the most prevalent. When testing human subjects without symptoms of diabetes mellitus, the finding of glycosuria is usually the expression, not of diabetes, but of alimentary glycosuria or of a low renal threshold for glucose. The diagnosis of diabetes mellitus depends upon demonstration of abnormal concentrations of glucose in blood, not in urine, the diagnostic feature being an excessively high and prolonged elevation of plasma glucose after ingestion of glucose (glucose 'tolerance' test).

Ketones

Ketones (hydroxybutyric acid, acetoacetic acid and acetone) are absent from normal urine. They appear during starvation or uncontrolled diabetes mellitus indicating excessive dependence upon fat as an energy source. Ketones enter urine readily at low blood plasma concentrations.

The traditional test, that of Rothera, utilising nitroprusside, is sensitive mainly to acetoacetic acid. Modern convenient forms include tablets (Acetest) and dip strips (Ketostix, Labstix and other multiple strips). The purple reactions given by both are only semi-quantitative. Phenylketones and L-DOPA metabolites in large amounts, phenolphthalein and sulphobromophthalein can produce false positive results.

Gerhardt's test, which utilises the reaction between acetoacetic acid and ferric chloride solution (10 per cent $FeCl_3$ in 2N HCl), is not available in dip strip form. The solution is stable and can be kept on the ward for long periods. When added dropwise to 10 ml urine in a test tube a reddish colour develops with acetoacetic acid. A similar colour forms in the presence of aspirin metabolites, salicylates and L-DOPA. Acetoacetic acid alone can be boiled off by heating the urine, after which Gerhardt's test is characteristically negative. This test is less sensitive to acetoacetic acid than the nitroprusside tests but it gives useful coloured reaction products with certain metabolites (phenylpyruvic acid — green/yellow; homogentisic acid — brief blue/green) or drugs (phenothiazines — red/brown).

Haem pigments

Red urine is usually due to the presence of blood. Blood may occur in urine as intact erythrocytes (haematuria) or, less commonly, as free haemoglobin in solution (haemoglobinuria), or both. Haemolysis in urine, especially in hypotonic or alkaline urine standing at room temperature, converts haematuria at least in part to 'haemoglobinuria'. The macroscopic appearances of haematuria, ranging from opalescent 'smoky' brownish-red urine with small amounts of blood to frankly red urine with gross haematuria, are often characteristic. Accuracy requires the positive identification of any red cells present in red urine by microscopy of a drop of the urine in a wet-film preparation. Minimal haematuria may be detectable only by microscopy or chemical test. Haematuria has many causes ranging from neoplasms of bladder or kidney to glomerulonephritis and haemorrhagic diatheses. During menstruation the urine from females may contain some blood from extraneous sources.

Haemoglobinuria and myoglobinuria are states with free haem pigments in urine. Unlike haematuria, in neither case can the pigment be sedimented using a bench centrifuge. True haemoglobinuria is urinary pigment which earlier was released into the blood plasma (haemoglobinaemia) following substantial lysis of erythrocytes from various causes. Haemoglobin is freely excreted by glomerular filtration once the binding capacity of serum haptoglobins is exceeded. Myoglobinuria, stemming remotely from disrupted striated muscle cells, results in brownish-red urine resembling haemoglobinuria or haematuria. Haemoglobinuria and myoglobinuria give identically positive chemical tests for 'blood'. Both are detectable only by chemical tests at the clinical level; microscopy is contributory only in the negative sense. Precise identification, by chromatographic or electrophoretic methods, is important in pointing to the source abnormality in muscle or blood. Moreover, myoglobin, although freely excreted by glomeruli at minimal plasma levels, unlike haemoglobin, is damaging to renal tubules and can induce oliguric renal failure.

Chemical tests for 'blood' depend upon the peroxidase-like action of free haemoglobin. Myoglobin reacts likewise. The peroxidase-like activity catalyses the reaction between peroxide and a chromogen orthotolidine to form blue oxidised orthotolidine. Hemastix contains these reagents, as does Labstix, and both can detect the haemoglobin in as few as five to ten intact erythrocytes per microlitre of urine. Positive chemical tests for haemoglobin with negative microscopy for erythrocytes suggests haemoglobin-uria or myoglobinuria. A positive chemical test on urine of normal appearance is usually found to be due to microscopic haematuria.

Bile pigments

Normal urine contains no bilirubin and only minimal amounts of the colourless chromogen urobilinogen and its brown oxidation product, urobilin. The finding of these substances in urine implies abnormality in the bile pigment pathway for the metabolic degradation of haem. In the interpretation of the urinary findings the state of the faecal pigment judged by colour (brown = bile pigment present; clay coloured = reduced bile pigment) and the overall arrangement of the bile pigment pathway must be known (Figure 4.22).

Haem catabolism releases the yellow pigment bilirubin, which circulates unconjugated and protein-bound in blood plasma. Hepatocellular activity extracts bilirubin from plasma and secretes it in water-soluble conjugated (glucuronated) form into bile, which enters the gut. Bacterial action in the gut lumen reduces bilirubin to colourless substances collectively termed urobilinogen (also called stercobilinogen). Exposure to oxygen converts urobilinogen to brown urobilin. A small quantity of urobilinogen is normally absorbed from the gut and it is excreted by the liver in bile with a little being excreted in the urine. With a normal rate of haem breakdown and an unimpaired excretion pathway, bilirubin and urobilin are absent from fresh urine and only a minimal amount of urobilinogen is present. Even when present in excess, urobilinogen, being colourless, is invisible. It is oxidised, on exposure to light and oxygen, to urobilin, which causes the urine to darken in colour and acquire the orange-brown hue familiar in stale urine. Urobilin in urine indicates secondary change in urobilinogen after voiding and is of little value in suggesting excess of urobilinogen.

Three characteristic abnormal patterns are recognised. Bilirubin without any accompanying urobilinogen in urine and pale stools is

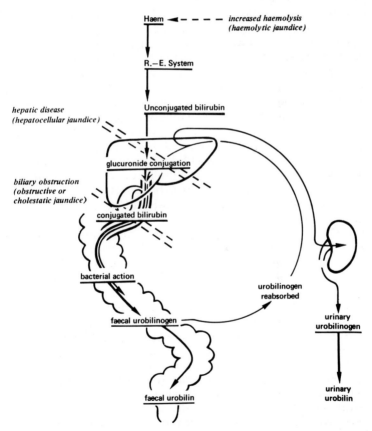

Figure 4.22. *Bile pigment pathway and enterohepatic circulation.*

associated with jaundice resulting from obstruction of the bile duct system (obstructive or cholestatic jaundice). Urine containing an excess of urobilinogen associated with jaundice (usually mild) and brown or even dark-brown stools is the combination of findings which results from abnormally rapid lysis of red blood cells (haemolytic jaundice). The third pattern is less common and consists of urine with excess of bilirubin and urobilinogen jaundice and normal or pale stools and jaundice (hepatocellular), which can stem from hepatic parenchymal disorders other than the subgroup which mimic cholestasis. Concomitant upsets in blood plasma enzyme activities (alkaline phosphatase, aminotransferase) are helpful in identifying the exact pattern in individual patients.

In urine, bile pigment, that is, conjugated bilirubin, generally causes a greenish-yellow or brown colour. The possibility that the colour is not simply the result of ordinary urochrome pigment in concentrated urine is decided by testing formally for bilirubin using a diazo reaction-based test, usually in the form of proprietary reagent (Ictotest, Ames). Fresh urine must be used since biliverdin, the oxidation product of bilirubin, does not react positively with the diazo reagents. Ictotest is two to four times more sensitive than the bilirubin-sensitive areas in the Ames dip strips (e.g. Bili-Labstix). The sensitivity of Ictotest is advantageous since any bilirubin in urine is abnormal and, because the renal threshold for conjugated bilirubin is low, some bilirubin can appear in urine with even slight conjugated-type hyperbilirubinaemia and before jaundice is clinically obvious. The finding of any positive result to Ictotest requires explanation in practice. False positive reactions are rare but may occur with chlorpromazine metabolites in large amounts. Bile pigment in urine to these tests is abnormal and an indicator of an excess of conjugated bilirubin in the blood plasma, that is, an expression of obstructive or hepatocellular jaundice. Urobilinogen in excess in urine is detected using Ehrlich's aldehyde reaction in the form of a dip strip (Urobilistix, Ames, or appropriate section of a multireagent strip).

On occasion, depending on the diagnostic possibilities, unusual tests are indicated. It is axiomatic that any unusual appearance observed in urine should be identified. Only in this way will uncommon but clinically significant substances be recognised. A good example is the red port-wine colour of the urinary pigments, porphyrins, which occur in porphyria, a group of disorders of haem synthesis. Both urobilinogen and the colourless porphyrin precursor, porphobilinogen, give a red reaction with Ehrlich's aldehyde reagent. Equal parts of fresh urine and Ehrlich's reagent are mixed in a test tube. Both urobilinogen and porphobilinogen produce red-pink colours within two to five minutes. One ml saturated sodium acetate and two ml chloroform are added, and the tube shaken. The mixture is allowed to settle. Urobilinogen is extracted into the chloroform, which turns pink. No colour change in the chloroform is observed with porphobilinogen, which partitions in the aqueous fraction. Note that Urobilistix cannot differentiate between urobilinogen and porphobilinogen.

Unfortunately only a few of the abnormal substances which may occur in urine are observable with the naked eye or are detectable by routine tests. Some, for example phenylketonuria and porphobilinogenuria, require specific chemical procedures and the tests which should be applied to the patient's urine are indicated by the possibilities arising during the clinical appraisal. For example the cystine content of urine is of significance when cystinuria is suspected but the chemical test is applied only after recognising specific indications. The urine often contains the diagnostic clue when sought after!

Microbiological assessment of urine

The positive identification of infection in the urinary tract depends upon the isolation of micro-organisms by culture of carefully collected specimens of urine. The recognition of micro-organisms during microscopy of a wet film of urine or in Gram-stained urine sediment is meaningful in expert hands but less generally useful than culture methods. For these purposes urine is selected from the 'mid-stream' during voiding. The first part of the stream carries away bacterial commensals from the area of the external urinary meatus. Before voiding women should cleanse the vulva from before backwards using tapwater-moistened wool mops. Mid-stream urine is collected into a sterile tinfoil bowl while avoiding finger contact contamination. If there is any vaginal discharge the introitus should be occluded with a dry wool mop. Bed patients need to be aided by nursing staff in swabbing down and collecting urine cleanly into the receiving bowl. It is only occasionally necessary to resort to the insertion of a urethral catheter for the aseptic collection of a specimen of bladder urine.

Despite these precautions it is difficult to be sure that micro-organisms grown from urine derive from the bladder urine and not the outermost section of the urethra. Experimental evidence indicates that when the common pyogenic pathogens have colonised the bladder the number of micro-organisms present per ml of mid-stream urine, the 'colony count', is usually in excess of 10^5 when the urine has been collected and cultured in the standardised way. Urethral commensals and contaminant skin micro-organisms are present in the specimen urine in smaller numbers ($\leqslant 10^5$ per ml).

Definitive appraisal of the urinary tract for infection requires quantitative bacteriology, sometimes on several occasions. It is imperative that such urine specimens are taken in the careful way described and transmitted to the laboratory within the next two hours or stored at 4°C until sent there. Delays common in clinical conditions make it often preferable to undertake the initial inoculation of the culture medium with the freshly collected mid-stream urine specimen at the bedside or in the clinic. This is possible using specially prepared commercial culture medium-coated slides in sterile containers. Inoculated dip slides can be delivered without refrigeration to the laboratory during the ensuing 24 to 36 hours. Such dip slides fail to isolate *Mycobacterium tuberculosis* and some other uncommon or fastidious organisms such as *Chlamydia* and *Neisseria gonorrhoeae*, which call for special culture media when suspected.

The culture of micro-organisms on two occasions with colony numbers $> 10^5$ per ml urine is termed 'significant bacteriuria', even in the absence of symptoms when the finding suggests covert infection. Indirect evidence of infection such as pyuria and pus cell casts in urine is less than conclusive. Pyuria can occur without infection in analgesic nephropathy or for a few days after cure of infection by antibiotics. Pyuria in the absence of the common pathogens should also suggest the possibility of tuberculosis. The isolation of *M. tuberculosis* requires the examination by egg medium culture of three consecutive early morning (i.e. concentrated) urine specimens.

Microscopy of the urinary sediment (Figure 4.23)

A graduated tapered centrifuge tube is filled with freshly voided urine to the 10 ml mark and spun at about 2000 rpm for three minutes. The appearance of the solid pellet of sediment at the bottom of the tube is noted before the supernatant urine is decanted off and discarded. The sediment pellet, mixed with a little residual urine by tapping, is transferred to a slide by bulb (Pasteurtype) pipette and made into a wet-film preparation with a glass cover-slip. The freshly made preparation is placed upon the stage of a microscope. Reduced illumination is necessary because of the low refractility of the diagnostically important organised components of the sediment. The light is cut down by narrowing the diaphragm and lowering the condenser. The whole wet-film is surveyed using the low-power objective ($\times 10$), special features being inspected with the higher power (dry) objective ($\times 40$).

The important parts of the sediment are the casts and cells. Casts are aggregations of Tamm—Horsfall protein with elongated

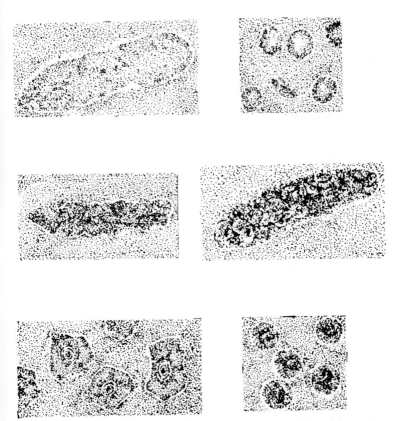

Figure 4.23. *Microscopic appearance of urinary sediments including (left to right) hyaline cast, erythrocytes, granular cast, pus cell cast, epithelial cells and leucocytes.*

cylindrical characteristics indicative of their origin in renal collecting ducts or nephrons. Cells may originate at glomerular level or more distally. Many of the cells in normal urine stem from the uroepithelium of the urinary passages including the bladder. Normal subjects excrete up to 15 hyaline casts, 500 erythrocytes and 2000 leucocytes per ml of urine. Note the excess of WBC over RBC. The normal sediment may contain up to two red blood cells per high-power field and up to three leucocytes. Casts on the other hand are rare in normal urine but one hyaline cast in 10 to 15 high-power fields would be acceptable. Disease changes both the number and variety of the cells and casts found in the sediment. For example orange-brown stained red blood cell-containing casts are common in all forms of active glomerulitis. Leucocytes are common in the presence of urinary tract infections. Leucocyte-containing casts are highly suggestive of infection at renal level and may be helpful in recognising both acute and chronic forms of pyelonephritis. In urine from women, contaminating vaginal squamous cells and leucocytes are common and these must be discounted for diagnostic purposes. With the exception of the flat hexagonal crystals of cystine in cases of cystinuria, crystals in the sediment are of little importance.

FURTHER INVESTIGATIONS

Gastrointestinal Tract

Radiology

Plain x-ray. The plain x-ray of the abdomen can be an extremely valuable investigation. The radiograph should be looked at for the presence of abnormal gas shadows, calcification and organ enlargement. In patients with intestinal obstruction the site of the obstruction can often be determined by the pattern of small-intestinal gas in the segment of the intestine above the obstruction and the absence of gas in the intestine below the obstruction. X-rays should be taken in both the erect and the supine position when the obstructed intestine is shown to contain air—fluid levels. In perforation of a viscus, such as perforation of a peptic ulcer, air may be seen in the erect abdominal film underneath the diaphragm. Air within the liver is an important radiological sign. If the air is confined to the area around the hilum of the liver then it is likely to be in bile ducts, perhaps as a result of a choledochoduodenal fistula. Air which is distributed throughout the liver shadow, perhaps reaching the periphery, is seen in a portal bacteraemia and is most often associated with vascular lesions of the small intestine. Calcification on the plain x-ray is again useful. Some gallstones are radio-opaque as are most renal calculi. It is sometimes difficult to distinguish between calcification in abdominal glands and calcification in relation either to the gallbladder or to the kidney. Calcification within the liver is associated with hydatid disease and some hepatic tumours may have calcium deposited within them. Calcification at the head of the pancreas is a useful diagnostic sign of chronic pancreatitis.

Contrast studies. A barium meal examination is useful with respect to the anatomy of the stomach and the duodenum. Development of fibreoptic endoscopy, however, has shown that these radiological investigations are not always successful in detecting duodenal ulcers, nor are they inevitably abnormal in patients with carcinoma of the stomach or gastric ulcer. Barium enema examinations, particularly when air contrast study is included, define the anatomy of the colon and suggest the presence of colonic tumours, polyps and ulceration.

Arteriography and venography. Arteriography of the gastrointestinal vessels is of particular value in patients who are suspected of having tumours either within the liver or within the pancreas and is useful in patients who are bleeding from the gastrointestinal tract. Sometimes arteriography will reveal the site of the bleeding provided the patient is bleeding at the rate of at least five ml of blood per minute at the time when the investigation is done. Splenic venography is used to demonstrate the portal vein in patients with portal hypertension before a portacaval shunt is attempted. Splenic venography should not be undertaken in the patient who has ascites.

Fibreoptic endoscopy

The recent development of fibreoptic instruments has enabled the examiner to inspect directly the oesophagus, the stomach, the duodenum and proximal small intestine. A colonoscope has been developed which allows direct inspection of the colonic mucosa. The value of such investigations is undoubted, for example in patients who have x-ray negative dyspepsia, some 30 per cent prove to have a lesion on endoscopy. Endoscopy is also valuable in the patient who is bleeding provided the investigation is done within 24 to 48 hours of the patient's admission to hospital. Colonoscopy allows the whole of the colonic mucosa to be inspected and this is the best way of diagnosing colonic polyps. Retrograde cholangio-pancreatography using a side-viewing endoscope with cannulation of the pancreatic and bile ducts enables the anatomy and the site of any obstruction or abnormality within these ducts to be defined.

Liver scanning

Liver scanning is a valuable technique which allows tumours of more than five cm in diameter to be shown up as a negative shadow in the liver scan. Pancreatic scanning is also available but the investigation is of less value than the liver scan. A normal pancreatic scan indicates that the pancreas is normal whereas an abnormal pancreatic scan may be seen in a patient who has no pancreatic disease.

Ultrasound

Ultrasound is valuable for detecting cystic lesions within the liver and within the abdomen generally. The recent development of the real-time ultrasound apparatus, which detects small gallstones within the gallbladder and a normal portal vein, is an extremely exciting advance which promises considerable diagnostic potential.

Biopsy

The histological examination of tissue from the gastrointestinal tract provides important diagnostic information. Biopsies can be obtained under direct vision from the oesophagus, stomach, duodenum and colon at the time of endoscopy. Small intestinal biopsy can be undertaken using either a Crosby capsule or the Rubin multipurpose suction biopsy tube. The sample of small bowel mucosa is examined using both the dissecting microscope and the light microscope. Small bowel histology may be of diagnostic significance in coeliac disease, acanthocytosis, lymph-angiectasia, Whipple's disease and hypogammaglobulinaemia and is of help in many other intestinal diseases.

A needle liver biopsy is indicated under the following circumstances: in the diagnosis of hepatomegaly, in the diagnosis of primary and secondary liver tumours, in the diagnosis of unexplained fever, in the diagnosis of splenomegaly, in the differential diagnosis of intra- and extrahepatic cholestasis, and when a precise diagnosis is to be made in patients with suspected cirrhosis, hepatitis, drug jaundice and hepatic infiltrations. It is important that liver biopsy is not carried out in patients with ascites. The most widely used instrument is the Menghini needle which is very simple to handle but the Vim—Silverman needle, which requires more complex manipulation, may be used to advantage in cirrhotic livers. Both intestinal and hepatic biopsy material can be submitted for electron-microscopic examination which provides much insight into disease mechanisms.

Functional studies of the gastrointestinal tract

Acid secretion from the stomach is studied following the intravenous administration of pentagastrin. The pentagastrin test is useful to assess the completeness of a vagotomy and may also be of use in those patients who have x-ray negative dyspepsia where endoscopy is unavailable. There seems little point in doing acid studies in the patient who has been shown radiologically to have a duodenal ulcer for the overlap of gastric acid secretion between normal individuals and individuals with a duodenal ulcer is large.

Pancreatic function is best studied by a method in which the duodenum is intubated and pancreatic juice is collected following the stimulation of pancreatic secretion either by parenteral secretin or by the intraduodenal infusion of a standard fatty meal (Lundh test). The test is of value in diagnosing patients with chronic pancreatitis. Pancreatic juice may also be collected and the cells studied in an attempt to diagnose patients with carcinoma of the head of the pancreas.

Investigation of the small intestinal function starts with the blood studies. Patients with distal intestinal disease have low blood levels of vitamin B_{12} and patients with proximal intestinal disease have low levels of calcium, iron and folate in the blood. Studies of proximal intestinal function include the glucose tolerance test and the xylose test. Faecal fat excretion is measured when the patient is on a standard fat diet (100 grams per day) over a three-day period. Small intestinal structure can be investigated by biopsy of the small intestine.

Stools

The importance of estimating the presence of occult blood in the stools has already been mentioned. If the presence of ova or cysts is suspected in the stool then a fresh sample of faeces should be examined in the laboratory under the light microscope. In some patients with pancreatic disease undigested protein foods can also be seen in the stool. Fat globules are obvious in patients with steatorrhoea.

Renal System

Radiology

Plain x-ray. The inspection of a plain x-ray of the abdomen routinely includes a check for the normal faint shadow of each kidney, the psoas shadows and for abnormal radio-opacities within the area of the renal shadows or the line of the ureters, bladder or prostate. The length of each kidney should be measured, pole to pole, since this characteristic is meaningfully altered in disease. Normally this is 12 to 13.5 cm in adults with a maximum normal difference of 1.5 cm between kidneys.

Excretory urography. Overlying intestinal gas shadows may conceal the renal soft tissue shadows. It is often necessary to display diseased kidneys and the urinary tract by using a contrast medium which is excreted in the urine, i.e. excretory urography. Excretory urography, often referred to as an intravenous pyelogram (IVP), involves appreciable ionising radiation near the gonads which should be protected by lead shielding whenever possible and particularly in children. Furthermore, the examination should not be carried out during pregnancy other than in exceptional circumstances. Especial care should be taken not to order excretory urography inadvertently during the first weeks after conception. Ideally women in the reproductive phase of life should only be x-rayed during the 12 days following the beginning of a normal menstrual period.

In azotaemic conditions, that is when the glomerular filtration function is reduced, the contrast medium is excreted slowly and the display of the collecting system, urinary pelvis and ureters is correspondingly less distinct. Definition can be improved by utilising tomography and an increased dose of contrast medium per unit of body weight. Tomography is a radiological technique in which the radiographer selects one transverse plane, for example the plane in which the kidneys lie. Within that plane, the radiodense features are shown sharply on the x-ray film while other features before or behind the selected plane are blurred out.

Excretion of the contrast medium opacifies the renal parenchyma briefly (the nephrogram phase) and this is followed within the next few minutes after injection by filling for several minutes of the calyces, renal pelvis and ureter (the pyelogram phase). In renal insufficiency these phases appear more slowly and, unless a high dose of contrast has been given, with less density and definition. Assessment includes a check on cortical width between calyceal tips and capsule. Distortion and clubbing of minor calyces, with localised narrowing of the overlying cortex and depression of the adjacent capsule, are characteristic of chronic pyelonephritic scars. Chronic glomerulonephritis causes general shrinkage with observable narrowing of the cortex. If sufficiently large a renal mass characteristically produces a soft tissue shadow within the renal outline and distortion of the calyceal system which is spread around the mass seen as a 'filling defect'. Such masses are usually neoplasms, especially renal carcinoma, and in the later stages they are commonly also palpable in the flank. Some masses, a minority, prove to be fluid-filled unilocular cysts. The distinction can be made by angiography or by ultrasound recordings.

Retrograde pyelography in effect is an extension of the basic cystoscopy examination, ureteric catheters being inserted upwards under visual control from below to permit the later injection of contrast medium directly into the renal pelvis and calyceal system from below. The subsequent radiographic display of the collecting system is usually well defined irrespective of the level of renal function. The convenience of excretory urography, the avoidance of the risk of introducing infection into the urinary tract and the effectiveness of the high dose-tomographic technique have made the retrograde method uncommon in recent years. 'High dose' excretion urography combined with tomography will usually enable the important distinction to be made between obstructive uropathy with dilated urinary tract on the one hand, and intrinsic renal disease with shrunken kidneys on the other. Excretion of contrast medium normally takes place within 20 minutes of intravenous injection but in disease states additional x-ray film exposures must be taken between six and 24 hours after the intravenous injection has been given.

Excretory urography finally shows the bladder filled and opacified by the contrast medium. When bladder neck obstruction is suspected, e.g. in prostatic disease, a post-voiding film should be obtained. The remaining contracted bladder shadow is an indication of the residual urine volume associated with the obstruction. Filling defects may occasionally be detected in this way. Some bladder deformities are produced by adjacent extravesical masses, e.g. uterine fibroids. While detailed assessment of the bladder lining requires direct inspection by cystoscopy (see below), the components of the act of urination can be displayed during a micturating cystogram. In particular, this special investigation shows the efficiency of the ureterovesical sphincter mechanism in preventing back-flow of urine into the ureters.

Renal angiography. Selective renal arteriography is a specialised radiographic technique which is helpful when major renal vascular disease is suspected. This includes renal artery stenosis or thrombosis or renal arterial embolic disease. Renal vein thrombosis is usually a complication of renal amyloidosis and may be recognised by renal venography. Arteriography is also helpful in outlining the arterial supply adjacent to and within a renal mass, which may previously have been seen as a 'filling defect' during excretion urography within the nephrogram or creating displacement and distortion of the calyceal system. In general, neoplasms have a leash of abnormal vessels near to and within them while, by contrast, simple unilocular fluid-filled cysts have no demonstrable new vessel formation. Ultrasound is capable of differentiating between a fluid-filled cyst and a solid neoplasm. Furthermore, ultrasound is a non-invasive technique which unlike selective angiography does not involve the insertion of a catheter into a major artery.

Renal biopsy

Percutaneous biopsy with a special (e.g. Tru-cut, Travenol) needle and using a posterior approach below the 12th rib, is useful in the identification of specific renal diseases. On clinical grounds it is often difficult to recognise amyloidosis, multiple myeloma, polyarteritis nodosa or systemic lupus erythematosus affecting the kidneys without examining the microstructure of the glomeruli and vasculature. This is particularly so in tracing the pathological basis for persistent proteinuria or recurrent haematuria in the absence of a lesion in the urinary tract.

Renal biopsy is intrinsically more risky than rectal or possibly even percutaneous liver biopsy. The risk from haemorrhage or laceration of the biopsied kidney becomes prohibitive when both kidneys are known on radiological grounds to be small and contracted. These features indicate a chronic irreversible process. Such end-stage kidneys are technically more difficult to biopsy and the attempt to do so is imprudent. Moreover histopathological interpretation of the tiny specimen may be difficult and even inconclusive. Renal biopsy is particularly indicated when persistent azotaemia or proteinuria or both occurs in the presence of normally sized or enlarged kidneys. Radiological assessment is invariably employed before resorting to biopsy in order that obstructive uropathy/nephropathy is excluded beforehand. Excretory urography is also necessary before resorting to renal biopsy since it is essential to confirm that the patient has two functioning kidneys. It is also necessary to display the position of the kidneys in relation to adjacent skeletal reference points. Percutaneous biopsy is contra-indicated if only one kidney is functional although open surgical biopsy is then permissible since haemostasis can be assured and the possibility of inadvertent and unobserved laceration during biopsy hardly arises.

Cystoscopy

Endoscopic visualisation of the neck and interior of the urinary bladder is a diagnostic technique largely restricted to surgical urologists. It is the prime method for investigating the urinary tract below the vesicoureteric orifices. This approach is mandatory in most patients presenting with gross haematuria and if it is necessary to exclude bladder neck obstruction. For example, enlargement of the median lobe of the prostate is essentially intravesical and cannot be detected by transrectal palpation.

Isotope renography

Radioactive iodine-labelled iodohippurate given as a bolus intravenously can be used in combination with a pair of gamma detectors, one placed posteriorly over each kidney to give an additional measure of renal function. The right and left ratemeters and associated recorders display the change in local radioactivity. While the hippurate is predominantly excreted by renal tubular secretion, the resultant time—activity curves reflect the successive vascular, secretory and excretory phases of each kidney. This technique, while intrinsically similar to excretory radiography, is more quantitatively functional and the component phases are capable of more detailed analysis. However, the time—activity curve gives no information about the pathological macroanatomy of the kidney and collecting system.

Scintiscanning with ^{99m}technetium DTPA, a molecule filtered out by the glomeruli, is an isotope technique which combines some of the attributes of excretory urography with the quantitative and time course features of isotope renography. The expensive gamma camera employed is capable of relating the emitted radioactivity to the topography of each kidney.

Ultrasound scanning

The kidneys are prone to develop cysts as well as tumours. The former are fluid-filled and the latter are solid tissue masses. This physical difference can be exploited for diagnostic purposes by scanning using ultrasound, and this is now the procedure of choice once a space-occupying lesion has been detected by physical examination or radiology. Polycystic disease of the kidneys, a common cause of enlarged poorly functioning kidneys, is readily identified by ultrasound. Ultrasound technique can provide information about the macroanatomy of a non-functional kidney when radiological and scintiscanning techniques are unhelpful.

Functional studies of the renal system

These are usually limited to estimation of glomerular filtration rate and quantification of urinary protein excretion rate. While inulin clearances are required for accuracy in research, endogenous creatinine clearance (Ccr) affords a cheap but approximate measure of glomerular function. This is simply calculated as follows:

$$Ccr = \frac{U \times V}{P}$$

where U is creatinine concentration in urine, V is the urine output rate per minute and P is the plasma concentration of creatinine. P and U must of course be expressed in like units, for example in micromoles per ml, with V as ml urine secreted per minute.

Accurate timed collection of the urine sample is critical. The result is usually expressed as ml plasma 'cleared of creatinine' per minute. This approximates to the rate of glomerular filtration in terms of ml plasma water filtered through all the glomeruli per minute (GFR).

Impairment of GFR, with accompanying reduction in endogenous creatinine clearance and development of azotaemia, is common to a wide variety of pathological states both acute and chronic. These may operate (a) by reducing vascular perfusion of the glomeruli, as in saline depletion, arteritis and gram-negative bacteraemic shock, or (b) by alteration of glomerular structure as in the many forms of glomerulonephritis and amyloid disease, or (c) by destruction and infiltration of renal tissue, as in hypercalcaemia, renal polycystic disease and lymphoma, or (d) by obstruction of the urinary passages at ureteric or bladder level. Identification of which particular disease process is operating depends on other evidence including full clinical examination. Nevertheless radiographic examination is often decisive in the initial sorting-out process.

Tubular function cannot be checked by any single test. This is to be expected since tubular functions are multiple and varied. In the majority of patients the renal disease present affects glomeruli and thereby nephrons as a whole. Consequently measurements of GFR do reflect well the stage and rate of progress of the disease process. Tests of renal concentrating and diluting ability, which relate to the capability of the kidneys to conserve or to eliminate water respectively, are available but are used infrequently. Assessment of concentrating ability in particular can be used as a criterion of the normality of the kidneys if that is in question, since concentrating ability is among the first functions to suffer in most diseases. Renal concentrating function is usually normal if the specific gravity of a sample is greater than 1.026 after 24 hours' deprivation of fluids. Urine osmolality is a better criterion, the corresponding value being 900 mosmol. Tests demanding less co-operation on the part of the patient, involving the use of parenteral injections of antidiuretic hormone, are available. Some discretion is called for in the application of these tests. For example, they could afford little information but might cause distress to the patient with a low GFR and obvious azotaemia. The induced dehydration incidental to a water conservation (urine concentration) test can potentiate the renal toxicity of myeloma paraproteinuria and even the iodine-containing contrast media used in urography and cholecystography.

Rarely, the renal abnormality is a discrete lesion affecting one tubular function such as amino acid transport or hydrogen ion secretion. In such patients GRF is not reduced and azotaemia is absent. Appropriate tests of these individual functions exist, such as amino acid chromatography or urine and plasma, and acid-loading tests respectively.

FURTHER READING

Bouchier, I. A. D. (1977) *Gastroenterology.* 2nd edition. London: Baillière Tindall.

Brooks, F. P. (Ed.) (1978) *Gastrointestinal Pathophysiology.* 2nd edition. London: Oxford Medical Publications.

Edwards, D. A. W. (1976) Discriminatory value of symptoms in the differential diagnosis of dysphagia. *Clinics in Gastroenterology,* **5,** 49-59.

Gabriel, R. (1977) *Postgraduate Nephrology.* London: Butterworths.

Newsam, J. B. & Petrie, J. J. B. (1981) *Urology and Renal Medicine.* 3rd edition. Edinburgh, London: Churchill Livingstone.

Sherlock, S. (1981) *Diseases of the Liver and Biliary System.* 2nd edition. London: Blackwell Scientific Publications.

Sleisenger, M. H. & Fordtran, J. S. (1978) *Gastrointestinal Disease.* 2nd edition. Philadelphia, London: W. B. Saunders.

Staniland, J. R., Ditchburn, J. & de Dombal, F. T. (1972) Clinical presentation of the acute abdomen. *British Medical Journal,* **iii,** 393-398.

Wright, R., Alberti, K. G. M. M., Karran, S. & Millward-Sadler, G. H. (1979) *Liver and Biliary Disease.* London, Philadelphia: W. B. Saunders.

5 The Nervous System

J. A. R. Lenman

The ultimate aim in the examination of a patient with neurological symptoms is to ascertain whether any neurological disease is present, and if so, to establish its nature in order to institute appropriate treatment; but frequently the first step in diagnosis is to localise the anatomical site of the disorder. Once this is known its nature can often be determined from a knowledge of the natural history of the disease. It is important to distinguish between single and multiple lesions, since the former may be due to a tumour whereas multiple lesions may be consistent with a vascular or inflammatory process, or a system degeneration. Frequently a careful history and physical examination enable a precise diagnosis to be made, but in some instances this is only possible after recourse to special investigations.

Localisation of a lesion in the nervous system demands a firm grasp of how the nervous system is organised, i.e. anatomical structure, function and in particular the way in which specific disturbances of function affect the patient. An important principle in clinical neurological diagnosis is that of progressive dissolution of function. This was developed by Hughlings Jackson, who considered that in disease of the nervous system the more recently evolved functions may be the first to be lost. Disease of the nervous system can give rise to (1) negative symptoms due to loss of function of a diseased structure, and (2) positive symptoms due to release of lower centres from control by higher centres in the nervous system. Thus in hemiplegia, paralysis of a limb is a negative symptom due to damage to the motor pathway, whereas the increase in reflex activity of the paralysed limb is a positive feature resulting from release of the spinal reflexes from higher control. In practice the situation is complicated by the compensatory adaptations which take place in response to the injury.

Although the different parts of the nervous system interact together so that the system may function as a whole, it is useful to think in terms of certain broad divisions which can be studied independently in the clinical examination. Thus the *motor system* can be distinguished from the *sensory system* although motor and sensory phenomena interact continuously. The motor system can be considered further as comprising the lower motor neurone, which includes the motor nerve cells and their processes, and the upper motor neurone, which includes all the motor influences in the nervous system from the cortex to the anterior horn cell. Thus if a patient has weakness of one upper limb, demonstration that the lesion has the characteristics of a lower motor neurone lesion localises the lesion to the nerve cells in the cervical cord, the spinal roots or the peripheral nerves. If the weakness is upper motor neurone in type, the lesion may still be in the cervical cord but could also be located in the brainstem or in the contralateral cerebral hemisphere. The mode of presentation of the illness and the presence of other physical signs may further localise the lesion.

HISTORY

The history is a vital part of the neurological examination and it is essential to obtain a careful and accurate account of the patient's illness. The age of onset of the symptoms must be ascertained together with their duration, course and development. Each symptom described must be analysed in detail. Sometimes the patient may not be able to give a clear account of his illness. For example he may not be able to describe what has taken place during an episode of loss of consciousness, he may have no insight into a disturbance of personality, or he may be confused or unable to speak. In these instances it is necessary to obtain a history from a relative or some other person who has witnessed the relevant events.

Genetic factors are important and the presence of a relevant family history must be carefully sought. The social history is also important where emotional factors may be significant or where there is any question of the illness being related to exposure to tobacco, alcohol or industrial chemicals.

Among the more important neurological symptoms which may form the basis of the clinical problem are pain, headache, disturbances of consciousness or speech, ataxia and muscular weakness, and impairment of sphincter control.

Pain

Pain other than headache may be the presenting symptom of a neurological disease and is sometimes the only complaint. It may result from irritation or disease affecting peripheral nerves, nerve roots or the sensory pathways in the brain and spinal cord and may be of great localising significance. Pain can vary greatly in character: neuralgic pain may take the form of lightning stabs of agonising intensity; deep boring pains of a peculiar unpleasant quality may arise in the viscera or in the central pathways; and burning pain sometimes associated with numbness and tingling may be due to irritation of peripheral nerves or roots.

In disease affecting the peripheral nerves the pain may be localised in the distribution of a single nerve such as the trigeminal or may be widespread and affect the extremities symmetrically as in peripheral neuropathy. Pain accompanying lesions of the sensory nerve roots is characteristically localised in a segmental distribution along the dermatomes innervated by the affected roots. This radicular distribution may cause pain to be felt at a considerable distance from the irritative lesion. Root pain is aggravated by stretching or local pressure on the nerve root and is thus frequently aggravated by coughing, sneezing or straining or by manoeuvres such as straight leg raising.

Neuralgic pain, within the distribution of the fifth or eleventh cranial nerve is characteristically paroxysmal. It may be triggered by touching a particular area and in trigeminal neuralgia the pain is frequently initiated by talking, eating, swallowing or touching a trigger zone on the face. Pain due to involvement of the central pathways of the nervous system is characteristically continuous and unpleasant. One variety occurs following an infarct in the thalamus. However, the pains that follow an attack of herpes zoster, or that occur occasionally in syringomyelia and which sometimes follow section of the trigeminal nerve are also partly the result of disturbed central function. *Central pain* may be aggravated by emotional stress and has a peculiarly unpleasant character which may give rise to unusual distress.

Paraesthesiae are abnormal sensations frequently experienced in a limb as a result of peripheral nerve lesions or following disease of the central sensory pathways. They are readily produced by pressure on a peripheral nerve and are then known as ischaemic paraesthesiae. Release of the pressure is followed by a succession of abnormal sensations known as postischaemic paraesthesiae. Study of ischaemic and postischaemic paraesthesiae in patients with spinal cord disease has shown that most forms of paraesthesiae are transmitted by the ipsilateral pathway in the cord which transmits touch and proprioception. Sometimes patients with disease of the sensory pathways in the spinal cord experience a sensation like an electric shock in the limbs if the neck is flexed (Lhermitte's sign). In young patients this may be evidence of demyelinating disease; in older subjects it may be due to cervical spondylosis.

Sensory loss may not always be recognised by the patient and not infrequently is discovered only during the course of physical examination. Sometimes the patient is aware of a subjective sensation of numbness or his attention may be drawn to loss of sensation because he may burn himself through being unable to recognise a high temperature.

Headache

Headache is one of the commonest of all neurological problems and is one in which the careful analysis of the details of the history is particularly important. Headache may be secondary to disease of the structures in the head, or primary where there is no recognisable disease. Primary headache is classified as tension, vascular (migraine) and cluster. The duration of the headache may give a very clear idea of the seriousness of the underlying disease. Thus headache which occurs suddenly in an adult for the first time may be the result of an acute meningitis or intracranial haemorrhage, whereas headache which has been a recurring complaint over 20 to 30 years is very unlikely to be the result of a progressive disease process. On the other hand, headache which has been present over a period of weeks or months suggests an expanding intracranial lesion and requires careful investigation.

The site of the headache is important and is best understood by considering which structures in the head are sensitive to pain. The scalp and subcutaneous tissues, the muscles, the periosteum covering the skull, and particularly the arteries are all sensitive to pain. Within the skull the dura covering the base of the skull is sensitive to pain as are the veins which drain into the venous sinuses, and the more proximal parts of the larger arteries supplying the brain. On the other hand the brain itself and most of the dura are insensitive to pain.

Pain-sensitive structures both inside and outside the head receive their sensory innervation from the trigeminal, glossopharyngeal and vagus nerves or from the upper three cervical nerves. If headache is due to a lesion situated above the tentorium, pain is generally felt within the distribution of the first division of the fifth cranial nerve. If the lesion causing the pain is below the tentorium the pain may be referred in the distribution of the upper three cervical nerves or the ninth or tenth cranial nerves. Headache can thus arise as a result of disease affecting the teeth, sinuses, eyes, ears and cervical spine. The headache of a brain tumour or other intracranial expanding lesion is derived from traction on neighbouring structures and its site and distribution is helpful since it may be felt overlying the tumour or on the same side of the head as the tumour is situated. In migraine headache the discomfort is frequently unilateral and in temporal arteritis the pain may be limited to the locality of the temporal artery. In tension headache where the headache is frequently accompanied by contraction of the scalp the discomfort is frequently diffuse and may be felt symmetrically over the head. If the headache is always in the same situation an underlying structural lesion is suggested such as a vascular malformation or a stereotyped syndrome such as periodic migrainous neuralgia.

The duration of the headache and its frequency are important when the headache is periodic and recurrent. Migraine headaches may occur regularly but may be confined to particular times such as the premenstrual period, or they may occur at a particular time of life such as the menopause. They are sometimes absent during pregnancy. Periodic migrainous neuralgia or cluster headaches occur in cycles of a few weeks or months during which the headaches occur in paroxysms several times a day. Likewise the headache of raised intracranial pressure may come and go, whereas a tension headache occurs particularly at times of stress; sometimes it is present continuously.

The time of onset of headache is less frequently consistent. Migraine may be present on waking in the morning and the pain of periodic migrainous neuralgia will frequently waken the patient during the night. The mode of onset is particularly characteristic in classical migraine where episodes of headache may start with a clearly defined focal disturbance frequently as a visual disturbance.

Attention must be paid to aggravating factors. Aggravation of headache by sudden movements or changes in posture is particularly characteristic of headache due to raised intracranial pressure but may be present in headache of vascular origin and is frequently a feature of post-concussional headache. Hypoglycaemia and the ingestion of certain foods, particularly those containing tyramine such as chocolate and cheese, may bring on migraine headaches. Rest will generally relieve a vascular headache. The quality of the headache can also be helpful. Migraine headache may have a throbbing quality. Migrainous neuralgia may take the form of a severe boring pain and a tension headache is characteristically dull, pressing and band-like and is often described by the patient with a wealth of detail. The patient with a headache due to a raised intracranial pressure is frequently unable to describe the pain in explicit terms.

Unconsciousness, fits and faints

The recording of the history from a patient whose problem is episodes of altered or impaired consciousness is one of particular difficulty, since the patient may not be fully aware of what is happening. It is essential to obtain a history from someone who knows the patient or who has witnessed the attacks. Nevertheless, a great deal may be learned from the patient's own account of what has taken place. Frequently the patient may have been told what has taken place when he has been unconscious and, even without this information, what the patient remembers himself may be of great significance.

In a *fainting attack* loss of consciousness is due to a sudden reduction in the cerebral blood flow and the patient may remember feeling unwell for a minute or longer before the attack took place. The patient who faints is generally standing when he loses consciousness, whereas a fit may just as easily take place when sitting or lying in bed. The person who faints may be aware of losing consciousness and may remember falling to the floor.

The loss of consciousness in an *epileptic fit* on the other hand is characteristically instantaneous although it is sometimes preceded by a premonitory sensation or aura, and the patient is aware of doing something before the attack takes place but then finds himself recovering consciousness. A person who has a fit may bite his tongue and pass urine but incontinence of urine occasionally occurs during a fainting attack if the bladder is full. Likewise convulsive movements may take place during a fainting attack if the patient is prevented from lying horizontal. The circumstances in which the attack occurs are also important. An epileptic attack may occur at any time of the day or night without apparent cause whereas a syncopal attack may occur as a result of severe pain or emotional shock or following a severe bout of coughing or sometimes during micturition after rising in the night to pass urine.

Major seizures

These may be diurnal or occur during sleep. If a clear description of the convulsion is obtained the nature of the attack is seldom in doubt. Sometimes the patient gives a harsh cry at the onset of the fit. After falling to the ground the first phase of the convulsion is the tonic phase in which the arms are flexed at the elbows with the legs extended and respiration is arrested. After less than a minute the clonic phase occurs in which jerking movements of the muscles take place and during this phase the tongue may be bitten and incontinence of urine and sometimes faeces may occur. The whole fit is over in a few minutes; the patient then remains unconscious for up to about half an hour and recovers completely or goes to sleep for several hours. Frequently the attack is followed by prolonged headache. Sometimes there is a period of mental confusion and occasionally a period of automatic behaviour or automatism in which the patient carries out complex actions of which he has no subsequent memory.

Focal seizures

If these arise in the cortex of the precentral gyrus over the motor area they are known as *jacksonian motor seizures*. The convulsive movements occur in a characteristic order determined by the spread of the disturbance over the area of the motor cortex where the parts of the body are represented. The seizure may start at the thumb, spread to the index finger, up the arm and then to the face, finally affecting the body, the leg and foot. The episode is characteristically brief, seldom lasting more than a few minutes. Occasionally focal convulsive movements may continue for days at a time — epilepsia partialis continua. A focal fit may subside without loss of consciousness but may develop into a major convulsion.

A *focal sensory seizure* consists of numbness or tingling sensations which also spread over the body in the order in which the parts are represented over the sensory cortex. Focal seizures arising in the temporal lobe give rise to a transient disturbance of consciousness without falling or to an episode of automatic behaviour of which the patient has no recollection (psychomotor attack). Sometimes there is an aura which may be visual, gustatory or olfactory. In some patients a vivid experience of déjà vu may be followed by a generalised convulsion.

Petit mal

Petit mal attacks are episodes of minor epilepsy in which there is a brief lapse of consciousness lasting for perhaps half a minute of which the patient may be unaware and in which falling is unusual. Petit mal nearly always commences in early childhood and must be distinguished from attacks of minor epilepsy due to a focal disturbance arising in the temporal lobe.

Epilepsy is a symptom and not a disease entity. It is not sufficient merely to make a diagnosis of epilepsy without attempting to determine what it signifies in terms of underlying disease. Genetic and constitutional factors are often important and a full family history must be obtained. Other events of importance in the history include a difficult birth with instrumental delivery, prematurity with low birth weight, meningitis in infancy and a severe head injury. Epilepsy arising in adult life may sometimes be due to a brain tumour and careful search for other evidence of an expanding intracranial lesion is an essential part of the clinical study of patients with epilepsy.

Vertigo

Vertigo is a subjective sensation of abnormal movement in space which frequently includes a subjective feeling of rotation and may be associated with nausea and vomiting. It is important in obtaining a history from a patient who complains of attacks of 'giddiness' to establish that a sensation of movement is part of the patient's experience because light-headedness or a feeling of faintness without any sensation of movement is a very common symptom with little localising significance. True vertigo indicates disease affecting the labyrinth or its central connections. It is important to ascertain how long the patient has been subject to vertigo, the duration of the episodes and whether they are brought on by changes in posture or accompanied by nausea and vomiting, headache or impairment of consciousness. The presence of deafness suggests a cochlear lesion such as occurs in Ménière's disease; diplopia, facial paraesthesiae and dysarthria suggest disease affecting the brainstem.

Ataxia

If a patient presents with a history of giddiness careful questioning may reveal that the problem is not one of vertigo but of impaired postural control so that the patient walks unsteadily. If ataxia is due to disease affecting the cerebellum the patient is likely to walk with a reeling gait; if the lesion is one of the cerebellar hemispheres he may reel from side to side; with a midline lesion there is a tendency to fall in any direction and this is known as truncal ataxia. Ataxia also occurs in diseases affecting the sensory pathways in which there is loss of proprioceptive information. In this case the difficulty is prominent when walking in the dark and characteristically the patient walks on a broad base with poor control of leg movements.

Speech

If a patient describes an episode in which speech was disturbed it is necessary to determine whether the difficulty was one of word finding or comprehension *(dysphasia)*, or one in which the patient was able to formulate his thoughts into words normally but could not clearly articulate what he said *(dysarthria)*. If the speech disturbance has recovered when the patient is seen it may be difficult without questioning relatives or close associates to decide whether the disturbance was dysphasic or dysarthric. If the disorder persists careful examination may clarify the nature of the disturbance.

Control of Bladder and Bowels

Impaired control of micturition has considerable importance in diagnosis. Careful enquiry must be made for this symptom if it is not spontaneously complained of by the patient. Precipitancy or urgency of micturition is seen in disease affecting the spinal cord and must be distinguished from the precipitancy which occurs in urinary tract infections or from stress incontinence in the female patient. Incontinence of urine also occurs when the higher cerebral functions are impaired as a result of organic disease of the brain, particularly the frontal lobes. Retention of urine is a particularly important symptom of disease affecting the spinal cord or the conus medullaris. It also occurs in lesions affecting the roots of the cauda equina or the first sensory neurone as in tabes dorsalis. Incontinence due to precipitant micturition, as in cystitis, must be distinguished from chronic retention of urine with overflow incontinence.

Incontinence of faeces is also a feature of nervous system disease, particularly of the spinal cord.

ASSESSMENT OF MENTAL STATE, PERSONALITY AND INTELLECTUAL FUNCTIONS

The examination of the mental state of the patient begins as he enters the consulting room. The patient's appearance may be unkempt and his dress untidy. It may be apparent when he relates his history that his ability to communicate does not match his social status and apparent educational level. Sometimes the patient's own account may give little indication of any alteration in mental state or personality and he may be unaware that he is ill. In these circumstances great dependence is placed on an independent account obtained from a close acquaintance or relative of the patient. Adequate assessment is particularly difficult if the patient has dysphasia. Mental confusion or emotional disturbance also makes assessment difficult. It is very important to describe the patient's mental state at the first examination since future management may depend on an accurate assessment of any changes that have taken place.

Orientation

It is important to record whether the patient is orientated in time and place. This is conveniently established by asking him to give his name, age, his present location, and the date.

Emotional State

Patients who are depressed may have a sad expression with little mobility of facial expression. They may be slow and retarded in their responses or they may be agitated so that they break down easily and weep. A diagnosis of depression is suggested by loss of interest in previous activities, diurnal variation in mood and disordered sleep rhythms. A facile mental state in which the patient's emotional responses appear out of keeping with his real circumstances may be seen in frontal lobe disorders; it is not uncommonly present in multiple sclerosis where it may take the form of an irrational euphoria. Hysterical patients may show a bland indifference to their apparent disability. An exaggerated tendency to laugh or cry with little provocation may be a feature of pseudobulbar palsy, where there is bilateral involvement of the supranuclear motor pathways in the brainstem.

Personality

A change in personality may be early evidence of disease affecting the brain and an assessment is made of how far the patient's manner and behaviour are consistent with what is known of his previous life and social status.

Intellectual Functions

Detailed testing of intellectual function is a specialised procedure best carried out by a clinical psychologist but much can be learned from simple bedside testing by the physician. The primary purpose of the examination is not to measure the patient's intelligence but to discover whether there has been any deterioration in mental capacity. The underlying principle is to see how far tests of concentration, memory and reasoning capacity correspond with tests which indicate the patient's level of educational attainment. Tests which depend on learning and short-term memory, the ability to calculate or think in abstract terms may be affected early in organic disease of the brain whereas memory of the distant past and the patient's vocabulary may be retained until a late stage.

The patient's recent and remote memory can generally be assessed in the course of history taking. Some indication of his basic level of intelligence can be gained from determining the age at which he left school, his occupation and work record since taking up regular employment. Formal testing may be carried out by giving the patient the following series of tests to carry out.

1. The patient is asked to remember a simple sentence such as a name and address and repeat it at a later stage in the examination.

2. The patient is requested to name the Prime Minister and Leader of the Opposition and the President of the United States and give the names of six large cities in Britain or six capital cities. General knowledge questions of this kind should be chosen according to the patient's education.

3. The patient is asked to subtract seven serially from a hundred. This test is impaired not only if there is a specific difficulty in calculating but also in general intellectual impairment and in psychoneurotic states.

4. The patient is asked to explain the likeness between pairs of similar objects, such as 'orange' and 'banana' which are both fruits. This test depends on the ability to form generalisations and may be poorly performed if there is intellectual deterioration.

5. The patient repeats a set of digits forwards and in reverse order. An average individual should be able to recall seven figures forwards and five backwards. If there is failure of concentration due either to psychoneurosis or organic impairment the test may be inconsistently performed.

6. The patient repeats a complex sentence such as the Babcock sentence: 'There is one thing a nation must have to be rich and great, and that is a large and secure supply of wood'. This test may be poorly performed in dysphasia, organic intellectual loss and psychoneurosis. In organic intellectual loss the patient may fail to repeat it correctly even after many repetitions and in psychoneurosis the responses may be variable and inconsistent.

7. The patient is asked to interpret common proverbs or a fable. Failure to accomplish this may indicate a failure of abstract reasoning.

8. The patient is asked to explain the meaning of a dozen words of which some but not all are in common usage. The extent of a person's vocabulary correlates closely both with a patient's educational level and with innate intelligence.

The above tests normally reveal any marked degree of intellectual impairment although they do not necessarily distinguish between impaired performance resulting from a neurotic or depressive illness and that due to organic disease of the brain.

Speech

A disturbance of speech should become evident at an early stage in the examination. The patient has difficulty in expressing himself, his comprehension is impaired or his articulation is indistinct.

In studying disordered speech it is necessary to decide whether the patient's difficulty is due directly to a disturbance of speech function or is the result of severe mental confusion. Sometimes a patient is mute in that although evidently conscious he makes no attempt to speak. Mutism may occur in mental illness but it also results from disease affecting the third ventricle or the frontal lobes.

If the patient has a speech difficulty it is necessary to discriminate between dysphasia, which is a failure to understand the spoken or written word or to find the words and phrases necessary to communicate, and dysarthria, which is a difficulty in using the muscles necessary for articulation. Dysphasia shows clear evidence of disease affecting one cerebral hemisphere, usually the left, whereas dysarthria is a consequence of disease affecting the muscles of speech, their nerves or their central connections. If dysarthria is central in origin it commonly results from disease in the brainstem or the cerebellum but it may also occur in extrapyramidal disease such as Parkinson's disease.

Dysphasia

In nearly all right-handed adults and in more than 50 per cent of left-handed adults the left cerebral hemisphere is the dominant hemisphere for speech. In young children cerebral dominance is not well established and dysphasia is less liable to result from a hemisphere lesion. In older children the dysphasia is less likely to be permanent. Wernicke's area on the first temporal gyrus and the neighbouring parts of the temporoparietal cortex is the most important part of the brain in connection with the understanding of speech and word finding but Broca's area on the third frontal convolution is also necessary for verbal expression. Disease of the frontal lobe may therefore give rise to a pure *expressive dysphasia* in which the patient is able to understand spoken speech but cannot express himself in words. Disease of the temporoparietal areas gives rise to *receptive dysphasia* in which both the ability to understand speech and to find the words necessary to express oneself are impaired.

The mildest form of dysphasia is *nominal dysphasia*, when the patient is unable to name objects although still able to speak, form sentences and understand what is said. A frequent and normal form of nominal dysphasia is the mild difficulty in the recall of names which occurs in healthy subjects as a result of fatigue. The symptom is associated with other forms of dysphasia. When nominal dysphasia is severe spontaneous speech is slow and interrupted by pauses in which the patient searches for the appropriate word or phrase. This type of speech disturbance may occur as a result of lesions in a variety of situations but is most frequently due to disease in the temporoparietal region.

In *receptive dysphasia* there is usually difficulty in understanding words and sentences and also difficulty in word finding. The patient may be unable to monitor his own speech so that he makes frequent errors. In its milder forms this may involve the use of neologisms or made up words and incorrectly formed sentences. A severely affected patient talks an unintelligible jargon and the difficulty in understanding speech may be matched by an inability to read or write. In *conduction dysphasia*, where the pathway between Wernicke's and Broca's area is interrupted, the patient again makes errors in his speech but is able to understand both spoken and written language.

In pure *word deafness* the patient is unable to understand the spoken word but can understand what is written and can speak and write normally. This is a very rare form of receptive dysphasia and occurs in lesions of the first temporal gyrus. Excessive use of neologisms which occurs when comprehension is intact may be due to a lesion interrupting the connections between the sensory areas for speech and Broca's area.

Difficulties with reading *(dyslexia)* and writing *(dysgraphia)* occur particularly in disease of the posterior parietal lobe. In disease affecting the angular gyrus of the parietal lobe dysgraphia and dyslexia occur in association with an inability to calculate and to distinguish right from left (Gerstmann's syndrome).

In examining a patient with suspected speech disturbance it is useful to start by testing the ability to understand spoken words. A difficulty in this respect may be evident from the history but in formal examination it can be demonstrated by giving the patient verbal instructions such as 'put out your tongue' or 'close your eyes'. The patient's ability to express himself in speech is noted from his response to ordinary questions. Careful attention is given to difficulties he may have in expressing himself grammatically and in forming complete and adequate sentences. A further test is the ability to name common objects. It must be borne in mind that mild nominal dysphasia may only be revealed if the patient is presented with a sufficient number of objects to induce mild fatigue.

Having studied spoken speech the patient's ability to read, understand written words and to express himself in writing is evaluated. Lastly the ability to calculate may be tested by simple arithmetical sums using pencil and paper.

Dysarthria

Dysarthria or difficulty in the articulation of spoken words may be due to a peripheral lesion affecting the muscles used in speech or their neuromuscular junctions, or to disease affecting the nerve supply of these muscles or the structures in the brain which control and regulate the peripheral nervous mechanisms.

Peripheral causes of dysarthria include myositis and myasthenia gravis when a combination of hoarseness and palatal weakness gives the voice a nasal intonation. In myasthenia the voice may be initially normal but gradually deteriorates as fatigue develops.

In dysarthria due to disease affecting the lower motor neurone there is difficulty in pronouncing consonants; the particular difficulty depends largely on the muscles affected. If the palate is paralysed there is a nasal speech which affects particularly the consonants m, n and g. Paralysis of the tongue makes it difficult to use letters such as l, d, n and t and in facial paralysis there is difficulty with labials such as b, f, m, p and w. In a spastic dysarthria where the muscles of articulation are affected by a bilateral upper motor neurone lesion, as in pseudobulbar palsy, the slurring of speech affects predominantly the labials. In cerebellar disease speech is slurred and articulation is irregular both in the spacing of the words and in the pitch and volume of the sound produced and the speech may take on a scanning and explosive quality. In Parkinson's disease speech becomes monotonous, lacking in emotional quality and with a marked diminution in voice volume. Palilalia, the constant repetition of a particular word or syllable, is also found. In some patients there is no difficulty in forming consonants but the patient is not able to produce any volume of sound. Complete aphonia occurs when the vocal cords are paralysed but partial difficulties of phonation are seen both in cerebellar dysfunction and in Parkinson's disease.

The examination for dysarthria consists of careful listening to the patient's speech during the taking of the history, paying careful attention to the volume and clarity of speech and to the ease with which particular consonants are pronounced. If there is evident difficulty it is useful to ask the patient to repeat certain test phrases such as 'British constitution' and to read a passage from a book or count aloud.

AGNOSIA AND APRAXIA

Whereas disturbance of speech and impairment of mental function may be recognised during the taking of the history and may be further analysed at an early stage in the examination, other defects of higher cortical function, such as agnosia and apraxia, may be difficult to recognise unless specifically sought. The detailed testing of these functions is best deferred until the general physical examination has been completed and is suitably carried out in several sessions, since fatigue may affect the patient's performance. Severe degrees of agnosia and apraxia, however, may become apparent during the testing of the motor and sensory functions.

Agnosia is failure to recognise a sensory impression in the absence of any impairment of sensation. *Apraxia* is inability to carry out an organised movement in the absence of paralysis or incoordination. Both disorders are evidence of imperfect function of the cerebral cortex, particularly the parietal lobe. The posterior portions of the parietal lobe are concerned with the ability to recognise both tactile perceptions, sight, and hearing, and the initiation of motor activity.

Whereas both parietal lobes are concerned with the perception and recognition of tactile and other sensations, the left posterior parietal lobe subserves language function and the right is important for the perception of space and the body image. The posterior parietal lobe, particularly of the dominant hemisphere, is also concerned with the initiation and development of voluntary movement. Lesions of either parietal lobe may therefore be associated with tactile agnosia. Disease of the left parietal lobe is also associated with visual agnosia and dyslexia, whereas disease of the right parietal lobe may be accompanied by spatial disorientation and defective appreciation of the body image. Apraxia is due to disease of either parietal lobe but particularly that of the dominant hemisphere.

In the examination of parietal lobe functions allowance must be made for the fact that the patient may have little insight into his disability, may be easily distractable and tire easily. For this reason the tests should be performed in quiet private surroundings and should be discontinued when the patient shows signs of fatigue. They may need to be repeated in several short sessions.

Examination for Agnosia

Tactile agnosia

Failure to recognise an object by touch is due to sensory impairment following a lesion of the peripheral nerves or sensory pathways, or due to a defect of the sensory cortex so that the patient is unable to appreciate characteristics of an object such as texture and shape. Tactile agnosia implies failure of recognition when both peripheral and cortical sensation are intact. It occurs particularly in lesions of the contralateral supramarginal gyrus. If the lesion is left-sided the disturbance of function may be bilateral. The patient is asked to identify with his eyes closed a variety of objects placed in either hand. He should be asked to describe the texture, shape, use and to compare what is felt in each hand. If he fails to recognise an object by touch in the one hand he should feel it in the other and if he is still unsuccessful he should be asked to look at it.

Visual agnosia

Failure to recognise objects by sight when they can be recognised in other ways is known as visual object agnosia. Usually the disability is limited to the recognition of small objects while the ability to recognise faces and large objects remains. Sometimes visual agnosia includes an inability to recognise and match colours and a specific disability to recognise familiar faces *(prosopagnosia)*. Visual agnosia occurs in lesions of the second and third convolutions of the left occipital lobe. It is tested by asking the patient to identify a number of common objects or by giving him a series of colours to match.

Auditory agnosia

This is a rare disorder in which the patient is unable to recognise sounds although hearing is intact.

Body image and spatial perception

Disease of the right or non-dominant hemisphere gives rise to spatial disorientation. In severe cases the patient may be unaware of the left half of space and unaware of the left half of the body *(autotopagnosia)*. If the patient is hemiplegic he may deny that the limbs are paralysed *(anosognosia)* or that the paralysed limbs belong to him. If there is a lesion of the major hemisphere speech disturbance may make examination difficult, but it may be possible to show that the patient is unable to identify any part of the body. In lesions of the left angular gyrus there is finger agnosia, agraphia, acalculia and right—left disorientation *(Gerstmann's syndrome)*.

The patient is asked to touch and identify different parts of his body and to identify his right and left hand several times in succession. He should be observed while dressing, which becomes very difficult when there is unilateral neglect and he may fail to put on a sock or shoe on the affected side. A sensitive test for unilateral neglect is to apply tactile stimuli to either side of the body separately and simultaneously. If there is tactile inattention the patient will be unaware of the stimulus to the affected side when both sides are touched at the same time. In the same way a patient may be shown to have an attention hemianopia: he can identify the examiner's moving finger in either the right or the left visual field when either finger is moved independently, but fails to notice the finger on one side when both are moved simultaneously. A further test is to ask the patient to draw a map or a clock face and if there is unilateral neglect one side of the picture may be left out or inadequately drawn. The patient may bump the affected side when walking through a door.

Examination for Apraxia

Disease of the parietal lobe leads to inability to carry out organised actions even when there is no loss of muscle power or coordination. If disease affects the dominant hemisphere this may lead to apraxia affecting the limbs of both sides of the body, whereas disease of the right parietal lobe gives rise to left-sided apraxia only. A lesion affecting the corpus callosum may block the passage of impulses from the left supramarginal gyrus to the right parietal cortex resulting in left-sided apraxia.

A patient with apraxia may perform automatic acts such as shaking hands or taking a pen out of his pocket without difficulty but fails to perform correctly on direct command *(ideomotor apraxia).* A more complex disturbance arises when simple individual actions are effected but there is inability to perform a task which requires several sequential actions. Thus a patient may take a pen out of his pocket, hold it in his right hand, open a pad of notepaper on the table in front of him and write, but when asked to write his name and address he is unable to perform the necessary actions in sequence *(ideational apraxia).*

To test for the presence of apraxia it is necessary first to establish that the patient has no weakness, sensory impairment or inco-ordination which could interfere with his actions and that he is able to understand what is said to him. Simple instructions are then given such as to put out the tongue, shake hands, make a fist or use a pencil. More complex instructions follow, such as to show how he would set about writing a letter. Care must be taken to differentiate the patient who has difficult in doing things to command from one who is able to perform actions automatically when they arise spontaneously.

Dressing disability has been described in connection with a disturbance of body awareness *(dressing apraxia).* It is due to agnosia for one half of space or of the body and is particularly likely to occur when disease affects the non-dominant hemisphere.

Constructional apraxia is a complex disturbance in which there is inability to reproduce simple patterns. It occurs in disease affecting either parietal lobe but is particularly severe when the non-dominant parietal lobe is affected. A woman with constructional apraxia may give a history that she has become unable to lay the table for a meal. The simplest test is to ask the patient to copy simple drawings with a pencil and paper. He may then be asked to copy designs made by arranging matchsticks or solid blocks which have one side coloured (Koh's blocks).

PHYSICAL EXAMINATION

Since the purpose of a physical examination is to clarify the problems stated in the history, it is logical to begin by studying the part complained of by the patient. Thereafter the examination must follow a strict sequence and, although there is no particular merit in following a specific order, it is particularly important that the neurological examination is fully systematic, otherwise essential details may be overlooked.

Emphasis has already been placed on the general appearance of the patient, his gait, dress and manner and the presence or absence of involuntary movements. *Gait* in a number of patients may be observed early in the examination but its detailed study will be considered later. A useful pattern to follow in the routine examination is to start by examining the cranial nerves and then proceed to a neurological examination of the limbs including gait, posture and the determination of motor and sensory functions.

Prior to examining the cranial nerves the *head and neck* should be carefully inspected. A large bulging skull suggests hydrocephalus, whereas a skull which tapers upwards may suggest oxycephaly. In acromegaly the bones are particularly prominent with a high forehead, large jaw, ears and nose and coarsening of the skin. Where there is a very short neck and the head appears extended this may indicate basilar impression or platybasia in which the angle between the basilar part of the occipital bone and the basisphenoid is widened to more than 140°. The head should be palpated for any skull defect or bony swelling. In infants the skull circumference is measured and the anterior fontanelle examined to decide whether it is open, enlarged or unusually tense. Percussion of the head may be helpful in children since an unusually high-pitched note may be noted in hydrocephalus and in such infants transillumination of the skull sometimes indicates the size of the ventricles. Auscultation is performed over the frontal bones, the occipital regions, over the closed eyes and over the neck since a bruit may sometimes be heard over a vascular malformation or a stenosed vessel in the neck. Where meningeal irritation is suspected the patient must be tested for *neck rigidity.* In order to do this the hands are placed underneath the occiput and the head raised forwards until it encounters resistance or the chin rests on the chest. *Kernig's sign* is elicited by flexing first one hip and then the other and then extending the knee. There is limitation of movement and pain in meningeal irritation. The sign can be misleading in infants with lax ligaments and in the elderly patient who has limitation of joint movement. In *Brudzinski's sign* flexion of the neck is followed by flexion of the thighs and legs. Where a lumbar or lumbosacral disc lesion is suspected the extended lower limb on the side of the lesion is raised and it is noted how many degrees of elevation give rise to pain (pain on straight leg raising — Lasègue's sign). If a lesion affects the upper lumbar roots pain may be elicited by flexing the knee when the patient is lying prone and hyperextending the hip.

In the preliminary inspection of the patient a careful examination must be made of the skin. Important signs to note are café-au-lait patches and subcutaneous swellings which may indicate neuro-fibromatosis (Figure 5.1), swollen discoloured patches particularly on the cheeks which may indicate tuberose sclerosis and naevi on the face which may be associated with vascular malformations in the brain as in Sturge—Weber disease.

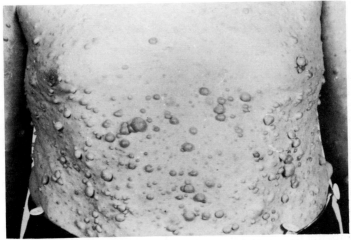

Figure 5.1. *Cutaneous neurofibromas in a patient with multiple neurofibromatosis.*

The olfactory nerve

The first cranial nerve is concerned with the sense of smell. Impairment or loss of smell is rarely the result of a lesion of the nerve itself but is usually the consequence of local inflammation of the nasal mucosa. For this reason careful examination of the nose is necessary.

To test the sense of smell the patient should be given a number of common or familiar odours to identify. Suitable substances are coffee, almonds, lemon, peppermint, soap or orange peel. The use of pungent odours such as ammonia which also stimulate the fifth nerve may give misleading results. Bilateral impairment of smell may be a complication of head injury. Unilateral impairment of smell may exist without the patient knowing about it and may only be discovered by careful testing of smell in each nostril separately. The recognition of unilateral anosmia is important since it may indicate a tumour such as a benign olfactory groove meningioma compressing the olfactory bulb or the olfactory tract.

The second cranial nerve

See Chapter 6.

The third, fourth and sixth cranial nerves

These three nerves supply the muscles that move the eyeball. The fourth or trochlear nerve supplies the superior oblique muscle and the sixth or abducens nerve the lateral rectus. The remaining muscles are supplied by the third or oculomotor nerve. The oculomotor nerve is also the main elevator of the upper eyelid and carries the parasympathetic nerve fibres responsible for pupillary constriction. Since the eyes are normally moved together in conjugate gaze, complex arrangements exist in the central nervous system to bring about reciprocal innervation between the muscles that move the eyes and a major structure links the nuclei of the third, fourth and sixth nerves, viz. the posterior longitudinal bundle.

Disorders of ocular movement. To test the external ocular movements the patient follows a fine point laterally to either side and upwards and downwards both when the gaze is directed forwards and when the eyes are deviated to one side. The test object should be held not less than 50 cm away from the patient so that binocular fixation is possible. With the patient looking forwards it is then brought nearer to the patient so that convergence also can be tested. After the patient's ocular movements are tested the patient is instructed to move his eyes voluntarily both laterally and vertically. This is necessary because rarely conjugate gaze is preserved for reflex fixation but lost for voluntary movement. Examining in this way tests firstly the integrity of conjugate eye movement; secondly, the presence or absence of squint of diplopia; and thirdly, nystagmus.

Conjugate movement of the eyes. Conjugate movement of the eyes depends on an intricate system of reciprocal innervation so that when one eye is abducted the other is adducted. Contraction of the one lateral rectus is accompanied by contraction of the opposite medial rectus and relaxation of the contralateral lateral rectus. This mechanism depends on connections in the brainstem between the nuclei serving eye movements on the two sides which are centred mainly in the posterior longitudinal bundle. Higher centres for conjugate movement exist in the frontal lobes, in the occipital region and probably also in the upper part of the brain stem. A lesion of the posterior part of the frontal lobe causes paralysis of conjugate gaze to the opposite side. The descending pathway crosses in the brainstem and a lesion in the brainstem may cause paralysis of conjugate gaze to the affected side.

There is a centre for conjugate vertical gaze in the upper part of the mid-brain and lesions in this situation may give rise to paralysis of vertical gaze. Paralysis of upward gaze (Parinaud's syndrome) is characteristically due to a lesion of the upper part of the mid-brain; it may occur as a result of tumours of the pineal gland and also as a result of vascular lesions and encephalitis.

Disturbance of lateral conjugate gaze arises following irritative lesions in which the eyes are deviated to the opposite side, away from the lesion. In a destructive lesion of the frontal cortex or internal capsule there is paralysis of gaze to the opposite side of the lesion and the patient may look towards the side of the lesion. There is ipsilateral paralysis of conjugate gaze if the lesion is lower down in the brainstem.

A disturbance of conjugate eye movements is therefore of considerable localising significance. Although it may not be posssible to decide the exact site of the lesion the deficit is invariably in the central nervous system and cannot be due to a lesion of the cranial nerve nuclei or of the cranial nerves innervating the eye muscles.

Squint and diplopia. Squint can be broadly categorised according to the age at onset. Adult squint is almost always related to a neurological disorder and is therefore usually of paretic origin, whereas squint of congenital or childhood onset (concomitant squint) is more often non-paralytic, arising from failure in the normal development of the binocular visual system. In clinical practice it is often difficult to be certain whether a squint is present, particularly in children. Acquired squint in the adult nearly always presents with a complaint of diplopia and the angle of squint is apparent on inspection.

The first step in the detection of squint at any age is examination of the corneal light reflexes. The patient is asked to look directly at a flashlight which is held approximately one third of a metre away. The position of the corneal light reflections in each eye is compared. The reflex is almost central in the normal non-squinting or 'fixing' eye, but is relatively eccentric in the squinting eye.

The cover test is now performed to verify the presence of any squint. The technique is as follows:

The examiner sits directly opposite the patient, who is instructed to look *directly* at the flashlight. The straight or 'fixing' eye is then completely covered with a card or the examiner's hand and the behaviour of the *uncovered* eye is observed.

If squint is present, *the squinting eye moves* to look at the light. In the case of convergent squint the squinting eye moves out (right eye, Figure 5.2a). In divergent squint the eye moves in to fixate the light (Figure 5.2b).

If the squint has become firmly established in one eye (uniocular squint), on taking away the cover there is movement back to the original squint. It is only in neglected uniocular squint, when the squinting eye becomes profoundly suppressed (amblyopia), that no movement is observed, despite the presence of squint, giving a false negative result: hence the importance of the early detection of uniocular squint by routine cover testing in the very young child from the age of six months onwards. Any child, particularly with a strong family history, who appears to have a squint confirmed by cover testing, must be referred for specialist examination by the ophthalmologist to exclude the presence of any ocular pathology such as cataract or other congenital abnormalities (focal choroiditis or tumour).

Adult, paretic or acquired squint is detected in the same manner and confirmed by cover testing. The characteristic feature of adult paretic squint is variability of angle of squint with the direction of gaze. The squint is greatest in the direction of action of the weak muscle, causing limitation of ocular movement in that direction. Testing the full range of ocular movement will reveal ocular muscle weakness.

On changing the direction of gaze the patient is subjectively aware of changing separation of the diplopic images. This forms the basis of the red/green diplopia test to elicit the specific extraocular muscle or muscle group involved.

Figure 5.3 illustrates the binocular pairing of extraocular muscles in the cardinal directions of gaze. The patient is fitted with transparent coloured goggles, red in front of the right eye and green

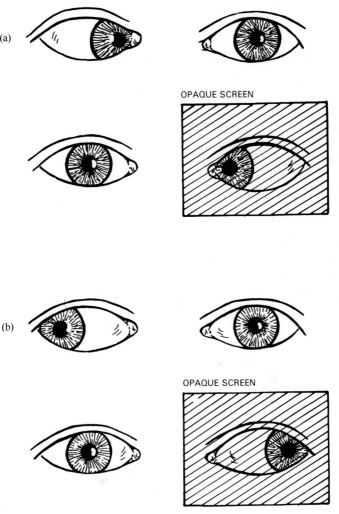

Figure 5.2. *The cover test. The* non-*squinting (fixing) eye is covered: observe the* uncovered *eye. Movement means squint is present; there is no movement in the absence of squint. (a) Right convergent squint. (b) Right divergent squint. Courtesy of Dr W. M. Haining, Dundee.*

before the left eye, and is asked to look straight ahead at a flashlight held at approximately one third of a metre away, to establish the presence of diplopia. If diplopia is present it is described as seeing red and green lights.

The light is then moved in the six cardinal directions of gaze shown in Figure 5.3. The patient is asked to indicate in which direction the two lights are widest apart and also the colour of the *'furthest out'* light. The paretic extraocular muscle is identified by two rules:

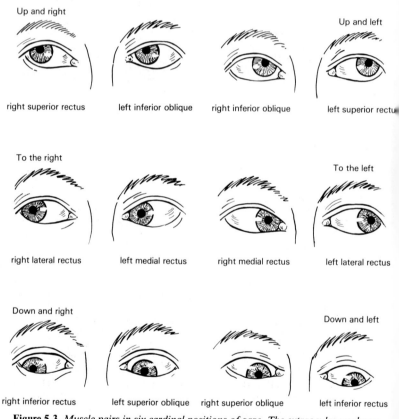

Up and right

right superior rectus   left inferior oblique   right inferior oblique   Up and left / left superior rectus

To the right

right lateral rectus   left medial rectus   right medial rectus   To the left / left lateral rectus

Down and right

right inferior rectus   left superior oblique   right superior oblique   Down and left / left inferior rectus

Figure 5.3. *Muscle pairs in six cardinal positions of gaze. The extraocular weakness of any movement can be defined in terms of the muscles or cranial nerves involved, as follows: lateral rectus — VIth nerve; superior oblique — IVth nerve; the remainder — IIIrd nerve. Courtesy of Dr W. M. Haining, Dundee.*

The 'furthest out' image belongs to the paretic eye; and maximum separation of the diplopic images is in the direction of action of the paretic muscle.

Nystagmus. Nystagmus is involuntary rhythmical movement of the eyes. It occurs as a normal fixation response when a person looks out of a railway carriage window and moves his eyes repeatedly to follow the passing scene. This physiological variety of nystagmus has been termed *optokinetic nystagmus* and it may be studied by asking the subject to observe an image on a rotating drum. The to and fro movement of the eyes includes a quick and a slow phase and in the case of the traveller looking out of the carriage window the quick phase is in the direction in which the train is moving. Nystagmus also occurs in healthy subjects as a result of stimulation of the labyrinths in the inner ear, either by rotation of the subject in a rotating chair or by instillation into the ear of warm or cold water. In clinical practice nystagmus is a valuable physical sign since it may denote a failure of the postural control of eye movements.

In testing for nystagmus the patient is instructed to look at a test object which is held in the midline and it is noted whether nystagmus is present on forward gaze. The target is then moved to the right, to the left and upwards and downwards. The extremes of lateral gaze must be avoided because jerking movements of the eyes occurs in healthy subjects on extreme lateral deviation of gaze. The target must be held not less than 50 cm away from the patient to ensure proper fixation. The position of gaze is maintained for at least five seconds as nystagmus may not develop immediately. Nystagmus which is not well sustained is of doubtful significance. In certain circumstances it is necessary to decide whether a sudden change in posture may evoke or modify nystagmus. Generally nystagmus is not accompanied by a subjective awareness of movement although it may occur with vertical nystagmus when the patient may be aware of the nystagmus (oscillopsia).

Nystagmus may be either pendular or jerking. *Pendular nystagmus* consists of a regular rapid deviation of the eyes to either side of the fixation point. It may be present on forward gaze and is sometimes accentuated on looking to either side. Characteristically it is due to poor vision and may be seen in individuals with severe myopia, defects of macular vision or albinism and as a congenital ιbnormality in individuals with normal vision. Miner's nystagmus is pendular in type and has been attributed to defective macular vision as a result of working in poor illumination.

In *jerking nystagmus* there is a slow movement of the eyes to one side which is corrected by a rapid jerking movement in the reverse direction. Jerking nystagmus may be horizontal, vertical or rotatory. It may be produced by stimulation of the labyrinth by rotating the subject or by caloric stimulation. In this event the direction of the slow phase depends on the direction of endolymph movement produced by the procedure and is the same regardless of direction of gaze. It is often accompanied by vertigo and nausea. Nystagmus of this kind may be seen in acute lesions affecting the labyrinthine system. Although the slow phase of the nystagmus is the one which is produced by the action of the labyrinths, by convention the direction of the nystagmus is always taken as the direction of the quick phase. If one labyrinth is damaged the quick phase of the nystagmus is towards the unaffected side.

Nystagmus also develops from disease affecting the central connections of the labyrinths, in disease of the cerebellum or disorders of the vestibular connections in the brainstem and cervical cord. In central nystagmus the quick phase is frequently in the direction of gaze to that if the patient looks to one side there is a slow drift of the eyes to the midline and a corrective jerk back towards the fixation point. Disease of the brainstem also gives rise to vertical nystagmus in which the movements of the eye are in an upwards and downwards direction. Ataxic nystagmus, also known as dissociated nystagmus or internuclear ophthalmoplegia, occurs with lesions affecting the posterior longitudinal bundle. It is characterised by paresis of the adducted eye and a coarse jerky nystagmus of the abducted eye. Although it can occur in a variety of conditions it is particularly characteristic of multiple sclerosis (Table 5.1).

Table 5.1. *Central and peripheral nystagmus.*

Peripheral nystagmus	Central nystagmus
Conjugate so that each eye is affected equally	May be conjugate or dissociated so that one eye, such as abducted eye may be predominantly affected
Unidirectional	May be direction changing with quick phase in direction of gaze
Enhanced by loss of fixation	Abolished by loss of fixation
Horizontal or rotatory	Horizontal, rotatory or vertical
Usually transient and associated with vertigo	May be persistent and unaccompanied by vertigo

Sometimes nystagmus is only evoked by placing the patient in a particular position (positional nystagmus). To test for this the patient sits on a bed or couch with his head turned 30° to 40° to one side. He is then moved into the horizontal position until he is supine with his head over the couch. If positional nystagmus is present he will develop nystagmus and experience vertigo after a short latent period. This may last for perhaps half a minute or may continue indefinitely. The first type is known as benign positional vertigo or nystagmus and is due to a lesion of the otolith organ sometimes following a head injury or as a result of infection or vascular disease. The persistent form of nystagmus is due to a central lesion in the posterior fossa. A rare form of nystagmus is so-called *see-saw nystagmus* which is a spontaneous nystagmus in which one eye moves upwards while the other moves down and occurs in lesions in the suprasellar region rostral to the third ventricle.

A useful special procedure which has helped in the analysis of nystagmus is the technique of *electronystagmography*. The nystagmus is demonstrated by recording the corneoretinal potentials with electrodes placed close to the inner and outer canthi. Eye movements give rise to potential changes which can be recorded by a pen recorder arranged so that an upward deflection refers to deviation to the right and a downward deflection to deviation to the left. This technique provides a written record of the nystagmus and is particularly helpful in connection with caloric testing. It also helps to distinguish a central from a peripheral nystagmus because peripheral nystagmus can be recorded in this way when fixation is abolished by eye closure or by recording in darkness, whereas central nystagmus is only present when the eye is open and fixating. The recording of optokinetic nystagmus with a rotating drum may also be clinically useful. Thus if blindness is suspected the presence of optokinetic nystagmus induced in this way is proof that vision is intact. In man optokinetic nystagmus depends on the integrity of the cerebral hemispheres, in particular the parietal and temporal lobes and it may be absent or difficult to elicit in lesions affecting the parietotemporal cortex.

The pupils and their reactions. The size of the pupil is controlled by autonomic nerves which act on the sphincter and dilator muscles. The parasympathetic nerves supplying the sphincter muscle are carried in the third cranial nerve and the postganglionic fibres arise in the ciliary ganglion. The dilator muscle is supplied by the sympathetic and the postganglionic fibres arise in the superior cervical ganglion. The sympathetic pathway has a very long course. The central pathway descends through the brainstem and the cervical cord to emerge from the cord at the upper thoracic segments and enters the cervical sympathetic chain. Postganglionic fibres pass along the internal carotid artery to the cavernous sinus plexus and are carried along the first division of the trigeminal nerve, leaving the nasociliary branch as the long ciliary nerves which pass to the dilator muscle in the iris.

In the examination of the pupils their size, shape and symmetry are noted. The light reflex is tested by suddenly shining a bright beam of light into one side of the eye which causes the pupil to contract briskly. Care is taken not to approach from the front as this may produce a convergence reaction. If the other eye is covered to shield it from the light of the torch it will be seen that its pupil will also contract briskly; the consensual reaction to light. The light reflex should be elicited separately in the two eyes. The reaction to convergence on the other hand is tested simultaneously in the two eyes. The patient is asked to look at a distant object and then the examiner's finger or a test object such as a pencil is brought about 9 to 12 inches in front of the patient's nose and he is asked to look at this. This should be followed by constriction of the pupils which dilate again when he looks into the distance.

In assessing the significance of pupillary abnormalities it must be recalled that local disease in the eye such as adhesions following iritis may cause the pupil to be small and irregular and react poorly to light. Sometimes direct injury to the eye may be followed by dilatation of the pupil. Otherwise a constricted pupil is evidence of a lesion of the sympathetic pathway anywhere along its course. If it is present bilaterally it generally means a lesion in the brainstem such as a pontine haemorrhage, but may be due to the action of drugs, for example morphine.

A complete sympathetic paralysis on one side gives rise to *Horner's syndrome* which consists of a constricted pupil with a mild degree of ptosis, enophthalmos and impairment of sweating on the same side of the face. The ptosis is incomplete since only the smooth muscle fibres of the lids and not the striated levator palpebrae are affected. Horner's syndrome may result from lesions anywhere in the sympathetic pathway to the eyes and face. In the upper brainstem it may result from pontine or midbrain haemorrhage and in the medulla from infarction as in the lateral medullary syndrome. In the cervical cord it is seen in intramedullary lesions, particularly syringomyelia. As it leaves the cord in the first dorsal root the sympathetic may be damaged by trauma and bronchial carcinoma may give rise to Horner's syndrome by involving the sympathetic outflow. In the neck the cervical ganglia may be exposed to trauma or infiltration by tumour. If the sympathetic fibres are affected as they are carried in the internal carotid artery ptosis and miosis occur but sweating is unaffected since fibres to the face pass in the external carotid artery *(Raeder's syndrome)*.

A dilated pupil suggests a parasympathetic lesion either in the midbrain, or along the course of the third cranial nerve or in the ciliary ganglion. Following a head injury the development of dilatation of the pupil may be the first evidence of pressure on the third cranial nerve as a result of increase of intracranial tension and tentorial herniation. A dilated pupil on one side is often due to a vascular lesion in the midbrain or an aneurysm of the carotid artery. It may occur because there has been prior instillation of atropine drops in the eye. Failure of the pupil to react to light may be due to a lesion in either the afferent or the efferent part of the light reflex. With a lesion in the afferent pathway the consensual reaction of the other pupil will be lost. With a lesion on the efferent pathway a light shone in the other eye will not produce constriction of the affected pupil.

The *Argyll Robertson pupil* is characteristically small and irregular in shape. It does not react to light but does react to accommodation and may be associated with atrophy of the iris. It reacts sluggishly to mydriatics. It is frequently present in neuro-syphilis in which however it may be present in an incomplete form. The exact site of the lesion in the Argyll Robertson pupil is not known but is probably in the midbrain close to the third nerve nucleus in the afferent portion of the reflex arc. Apart from neurosyphilis it is sometimes seen in other disorders of the brain-stem and may be seen in either complete or incomplete form in diabetes mellitus.

The *myotonic or Holmes—Adie pupil*, unlike the Argyll Robertson pupil, is characteristically large. It reacts extremely sluggishly both to light and to accommodation but on sustained convergence prolonged constriction may occur. Brisk constriction may be brought about by a minute dose of mecholyl in two and a half per cent solution. It is likely that the abnormality is due to parasympathetic denervation of the pupil, the site of the lesion being in the ciliary ganglion and the pupil showing denervation hypersensitivity. It is an important sign to recognise because although it occurs in association with other signs in the central nervous system, such as absent knee and ankle jerks, it gives rise to no symptoms other than occasional blurring of vision and is not associated with progressive disease of the nervous system.

The fifth cranial nerve

The fifth cranial nerve or trigeminal nerve is divided into three divisions, the first or ophthalmic, the second or maxillary and the third or mandibular division. All three divisions contain sensory fibres which have their first cell station in the Gasserian ganglion from which the sensory root passes to enter the lateral aspect of the pons. The third or mandibular division also contains motor fibres to supply the muscles which move the jaw. The greater part of the face receives its sensory supply from the fifth cranial nerve which also supplies the anterior two thirds of the tongue, but the angle of the jaw is supplied by the upper cervical segments (see Figure 5.20).

In the examination of the fifth nerve sensory testing is carried out in all three divisions of the nerve, testing for pain, light touch and temperature and it may also be necessary to test over the anterior two-thirds of the tongue. Wasting and weakness of the temporalis and masseter muscles is revealed by inspection and palpation. Power is tested by asking the patient to open the jaw. If there is marked weakness there is deviation to the weaker side and moderate weakness may be detected if the patient attempts to open the jaw against resistance.

The *corneal reflex* consists of blinking of both eyes when the cornea of one is touched. Both eyes should be tested and the procedure is to touch the cornea lightly while the patient is looking to one side. The cornea may be touched with a wisp of cotton wool or fine tissue. Loss of the corneal reflex may be evident before any other signs of fifth nerve deficit are present and is of value in the early detection of a tumour of the lateral recess such as an acoustic neuroma. The corneal reflex is distinct from the conjunctival reflex, which has a similar afferent and efferent pathway but is not always present in healthy subjects. To elicit the *jaw jerk* the patient opens his mouth slightly and the examiner places his forefinger on the chin below the lower lip. The examiner then taps the finger lightly with a percussion hammer. In the healthy subject the jaw jerk can only just be elicited but in the presence of an upper motor neurone lesion above the level of the pons the reflex may be exaggerated. The trigeminal nerve also subserves the afferent pathway for the *blink reflex*. The efferent arc is by the facial nerve and the reflex response of blinking is evoked by a light tap to the forehead (glabellar tap). In a healthy subject this reflex habituates rapidly but in Parkinson's disease repeated stimuli continue to evoke a response.

The seventh cranial nerve

The facial nerve arises from a nucleus in the pons and runs a long course in the facial canal of the temporal bone to supply the muscles of facial expression. It also supplies the stapedius muscle and for part of its course travels in close association with the nervus intermedius which carries fibres derived from the chorda tympani subserving taste in the anterior two-thirds of the tongue. The frontalis muscle which normally moves symmetrically on either side is represented on both sides of the motor cortex and consequently an upper motor neurone lesion affecting the facial nerve on one side tends to leave movement of the forehead muscles intact while the rest of the facial muscles are paralysed. The central pathways for emotional and voluntary movement are different and for this reason in an upper motor neurone lesion of the facial nerve emotional movements of facial expression are frequently intact when voluntary movement involving all the facial muscles is impaired. The converse may also occur so that voluntary movement is preserved but emotional movement is lost.

On examination of the facial nerve, inspection may show facial asymmetry, wasting of the facial muscles, twitching, fasciculation or involuntary movements, poverty of facial expression and drooping of the angle of the mouth on the affected side. In the formal examination of facial movements the patient is asked to bare his teeth and in doing this it is helpful if the examiner does the same thing to show the patient what is required. Next the patient is asked to puff out his cheeks and purse his lips, as when whistling, and to open his mouth. All these movements are defective in either upper or lower motor neurone lesions. The upper part of the face is tested by asking the patient to close his eyes, screw them up tightly and hold them tightly closed when the examiner attempts to open them. Lastly the patient is asked to raise his eyebrows and this will be defective in a lower motor neurone lesion but may be intact in an upper motor neurone lesion.

To test the sense of taste the patient is asked to protrude his tongue, the tip of which can be held gently, and test substances are applied to either side of the tongue. In between each test the patient should wash his mouth with water. Since there are only four primary tastes —sweet, salt, sour and bitter — testing of taste is carried out adequately with four flavours viz., sugar, salt, vinegar and quinine. If an electrical current is passed through the tongue this will give rise to a metallic taste, and the threshold of taste can be measured by an instrument known as a gustometer, which enables one to pass a measured current into the tongue. A normal subject tested in this way will detect a current of the order of $20\,\mu A$. A very simple technique is to use two leaves of copper and zinc soldered together at one end. If the two ends are applied by the examiner to the tongue this will give rise to a small electric current and a metallic taste will be noted if taste sensation is intact.

An *upper motor neurone facial palsy* can be recognised by the fact that only the muscles of the lower part of the face are affected and facial movements may be intact following an emotional stimulus when they are lost for voluntary movement. A *lower motor neurone lesion* affects all the muscles of the face supplied by the facial nerve on the side of the lesion. If the lesion affects the geniculate ganglion or the part of the nerve between the ganglion and its junction with the chorda tympani taste also may be lost on the affected side. Upper motor neurone lesions of the facial nerve occur commonly in cerebral vascular accidents, in cerebral tumours and sometimes in demyelinating disease. Loss of emotional movements in both sides occurs frequently in Parkinson's disease and on one side in lesions affecting the thalamus. A lower motor neurone facial palsy is most commonly the result of Bell's palsy but it can be due to any lesion affecting the nerve between the nucleus in the pons and the muscles it supplies including tumours of the cerebellopontine angle, fractures of the petrous bone, tumours of the parotid or sarcoidosis. Bilateral palsy of the facial nerve occurs in peripheral neuritis, encephalitis, motor neurone disease and leukaemia. In muscular dystrophy there is frequently weakness of the muscles, particularly those supplying the orbicularis oris and the orbicularis oculi which results in a characteristic myopathic facial expression and an inability to purse the lips in a whistle.

The eighth cranial nerve

The eighth or acoustic nerve comprises two divisions, the cochlear nerve and the vestibular nerve. The fibres of the cochlear nerve arise from bipolar cells in the spiral ganglion of the cochlea and pass centrally to end in the cochlear nuclei of the medulla. The vestibular nerve arises from bipolar cells in the vestibular ganglion and again the central termination is in the medulla in the vestibular nuclei.

In testing the cochlear division the first aim is to ascertain whether or not deafness is present, and secondly to determine the cause of the deafness. Deafness is of two types. In *conductive deafness* there is malfunction or obstruction of the external or middle ear; in *perceptive deafness* there is impaired function of the receptors of the cochlea or a lesion affecting the eighth nerve. It is important to distinguish cochlear deafness from retrocochlear deafness due to a lesion of the eighth nerve.

Both the history and the mode of speech of the patient may be helpful in recognising the nature of a patient's deafness. Thus a patient with *conductive deafness* may find that it is possible to hear and understand speech better in noisy than in quiet surroundings. This is known as paracusis and is particularly characteristic of otosclerosis. In *perceptive deafness* on the other hand the patient may be abnormally sensitive to small increases in the loudness of sound and may complain that persons who talk to him in a normal voice are shouting. This is due to the recruitment of loudness phenomenon which is particularly characteristic of deafness due to cochlear lesions. In perceptive deafness the hearing loss may affect predominantly the higher frequencies so that in rapid speech the high-pitched sounds of consonants may be missed and the patient may have difficulty in understanding speech unless he is spoken to slowly. In conductive deafness the patient may hear his own speech clearly by bone conduction even when he speaks quietly. He thinks he is talking loudly and for this reason a patient with conductive deafness may speak abnormally quietly. On the other hand a patient with perceptive deafness may hardly hear his own speech and consequently may tend to shout during conversation.

To test hearing the patient is asked to repeat words whispered to him when his eyes are closed and one ear occluded. A patient with intact hearing should be able to recognise the whispered voice at a distance of three feet. Other simple tests are to ask the patient if he can hear a watch ticking at 30 inches (75 cm) from the ear or if he can appreciate the noise of a tuning fork vibrating at 256 Hz. If deafness is present the external ear should be examined by means of an electric auriscope to make sure that it is not occluded by wax and that there is no injury to the tympanic membrane. The healthy drum is pinkish grey in colour and the malleus can be seen situated nearly vertically across the tympanic membrane.

The detailed analysis of hearing is best carried out by means of an audiometer but simple bedside tests can be undertaken with a tuning fork. *Rinne's test* is performed by placing a vibrating tuning fork at 256 or 512 Hz over the mastoid bone. The patient is asked to indicate when the sound is no longer heard. The tuning fork is then removed and the vibrating end held close to the external ear and in the healthy subject the sound will again be heard since air conduction is normally better than bone conduction. In conductive deafness bone conduction is better than air conduction whereas in perceptive deafness both air and bone conduction may be equally affected. In *Weber's test* the tuning fork is applied to the forehead or to the vertex and the patient is asked to say where he hears the sound. In the healthy subject the sound is heard in the midline but in perceptive deafness the sound will be heard less well on the affected side. In conductive deafness on the other hand the sound is better heard in the affected ear; this is because in conductive deafness the sound is transmitted by bone conduction equally well on either side but on the healthy side sound may be masked to some extent by the background noise in the room which is transmitted by air conduction.

A more detailed analysis of hearing can be undertaken using a *pure tone audiometer.* This is an instrument which produces musical notes of varying pitch and intensity. By this means the hearing loss in decibels can be measured throughout the auditory frequency band both for air conduction and bone conduction. In this test perceptive deafness will be found to affect the higher frequency bands selectively. *Speech audiometry* is a further valuable test which will not only distinguish perceptive from conductive deafness but also discriminates between end organ and nerve deafness. The procedure is to play back tape recorded speech at different sound intensities and the percentage of words recognised at each sound intensity is recorded. In cochlear deafness, although word recognition improves to some extent as sound intensity increases a point is soon reached where increasing the sound intensity further leads to a deterioration in word recognition.

A number of refined tests using the pure tone audiometer will also discriminate between end organ and nerve deafness. One of these is *recruitment of loudness.* In this the patient is presented with sound in each ear, the intensity of which is progressively increased in loudness. When recruitment is present loud noises are experienced as equally intense in the two ears but soft noises are heard less acutely in the affected ear. Recruitment of loudness is an indication of cochlear deafness and is characteristically present in Ménière's syndrome but absent when deafness is due to an acoustic neuroma. The mechanism of recruitment is not fully understood.

A limitation on the recruitment test is that it is only helpful if deafness is largely confined to one ear. Several other tests however have been developed which depend on the fact that in cochlear deafness relatively small increments in sound intensity will produce a relatively large increase in the sensation of loudness. In the *short increment sensitivity index* (SISI) the ability of the subject to appreciate increases of about one decibel in the loudness of a continuous tone is tested and this is a helpful test in the presence of bilateral disease. Tone decay occurs in perceptive deafness and is particularly marked in nerve deafness. Bekesy audiometry depends on the phenomenon of tone decay or adaptation so that the intensity of a pure tone appears to fall when listened to continuously (Table 5.2).

The vestibular division of the eighth nerve cannot be readily tested at the bedside. The patient can however be tested for nystagmus both in the resting position and following a sudden change in posture as detailed in a previous section. The integrity of

Table 5.2. *Conductive and perceptive deafness.*

Conductive deafness
Speech may be better heard in noisy surroundings (paracusis)
Bone conduction better than air conduction (Rinné)
Bone conduction lateralised to deaf ear (Weber)
Amplification of speech increases intelligibility (speech audiometry)

Perceptive deafness
Patient may be abnormally sensitive to small increases in sound — people seem to be shouting
High frequencies predominantly affected so that speech may be poorly understood
Bone conduction lateralised to normal ear (Weber)
Amplification of speech above a certain level decreases intelligibility (speech audiometry)

Cochlear deafness	*Nerve or retrocochlear deafness*
Recruitment present	No recruitment
Increase in short increment sensitivity (SISI)	Short increment sensitivity normal (SISI)
Little tone decay	Marked tone decay

one labyrinth can be studied in the laboratory procedure of *caloric testing* in which cold and warm water are successively instilled into each ear and the duration of the resulting nystagmus is recorded. If the patient lies with his head elevated 30 degrees the lateral semicircular canal is vertical; warm water in the ear will produce an upward flow of endolymph and cold water a downward flow. Thus warm water (44°C) will give rise to nystagmus with a quick phase toward the side stimulated and cold water (30°C) nystagmus with the quick phase toward the opposite side. Failure to produce nystagmus by stimulating one side is known as canal paresis and indicates malfunction of one labyrinth. A second abnormality is directional preponderance which means that nystagmus in one direction is more prolonged than nystagmus in the other. Directional preponderance can be caused either by peripheral or by central lesions.

The ninth cranial nerve

The ninth or glossopharyngeal nerve has a small motor supply to the stylopharyngeus muscle and also an autonomic supply to the parotid gland. Its peripheral function is a sensory one conveying ordinary sensation from the posterior third of the tongue and the pharynx and also the middle ear and the eustachian tube. It also carries taste sensation from the posterior third of the tongue. It is difficult to test for taste in this distribution in isolation and the usual test for the integrity of the ninth nerve is to ascertain if the patient is aware of sensation on the posterior wall of the pharynx. Normally a person will gag if this area is touched and loss of the gag reflex results from damage to the afferent arc subserved by the glossopharyngeal nerve.

The tenth cranial nerve

Motor fibres of the tenth cranial or vagus nerve arise from the nucleus ambiguus and in addition autonomic fibres are derived from the dorsal motor nucleus in the medulla. Sensory fibres carrying visceral sensation arise from the nodose ganglia and terminate in the tractus solitarius of the medulla. The motor supply is to the palate, larynx and pharynx and the autonomic supply to the heart, bronchi and the gastrointestinal tract. A patient with a lesion of the vagus nerve has a hoarse voice if there is vocal cord paralysis and a nasal voice if the palate is paralysed. He may have difficulty in swallowing his saliva. The muscles supplied by the tenth as well as the eleventh and twelfth nerves are represented bilaterally in the cortex and are concerned with bilateral movements. Supranuclear lesions therefore produce little disability unless they are bilateral when a pseudobulbar palsy results.

To test the functions of the nerve the patient is asked to open his mouth and say 'Ah'. If necessary a tongue depressor is used to depress the tongue. In the healthy subject the uvula will be central and the palate will move upwards equally on either side. If there is unilateral paralysis the palate will be drawn to the healthy side which will also rise higher than the paralysed side. Bilateral paralysis will result in no visible movement of the palate which may hang low.

If hoarseness is present the vocal cords should be examined. This can be done using a laryngeal mirror but the technique requires special skill and is best undertaken by an experienced examiner. In unilateral abductor paralysis the affected cord lies close to the midline and fails to abduct on inspiration; it is generally due to a lesion of the recurrent laryngeal nerve. In unilateral total paralysis the cord lies in mid-abduction but is pulled to the abnormal side on phonation. This also may be due to a recurrent laryngeal nerve lesion but is more likely to be due to a severe lesion of the trunk of the vagus or of the nucleus ambiguus. Bilateral lesions are less common; in total paralysis phonation is impossible and in abductor paralysis the cords lie close together and do not abduct on inspiration so that severe respiratory distress may result. Phonation may also be lost if the adductors are paralysed but this is usually hysterical and adduction may still occur in coughing.

The eleventh cranial nerve

The spinal accessory nerve arises from the cervical cord in the upper five segments to enter the skull through the foramen magnum and leave it through the jugular foramen to supply the sternomastoid and trapezius muscles. A cranial portion of the accessory nerve arising from the caudal part of the nucleus ambiguus is described and these fibres join the vagus nerve.

To test the sternomastoid the patient is asked to turn his head to one side against resistance when the contralateral sternomastoid will contract. The patient is then asked to bend his head forwards with the examiner's hand placed on the forehead to resist this manoeuvre and both muscles will contract. The trapezius is tested by asking the patient to raise his shoulders against resistance of the examiner's hands which are placed on top of the shoulders. Bilateral weakness of the sternomastoid occurs in muscular dystrophy, in motor neurone disease and particularly in dystrophia myotonica. Bilateral weakness of the trapezius may be seen in motor neurone disease or poliomyelitis. Syringomyelia, tumours of the jugular foramen and infections such as poliomyelitis can give rise to unilateral abnormalities.

The twelfth cranial nerve

The fibres of the twelfth or hypoglossal nerve arise from a nucleus on the floor of the fourth ventricle in the medulla, leave the skull through the hypoglossal canal and innervate the intrinsic muscles of the tongue on the same side. It is tested by asking the patient to protrude the tongue and move it from side to side. The tongue is also inspected when resting on the floor of the mouth; in this position wasting, fibrillation and fasciculation may be observed. The tongue is the only site in the body where the fine movements of fibrillation can be seen through the intact skin. If there is a unilateral lower motor neurone lesion, in addition to wasting being present on the affected side, the tongue deviates towards the affected side when it is protruded (Figure 5.4). In a bilateral upper motor neurone lesion movement of the tongue may be difficult and slow. If myotonia is suspected the tongue should be tapped sharply with a blunt point when a local contraction may be observed. Again, with an upper motor neurone lesion affecting the nerve on one side, the tongue may deviate on protrusion but this deviation is less marked than with a lower motor neurone lesion. Sometimes if there is facial palsy the tongue may appear to deviate to one side but this is a result of asymmetry of the mouth.

Examination of Motor Functions

It is useful to distinguish between the motor and the sensory systems although all nervous activity is derived from the interaction of afferent and efferent signals so that motor and sensory functions are inextricably related. When undertaking a clinical examination, however, it is helpful to consider them separately. In the study of motor functions in the systematic examination of the patient an orderly sequence is adopted, considering first posture and gait, and then muscle power, tone and coordination.

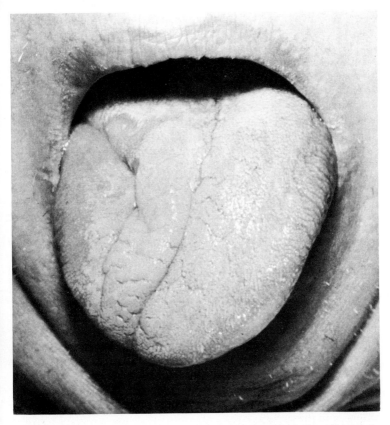

Figure 5.4. *Weakness and wasting of right side of tongue in a lesion affecting the hypoglossal nerve.*

A helpful concept in motor function is that of the upper motor neurone and the lower motor neurone. The *lower motor neurone* consists of the motor nerve cells in the brain or spinal cord and their processes, and therefore includes the peripheral nerve fibres which pass to the musculature of the body. The *upper motor neurone* comprises all the pathways and sources of impulses in the brain and the spinal cord which act on the lower motor neurone (Table 5.3). Another division which has been introduced into the concept of the central pathways of the motor system is that between the pyramidal and the extrapyramidal motor systems. This is to some extent an artificial distinction but is nevertheless clinically useful.

The *pyramidal or corticospinal system* is a system of pathways which arise from the motor area of the cortex to pass uninterrupted to nerve cells in the brainstem and spinal cord; it has a major role in initiating voluntary movement. The *extrapyramidal system* consists of descending pathways and circuits which pass from various parts of the brain to end in nuclei situated deeply in the brain such as the basal ganglia and the reticular formation. These give off relays which may descend to act on structures at a spinal or brainstem level. In addition the *cerebellum* plays an important part in the control and regulation of voluntary movement.

Table 5.3. *Paralysis due to lesions affecting upper and lower motor neurone.*

Upper motor neurone	Lower motor neurone
Paralysis extensive or localised	Paralysis localised to segmental or peripheral nerve distribution
Little wasting	Marked wasting
Increase in tone (spasticity or rigidity)	Decrease in tone
Fasciculation absent	Fasciculation may be present
Tendon reflexes increased	Tendon reflexes diminished
Extensor plantar response (Babinski's sign)	Flexor plantar response
Electrophysiological tests normal or nonspecific	Electrophysiological evidence of denervation or impaired nerve conduction

It is in the consideration of the motor system that Hughlings-Jackson's concept of the progressive dissolution of more recently evolved functions is particularly important along with his concept of positive and negative signs. Thus a lesion of the lower motor neurone will produce paralysis with loss of reflex activity — a purely negative sign — whereas in an upper motor neurone lesion there may also be paralysis but reflex activity can be enhanced due to destruction of inhibitory pathways — a positive sign. Damage to the pyramidal system characteristically produces spasticity in which the resistance to passive movement is most noticeable at the onset of movement, disappearing as the movement is increased. This is described as 'clasp-knife' rigidity. The tendon reflexes are characteristically exaggerated. In disease of the extrapyramidal system on the other hand the abnormality of tone is a rigidity which remains uniform throughout the whole range of movement. Other disorders of movement are important in disease of the extrapyramidal system, in particular bradykinesia or a generalised slowness or poverty of movement and a number of involuntary movements such as tremor, choreiform movements and athetosis. The association of tremor and rigidity in extrapyramidal disease produces the effect of 'cog-wheel' rigidity. Some of the features of lesions of the cortico-spinal pathway at different levels are shown in Table 5.4.

The examination of gait

The general character of a patient's gait is noted as he enters the room. If the patient is in bed at the time of examination and is able to walk it is necessary to observe his gait before the end of the examination.

In a *hemiplegic gait* the upper limb of one side is held flexed and stationary; flexion of the knee and hip is reduced so that the foot is not lifted off the ground and the hip on the affected side is swung outwards as the patient walks. With mild spastic weakness of one side the patient simply drags the affected foot and scuffs the toe as he walks. In *Parkinson's disease* the patient shuffles with small steps often leaning forwards with flexion of the hips and knees and has great difficulty in making any change in direction. With marked *spasticity of the lower limbs* the patient drags his feet but the legs may be forced to cross each other by adductor spasm giving rise to a 'scissors' gait. With severe *foot drop* the patient lifts the foot high to keep the toe off the ground. A similar high steppage gait occurs when there is marked loss of position sense but here the patient is also unsteady and tends to walk on a broad base. With *cerebellar ataxia* the patient may reel as he walks and sway to either side. With weakness of the pelvic girdle as in *muscular dystrophy* the proximal weakness is compensated by movements of the trunk and swinging of the pelvis so that the patient appears to have a 'waddling' gait. In *hysteria* many bizarre abnormalities of gait may appear. These are characteristically inconsistent and the gait may return almost to normal when the patient is unaware that he is being watched.

Although gross abnormalities of gait are obvious as soon as the patient walks, minor abnormalities may only be detected with careful testing. If the patient is asked to walk in a straight line with his heel against his toe, mild degrees of unsteadiness become

Table 5.4. *Localisation of lesion in corticospinal pathway: some characteristic features.*

Site	Neurological deficit
Cortex	
Wide surface distribution of motor representation	Monoplegia
Presence of excitable neurones	Focal epileptic seizures
Corona radiata and internal capsule	
Converging motor fibres	Contralateral hemiplegia with facial paralysis — in mild lesions fine movements of fingers affected first
Proximity of sensory pathways and optic radiation	Loss of sensation, homonymous hemianopia
Midbrain	
At this level and below cranial nerves on side of lesion may be affected together with adjacent sensory pathways and connections with cerebellum	Contralateral hemiplegia and facial paralysis. Ipsilateral III N. palsy (Weber's syndrome). Contralateral tremor (Benedikt's syndrome). Paralysis of upward gaze and ataxia (Nothnagel's syndrome).
Pons	Contralateral hemiplegia. Ipsilateral VI N. lesion and paralysis of conjugate gaze (Foville's syndrome). Ipsilateral VII N. palsy (Millard—Gubler syndrome).
Medulla	Contralateral hemiplegia without facial weakness. Ipsilateral paralysis of tongue, palate or vocal cords. In lateral medullary syndrome (post. inf. cerebellar artery) there is vertigo, ipsilateral ataxia, loss of pain and temperature sensation on face on affected side and contralateral side of body with dysphagia and dysarthria.
Spinal cord	
At this level motor neurones at level of lesion and long tracts below lesion are affected	Lower motor neurone weakness at level of lesion with upper motor neurone type of paralysis and sensory loss below level of lesion.

evident. If the patient is made to walk briskly for a reasonable distance, loss of associated movements such as swinging of the arms becomes apparent and this is an early sign of Parkinson's disease. Other tests include walking on heels and on tip-toe and hopping on one foot which are poorly performed when there is any disturbance of balance. These tests are also useful to detect weakness of the plantar flexors.

After testing gait the patient is asked to stand with his feet together. Inability to do this with the eyes open suggests trunk ataxia and the patient may have a tendency to sway particularly in a backwards direction. Ability to maintain posture with the eyes open but not when the eyes are closed indicates loss of position sense due to posterior root dysfunction as in tabes dorsalis (Romberg's sign), or a lesion of the ascending sensory pathways.

Muscle tone

Muscle tone in the clinical sense refers to the resistance which a muscle imposes to passive movement of the limb. It depends on the excitability of reflexes affecting the limb musculature, particularly the stretch reflex. These reflexes become hyperexcitable in the presence of disease affecting the upper motor neurone and diminished in lesions of the lower motor neurone.

The hypertonus of an upper motor neurone lesion may be either spasticity which is due to a lesion of the corticospinal system or rigidity which is seen particularly in Parkinson's disease and other disorders of the extrapyramidal system. Spasticity affects either the flexors or the extensors predominantly; generally in the upper limbs the flexors are affected and in the lower limbs the extensors. The resistance is most marked at the onset of a passive movement and then may give way as the force is maintained, i.e. 'clasp-knife' effect. Rigidity affects equally the flexors and the extensors of the limb and is felt equally throughout the whole range of movement, i.e. 'plastic' or 'lead-pipe' rigidity. When rigidity coexists with tremor it has an irregular quality, i.e. 'cog-wheel' rigidity. Often rigidity is most marked in the distal muscles particularly in the upper limbs where it may be felt on movement of the metacarpophalangeal joints or the wrists before it is evident at the elbows.

Hypotonus occurs when the reflex arc is interrupted as in a lower motor neurone lesion such as a peripheral nerve lesion or in a peripheral neuropathy.

The expression muscle tone frequently gives rise to confusion because the word tonus is also used to refer to postural tone in which there is a continued contraction of the muscles involved in maintaining the body posture. Electromyography however has clearly shown that when a muscle is completely relaxed no fibre contraction occurs. Provided relaxation is maintained contraction only takes place if the limb is moved passively. Muscle tone should be tested in all four limbs with the patient lying in a comfortable position. The fingers of one hand are first moved passively and then the more proximal joints and these must be moved through a full range of movement, the same procedure being gently carried out in the lower limbs.

Coordination

In the conscious and cooperative patient it is useful to test for the coordination of limbs before formally testing for muscle power. Failure to perform a coordinated voluntary movement is due to disturbance of function affecting the cerebellum and its connections in the brainstem or to loss of position and joint sense. Tests of coordination are also likely to be performed poorly if there is severe muscular weakness. Lesions of the corticospinal system and extra-pyramidal lesions give rise to difficulty in coordination, particularly in the performance of fine voluntary movements.

In testing for coordination the patient is asked first to hold both arms outstretched in front of him and to maintain this posture both with the eyes open and with the eyes closed. If one arm should drift downwards this is frequently a sign of muscle weakness but may also indicate loss of postural sensibility. Loss of postural sensation is also accompanied by upward and outward displacement of one or both arms and involuntary rotation of either limb. In cerebellar disease the affected arm tends to overshoot its position when it is outstretched and frequent corrective movements are necessary to maintain the posture. If the limb is tapped or moved passively it may oscillate before returning to its resting position. When the arms are outstretched careful notice must be taken whether there is any postural tremor or whether slow involuntary movements of the hands and fingers take place indicating dystonia.

The patient is then asked to perform the finger—nose test. This is done by moving the arms to full abduction and instructing the patient to touch the tip of his nose with the tip of the index finger. It is helpful in this test for the examiner to illustrate to the patient exactly what is intended. In cerebellar disease this test is performed with poor coordination and the finger may oscillate as it reaches the nose, i.e. intention tremor. With loss of postural sensibility the test is performed without difficulty with the eyes open but when the eyes are closed the finger may fail to find the nose or find it with difficulty. Further tests of coordination in the upper limbs are to ask the patient to tap the dorsum of one hand rapidly with the palm of the other, to rotate the wrist rapidly in alternate directions, and to touch each finger in turn with the thumb of the same hand. The first two tests may be markedly impaired in cerebellar disease and the inability to perform rapid alternating movements of the wrists is known as dysdiadochokinesis. Loss of fine movement of the hand is due to loss of postural sensibility, or to cerebellar disease but is not uncommonly the result also of disease affecting the motor pathway of the corticospinal system.

To test coordination in the lower limbs the patient is asked to place the heel of one foot on the knee of the opposite leg and slide the heel accurately up and down the shin to the ankle and back to the knee. This test is poorly performed in cerebellar ataxia or loss of postural sensibility but also if there is severe muscular weakness. In disordered postural sensibility it will be affected particularly if the eyes are closed. The test can be refined by asking the patient initially to touch the examiner's forefinger with his toe and then move the heel to his opposite knee and complete the test.

Muscle power

Prior to formal testing for muscle power much will have been learned in the preliminary examination of the patient. Thus as the patient walks into the consulting room weakness of one or other lower limbs may be apparent from the gait and of the upper limbs from the posture in which the limbs are held. If the patient is confined to bed it will be apparent whether the patient has difficulty in performing normal functions such as feeding himself and the tests for coordination described above will illustrate whether there is any gross impairment of muscle power. The findings should be recorded in explicit terms which can be understood by another examiner on a different occasion. Weakness of a lower limb may be so severe that the patient is unable to raise the limb off the bed or can do so but not against resistance; or the weakness may be confined to a single muscle group such as the muscles responsible for dorsiflexion of the ankle. In recording muscle power the scale adopted by the Medical Research Council is useful:

5 — Normal power.
4 — Ability to carry out full range of movement but not against resistance.
3 — Ability to carry out movement against gravity but not against additional resistance.
2 — Ability to carry out a movement but not against gravity.
1 — Ability to produce visible or palpable contraction of a muscle but no movement of the joint.
0 — Total paralysis.

In the examination of muscle power it is appropriate to test the power of muscle groups which move individual joints. Thus in the upper limb one may test abduction and adduction of the shoulder, flexion and extension of the elbow, flexion and extension of the wrist and of the fingers. In the lower limbs flexion, extension adduction and abduction of the hip, flexion and extension of the knee, dorsi and plantar flexion, eversion and inversion of the ankle and dorsi and plantar flexion of the toes, particularly the great toe, are tested. Flexion and extension of the neck should also be tested and the trunk muscles are tested by asking the patient to sit up in bed with the arms folded. If the patient lies recumbent and attempts to lift his head against resistance upward or downward, shifting of the umbilicus may indicate weakness of either the upper or the lower abdominal muscles.

There is considerable variation between the power of the muscles at different joints and experience will show which voluntary movements the examiner can expect to overcome. Abduction of the shoulder can be overcome relatively easily but if the arm is extended it is difficult to overcome the contraction of the triceps muscle. However, if the arm is flexed and the patient attempts to extend it against resistance, relatively minor degrees of weakness may be detected. Likewise in the lower limb if the knee is extended it is not possible to overcome the quadriceps muscle except in the presence of severe weakness, but if the knee is flexed and the patient attempts to extend it against resistance relatively minor degrees of weakness will be detected. At the ankle dorsiflexion can be overcome by the examiner if only a mild degree of weakness is present but plantar flexion is a powerful movement and can only be overcome when there is severe weakness. A sensitive test for weakness of plantar flexion is to ask the patient to stand and hop on the ball of one foot. At certain joints if movement is restricted for any length of time marked stiffness may develop and if active movement is limited at a joint it is important to test the range of passive movement. This applies particularly to the shoulder joint where a pericapsulitis following immobilisation readily gives rise to a frozen shoulder.

In the examination of muscle power attention must be given both to the segmental supply of the muscles affected and to the peripheral nerves which supply them. The principal spinal segments which innervate the muscles moving the joints of the limbs are shown in Table 5.5.

Table 5.5. *Segmental innervation of the muscles to joints.*

Adduction of shoulder	C5
Abduction of shoulder	C5
Flexion of elbow	C5
Extension of elbow	C7
Flexion of wrist	C6,7,8
Extension of wrist	C6,7
Finger movements	C8, T1
Flexion of hip	L1,2,3
Extension of hip	L5, S1
Adduction of hip	L5, S1
Abduction of hip	L4,5, S1
Flexion of knee	L4,5, S1,2
Extension of knee	L3,4
Dorsiflexion of ankle	L4,5
Plantar flexion of ankle	S1
Inversion of ankle	L4
Eversion of ankle	L5, S1
Dorsiflexion of toes	L5

If any serious question arises that there may be a peripheral nerve lesion it is necessary to make a systematic examination of the muscles which may be affected. Detailed instructions for this may be found in the Medical Research Council War Memorandum No. 7 entitled *Aids to the Investigation of Peripheral Nerve Injuries*. Selected muscles in the upper and lower limbs together with their nerve supply and mode of testing are shown in Tables 5.6 and 5.7. The distinction between a segmental and a peripheral nerve lesion is usually made by careful muscle testing supplemented by the findings on a sensory examination. For example, if there is wasting of the thenar muscles of one hand, sparing adductor pollicis, the

Table 5.6. *Muscles of upper limb.*

Muscle	Nerve supply	Segments	Method of testing
Trapezius	Spinal accessory	C3,4,5	Patient elevates shoulder against resistance and braces it backwards.
Serratus ant.	Nerve to serratus anterior	C5,6	Patient pushes arms forwards. If weakness present winging of scapula occurs.
Rhomboids	Nerve to rhomboids	C4,5	With hand on hip arm is braced back against resistance. Muscle is felt over upper medial edge of scapula.
Supraspinatus	Suprascapular nerve	C5	Arm is abducted from side of body against resistance
Infraspinatus	Suprascapular nerve	C5,6	With elbow at side flexed forearm is moved backward against resistance. Muscle is felt over body of scapula.
Pectoralis major	Lateral and medial pectoral nerves	C5,6,7,8, T1	With arms raised to 60° patient brings hands together against resistance.
Latissimus dorsi	Nerve to latissimus dorsi	C6,7,8	Muscle is felt below posterior axillary fold when patient coughs.
Deltoid	Circumflex nerve	C5,6	With arm abducted 60° patient abducts arm against resistance.
Biceps	Musculo-cutaneous nerve	C5,6	Supinated arm is flexed against resistance.
Triceps	Radial nerve	C7,8	Flexed arm is extended against resistance.
Ext. carpi radialis	Radial nerve	C6,7,8	Wrist is extended to radial side against resistance.
Ext. digitorum	Radial nerve	C7,8	Fingers are extended at metacarpophalangeal joints against resistance.
Flexor carpi radialis	Ulnar nerve	C6,7	Wrist is flexed toward radial side against resistance.
Flexor digit. sublimis	Median nerve	C7,8, T1	With proximal phalanx fixed interphalangeal joint is flexed against resistance
Flexor pollicis longus	Median nerve	C8, T1	Terminal phalanx of thumb is flexed against resistance.
Abd. pollicis brevis	Median nerve	C8, T1	Thumb is abducted from palm against resistance.

Table 5.6. *Continued*

Muscle	Nerve supply	Segments	Method of testing
Ext. pollicis longus	Radial nerve	C6,7	Terminal phalanx of thumb is extended against resistance.
Opponens pollicis	Median nerve	T1	Thumb is opposed against 5th finger.
Adductor pollicis	Ulnar nerve	T1	Paper is held between thumb and palmar aspect of index finger.
1st palmar interosseus	Ulnar nerve	T1	With hand flat on table index finger is adducted against resistance.
Abd. digiti minimi	Ulnar nerve	T1	With back of hand on table little finger is abducted against resistance.
Opponens digiti minimi	Ulnar nerve	T1	With fingers extended little finger is carried in front of others.

cause is likely to be a lesion affecting the median nerve. An ulnar nerve lesion on the other hand may affect all the intrinsic muscles except those of the thenar eminence. If both groups of muscles are affected the disease process is more likely to be one affecting the first dorsal segment, implicating either the anterior horn cells in the spinal cord or the first dorsal root. Both an ulnar and a median nerve lesion are likely to give rise to sensory changes in the appropriate distribution but a lesion affecting the deep branch of the ulnar nerve will give rise to motor deficit only. The testing of certain of the intrinsic muscles of the hand is illustrated in Figures 5.5. to 5.12.

The Reflexes

Absence of a reflex is due to a lesion affecting either the afferent or the efferent part of the arc. Reflexes are exaggerated if there is a lesion of the upper motor neurone affecting pathways which function to diminish the excitability of the reflexes concerned. In spinal shock, however, an upper motor neurone lesion causes temporary reduction in reflex activity. Certain reflexes such as the pupil reactions, the corneal reflexes and the jaw jerk have already been described in appropriate sections. The tendon reflexes and the superficial reflexes provide an important part of the clinical examination.

Table 5.7. *Muscles of lower limb.*

Muscle	Nerve supply	Segments	Method of testing
Iliopsoas	Femoral nerve	L2,3	With patient supine thigh is flexed against resistance.
Quadriceps femoris	Femoral nerve	L2,3,4	Flexed knee is extended against resistance.
Adductor muscles	Obturator nerve	L2,3,4	Thigh is adducted against resistance.
Gluteus maximus	Inf. gluteal nerve	L5, S1	With patient prone knee is raised against resistance.
Hamstrings	Sciatic nerve	L4,5, S1,2	With patient prone knee is flexed against resistance.
Tibialis anterior	Deep peroneal nerve	L4,5	Ankle is dorsiflexed against resistance.
Gastrocnemius	Posterior tibial nerve	L4	With patient prone ankle is plantar flexed against resistance.
Tibialis posterior	Posterior tibial nerve	L4	Foot is inverted against resistance.
Peroneal muscles	Superficial peroneal nerve	L5, S1	Foot is everted against resistance.
Ext. digitorum longus	Deep peroneal nerve	L5	Toes are dorsiflexed against resistance.
Ext. hallucis longus	Deep peroneal nerve	L5, S1	Toes are dorsiflexed against resistance.
Ext. digitorum brevis	Deep peroneal nerve	S1	Great toe is dorsiflexed against resistance.

Tendon reflexes. A tendon reflex is a reflex contraction of a muscle occurring in response to a brisk tap on the tendon. It is an example of the phasic stretch reflex. In testing the reflexes it is essential that the patient is comfortable and relaxed. An efficient tendon hammer should be used with a long and flexible handle and a rubber ring at the base. It is important that the elicitation of a reflex is carried out with the care given to a quantitative test and the tendon hammer should be allowed to swing lightly on the tendon to deliver as

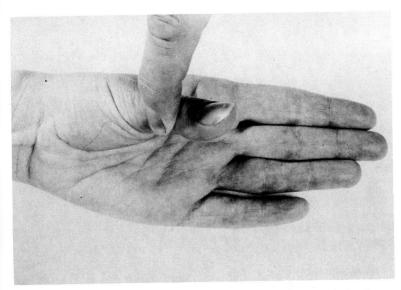

Figure 5.5. *Method of testing for weakness of abductor pollicis brevis (median nerve).*

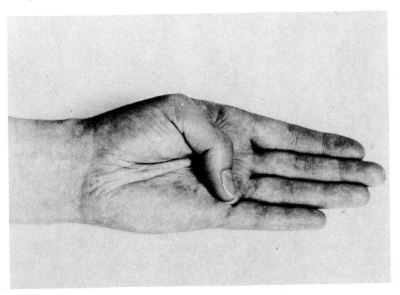

Figure 5.6. *Method of testing for weakness of opponens pollicis (median nerve).*

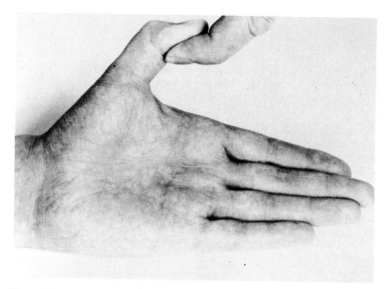

Figure 5.7. *Method of testing for weakness of flexor pollicis longus (median nerve: anterior interosseous branch).*

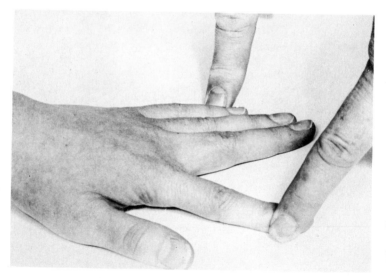

Figure 5.8. *Method of testing for weakness of first dorsal interosseous (ulnar nerve).*

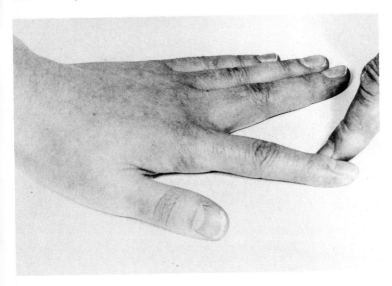

Figure 5.9. *Method of testing for weakness of first palmar interosseous (ulnar nerve).*

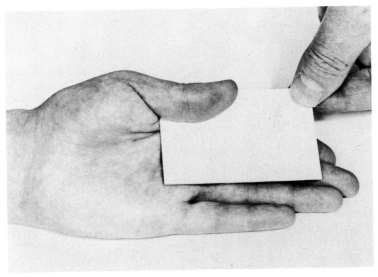

Figure 5.10. *Method of testing for weakness of adductor pollicis (ulnar nerve).*

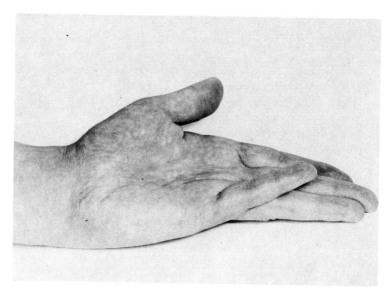

Figure 5.11. *Method of testing for weakness of opponens digiti minimi (ulnar nerve).*

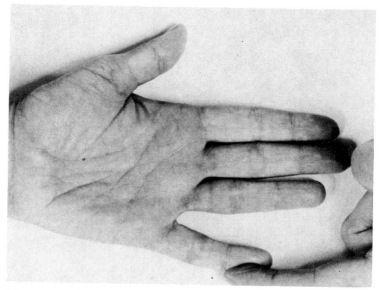

Figure 5.12. *Method of testing for weakness of abductor digiti minimi (ulnar nerve).*

uniform a blow as possible. More important than general exaggeration or diminution of the reflexes is their symmetry or asymmetry and with each reflex care should be taken to compare the response obtained on the two sides.

Biceps jerk. The biceps is supplied by the musculocutaneous nerve with a segmental innervation of C5,6. The arm is held flexed with the forefinger over the biceps tendon and the finger is struck with the hammer.

Supinator jerk. The brachioradialis muscle is supplied by the radial nerve with a segmental innervation of C5,6. The reflex is elicited by striking the lower end of the radius and the response is flexion of the forearm.

Triceps jerk. The triceps muscle is supplied by the radial nerve with a segmental innervation C6,7,8. The arm is held flexed to a right angle and the triceps tendon is tapped above the elbow.

Sometimes when the supinator jerk is tested the reflex is absent but flexion of the fingers occurs. This sign is known as an *inverted supinator jerk* and indicates a lesion affecting the cervical cord in which there is a lower motor neurone lesion at the fifth cervical segment. It also indicates that there is an upper motor neurone lesion affecting the reflexes below this level. There is sometimes an associated inverted biceps jerk which has the same significance.

Finger flexion reflex. This is tested by having the patient's fingers flexed and supported by the examiner's own fingers. The patient's fingers are struck with the hammer and if the reflex is present there is slight flexion of the patient's fingers. This reflex implicates segments C6,7,8 and T1 and it is not normally elicited in the absence of an upper motor neurone lesion. Its significance is similar to that of the Hoffmann reflex in which flexion of the thumb occurs when the patient's index or middle finger is flicked downwards between the examiner's finger and thumb (Figure 5.13).

The knee jerk. This is the quadriceps reflex the segmental innervation of which is L3,4 and the nerve supply is the femoral nerve. The hand is placed under the patient's knees which are held flexed and the patella tendon is struck lightly on each side (Figure 5.14). If the reflex is not easily obtained in the lying position it may be elicited when the patient sits on the edge of the bed with his legs hanging free.

The ankle jerk. This reflex involves the contraction of the gastrocnemius muscle supplied by the posterior tibial nerve with a segmental innervation of S1. The patient's legs should be laterally

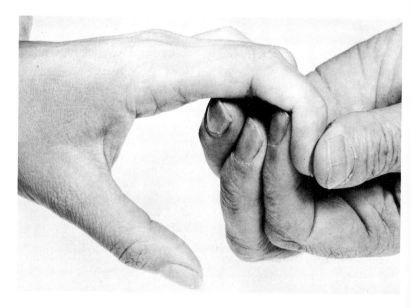

Figure 5.13. *Method of eliciting Hoffmann's sign.*

rotated with the knee slightly flexed. The foot is held and slightly dorsiflexed and the Achilles tendon is struck (Figure 5.15). If the reflex is difficult to obtain the patient may kneel on a chair with the ankles protruding over the edge and the tendon is tapped while the foot is slightly dorsiflexed by the examiner. A further method is to have the patient lying prone in bed with the knees bent to a right angle and the foot held with light pressure. It is important that the tension the examiner exerts on the foot should be adequate without overstretching the tendon. Failure to employ the correct technique is a common cause for inability to obtain the ankle jerks.

If the tendon reflexes are difficult to obtain it is important to carry out the procedure of reinforcement. In the lower limbs Jendrassik's manoeuvre is applied in which the patient holds his hands together and tries to pull them apart at the moment that the tendon is stretched. For the upper limbs the same effect may be achieved if the patient clenches his teeth or clenches the fist of the hand that is not being tested.

If marked exaggeration of a tendon reflex is present the reflex may be clonic so that repetitive contractions of the muscle occur

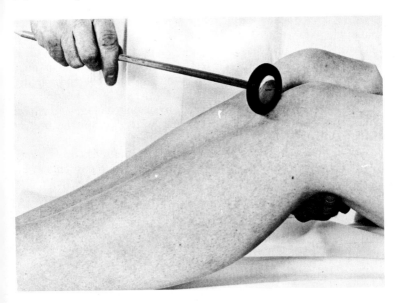

Figure 5.14. *Method of eliciting knee jerk.*

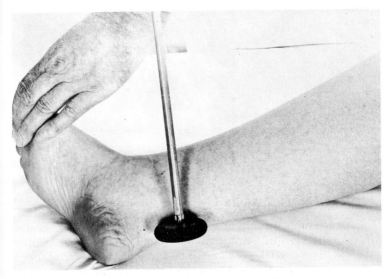

Figure 5.15. *Method of eliciting ankle jerk.*

until the stretch is relieved. *Clonus* is readily tested for in the knee and ankle. At the knee it may be obtained if the leg is held extended and firm downward pressure is placed on the patella. At the ankle it may be present when the ankle jerk is elicited in the normal manner or alternatively it may be brought out by forcibly and rapidly applying pressure on the foot to dorsiflex the ankle. When doing so it is important that the knee is flexed. In sustained clonus repetitive contractions will continue for so long as tension on the muscle tendon is maintained.

Apart from reflexes being exaggerated or diminished they may sometimes be excessively prolonged. This occurs particularly in myxoedema where there is a delay in relaxation.

In documenting the reflexes it is useful to apply a numerical scale, for example the figure 2 is used to indicate a normal reflex, 1 a diminished reflex, 3 an exaggerated reflex, 4 clonus, and 0 for absent reflexes (Table 5.8).

Table 5.8. *Scheme for recording examination of reflexes.*

	Right	Left
Triceps	2	2
Biceps	2	2
Supinator	2	2
Hoffmann	0	0
Abdominal	+ + + +	
Knee	2	2
Ankle	2	2
Plantar	↓	↓

4 = clonus.
3 = exaggerated reflex.
2 = average reflex response.
1 = diminished reflex.
0 = absent reflex.

The superficial reflexes. These include the abdominal reflexes, the gluteal reflexes, the cremasteric and anal reflex and the plantar response. These reflexes are of particular interest because, although their absence may signify a lesion affecting the lower motor neurone in the affected segments, abnormalities in these reflexes can also provide useful information regarding the presence or absence of an upper motor neurone lesion. The abdominal, gluteal, cremasteric and anal reflexes are all comparable responses although the abdominal reflex is the most important of this group as a clinical test.

Abdominal reflex. Light strokes are applied over each of the four quadrants of the abdomen with a blunt point such as a pencil, key or an orange stick. It is important that the patient should be lying supine and relaxed. If the reflexes are present brisk contraction of the underlying muscles takes place. The upper reflexes are subserved by segments T9—T10 and the lower by T11—T12. In healthy individuals the reflex may sometimes be difficult to obtain. This is particularly so if the patient is obese, if the abdomen is scarred, or the patient has had multiple pregnancies. Particular attention should be paid to asymmetry of the reflex response since its absence on one side may be strong evidence of an upper motor neurone lesion. Fatiguability of the abdominal reflexes is a sign that must be interpreted with caution but it is of importance as it may indicate early disease of the corticospinal tracts and is particularly likely to occur in demyelinating disease.

The cremasteric reflex. This is elicited by stroking the inside of the thigh when the ipsilateral testis will move upwards.

The gluteal reflex. This is the brisk contraction of the gluteal muscles following stroking of the overlying skin.

The anal reflex. This is contraction of the external sphincter when the skin around the anus is stroked.

Any of these reflexes may be absent in the presence of an upper motor neurone lesion and it has been held that they depend on the integrity of a long loop pathway extending up the spinal cord into the brain. However, experimental studies on the abdominal reflexes have shown that the reflex time is consistent with a polysynaptic spinal reflex and there seems little doubt that the abdominal reflex following a painful stimulus is a simple polysynaptic withdrawal response. It does however habituate easily but even when habituated can still be elicited provided a sufficiently painful stimulus is employed. The response, which normally occurs to relatively light stimulation and which is absent in the newborn, would seem therefore to be dependent on a conditioning process which is lost when the pathway between the brain and spinal cord is interrupted.

The plantar response. This is a particularly important reflex because it may provide the most objective clinical evidence available of the presence of an upper motor neurone lesion. The plantar response is elicited by firmly scratching the outer surface of the sole with a blunt pointed instrument such as a key or the end of a percussion hammer. The stimulus should move forwards from the heel, along the lateral margin of the sole and curve towards the middle metatarsophalangeal joint. Since the plantar aspect of the foot is normally extremely sensitive great care must be taken to avoid applying too painful a stimulus since withdrawal of the foot may give rise to a false appearance of an extensor plantar response. The foot should be warm and the patient advised that the foot is about to be stimulated. When the test is carried out great care should be taken to compare the response on the two sides. In the healthy subject the great toe will flex and the other toes will also generally flex at the same time. The most critical sign to observe is the first movement of the great toe. The test may first be carried out with the knee slightly flexed and then repeated with the lower limb firmly extended.

In an abnormal plantar response, known as *Babinski's sign*, the great toe is dorsiflexed at the metatarsophalangeal joint while the other toes fan outwards and become dorsiflexed (Figure 5.16). Although the lateral border of the sole of the foot is in general the most effective site for eliciting an abnormal plantar response it is often readily elicited from stimulation of the medial border of the sole of the foot. In the presence of severe disease of the corticospinal system such as paraplegia it may be evoked by applying a painful stimulus to the skin often as high up as the thigh.

The plantar response is part of the primitive flexor response which occurs in response to a painful stimulus applied to the skin. Dorsiflexion of the toes is in physiological terms a flexor response since flexion of the limb includes any movement which tends to raise it off the ground. In the healthy subject application of a painful stimulus to the foot will produce flexion of the proximal part of the limb to withdraw it from the stimulus but will also give rise to local extensor reflexes in the foot which lead to a plantar flexion of the toes. With a lesion of the upper motor neurone however these local extensor reflexes are lost and the flexor reflex becomes so hyperactive that its field of excitation is enlarged and the response comes to include also dorsiflexion of the toes.

Primitive reflexes. In addition to the reflexes already described which are present in healthy adults a number of reflexes are normally present in early infancy and their absence at this stage or their persistence or reappearance at a later age may be of clinical significance.

The sucking reflex. This is present at birth and may persist during the first year of life. It is elicited by touching the corner of the mouth when sucking movements of the lips and tongue will take place. It is subserved by the fifth and seventh cranial nerves and in adults may be seen in pseudobulbar palsy if there is an upper motor lesion above the level of the seventh nerve nucleus in the pons. The clinical significance and pathways subserved are similar to those of the *snout reflex*, in which contraction of the lips occurs in response to a firm tap on the upper and lower lips on either side.

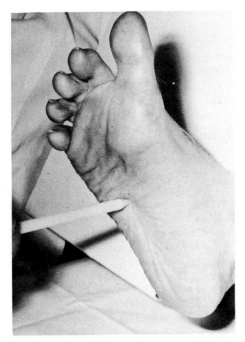

Figure 5.16. *Extensor plantar response (Babinski's sign).*

The Moro reflex. This is present from birth until the age of about three months. It is elicited by holding the baby in a supine position supporting the shoulders, back and buttocks with one hand and the head with the other. If the head is allowed to fall back suddenly while the rest of the body remains supported rapid abduction of the arms occurs and then the arms come together in an embracing movement. It may be absent on one side in the presence of a lower motor neurone lesion such as a brachial plexus palsy and if it persists beyond the age of six months it is indicative of cerebral disease.

The grasp reflex. This reflex is present in healthy newborn babies and normally persists for two to three months. It is elicited by placing the first and second fingers of one hand between the thumb and forefinger of the patient. The baby's hand will close on them, the hold increasing as the examiner attempts to withdraw his fingers. Persistence of this reflex may occur in cerebral disease and in adults it is found in disease affecting the frontal lobe or the corpus callosum.

The tonic neck reflexes. This reflex is present in babies up to the age of three to six months. If the patient is examined in the supine position rotation of the head to one side will produce extension of the arm on the same side with flexion of the contralateral arm and sometimes the contralateral leg. Its presence in adults signifies disease affecting the brainstem or the basal nuclei.

Involuntary Movements

In many patients with neurological disease involuntary movement is the presenting complaint and in some may be the sole physical sign. In others it is part of a widespread disorder. But even when involuntary movement is not the main problem its analysis may have an important bearing on diagnosis and on the management of the patient. The most immediately disabling variety of involuntary movement may occur during an epileptic seizure and the features of both generalised convulsions and focal seizures have been described in an earlier section. The mechanisms which underly the development of different varieties of involuntary movement are complex and in many instances imperfectly understood and the classification is in general clinical and descriptive. Important varieties of abnormal movement which may be noted in a clinical examination are as follows:

1. Tics and habit spasms
2. Myoclonus
3. Tremor
   a. static
   b. postural
   c. intention

4. Chorea
   a. generalised
   b. unilateral
5. Athetosis
6. Torsion dystonia

Tics and habit spasms

This expression covers a wide range of twitching or jerking movements, often bizarre and sterotyped, which may affect different
parts of the body but are usually confined to the face or the upper
limbs. In the face repetitive movements such as blinking, screwing
up the face and pursing of the lips may occur. These movements are
generally most marked when the patient is observed and less
evident during concentration. They are generally regarded as a
functional disorder and there is a clear association with anxiety and
tension. It is not at all certain, however, that there is not an organic
basis for at least some aspects of the condition. Thus a tic or habit
spasm may occur as a sequal to *Sydenham's chorea* and tics have
occurred in the course of *encephalitis lethargica*. A particularly
disabling tic is that which is present in the syndrome of *Gilles de la
Tourette* in which the affected child carries out repetitive movements and at the same time may swear or mutter obscenities under
his breath.

Myoclonus

Myoclonus refers to a sudden shock-like movement of a group of
muscles. Myoclonic jerks are frequently confined to relatively small
groups of muscles and a form which may occur in healthy subjects
is the sudden jerking of the lower limbs which sometimes takes
place when a person is falling asleep. Sometimes myoclonus may
involve many parts of the body and may occur repetitively either
spontaneously or in response to a sudden noise. This may be
unaccompanied by other evidence of disease and is known as
paramyoclonus multiplex or, if it occurs as a familial condition,
hereditary essential myoclonus. Myoclonus in response to startle
may be a feature of cerebral lipoidosis.

Periodic myoclonic jerks are not uncommon in patients subject
to epilepsy. Thus petit mal attacks may be accompanied by a
sudden myoclonic jerking of the upper limbs. In progressive
myoclonic epilepsy there are severe periodic myoclonic movements

and epileptic attacks and the patients develop cerebellar degeneration and eventually dementia. Myoclonic jerks may also be a feature, along with progressive dementia, of Jakob—Creutzfeldt disease. A type of myoclonic jerk affecting the trunk and the limbs which is followed by a coarse tremor may be a feature of *subacute inclusion body encephalitis.* Occasionally middle-aged or elderly patients develop a regular rhythmical movement of the palate and throat muscles, *palatal myoclonus.* This is due to a lesion affecting the olivary nuclei and central tegmental tract in the midbrain and may occur as an isolated non-progressive disturbance.

Tremor

A tremor is present in the healthy subject but this *physiological tremor* cannot normally be seen unless it is recorded with special transducers. In the adult it has a frequency of about 10 Hz but is slower in childhood and in old age. It is a postural tremor, being absent when the limb is at rest but present when the limb maintains a posture and it persists during a voluntary movement.

Many patients have a postural tremor which is not present when the limb is at rest but it is obvious when the arms are outstretched. These tremors may occur in severe anxiety, in patients who are fatigued or depressed, in thyrotoxicosis or chronic alcoholism, or in patients who have been exposed to drugs such as the amphetamines, the tricyclic antidepressants or mercury. The mechanism of these tremors is not clearly understood but it may be that in some instances they are exaggerations of physiological tremor. In chronic liver disease with hepatic encephalopathy when the arms are outstretched a *flapping tremor* of the wrists is sometimes seen, i.e. 'liver flap'. It is also found in CO_2 narcosis and uraemia. A similar tremor may be seen in Wilson's disease (hepatolenticular degeneration) in which the tremor is part of a widespread movement disorder and may be markedly aggravated by any attempt at voluntary movement.

Essential or *familial tremor* is a postural tremor which sometimes develops in childhood but may not appear until later. It may be inherited as autosomal dominant. This tremor does not interfere with fine movements but may be a considerable embarrassment to a patient if he is lifting a heavy object or one which requires careful balancing such as a cup and saucer. It is not as a rule progressive but may affect the arms and head and some patients find that it is relieved by alcohol. When severe this tremor may resemble that of

Parkinson's disease, but it has a higher frequency and is absent when the limb is relaxed.

The tremor of *Parkinson's disease* is a resting tremor which has a relatively slow frequency of 4 to 6 Hz. It may start at the fingers consisting of regular adduction and abduction of the thumb in relation to the other fingers i.e. 'pill-rolling' tremor. Gradually it affects the greater part of the limb including the proximal muscles and later may affect the tongue and sometimes the head. It disappears during sleep but is brought on by mental concentration or by emotion. If the patient has a history of tremor but the tremor is not present during the examination it may sometimes be evoked if the patient is asked to carry out an arithmetical calculation or spell a word in reverse order. Parkinsonian tremor is frequently abolished if the patient holds the arms outstretched or performs a voluntary movement such as the finger—nose test, but if it is severe the tremor will not be wholly abolished by posture and may even have an intention component. Generally a patient with this type of tremor has other features of Parkinson's disease such as rigidity of the limbs and a generalised slowness of movement (bradykinesia) with loss of facial expression. Tremor may be the first sign of Parkinson's disease and such patients may present diagnostic difficulty.

A slow coarse resting tremor which persists throughout a voluntary movement is sometimes seen in vascular disease of the brainstem and is due to a lesion of the red nucleus, i.e. red nucleus tremor. It may be present as a unilateral tremor in Benedikt's syndrome along with a third nerve palsy and cerebellar ataxia on the same side.

Intention tremor is a coarse tremor which is not present at rest or when maintaining a static posture but occurs during a voluntary movement and is readily demonstrated by the finger—nose test. It indicates a lesion of the cerebellum or its connections and is due to breakdown of the mechanism whereby the cerebellum acts as an error detector in the carrying out of a voluntary movement. Thus in the finger—nose test any deviation of the hand from its path is instantly corrected but in cerebellar disease this is not the case and the limb strays from its path to be returned by a coarse correcting movement.

Chorea

Choreiform movements are rapid, jerking, darting movements which affect the face, tongue and particularly the distal portions of the arm and leg. Chorea is associated with hypotonia of the limbs but the reflexes are not lost. When the limbs are extended the joints may be hyperextended. The patient may have great difficulty in maintaining the posture if the arms are held above the head with the palms forward. Chorea may be present in children in the uncommon condition of *Sydenham's chorea* which follows a streptococcal infection, usually of the throat. *Huntington's chorea* usually occurs in adults but may develop at any time of a person's life; there is also a progressive dementia. Hypotonicity is not a feature. The condition is inherited as an autosomal dominant. Chorea also develops following a vascular episode in middle age, i.e. *senile* or *arteriosclerotic chorea.* Chorea occurring on one side of the body is called hemichorea or *hemiballismus.* There is a rapid flail-like movement affecting the proximal joints of one arm throughout the waking hours. It may develop suddenly as a result of a vascular lesion of the subthalamic nucleus.

Athetosis

Athetosis is a slow writhing movement of the body in which the limbs move slowly and the body moves from one dystonic posture to another. It may affect the arms and the legs and the movements tend to disappear in sleep. Athetosis is most commonly a feature of cerebral palsy.

Torsion dystonia

This occurs in its most severe form as *dystonia musculorum deformans* which is a hereditary condition of either dominant or recessive inheritance. It is also seen in Wilson's disease. In its mildest form it occurs as *spasmodic torticollis*; in the severe form the movements include arching of the back and the neck with rotation of the neck and arms. At the same time more rapid movements are present such as turning of the neck, grimacing movements of the face and protrusion of the tongue. In spasmodic torticollis the head turns involuntarily to one side or sometimes backwards. It is not certain how far spasmodic torticollis is related to psychogenic factors but some patients show a mild form of torsion dystonia. Many individuals who do not have a fully developed dystonia show dystonic symptoms of which the commonest are grimacing movements of the face. These occur as an isolated feature in mild forms of Huntington's chorea; they may be a side-effect of L-dopa in the treatment of Parkinson's disease and occasionally occur in patients who have had prolonged therapy with phenothiazine drugs when the disorder may be irreversible.

Sensation

The testing of sensation is clarified by the vigorous analysis of sensory symptoms in the history and by careful observation of the patient during the earlier stages of the examination. Thus impairment of gait and the presence of Romberg's sign may provide evidence of sensory ataxia and impaired function in the finger—nose test may suggest impaired proprioception in the upper limbs. The presence of burn marks in the hands indicates impairment of pain and temperature sensation. The formal testing of sensation can be relatively difficult because a great deal depends on the cooperation of the patient and even the most careful and objective witness may become fatigued and give faulty answers during a prolonged examination.

A number of highly developed forms of sensation such as sight and hearing, smell and taste are subserved by special organs and comprise the special senses which are dealt with in the appropriate sections. In sensory testing one is concerned firstly with *exteroceptive sensation* which includes pain, light touch and temperature and *proprioceptive sensation* which includes position sense, the awareness of passive movement and vibration. Secondly it is necessary to consider the ability of a patient to recognise and interpret particular sensory stimuli. To do this requires a test for stereognosis, two point discrimination and the ability to localise stimuli to particular parts of the body. These functions are sometimes grouped together as cortical sensations.

The sensory system is organised so that the primary afferent pathway consists of the peripheral nerves which convey fibres carrying all the different modalities of sensation. Division of a peripheral nerve therefore produces total loss of sensation over the part of the body supplied by the nerve, the loss affecting all modalities equally. With partial lesions of peripheral nerves some modalities of sensation are affected selectively because touch, pressure and proprioception are conveyed by large myelinated rapidly conducting fibres whereas pain and temperature depend upon smaller more slowly conducting fibres some of which are unmyelinated. If disease of the peripheral nerves affects the more slowly conducting fibres first then there is relative loss of pain and temperature, whereas the converse will be true if the larger fibres are first affected. Moreover in some disorders the longer fibres are affected first so that sensory loss may be most marked in the periphery of the limb. After entering the spinal cord the fibres separate so that those conveying touch and proprioception pass up on the same side of the spinal cord as the first sensory neurone to synapse with the second sensory neurone in the medulla. Many of these fibres pass up the posterior columns but this is not the exclusive ipsilateral pathway for touch and position sense. Fibres carrying pain and temperature on the other hand cross over to the opposite side of the cord at or close to the level of entry and there synapse with the second sensory neurone which passes upward to the brain in the spinothalamic tract. Disease within the spinal cord may therefore affect one modality of sensation selectively since the fibres carrying different modalities are anatomically separated. A *dissociated anaesthesia* in which a particular modality of sensation is impaired is strong evidence of the lesion within the nervous system rather than in the peripheral nerves. Dissociated anaesthesia

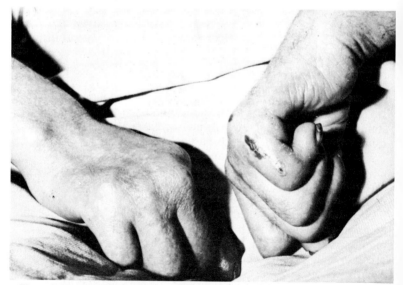

Figure 5.17. *Hands of a patient with syringomyelia showing wasting and marks on left hand where patient has sustained burns over analgesic area.*

Table 5.9. *Extramedullary and intramedullary cord lesion.*

Extramedullary	Intramedullary
Root pains common	Root pains exceptional
Early development of spastic paralysis	Late development of spastic paralysis
Atrophy and lower motor neurone signs strictly localised	Atrophy and lower motor neurone signs may be marked and extend for several segments
Brown—Séquard syndrome characteristic of lateral compression of cord	Dissociated anaesthesia with loss of pain and temperature may be conspicuous
Changes in CSF may occur early with manometric block and elevated protein	Changes in CSF occur late

is particularly likely to occur in the presence of intrinsic cord lesions such as syringomyelia (Figure 5.17) and intramedullary tumours (Table 5.9) and may be a striking feature in hemisection of the cord (Brown—Séquard syndrome) (Table 5.10 and Figure 5.18). The second sensory neurone ends in the thalamus where a third relay carries impulses to the sensory cortex in the parietal lobe.

Sensation from different parts of the body is carried in the spinal cord in an orderly manner. Thus in the posterior columns fibres from the lower half of the body are displaced medially by those which enter the cord at a higher level. In the spinothalamic tract on the other hand fibres from the lower part of the body are displaced laterally to lie superficial to those from the upper part.

In testing exteroceptive sensation it is necessary to know both the segmental distribution of the sensory nerves or dermatomes and the areas of skin which are supplied by individual peripheral nerves (Figures 5.19 and 5.20). There is, however, considerable overlap

Table 5.10. *Brown—Séquard syndrome (hemi-section of cord).*

Side of lesion	Contralateral side
Lower motor neurone weakness at level of lesion	No weakness
Upper motor neurone type weakness below level of lesion	
Loss of all sensation at level of lesion	
Loss of touch, position and vibration sense below level of lesion	Loss of pain and temperature sensation below level of lesion

between dermatomes. Representative sites of segmental innervation on the skin are given in Table 5.11.

In the hand the anatomical snuff box at the base of the thumb is innervated by the radial nerve, the tips of the first, second, third and lateral half of fourth fingers by the median nerve and the medial half of the fourth and the fifth finger by the ulnar nerve.

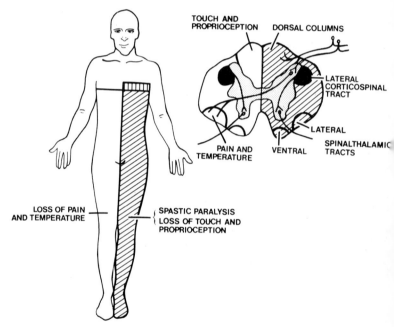

Figure 5.18. *Diagram to illustrate pathways affected in Brown—Séquard syndrome and distribution of paralysis and sensory impairment (Table 5.10).*

Since the spinal cord is shorter than the vertebral column the segmental level of a spinal lesion does not necessarily correspond with the level of a particular vertebra. Thus spinal segment C8 is opposite the seventh vertebra, T3 is opposite the first thoracic vertebra, T8 is opposite the fifth thoracic vertebra and all the lumbar and sacral segments are situated opposite the vertebrae from T11 to L1.

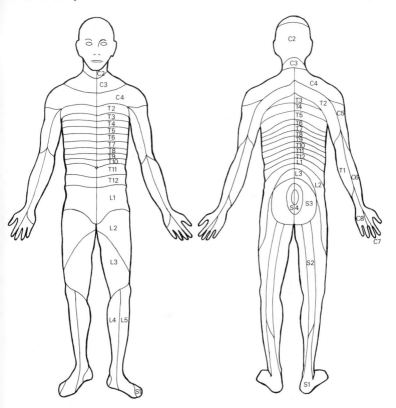

Figure 5.19. *Diagram to illustrate segmental innervation of skin.*

Pain sensation

This is tested with a pin, one end sharp and the other blunt, and the patient is asked if what he is feeling is sharp or blunt. After a general examination of the body, areas where abnormality is found are studied in detail. It is useful to move the pin from the area where sensation is impaired to where it is normal in order to map out the boundaries of the affected area. For increased accuracy the pin is then moved in the reverse direction from the area of intact to that of impaired sensation.

In addition to testing for *superficial pain* it is also important to test for *deep pain*. This is done by squeezing the muscles of the lower limb and also the Achilles tendon. Muscle tenderness is present in peripheral neuropathy, in polymyositis and sometimes following virus infections. Diminished tenderness is a feature of lesions of the posterior roots such as tabes dorsalis.

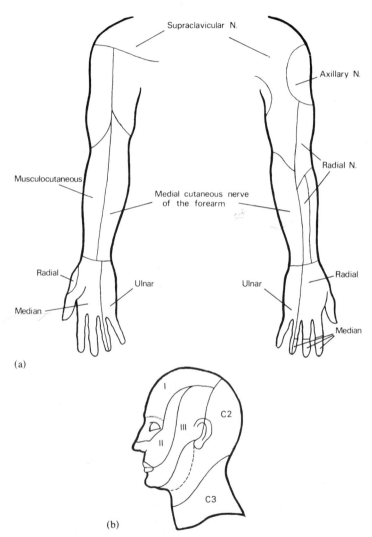

(a)

(b)

Figure 5.20. *Cutaneous nerve supply of* (a) *upper limbs and* (b) *head.*

Table 5.11. *Segmental innervation.*

C2	Occiput
C3	Lateral cervical area
C4	Tip of shoulder
C5	Lateral aspect of elbow
C6	Thumb
C7	Middle finger
C8	Little finger
T1	Inner aspect of elbow
T3	Axilla
T8	Costal margin
T10	Umbilicus
T12	Pubis
L1	Immediately below inguinal ligament
L3	Knee
L4	Medial surface of tibia
L5	Outer aspect of tibia to inner aspect of foot and great toe
S1	Lateral aspect of foot and little toe
S1—S5	Skin over buttocks and surrounding anus

Touch sensation

Touch sensation is examined in the same systematic manner as pain using a piece of fine cotton wool or soft tissue. The patient is asked to shut his eyes and say 'yes' every time he feels anything and it is impressed upon the patient that this is the only response required of him.

Temperature sensation

A cold object such as a tuning fork is used in the preliminary examination of the body but when areas of suspected sensory loss are discovered they should be tested with tubes containing either hot water (50°C) or cold water (17°C). The patient is asked to say whether he is being touched with the hot or the cold tube.

Position sense

In the upper limbs observation of the posture of the outstretched arms and the performance of the finger—nose test give valuable preliminary information. In formal testing the finger or toe is held along the lateral borders and moved upwards and downwards and the patient is asked to say in which direction the digit moves. If the digit is held in any other way unequal pressure subserved by touch fibres, rather than position sense, will indicate movement. Should position sense be impaired at the fingers or toes the examination should proceed proximally to test the ability to perceive movements at the ankle and wrist and if necessary at the elbow and knee.

Vibration sense

The ability to appreciate vibration depends on the integrity of rapidly adapting receptors in the skin and in the deeper tissues. It is a useful test because although vibration sense is carried in the ipsilateral part of the cord along with touch and proprioception it is not infrequently absent when position and joint sense is intact. In performing the test a tuning fork preferably of 128 Hz is first placed over the sternum so that the patient is able to recognise the vibrating stimulus. The tuning fork is then applied to the great toe and if an awareness of vibration is absent it is applied progressively upwards at the lateral malleolus, the knee and the iliac crest. It is important to be certain that the patient knows that he is feeling the vibration and the test can be made more accurate by stopping the vibration by holding the end of the tuning fork and asking the patient to say when it stops.

Cortical sensation

The ability to recognise and make judgements about the nature of the stimulus depends not only on intact sensation but also on the integrity of the cortex of the parietal lobe. *Stereognosis* is the ability to recognise an object by touching it and can be tested by placing an object such as a coin into the patient's hand when his eyes are closed. Inability to recognise the object is known as astereognosis.

Two point discrimination depends on the ability to discriminate between being touched by two points or a single point. This ability varies over different parts of the body. At the tips of the fingers a healthy subject should be able to recognise two points two to three millimetres apart, over the toes two to three centimetres apart, and over the skin of the back two points can only be recognised over a considerably wider separation. It is essential to use two blunt points. This is a valuable test because it is a highly sensitive index of the integrity of the peripheral sensory pathways and also tests cortical function. Other useful tests of cortical function include the ability to localise touch to a particular part of the skin, the identification of figures or letters which are written with the examiner's finger on the patient's skin and the ability to judge weights.

Sensory inattention or *extinction* should be looked for when the above tests are performed. A stimulus is applied to either side of the body separately and the patient is asked to state on which side it is felt. When both sides of the body are tested simultaneously the patient with a parietal lobe lesion may be aware of the stimulus only on the side represented on the healthy cerebral hemisphere. Sensory extinction is particularly liable to occur with lesions of the right parietal lobe. Disease affecting the left parietal lobe may give rise to finger agnosia, right/left disorientation, inability to calculate and difficulty in writing — Gerstmann's syndrome. It is essential when testing for cortical sensory loss to be certain that tactile sensation over the skin is intact, because if there is any sensory impairment tests of cortical function will be poorly performed and no longer have localising significance.

EXAMINATION OF THE UNCONSCIOUS PATIENT

Examination of the unconscious patient requires particular techniques and skills because the patient is unable to give any account of his illness and cannot cooperate fully in the examination. Although the content of consciousness depends on proper cortical function the maintenance of conscious awareness depends on the integrity of a relatively small mass of centrally placed cerebral tissue. This is the reticular activating system which extends caudally from the posterior diencephalon to the middle third of the pons. Direct injury to this part of the brain results in loss of consciousness but impairment or loss of consciousness can also result from disease above the tentorium if this causes displacement or ischaemia of the deep midline structures. The reticular activating system can also be involved in metabolic disorders of the brain as part of a general depression of cerebral function.

Structural disorders of the brain affecting either the cerebral hemisphere or the brainstem are associated with tumours, haemorrhage and infarct. Diffuse disorders include anoxic states and the effects of infection or toxic agents, of epileptic seizures or of concussion. After subarachnoid haemorrhage, coma due to diffuse depression of cerebral function may be present together with signs of focal cerebral injury. In the examination of an unconscious patient it is not therefore sufficient to consider primary disease of the nervous system but a careful search must also be made for signs of generalised disease which may affect cerebral function.

Because the patient cannot give any account of history it is important to ascertain the history so far as possible from relatives or other witnesses. It is necessary to know whether the coma was of sudden or of gradual onset and whether it developed without warning or was preceded by premonitory symptoms such as headache, mental change or weakness of the limbs. Other features in the history that are important include a history of previous episodes of unconsciousness, of epileptic fits or of trauma. General features in the history that may be helpful are a history of cough, loss of weight, infection in the ears or chest or a history of alcoholism or depression.

In the physical examination it is essential to establish and document the *level of consciousness*. Following a head injury or if there is raised intracranial pressure an alteration in the level of consciousness may be a major factor in determining management and adequate assessment necessitates repeated examinations sometimes over an extended period of time. The essential criterion in the assessment of conscious level is the response to stimuli and the patient's state can be described in the following terms:
1. Fully conscious, cooperative and able to give a clear history.
2. Drowsy but orientated for time, place and person.
3. Able to respond to simple questions.
4. Able to respond to commands such as 'Put out your tongue'.
5. Able to respond to painful stimuli.
6. Unresponsive to painful stimuli.
7. Totally unresponsive with tendon and corneal reflexes absent.

A *drowsy patient* is one who is responsive to verbal stimuli and shows only mild clouding of consciousness. A *confused patient* is disorientated. A *delirious patient* is restless, disturbed and perhaps hallucinated. A *stuporose patient* appears unconscious but is responsive to vigorous stimulation. A *comatose patient* does not respond to painful stimuli or only in the most primitive manner. In assessing the level of consciousness if a patient fails to respond to questions it is important to consider whether this is due to dysphasia and so to look for other evidence of a left hemisphere lesion such as right-sided facial weakness or hemiparesis. Chronic coma may give way to a vegetative state in which the patient lies with eyes open, apparently unaware, but showing primitive responsiveness.

Other states which should be recognised include *akinetic mutism* where the patient lies still and silent but appears to follow movements with his eyes, and the de-efferented state or *locked-in syndrome* in which the patient is totally paralysed except for vertical eye movements and blinking and although conscious is unable to communicate. Akinetic mutism may be due to disease affecting the diencephalon and the locked-in syndrome to a lesion in the ventral part of the pons. In *psychogenic unresponsiveness* the patient is mute and immobile and may show catatonia of the limbs which remain rigid in any position in which they are placed. This can be difficult to distinguish from organic states of coma or stupor.

General examination

A careful examination is made of the head for evidence of injury. The breath should be smelt for alcohol or acetone and the tongue inspected for scars which may have arisen from epileptic fits. Corrosion of the mouth may be a sign of poisoning and severe emaciation suggests malignant disease. Cyanosis indicates cardio-respiratory inadequacy, jaundice drug intoxication or hepatic dysfunction, and purpura a blood dyscrasia. Pigmentation of the skin occurs in Addison's disease and thinning of the hair in hypothyroidism. If the patient is cold it is essential to measure the body temperature with a thermometer capable of recording low temperatures.

The position of the body should be observed because neck retraction, arching of the back and turning away from the light often signify meningeal irritation. It is important to test for neck rigidity and Kernig's sign (resistance to extension of the knee when the hip is flexed). The ears should be inspected for bleeding or evidence of infection.

Pulse, blood pressure and respirations. The *pulse* is slow in raised intracranial pressure and in heart block. A rapid pulse is present in severe shock and a totally irregular pulse indicates atrial fibrillation and suggests the possibility of cerebral embolism.

A raised *blood pressure* is a sign of established hypertension but can also occur as an acute phenomenon in association with raised intracranial pressure when the pulse is slow. A low blood pressure occurs in shock.

The character of *respirations* is useful in the assessment of the comatose state. Cheyne—Stokes or periodic breathing (page 154) occurs in the deeply unconscious patient. It does not have localising significance although it may occur in disease affecting the diencephalon. Sustained hyperventilation is found in bilateral disease affecting the midbrain and pons and in the metabolic acidosis accompanying diabetes mellitus or uraemia. Disease of the pons and medulla may be associated with extreme slowing of respiration or with ataxic breathing in which the breathing becomes totally irregular, the respirations varying in both depth and frequency.

Central nervous system. In the neurological examination of the unconscious patient many of the tests which are carried out in a routine examination cannot adequately be performed since they depend on the cooperation of the patient. Attention should be directed to particular aspects which are helpful, such as the fundus oculi, the pupils, the external ocular movements, the reflexes and the movements of the body which occur either spontaneously or in response to stimulation.

The fundi must be carefully examined for papilloedema. Although the visual fields cannot be formally examined, if the patient is responsive to stimulation a menacing movement of the hand towards the eye on one side may produce a blink which will not occur if the movement is directed towards a hemianopic field.

The pupils. The size and symmetry of the pupils must be noted together with their reactions to light. Dilatation of one pupil is likely to be due to a third nerve lesion and pressure on the third cranial nerve as a result of downward shift of the brain must always be considered when unilateral dilatation of the pupil occurs in association with diminished consciousness. A lesion in the midbrain is likely to give rise to bilaterally dilated pupils whereas pinpoint pupils are seen in pontine lesions. Severe anoxia may give rise to fixed dilated pupils and the return of normal pupil reactions is an early sign of recovery from cerebral anoxia. Drugs such as morphine produce small pupils, and large pupils occur following the use of mydriatic drugs.

The ocular movements. The position of the eyes should be noted together with any spontaneous movement or deviation from the midline. In lesions in the midbrain the eyes have a fixed position looking straight ahead. A severe lesion affecting one hemisphere may give rise to conjugate deviation of the eyes towards the side of the lesion, whereas a lesion in the pons may cause deviation of the eyes towards the opposite side. Reflex eye movements following movement of the head or stimulation of the labyrinths should also be tested. These are normally suppressed in the intact waking subject, are released from inhibition during coma but are lost in lesions of the brainstem.

To test for the *oculocephalic (doll's head) reflex* the patient's head is turned from side to side and if the reflex is present the eyes will turn in the opposite direction to the movement of the head. This reflex is absent in the healthy waking adult, appears in states of unconsciousness but is lost if there is a lesion in the brainstem. The *oculovestibular reflex* is elicited with the head raised 30° above the horizontal and 1 ml of ice cold water is instilled into the ear. In the healthy conscious subject nystagmus is elicited with the quick phase toward the opposite side. In the unconscious patient tonic deviation of the eyes will take place toward the irrigated side but if the brainstem is damaged no movement of the eyes will occur.

Movement and sensation. Disease affecting the motor pathways in the cerebrum or the brainstem may give rise to hemiplegia or hemiparesis. If this is the case inspection of the patient may show facial asymmetry and there may be diminished movement of the limbs on one side. If both arms are raised and allowed to fall back the fall will proceed unchecked on the paralysed side; if the knees are flexed an unparalysed limb will retain its position but a paralysed limb will fall back and passively extend. The tone of the limbs is tested in the normal manner and will be diminished or increased depending on the acuteness of the lesion. Sensation is tested by observing any withdrawal responses which take place in the limbs following painful stimulation.

With disease of the cerebral hemispheres or of the brainstem a number of specific responses can be obtained following painful stimulation as for example by applying firm pressure to the orbital rim. In decorticate responses there is flexion of the upper limb with extension of the lower limb. Decerebrate responses, with opisthotonos and extension of both arms and legs occur in more caudally placed lower midbrain lesions.

Reflexes. The corneal reflex may be bilaterally absent in deep coma and should always be tested. Asymmetry of the tendon reflexes is a valuable sign of a focal intracranial lesion, but in deep coma the tendon reflexes may be bilaterally absent and the plantar responses extensor and so have no localising significance.

Investigation of a Patient in Coma

There is no substitute for the meticulous clinical assessment of the patient but wherever possible this is supplemented by appropriate laboratory and radiological investigations. Investigations which should always be carried out include examination of the *urine* for sugar, albumin and ketones, examination of the *blood* for urea, electrolytes and drugs and *x-rays of the skull and chest.* X-ray of the skull may demonstrate the presence of a fracture even in the absence of a superficial injury and may show displacement of the pineal and erosion of the sella turcica. X-ray of the chest may show evidence of a primary neoplastic lesion.

If there are signs of meningeal irritation the *cerebrospinal fluid* should be examined. A lumbar puncture should not be carried out before careful consideration because if there are signs of raised intracranial pressure there is a risk that withdrawal of CSF may lead to downward shift of the brain with coning at the tentorial incisura or the foramen magnum. *Electroencephalography* is of value in localising a supratentorial lesion and may provide essential information in encephalitis and post-epileptic states. The presence of a normal EEG in the absence of focal neurological signs may be consistent with a diagnosis of psychogenic unresponsiveness. Total absence of activity in the EEG over a period of 24 hours or longer is strong evidence of irreversible cerebral damage. Echoencephalography is a safe method of demonstrating a shift of midline structures and isotope scanning is a safe and effective method of detecting a focal intracranial lesion such as a tumour, infarct or blood clot. If a space-occupying lesion is strongly suspected *computerised axial tomography* (CAT scanning) is now the investigation of choice and invasive radiological techniques such as angiography are less frequently necessary.

EXAMINATION OF THE CHILD

The first year is regarded as the period of infancy and the first month of life as the neonatal period. With older children the principles and practice of neurological examination are essentially similar to those in the adult. In early childhood, however, particular problems arise. The child is not able to give a history and may cooperate only partially in the physical examination. The child, moreover, is undergoing continuous growth and maturation and therefore it is necessary to know what is to be expected of a child at its particular stage of development, bearing in mind that not all children reach particular milestones of development at the same time. If the child is backward, mentally disturbed or handicapped by deafness or visual impairment, patience and understanding are necessary to gain the patient's full cooperation. In a paediatric examination it is essential to obtain as much information as possible from the parents, not only about the illness of the child but also about details of the mother's pregnancy, the birth of the child and any relevant family history. Events of importance in the pregnancy include rhesus incompatibility, a history of diabetes mellitus, rubella or toxaemia of pregnancy. Relevant factors at the perinatal period include intrumental delivery, anoxia after birth or jaundice.

In young children the formal testing of muscle power and of sensation may not be possible and the significance of changes in the reflexes may be closely dependent on the state of maturation of the child. Other examinations such as that of the fundus oculi may require much patience and may need to be carried out in repeated brief sessions. The examination of the newborn calls for a special approach with emphasis on the study of muscle tone and posture and on the presence and character of reflexes which change during development. The estimation of intelligence in the newborn may be a matter of great difficulty and the recognition of mental backwardness may not be possible until the child's progress through the first year of life has been followed. Meningeal infection in babies is easily missed, particularly in the newborn since head retraction and signs of raised intracranial pressure, such as a bulging fontanelle, are relatively rare. Lumbar puncture should be carried out in a young infant who shows unexplained unwillingness to feed, unusual pallor or diminished activity.

The neonatal examination

The initial step in the examination of the newborn is to inspect the baby noting the colour and texture of the skin, its posture and the character of its cry. The infant is examined for deformities of the limbs and the presence of spina bifida or meningocele. The state of consciousness may be assessed by noting whether it is unresponsive or hyperactive and by testing reaction to stimuli such as gently pinching the skin. Twitching or convulsive movements may be recognised and localised paralysis of the face or limbs should be sought. The circumference of the head is measured, the tenseness of the fontanelles noted and the head and neck auscultated for bruits. Hearing may be tested by a sudden clap of the hands near one ear when the baby will blink and stare.

Muscle tone is tested in the first place by turning the head to either side to evaluate the resistance to passive movement. The baby is then pulled forward to a sitting position with its arms so that the tone of both the neck extensors and the sternomastoids is assessed. The limbs are then moved passively in all directions at each joint. If the child is held vertically above the bed and the legs remain extended, paresis of the limbs is suggested. In marked hypotonia it is sometimes possible to move the forearm towards the opposite shoulder and almost wrap it round the neck, i.e. the 'scarf' sign.

The tendon reflexes, with the exception of the triceps and ankle jerks, are normally present in the newborn but the plantar response may be extensor during the first year of life although only the great toe is dorsiflexed the other toes being plantar flexed or extended without any fanning movement.

A number of reflexes present in early infancy should be elicited as their absence, asymmetry, or abnormal persistence may be indicative of cerebral disease. Of these the sucking and grasp reflexes, the Moro response and the tonic labyrinthine reflexes have already been described. In addition to these the oculocephalic or doll's head reflex may be present in the first ten days of life. Other useful reflexes are the cardinal-points sign in which the angles of the mouth are stroked and the lip and tongue move towards the stimulating finger and the righting reaction in which the infant is placed squatting on its haunches on a firm surface and intermittent pressure on the feet results in extension of the legs and trunk. If the baby is held vertically and its feet allowed to touch the ground automatic marching movements will take place.

If at the end of the examination hydrocephalus is suspected transillumination of the skull is undertaken in a darkened room so as to outline the ventricles.

Assessment of the developing child

In the *first four weeks of life* the infant shows little visual attention and when raised to the sitting position there is almost complete head lag. After four weeks the eyes follow an object moved from side to side but not vertically and at six weeks smiling occurs. Automatic walking disappears at about the age of two months but at the age of six months the child again attempts to walk when the legs are alternately touched on the ground. At *four months* the head should cease to lag behind the body when the baby is pulled up into the sitting position and at *six months* the baby lifts the head when supine and can sit up unaided. At this time the baby starts to crawl and at ten months he should be able to stand without support, use the thumb and index finger in opposition and say 'ma ma'. The age at which a child learns to walk is very variable but independent walking occurs at any time after the age of twelve months.

The triceps and ankle jerks which are absent at birth are generally present at about the age of four months. Many of the primitive reflexes such as the Moro response become modified and disappear during the first six months. At about six to eight months a further transient reflex — a Landau response — may be obtained. In this the baby is supported in the prone position and when the head is flexed the legs flex; likewise extension of the head is accompanied by extension of the legs.

The significance of deviation from the normal examination requires further study and in many cases the clinical diagnosis of an infant with signs of neurological deficit requires observation over an extended period as well as ancillary methods of investigation. Common causes of neurological disability in childhood are hydrocephalus, spina bifida and the different varieties of cerebral palsy. In cerebral palsy, which is essentially a non-progressive failure of cerebral development, it is important to distinguish the milder forms of disordered cerebral function which may present as clumsiness or difficulty in reading from mental backwardness or a behaviour disorder. Likewise the severer forms where there is severe spasticity, athetosis or ataxia must be differentiated from other forms of neuromuscular disorder in infancy, any of which may present as a 'floppy baby syndrome'. Hypotonia in infancy, moreover, is not always the result of a primary neuromuscular disorder but may be associated with recovery from an acute infection, malabsorption or congenital heart disease. Many of the cases of severe hypotonia, however, are examples of infantile progressive spinal muscular atrophy or the Werdnig—Hoffmann syndrome and in these cases the diagnosis is clarified by electromyography. Muscular dystrophy also develops in very early childhood and in the common Duchenne variety, where there is severe proximal weakness and sometimes pseudohypertrophy of the calf muscles, the child may display the classical physical sign of rising to his feet from the supine position by turning to the prone position and climbing up its legs (Gowers' sign). A very similar presentation may occur with certain varieties of spinal muscular atrophy which tend to occur at a later age than Werdnig—Hoffmann disease and electromyography and muscle biopsy may be of great value in distinguishing these disorders and in identifying cases of congenital myopathy which may present with mild apparently non-progressive hypotonia.

FURTHER INVESTIGATIONS

In many neurological disorders it is possible to arrive at the diagnosis on the basis of a careful clinical examination alone. Thus it may be evident that a patient with a long history of convulsions in whom physical examination shows the limbs on one side to be spastic and relatively underdeveloped is likely to have epilepsy secondary to an infantile hemiplegia. Similarly a patient with recurrent hemicranial headaches preceded by transient visual disturbances in the form of flickering lights in one half field and with no focal signs on neurological examination is clearly suffering from classical migraine. In other instances examination may provide evidence of a structural lesion localised to a single site in the brain and contrast radiology may be necessary to identify and clarify the nature of the lesion. Many neurological disorders are the direct result of disease elsewhere in the body and in these circumstances a complete general medical investigation is necessary to establish the diagnosis. An important consideration in neurological diagnosis is that a number of neurological investigations are unpleasant for the patient and not without hazard. Therefore it is advisable always to proceed initially with the simpler tests only proceeding to more elaborate methods of investigation when it is clear that they are necessary to provide information essential for the well-being of the patient.

General Investigations

Examination of the *urine* and the *peripheral blood* are essential parts of the examination of a patient with neurological symptoms. Where indicated specific biochemical and bacteriological tests are undertaken. The comparative rarity of neurosyphilis emphasises the need to carry out the Wasserman and other appropriate serological tests for syphilis in any patient in whom the clinical picture is out of the ordinary. The application of special tests of eighth nerve function has been elaborated in a previous section.

Lumbar Puncture

The examination of the cerebrospinal fluid is of great value in neurological diagnosis and specimens can readily be obtained by the technique of lumbar puncture. A needle is inserted into the lumbar subarachnoid space usually between the second and third or third and fourth lumbar vertebrae. When this is done with the patient horizontal the pressure of the CSF can be measured. A pressure of more than 200 mm of CSF in a relaxed patient suggests the presence of raised intracranial pressure. If there is clinical evidence of raised intracranial pressure it is advisable not to perform a lumbar puncture on account of the danger of a tentorial or medullary impaction. Should the pressure be elevated on manometry great care must be exercised to withdraw no more than a few drops of CSF. In the healthy subject compression of the jugular vein produces a brisk rise in CSF pressure, but this rise is not transmitted to the lumbar theca in a lesion compressing the spinal subarachnoid space (Queckenstedt's test). If lumbar puncture is not possible for any reason spinal fluid can be obtained by means of a needle inserted into the cisterna magna. This is a hazardous procedure since if the needle is inserted too far it may enter the medulla.

In *subarachnoid haemorrhage* the spinal fluid is uniformly bloodstained; red cells may be found in the CSF for as long as a week after a single haemorrhage. If the fluid is centrifuged the supernatant CSF will be yellow in colour (xanthochromia) providing confirmatory evidence that the blood in the CSF is the result of haemorrhage and not a contaminant from a traumatic puncture. Xanthochromia appears within 24 hours of a haemorrhage and may persist for as long as ten days. It is sometimes seen if there is an intracranial or subdural haematoma. In *infections* of the central nervous system there is usually a marked increase in the white cell count and in bacterial infections this may be accompanied by a fall in the sugar content. *Tumours* of the brain and spinal cord may sometimes be associated with an elevation in the CSF protein content which can be particularly high if the tumour is a neurofibroma. In cord compression with a spinal block the protein below the level of the block may be many times the normal value and the fluid is xanthochromic — Froin's syndrome. In multiple sclerosis and in neurosyphilis elevation in the gamma globulin fraction of the total protein may occur.

Electroencephalography

The electroencephalograph (EEG) records the electrical activity of the brain through the intact skull by means of surface electrodes arranged in rings over the scalp so that the potential changes can be recorded on moving paper after amplification. The use of eight to sixteen amplifying channels enables the changes occurring in widely separate areas to be recorded simultaneously.

In infants the EEG consists largely of slow activity of less than 3.5 Hz (delta activity) which is replaced during growth and maturation by increasing amounts of theta activity (4 to less than 8 Hz). In the waking adult a rhythm of 8 to 13 Hz (alpha rhythm) is recorded from the postcentral areas when the eyes are closed but disappears during visual attention and faster beta rhythms (14 to 22 Hz) may be recorded from the frontal regions (Figure 5.21). During sleep the alpha rhythm disappears to be replaced by slow activity.

The EEG is of great value in the study of epilepsy, the characteristic feature of which is the appearance of paroxysmal spike discharges (Figure 5.22). If these are widespread, as in the case of the 3.5 Hz spike and slow wave discharge of petit mal, this suggests that the cells giving rise to the epileptic discharge are situated in deep midline structures, whereas a focal spike discharge localised to one situation suggests that the epilepsy may arise from a cortical focus. Great caution is necessary in interpreting the findings since in many epileptic subjects the inter-seizure record shows no abnormality while paroxysmal discharges occur in a significant proportion of the healthy population.

Slow activity is the characteristic change recorded from brain cells where the metabolism is disturbed and may therefore be recorded from cerebral tissue overlying a tumour or a cerebral infarct. The slow activity recorded from the neighbourhood of a tumour may become more prominent with the passage of time whereas serial records may show that the changes associated with a vascular lesion undergo resolution. A tumour if large enough may give rise to an area of relative electrical silence and a subdural

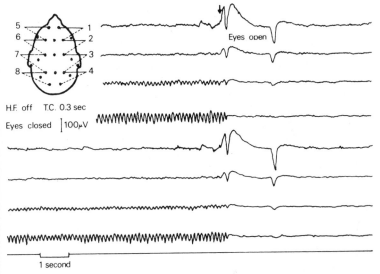

Figure 5.21. *Electroencephalogram of healthy subject. Alpha rhythm disappears on eye opening. Eye movement artefacts recorded immediately after eye opening and 2 seconds later.*

haematoma overlying part of the brain gives rise to a reduction in amplitude of the background rhythms on the affected side. In metabolic and degenerative disorders of the brain the EEG can show widespread abnormalities and serial records are of value in illustrating the evolution of the disorder. Although diffuse abnormalities are in many cases nonspecific, occurring in a wide variety of disorders such as encephalitis, raised intracranial pressure, cerebral abscess, vitamin B_{12} deficiency, or cerebral atrophy, there are a number of conditions, such as subacute encephalitis, hepatic coma and Jakob—Creutzfeldt disease in which highly characteristic bizarre slow wave complexes can be recorded. Moreover the EEG is a highly sensitive index of the acuteness of a cerebral disturbance and where it is important to assess the severity of cerebral damage it may be helpful, particularly if serial records are taken, in assessing the prognosis. A major advance in EEG has been the development of techniques to record potentials evoked from the brain by sensory stimulation. A particularly valuable

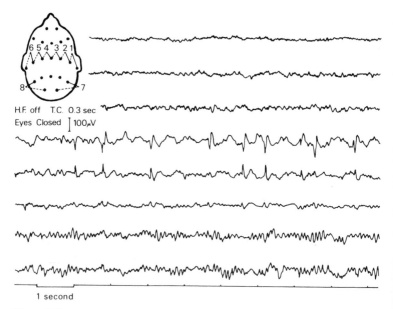

Figure 5.22. *EEG recorded from a child aged 7 years with history of epileptic attacks showing left-sided focal spike discharge. The discharges show reversal of phase about the electrode which is common to channels 4 and 5.*

method is the recording of evoked responses to a changing visual (reversing checker board) pattern since the well-defined response is delayed in lesions of the visual pathway (Figure 5.23).

An important feature of the electroencephalogram is that the technique is entirely harmless to the patient. It must be emphasised however that it is a physiological technique and as such it gives physiological information and only helps in diagnosis if evaluated in association with the clinical findings. Moreover, although abnormal findings in the EEG may provide information of particular value and interest a normal EEG in no way excludes organic disease.

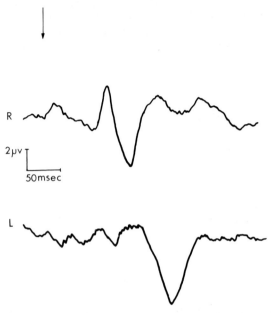

Figure 5.23. *Illustration of visual evoked response to stimulus from reversing checker board pattern recorded from patient with history of left optic neuritis. Arrow indicates time of stimulus. Positive deflection downwards. Electrodes placed to record from 5 cm above inion to vertex. Upper trace right eye; lower trace left eye.*

Electrophysiology of Peripheral Nerve and Muscle

Electromyography is the study of the electrical activity of skeletal muscle. The most widely used clinical method uses concentric needle electrodes which are inserted into muscle. The apparatus measures the potential difference between the shaft and the insulated core of the electrode and potential changes in the muscle are displayed after amplification on an oscilloscope screen. Healthy relaxed muscle is electrically silent but after denervation low amplitude short duration potentials which represent the spontaneous contractions or fibrillation of denervated fibres are recorded. Their identification is strong evidence that the innervation of a muscle has been interrupted. During a voluntary contraction motor unit potentials are recorded which represent the summated potentials derived from many muscle fibres contracting nearly synchronously. During a strong contraction so many motor units are recruited that the individual potentials cannot be separately identified and the appearance is known as an interference pattern (Figure 5.24).

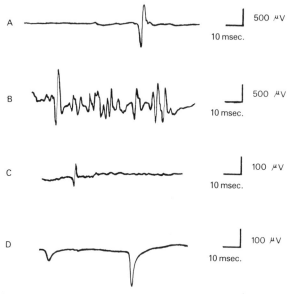

Figure 5.24. *Examples of electromyogram recorded with concentric needle electrode. (A) Motor unit action potential during weak contraction of healthy muscle. (B) Interference pattern on strong contraction of healthy muscle. (C) Fibrillation potential in denervated muscle. (D) Positive sharp wave in denervated muscle. In each trace positive deflection downwards.*

In primary disorders of muscle such as the muscular dystrophies the motor units lose a proportion of their constituent fibres and the potentials have a short duration and appear broken up and poly-phasic but because the total number of units is not markedly reduced the interference pattern is preserved. In neuropathies, on the other hand, the total number of units is markedly reduced and there is no interference pattern, single units being clearly identifiable even during a maximal contraction. In peripheral neuropathies the motor unit potentials also appear broken up and polyphasic but tend to be of longer duration than in the myopathies. In disease affecting the anterior horn cells where some neurones have died there is a tendency for the axons of the surviving neurones to send out peripheral sprouts to reinnervate denervated muscle fibres so that motor units of large size are formed and very high amplitude motor unit potentials can be recorded.

A second method of demonstrating the presence of denervated muscle depends on the differing excitability of nerve and muscle. A nerve is readily activated by weak stimuli of short duration whereas muscle requires stimuli of either longer duration or greater intensity. Since muscle is normally stimulated through its motor nerve the application of a weak stimulus to the skin overlying a muscle will generally excite it through its nerve. If however the muscle has lost its nerve supply it will only be activated if the stimulus is strong enough to stimulate the muscle directly. Using an electronic stimulator capable of delivering pulses of known intensity and duration the excitability of a muscle can be recorded in the form of an intensity duration curve. This is a simple technique which without needle puncture will identify denervated or partially denervated muscle.

The conduction velocity along a nerve can be measured by applying stimuli to the nerve and measuring the time interval before an evoked potential is recorded from the muscle it supplies. With local pressure over a nerve as in the carpal tunnel syndrome there may be slowing of nerve conduction across the compressed area and in some varieties of peripheral neuropathy where the principal change in the nerve fibre is one of segmental demyelination, substantial slowing of nerve conduction velocity occurs.

The value of these tests is enhanced if more than one technique is used. Thus if a patient with weakness of the lower limbs had electromyographic evidence of partial denervation in the affected muscles with slowing of nerve conduction the probable diagnosis is one of peripheral neuropathy, whereas if nerve conduction velocity is normal, there is no evidence of denervation and the electromyograph shows polyphasic potentials with a full interference pattern the condition is more likely to be a myopathy. If a patient with wasting of the small muscles of the hands has fibrillation potentials in the lower limbs the condition is not due to a lesion localised to the cervical cord but is more probably a generalised disorder such as motor neurone disease.

Gamma-encephalography

If a suitable isotope such as ^{99m}technetium is injected intravenously and the radioactivity over the skull is scanned areas of increased vascularity and tumours may appear as areas of increased radioactivity. This technique, which like the EEG is harmless to the patient, is extremely useful in localising tumour tissue (Figure 5.25) although it will also show an increased uptake if there has been an infarct.

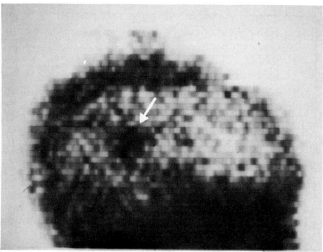

Figure 5.25. *Technetium brain scan recorded in patient to show secondary deposit from bronchial carcinoma. Arrow indicates site of increased uptake of technetium.*

A particular application of the method is the RISA scan in which radioiodinated serum albumin is injected into the lumbar theca. In the healthy subject it passes rapidly over the surface of the cerebral hemisphere, but in the presence of communicating hydrocephalus it enters the ventricular system where it may persist for as long as 48 hours after the injection.

Radiology

Although contrast radiography is frequently necessary to reach a definitive diagnosis of a neurological lesion a great deal of useful information can be obtained from careful study of plain x-ray films. Thus a plain film of the chest may reveal a bronchial carcinoma which may be the source of metastases in the brain or of a non-metastatic neuropathy associated with carcinoma. Plain films of the skull may show intracranial calcification, bony overgrowth due to a meningioma, decalcification of the sella due to raised intracranial pressure, enlargement of the sella by a pituitary tumour (Figure 5.26), enlargement of the internal auditory meatus by an acoustic tumour or shift of the calcified pineal. X-rays of the spine may show bone destruction by secondary deposits or erosion by a benign neurofibroma, congenital lesions such as spina bifida, or the degenerative changes of cervical spondylosis.

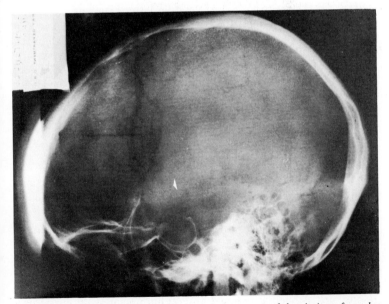

Figure 5.26. *Plain x-ray of the skull to show enlargement of the pituitary fossa due to a pituitary tumour in a patient who complained of impairment of vision and on examination had a bitemporal field defect.*

The methods of contrast radiology include air encephalography, ventriculography, angiography and myelography. These methods all involve varying degrees of discomfort to the patient and are not free from hazard. They should only be carried out if there is no other way to obtain an accurate diagnosis. In *lumbar air encephalography* the ventricles are outlined by air injected into the lumbar theca. It is a safe and effective method of demonstrating tumours both above the tentorium and in the posterior fossa. It also demonstrates hydrocephalus and cerebral atrophy but it should not be performed where there is raised intracranial pressure. There are sometimes adverse reactions in patients with dementia. In raised intracranial pressure *ventriculography* either with air or myodil may be performed by the neurosurgeon by direct ventricular puncture.

In *angiography* dye is injected either into the carotid or vertebral circulation or through the femoral artery to demonstrate the aortic arch. It is an extremely useful method of demonstrating cerebral tumours, the character of the tumour circulation sometimes giving information regarding the nature of the growth. It is an essential method for the investigation of vascular lesions such as aneurysms or vascular malformations or to demonstrate stenosis of a major vessel. Angiography is less distressing to the patient than air encephalography but carries a slightly greater hazard particularly with studies of the vertebral circulation.

Myelography is an essential investigation when there is evidence of spinal cord compression. The contrast medium is injected by the lumbar route, or if necessary by the cisternal route, and the flow of contrast is observed while the patient is screened on a tilting table.

Computerised axial tomography (CAT scan)

In this relatively new technique the cranium is scanned by a narrow beam of x-rays which is directed to examine successive horizontal slices of brain. The apparatus measures the transmission of the beam through areas of different density and by means of a computer it is possible to construct a picture of the internal structures of the brain which is displayed on a cathode ray oscilloscope and photographed. This is a non-invasive technique which not only can accurately localise tumours and other space occupying lesions such as haematoma and abscess but may make it possible to define vascular lesions and differentiate haemorrhage from infarct (Figures 5.27, 5.28, 5.29 and 5.30).

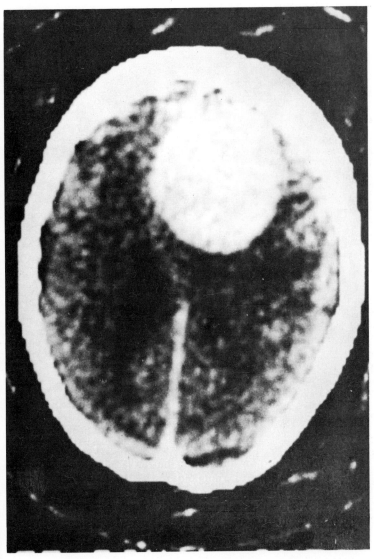

Figure 5.27. *CAT scan showing right frontal meningioma.*

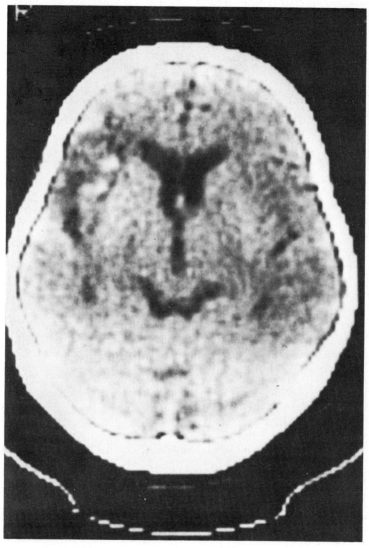

Figure 5.28. *CAT scan showing left-sided haemorrhagic infarct.*

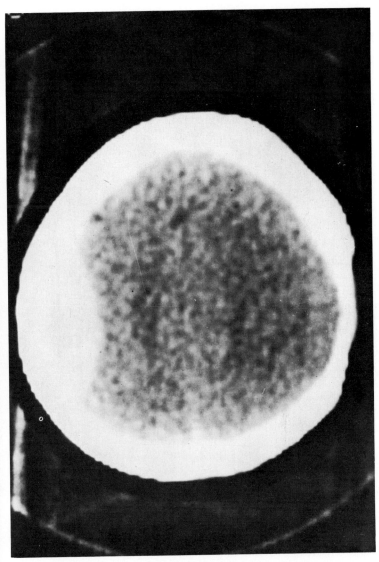

Figure 5.29. *CAT scan showing left-sided extradural haematoma.*

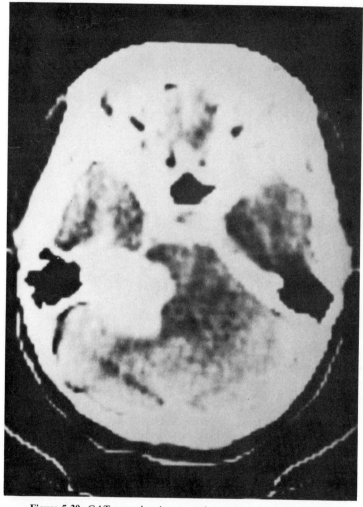

Figure 5.30. *CAT scan showing acoustic neuroma in posterior fossa.*

FURTHER READING

André-Thomas, Chesni, Y. & Dargassies, S. A. (1960) *The Neurological Examination of the Infant.* Little Club Clinics in Developmental Medicine No 1. London: National Spastics Society.

Ballantyne, J. (1970) *Deafness.* 2nd edition. London: Churchill.

Bickerstaff, E. R. (1980) *Neurological Examination in Clinical Practice.* 4th edition. Oxford: Blackwell.

Brain, W. R. (1965) *Speech Disorders.* 2nd edition. London: Butterworth.

Critchley, M. (1953) *The Parietal Lobes.* London: Arnold.

Geschwind, N. (1970) The organization of language and the brain. *Science,* **170,** 940-944.

Hallpike, C. S. (1965) Clinical otoneurology and its contributions to theory and practice. *Proceedings of the Royal Society of Medicine,* **58,** 185-196.

Kiloh, L. G., Osselton, J. W. & McComas, A. J. (1972) *Clinical Electroencephalography.* 3rd edition. London: Butterworth.

Lenman, J. A. R. & Ritchie, A. E. (1977) *Clinical Electromyography.* 2nd edition. London: Pitman.

Mayo Clinic & Mayo Foundation (1976) *Clinical Examinations in Neurology.* 4th edition. Philadelphia: W. B. Saunders.

Medical Research Council (1954) *Peripheral Nerve Injuries.* MRC Report No. 282. London: HMSO.

Paine, R. S. & Oppé, T. E. (1966) *Neurological Examination in Children.* Clinics in Developmental Medicine 20/21. London: Heinemann.

Peterson, H. O. & Kieffer, S. A. (1972) *Introduction to Neuroradiology.* New York: Harper.

Plum, F. & Posner, J. (1980) *The Diagnosis of Stupor and Coma.* 3rd edition. Philadelphia: Davis.

Reed, H. & Draace, S. M. (1972) *The Essentials of Perimetry.* 2nd edition. London: Oxford University Press.

Robertson, M. A. H. (1970) A simple instrument for testing the sense of taste. *British Medical Journal,* **ii,** 109.

6 The Eye and Visual System
W. M. Haining

Included in this section is an outline of how to examine the eye, the primary objectives being to enable the doctor to detect serious and often *asymptomatic* eye disease at an early stage, to make a preliminary evaluation of the patient with an eye *complaint*, and then to decide whether to provide treatment or alternatively refer the patient to an ophthalmologist with the appropriate degree of urgency. In order to achieve these objectives it is essential to be familiar with common symptoms of eye disease and the techniques of eye examination.

CLINICAL HISTORY

Questioning should be directed towards eliciting from the patient a description of: loss of vision, visual distortion, double vision (diplopia), ocular discomfort or pain, redness, watering, or discharge from the eye.

Visual loss may involve one or both eyes, be of gradual or sudden onset, and affect the central area or peripheral visual field. Unilateral central visual distortion usually indicates a macular disorder. 'Floaters' (vitreous opacities) are common in myopes or following small retinal bleeds in vascular disorders or after blunt trauma. Shadows progressively obscuring part of vision after premonitory flashes of light indicate retinal detachment.

Double vision can be a monocular symptom, for which cataract

367

is the commonest cause. Binocular diplopia is described under 'Squint' (see page 287).

Watering eyes (lacrimation) per se indicates blockage of tear outflow to the nasal cavity via the nasolacrimal duct. This occurs in the very young (congenital atresia) and in the aged (recurrent tear sac infections) often with a mucoid or mucopurulent discharge. Lacrimation and discharge, associated with a red eye and ocular discomfort, connotes conjunctivitis. Corneal ulceration may arise either from secondary infection of an epithelial abrasion or as a primary bacterial and viral infection.

Progressively severe *ocular pain* with profound visual loss of sudden onset is acute glaucoma until proved otherwise. Lancinating pain in the eye with nausea, 'blinding' headache, shimmering lights, and sometimes transient ipsilateral partial loss of vision describes ocular migraine. Any recurrent or prolonged visual field loss warrants a full neurological examination.

The family history is often relevant in, for example, children with squint and adults in whom glaucoma is suspected. The general medical history is pertinent because a number of ocular disorders are manifestations of systemic disease. The patient should be questioned specifically about current topical and systemic medication, and the use or abuse of tobacco and alcohol (toxic amblyopia).

INSPECTION OF THE EYES

During the history taking the general external appearance will have been observed. A detailed inspection is now performed for the visual symmetry of both eyes and eyelids, comparing ocular prominence or recession, and assessing any displacement or squint.

Drooping of either eyelid (ptosis) may be congenital or acquired, as evidence of a neurological disorder. Protrusion of the eyes (proptosis) may occur in healthy subjects, but when accompanied by lid retraction and lid lag it suggests the presence of dysthyroid exophthalmos, which may be associated with oedema of the lids and conjunctiva, and paralysis of extraocular muscles. Unilateral proptosis may indicate the presence of uncorrected axial myopia, thyroid disease or orbital tumour.

A pocket hand light is now used to examine the eyes. Asymmetry of the reflected corneal highlights may suggest the presence of squint and a cover test should be performed (Figure 6.1). This is a

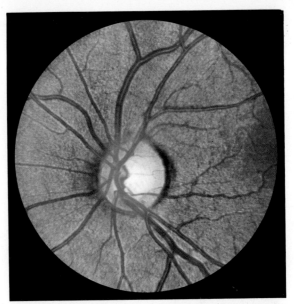

Plate 6.1

A normal left fundus showing the optic nerve head, which is pinker along the nasal margin, with a paler central physiological cup. Vessel entry is nasal to the cup; the veins are darker and nasal to the anterioles. The densely shaded macula is temporal to the disc; overall pigmentation is darker than average.

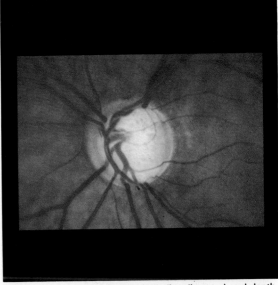

Plate 6.2

In glaucoma the physiological cup enlarges in area ($> \frac{1}{3}$ disc diameter) and depth. The excavation of the disc margin below and above partially obscures the vessels, with notching of the disc rim; the main vessels are shifted nasally.

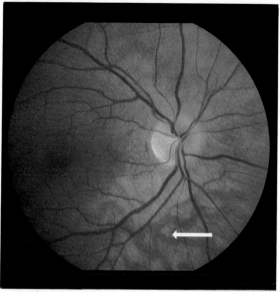

Plate 6.3

A normal right fundus. The patient is blonde with a lightly pigmented fundus background and the choroidal vessels are clearly visible (white arrow). The shaded macular area is centred two disc diameters temporal to the optic nerve head.

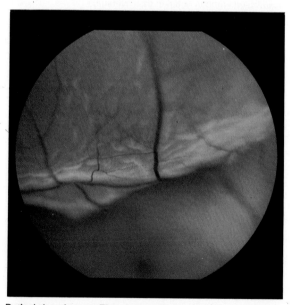

Plate 6.4

Retinal detachment. The upper retina is deeply detached, undulating with ocular movement. The detached retina is dull grey with dark retinal vessels. Normal retinal background is out of focus.

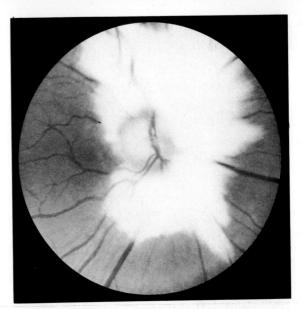

Plate 6.5

Congenital opaque nerve fibres. Extensive myelination of the juxtapapillary nerve fibre layer. Note the crisp feather-like edge of the affected area, in contradistinction to the fuzzy appearance of pathological juxtapapillary conditions.

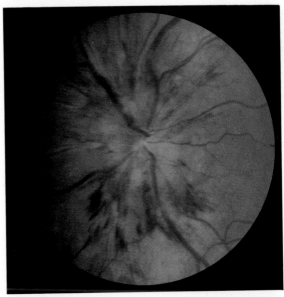

Plate 6.6A

Acute papilloedema, with gross disc swelling, loss of the physiological cup and venous distension. The superficial radial streak haemorrhages are confined to the peripapillary zone. See also Plate 6.9.

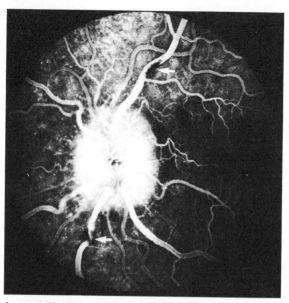

Plate 6.6B

Acute papilloedema. Fluorogram shows distended superficial disc capillaries leaking dye into optic nerve head. Early haemorrhages show up against fluorescent venous blood column (white arrows).

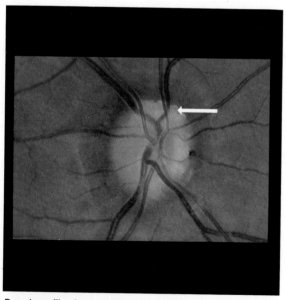

Plate 6.7

Pseudopapilloedema, caused by hyaline bodies of the nerve head. The arrow indicates the nodular elevation at the superior portion of the disc. Fluorography does not show dye leakage.

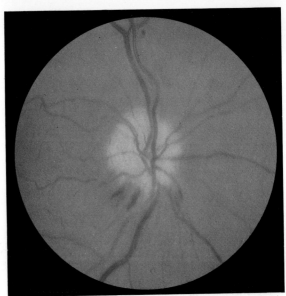

Plate 6.8

Pale papilloedema is *not* associated with raised intracranial pressure. The disc is swollen and greyish white in colour due to ischaemic capillary closure and oedema of the optic nerve head. Peripapillary haemorrhages are also present. There is profound visual loss.

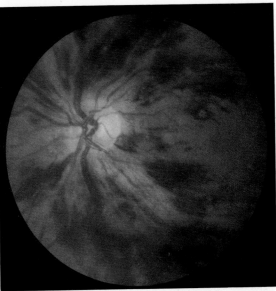

Plate 6.9

Central retinal vein occlusion. Venostasis is evident from abnormally distended veins. The optic nerve head is minimally swollen but widespread superficial and deep retinal haemorrhages extend out to the periphery.

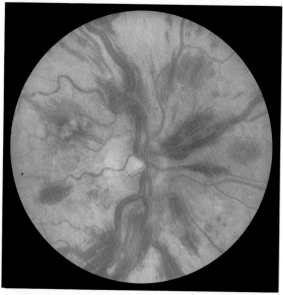

Plate 6.10

Hyperviscosity syndrome. Generalised venostasis resulting in marked dilatation of retinal veins, with superficial and deep retinal haemorrhages. A similar picture is seen in other hyperviscosity states.

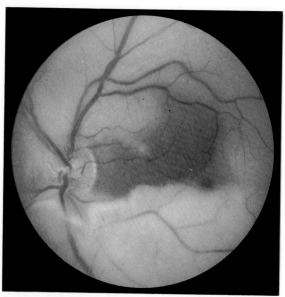

Plate 6.11

Central retinal artery occlusion. The arterioles are narrow but the striking feature is the overall retinal pallor, denoting ischaemic retinal swelling. Note the presence of a patent cilioretinal artery (present in 20 per cent of normal eyes), which supplies the central area of retina.

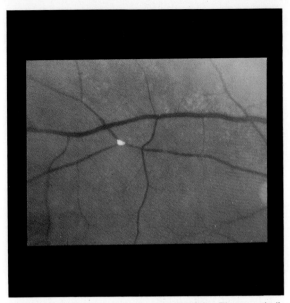

Plate 6.12

A Hollenhorst plaque is seen at the bifurcation of an arteriole. These embolic particles are composed of cholesterol derived from the carotid artery system.

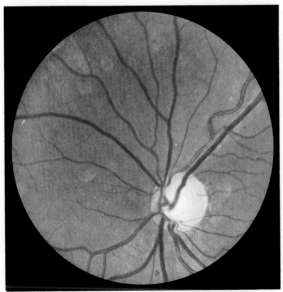

Plate 6.13

Primary optic atrophy after central retinal artery occlusion is demonstrated by a flat white optic nerve head with sharp edges, but no excavation of disc tissue.

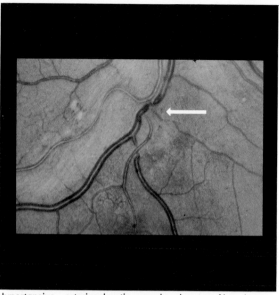

Plate 6.14

Hypertensive—arteriosclerotic vascular changes. Note 'copper wire' colour of the arterioles, and extreme nipping of the vein at the arrowed arteriovenous crossing. The soft exudates are a sign of hypertension.

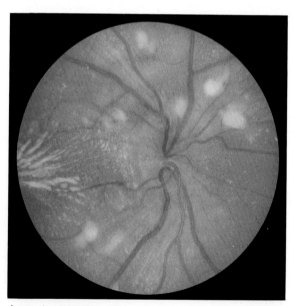

Plate 6.15

Acute hypertension. The principal features are attenuated arterioles, many scattered cotton wool patches, and retinal oedema with a 'star figure' of hard exudates at the macula.

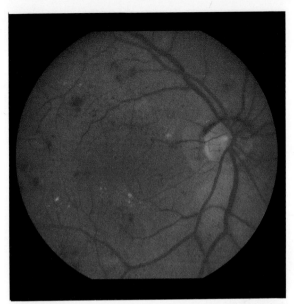

Plate 6.16

Diabetic background retinopathy. Microaneurysms and small dot and blot *intra*retinal haemorrhages are visible, together with scattered isolated hard exudative lesions. Fluorescein angiography demonstrates many more micro-aneurysms than are visible by ophthalmoscopy.

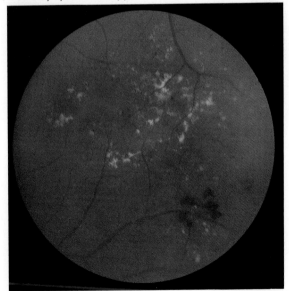

Plate 6.17

More advanced mixed diabetic retinopathy, with extensive confluent hard exudates in circinate configuration. The cluster of globular haemorrhages (bottom right) are in the preretinal plane, arising from immediately subjacent new vessels.

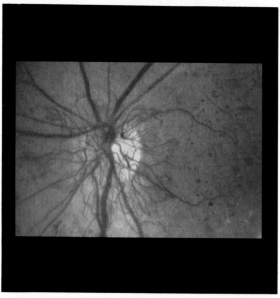

Plate 6.18

Proliferative diabetic retinopathy. Widespread microangiopathy to the right of the picture, with an advanced neovascular membrane arising from the optic disc and projecting forward into the vitreous gel.

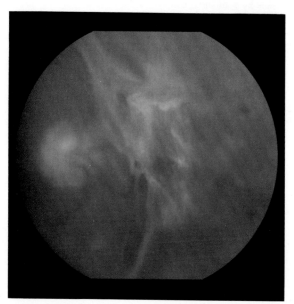

Plate 6.19

Retinitis proliferans. Diffuse bleeding into the vitreous from new vessel formation settling downwards obscures the view of the optic disc. There is also intravitreal fibrosis following a previous vitreous haemorrhage.

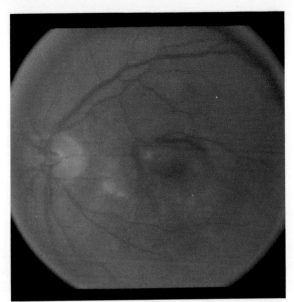

Plate 6.20

Senile macular degeneration. The central dark raised area is a sign of new vessel growth from the subjacent choroid. The surrounding streak haemorrhages indicate bleeding from these vessels, breaking into the retina.

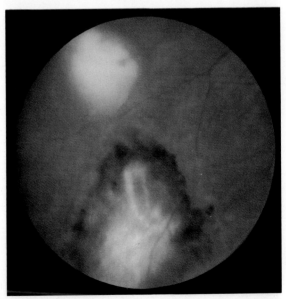

Plate 6.21

Focal choroiditis. The dark fringed lesion inferiorly is a healed scar from previous *Toxoplasma* infection. The pale fuzzy area above is typical of active focal choroiditis obscured by overlying exudate.

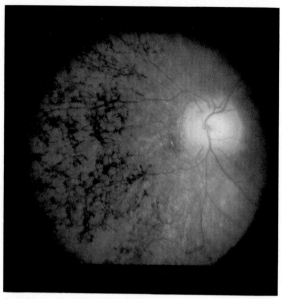

Plate 6.22

Retinitis pigmentosa. The appearance of advanced degeneration is one of widespread 'bone-spicule' pigmentation, with gross narrowing of the vessels and optic disc pallor.

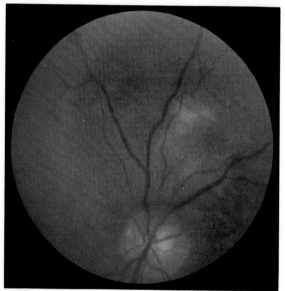

Plate 6.23

Choroidal melanoma. An extensive mottled grey raised lesion, adjoining the optic disc. The pale central area suggests rapid growth and incipient forward extension.

Plates reproduced by kind permission of The Upjohn Company.

simple diagnostic test used to establish unequivocally the presence or absence of squint. The test is described in detail on page 288 (under 'Squint and Diplopia').

The size, shape and symmetry of the pupils are compared and reactions to light and accommodation are checked, as described previously (Chapter 5).

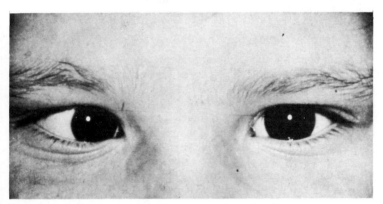

Figure 6.1. *Right convergent squint seen by corneal reflections. A cover test confirms the presence of squint.*

EXAMINATION

In order to undertake a thorough examination of the eyes, the following basic equipment is required:
1. A 6 metre or 3 metre Snellen test card (children and illiterates 'E' test) to assess and record visual acuity.
2. A hand lamp with prefocused bulb to provide focal illumination.
3. A simple 20 dioptre hand magnifier or binocular magnifier to give adequate magnification.
4. Diagnostic eye drops:
   Sodium fluorescein 2%
   Normal saline
   Amethocaine 1%
   Phenylephrine 10%
   Tropicamide 0.5%
   Cyclopentolate 0.5-1%
   Pilocarpine 2%

5. A direct ophthalmoscope for fundoscopy
6. An applanation tonometer to measure intraocular pressure.

Although the range of equipment in an eye clinic is much more extensive, using the items listed, a comprehensive ocular examination can be performed which will give a diagnosis and therefore a decision as to the management of the case.

Visual Function

Visual acuity testing

The first step in the examination of the eye is the subjective assessment of visual acuity. This is the simplest and most informative measure of visual function and should be tested and recorded in every patient presenting with an ocular complaint.

The Snellen 6 metre test chart is used in daylight or normal room lighting. The patient is seated 6 metres away from the chart. Each eye is tested separately, covering the other eye with a piece of card or paper. The visual acuity is recorded as a fraction. The denominator is the standard test distance in metres at which the chart is read (6 metres). The numerator indicates the size of letter which the patient can read. Normal visual acuity is 6/6 although the healthy young adult easily achieves 6/5 or 6/4. 'Half normal' vision is 6/12, which means that the patient can read letters only twice the size of the letters read by a patient with normal vision.

When a 6 metre test distance is not available a *reduced* 3 metre Snellen chart (reduced Snellen test type by Theodore Hamblin Limited, Langham Place, London) is used. The acuity is still recorded with a number 6, even at the reduced test distance of 3 metres. The 'reduced' size of the letters on the test chart compensates for the shorter working distance. If the patient is unable to read any letter on the Snellen chart, the visual acuity is expressed as the ability to count fingers (CF), to see hand movements (HM) or to perceive light (PL).

The patient's usual distance glasses should be worn during testing because the aim is to detect changes in visual acuity which are *not* corrected by spectacles.

The common types of refractive error may result from abnormal variation in the axial length of the eyeball (axial myopia and hypermetropia) (see Figure 6.2).

(a) In axial myopia, prefocused light rays are correctly focused on the retina by a concave lens (see Figure 6.2a).

(b) In hypermetropia, postfocused rays are brought forward to the retinal plane by a convex lens (see Figure 6.2b).

Astigmatism from differing corneal curvatures may co-exist with axial refractive errors (myopia or hypermetropia). Presbyopia appearing in middle age is a progressive failure of near-point focusing from loss of crystalline lens elasticity, requiring supplementary convex spectacle lens correction (cf. hypermetropia). A simple method of excluding refractive error as a cause of visual defect is to have the patient repeat the unaided sight test, viewing the chart through a 'pinhole' (see Figure 6.3). If the performance is improved a refractive error is present.

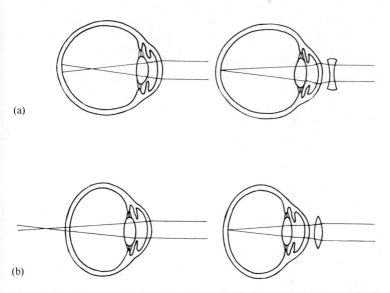

Figure 6.2. *(a) The myopic (short-sighted) eye. (b) The hypermetropic (long-sighted) eye.*

Visual acuity testing in young children and illiterates requires a different approach. In the case of preschool children and non-literate adults either the 'E' test or the Sheridan—Gardiner test can be used. For the 'E' test a large cut-out letter 'E' is held by the patient. The examiner stands 6 metres from the patient and holds up a series of cards, each of which has a single letter 'E' corresponding in decreasing size to a line of the Snellen chart. Each card is held in different positions, e.g. upright, sideways, inverted, and the patient is asked to hold his letter 'E' in the same orientation as on the examiner's card. Each eye is tested separately as before. In the Sheridan—Gardiner test, the examiner shows individual letter cards of progressively decreasing Snellen size and the patient points to the corresponding letter on a composite card.

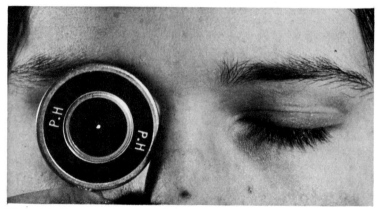

Figure 6.3. *The pinhole test to exclude refractive error as a cause of visual deficit.*

Visual field testing

Disease can affect the visual pathway anywhere from the retina back to the visual cortex. Examination of the fields of vision can detect field loss, which can often localise the site of the disease process. A history of visual field loss can be quickly assessed by the simple confrontation method. The basis of the confrontation test is to compare the patient's visual field with that of the examiner. The test can be performed rapidly with weak or unco-operative patients. In essence, the subject closes one eye, looking directly with the other eye into the corresponding eye of the examiner. The subject signifies as soon as he can see the doctor's fingers moving inwards from the periphery along horizontal and vertical lines and diagonal quadrants. Each eye is tested separately and the examination routine is as follows.

The examiner sits opposite to the subject, who is asked to look directly at the examiner's eye. The non-tested eye is completely covered by the *patient* using the palm of the hand. If necessary, the subject's head is tilted to avoid obstruction from a prominent nose or overhanging eyebrows. If spectacles are worn by the patient these should be removed before commencing the examination. The examiner's moving fingertip is brought into the patient's seeing field along a temporal horizontal *arc*, as shown in Figure 6.4, and in the same way along the upper and lower temporal quadrants to

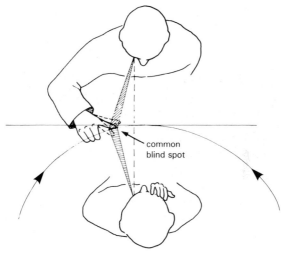

Figure 6.4. *The confrontation test of visual fields. The technique is fully described in the text.*

detect any defect at the extreme periphery. Testing from all other directions is performed along a plane midway between subject and examiner, who uses right and left hands alternatively. If there is any doubt about the accuracy of the patient's response, the patient's physiological blind spot is compared with that of the examiner because both blind spots are projected to the same point in space (Figure 6.5). With practice and a co-operative patient, the physiological blind spot can be spatially plotted, using a small object such as a hat pin or a cotton bud.

The blind spot is found to be enlarged in papilloedema or early glaucoma. Binocular visual field testing by confrontation is used when a parietal lobe lesion is suspected. The patient keeps both eyes open and the examiner, holding out both hands in the outermost part of each field, moves the fingertips of both hands simultaneously. If a parietal lesion is present, the patient can perceive movement only in the normal field (visual inattention).

There may be a complaint of a central 'hole' or scotoma in the vision. The patient is instructed to find the scotoma subjectively. The observer can then delineate the extent and shape of the defect, always moving the fingertip or test target from the centre of reduced vision towards the junction with normal vision.

The type of field loss may indicate a possible cause. For example, a central scotoma (Figure 6.5a) may be due to axial *ischaemia* of the optic nerve, central intrinsic glioma or demyelinating plaque. Toxicity from drugs or tobacco/alcohol abuse may cause a paracentral defect involving macular and disc (centrocaecal scotoma).

A typical finding in glaucoma is an arcuate scotoma arching across the visual field from the blind spot across to the temporal side, first below and then above. If undetected this can slowly extend outwards to involve the extreme peripheral field. Finally, with central field constriction, the vision is extinguished (Figure 6.5b).

The fibres from the nasal half of each retina cross at the chiasma; lesions in the region therefore give a bitemporal hemianopia. This starts asymmetrically in one upper temporal quadrant, most commonly caused by pressure from a pituitary tumour impinging eccentrically on the chiasma from below. (Inferior chiasmal nerve fibres project on the *upper* visual quadrants.) Retrochiasmal lesions in the optic tracts, radiations or visual cortex cause a homonymous hemianopia. Optic tract involvement is rare and defects are characteristically incongruous (i.e. hemianopia is not identical in each eye). Radiation and central lesions are characteristically congruous (Figure 6.5c). Differential localisation of lesions behind the chiasma is outlined in Table 6.1.

The detection and recording of central visual field loss requires the use of a Bjerrum tangent screen or, for comprehensive coverage of the central and peripheral field, the Goldman recording perimeter.

The *Bjerrum screen* is used to plot out in detail any defect of the central visual field out to 30 degrees from the central fixation point. It consists of a wall-mounted black matt screen with a white central fixation spot, and is marked into five degree concentric circles. The patient is seated one or two metres from the screen with one eye covered, looking directly ahead at the central spot with the uncovered eye. White and coloured test objects, from 2 to 20 mm in diameter, are introduced from the periphery inwards. The healthy

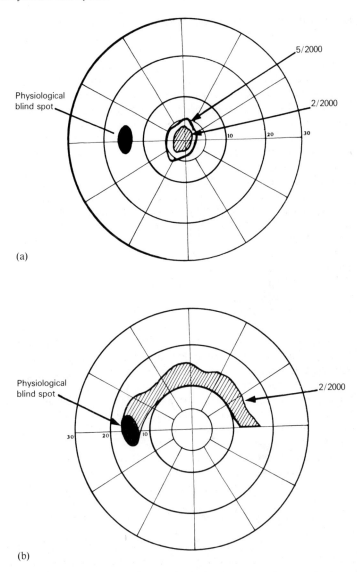

Figure 6.5. *(a) A central scotoma characteristic of axial optic nerve lesions. (b) An arcuate scotoma typical of glaucoma.*

subject will see a 2 mm test target at 30 degrees from fixation. Accuracy of central spot fixation is essential and this should be checked by charting out the physiological blind spot 15° temporal to fixation, using a 20 mm white target. Non-reflecting matt black pins are placed in the screen to record the blind spot and where targets come into view. Coloured targets reflect less light, size for size, providing a wider range of variable stimuli.

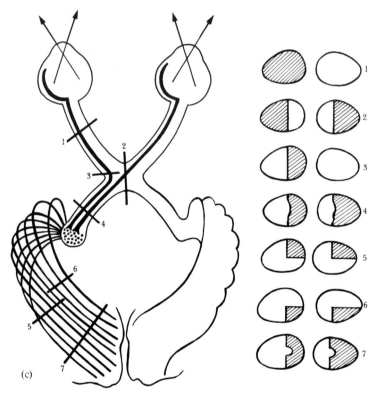

(c)

Figure 6.5 (contd.). *(c) Types of field defect caused by lesions affecting different parts of the visual pathway. 1, Left optic nerve: loss of vision in left eye. 2, Optic chiasma: loss of vision in temporal fields (bitemporal hemianopia). 3, Lateral edge of chiasma: loss of vision in nasal field. 4, Left optic tract: loss of vision in right homonymous field (incongruous). 5, Inferior fibres of left optic radiation in temporal lobe: right upper quadrant field defect. 6, Superior fibres of optic radiation in parietal lobe: right lower quadrant hemianopia. 7, Left occipital cortex: right homonymous hemianopia with macular spring.*

The Bjerrum screen is particularly useful to detect early enlargement of the blind spot (papilloedema) and small central, paracentral or arcuate scotomas.

The *Goldman bowl perimeter* covers the entire visual field, which extends to about 100° temporally, 60° nasally, and 75° downwards and upwards. The observer views the accuracy of patient fixation through a telescope at the rear of a dimly illuminated bowl. Test 'spots' of variable size, luminosity and colour are projected into the bowl and moved from periphery to centre. The patient presses a buzzer at the moment of sighting the illuminated spot, and the field is recorded on a special chart. The controlled variability of test spot and stimuli quantitates the density of field loss as well as delineating the shape and size of the field defect. The constancy of test conditions permits valid comparison of serial perimetric recording.

Table 6.1. *Lesions in optic tract and radiations*

Optic tract	Optic radiation
Field defect incongruous	Field defect congruous
Central vision loss in hemianopic field	Central vision preserved 5° around fixation point (macular sparing)
Optic atrophy may be present	No optic atrophy
Pupil reaction lost if light shone in hemianopic field (Wernicke's reaction)	Pupil reaction intact
Patient aware of the visual defect	Patient unaware of the visual defect

Anterior Segment Examination

The 'anterior segment of the eye' here refers to those parts of the eye which can be directly examined, namely, the cornea, circumcorneal area, anterior chamber, iris, lens and anterior vitreous. The eye responds to inflammation and trauma by microscopic changes, requiring magnification and focal illumination to be clearly seen. In practice a hand flash light with a prefocused bulb when used in conjunction with a ×6 magnifier reveals sufficient micropathology to make a differential diagnosis.

The examination is performed focusing the filament of the bulb onto the cornea (by extending sleeve), the hand light is held in the right or master hand, gently elevating the upper lid with the other hand and viewing the enlarged image through the magnifying lens held in the left hand or attached to the right (Figure 6.6). Prior to

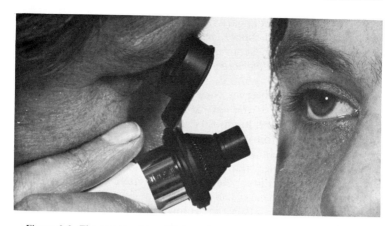

Figure 6.6. *The combined hand light and ×6 magnifier (after Barrie Jones).*

commencing the examination a drop of sodium fluorescein 2 per cent is instilled from a unidose applicator followed by several drops of saline (sodium chloride 0.9 per cent) to wash away excess dye. Areas of corneal and conjunctival epithelium damaged by viral inclusions or bacterial toxins are stained green (fluorescing in blue light).

Patients frequently complain of having a 'bloodshot' eye or 'red eye'. This presenting feature may be due to a condition which requires urgent referral to a hospital eye department, or at the other extreme may require little or no treatment at all.

It is necessary to become competent in examining the ocular anterior segment as described to differentiate between the serious and not so serious causes of 'red eye'. The principal causes of 'red eye' are

1. Subconjunctival haemorrhage
2. Episcleritis
3. Corneal ulcer
4. Acute iritis
5. Acute glaucoma

In addition to the complaint of 'red eye', the patient may be aware of:

Visual loss
Ocular discomfort and pain
Photophobia
Discharge from the eye

The preliminary examination should be directed towards the orientation and comparative evaluation of symptoms in relation to the known possible causes. The nature and degree of any visual loss should be determined and recorded. This is important since, not infrequently, patients are unaware of any uniocular visual deficit.

Acute pain, photophobia, lacrimation and discharge indicate a traumatic corneal epithelial abrasion commonly associated with a foreign body under the top lid (Figure 6.7). Ocular discomfort is often described as an irritation or grittiness, which is characteristic of conjunctivitis and not uncommonly associated with the occurrence of subconjunctival haemorrhage, whereas pain is not a feature of these conditions. Moderate pain in the eye will usually be reported in corneal ulcer, episcleritis and acute iritis. Pain of great

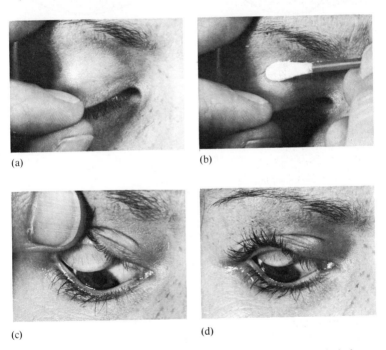

(a)   (b)

(c)   (d)

Figure 6.7. *Everting the top lid. (a) With patient looking downwards, the lashes are grasped between thumb and forefinger, the eyelid pulled down and away from the eyeball. (b) The applicator tip is gently pressed against the upper lid as shown, the lid margin turned up and everted, simultaneously increasing applicator pressure to flip over the lid. (c) The thumb maintains everted position. (d) The lid simultaneously returns to normal position on instructing the patient to look upwards.*

severity is always an indication of acute glaucoma until proven otherwise.

The topographical distribution of inflammatory *redness* is an important differential sign, as depicted schematically in Figure 6.8. (a) Uniform dense redness with a discrete often scalloped posterior margin but with no accompanying inflammatory feature is the unmistakable appearance of subconjunctival haemorrhage. There is often a history of minor trauma or of rubbing the eye in response

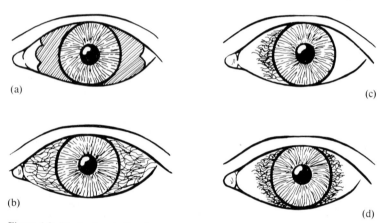

Figure 6.8. *The 'red eye': distribution of 'redness' in relation to the principal causes. (a) Subjunctival haemorrhage. (b) Generalised inflammation. (c) Segmental injection. (d) Circumcorneal injection.*

to a feeling of irritation or grittiness — particularly in the elderly arteriosclerotic patient. However, never ignore the possibility of serious concussional or penetrating injury in such patients. Where there is no clearly defined posterior margin to the haemorrhage, intracranial bleeding tracking downwards should never be forgotten as a possible cause. (b) Generalised superficial conjunctival small vessel engorgement indicates conjunctivitis. (c) Segmental injection occurs typically in episcleritis. (d) Circumcorneal injection arises from deep ciliary vessel engorgement, which occurs in acute glaucoma, acute iritis and corneal ulceration.

Discharge from the eye may be watery in nature, indicating either viral or allergic conjunctivitis. Bacterial conjunctivitis causes purulent discharge. Reflex watering occurs in acute glaucoma, iritis and corneal ulcer.

The preliminary examination should give good indication of the possible cause of a 'red eye' (Table 6.2). The specific diagnosis can now be made using the methods described of fluorescein staining, focal illumination and magnification. Finally, the intraocular pressure is measured by applanation tonometry.

The pattern of corneal staining can identify the infecting organism, e.g. a branching appearance indicates herpes simplex virus ('dendritic ulcer').

Table 6.2. *Summary of preliminary examination*

Condition	Vision reduction	Photophobia	Pain	Inflammation	Discharge
Subconjunctival haemorrhage	None	No	No, or grittiness	None, eye is uniformly red	None
Conjunctivitis	None	No	No, or grittiness in allergic conjunctivitis	Generalised	Watery: viral or allergic Purulent: bacterial
Episcleritis	None	No	Moderate	Segmental injection	None
Corneal ulcer	Yes	Yes	Moderate	Circumcorneal injection	Reflex watering
Acute iritis	Yes	Yes	Moderate	Circumcorneal injection	Reflex watering
Acute glaucoma	Yes	Yes	Severe, usually of sudden onset	Circumcorneal injection	Reflex watering

The shape and appearance of the *pupil* is now noted, focusing the flashlight bulb image on the iris. A small irregularly shaped immobile pupil occurs in acute iritis due to inflammatory adhesions of the sphincter to the anterior lens capsule (synechiae). A mid-dilated pupil which is often vertically oval occurs in acute glaucoma. The pupil does not react to light due to iris sphincter oedema resulting from the high intraocular pressure. The pressure can be roughly estimated by palpating the eyeball between index fingertips (Figure 6.9). However, an accurate reading of intraocular pressure can be obtained by carrying out instrumental measurement (see below).

A definitive differential diagnosis of the serious conditions causing 'red eye' can be made following the schedule in Table 6.3.

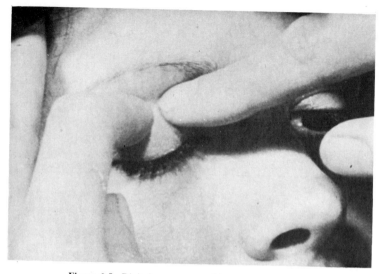

Figure 6.9. *Digital assessment of intraocular pressure.*

Applanation Tonometry

It is appropriate at this stage to consider the measurement and recording of intraocular pressure in the diagnosis of glaucoma or abnormally raised intraocular pressure (IOP). The two commonest manifestations of pathologically raised IOP are acute congestive glaucoma and chronic open angle glaucoma.

Accurate measurement of IOP can be most readily made by using a Perkins hand held applanation tonometer (Figure 6.10). The principle of this method of IOP measurement is the application of an increasing measured force to the anaesthetised anterior corneal surface until 'applanation' or paratangential flattening of the external corneal curve is observed over the area of the applied force.

Sodium fluorescein 2 per cent and a drop of amethocaine 1 per cent are instilled to both eyes. The blue light is switched on by turning the thumb wheel until the pressure loading scale is set above zero. The heel of the examiner's left hand is rested on the patient's brow and the tonometer held in the right or master hand. The doubling prism is gently laid on the fluorescein-stained corneal tear film (Figure 6.11). The prism-separated hemicircles of fluorescein-

Table 6.3. *Summary of further examination*

Condition	Cornea	Pupil shape	Pupil response to light	Hardness
Episcleritis	Clear	Normal	Normal	Normal
Corneal ulcer	Fluorescein staining	Normal	Normal	Normal
Iritis	May be hazy	Small irregular	May be no response	Normal
Glaucoma	Hazy opacity	Mid-dilated vertical oval	No response	Hard

stained tear meniscus are brought together by increasing the loading pressure on the prism. This is done by turning the thumb wheel until the *inner* ends of the hemicircles just touch with each eye pulsation (Figure 6.12). At this point the tonometer is removed from the eye and the scale reading noted, and multiplied by ten to give the IOP in mm Hg. The procedure is then repeated for the fellow eye. The upper limit of normality is generally taken to be scale reading 21, equivalent to 21 mm Hg intraocular pressure. The IOP shows a normal diurnal variation of 6 mm Hg. Serial follow-up measurements should therefore be done at the same hour on each occasion.

The tonometer provides an investigative tool in general practice to differentiate acute congestive glaucoma from the other causes of 'red eye'.

Acute congestive glaucoma

The clinical picture of acute congestive glaucoma (syn. acute angle closure glaucoma) is sudden onset of severe pain in and around the eye, with profound visual loss. Pain may be so severe that the patient is nauseated or even vomiting and is in a state of shock. The appearance of the eye has been previously described (Tables 6.2, 6.3). This condition constitutes perhaps the most serious emergency in ophthalmology, requiring immediate admission to hospital, firstly to normalise the IOP in the affected eye before vision is irreversibly lost, and secondly to prevent a similar incident occurring in the fellow eye, which is equally at risk. Acute attacks are often heralded by bouts of raised IOP manifested by the subjective appearance of coloured haloes around street lamps at

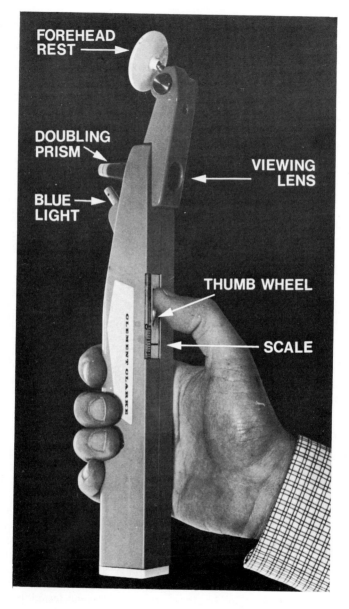

Figure 6.10. *The Perkins hand held applanation tonometer.*

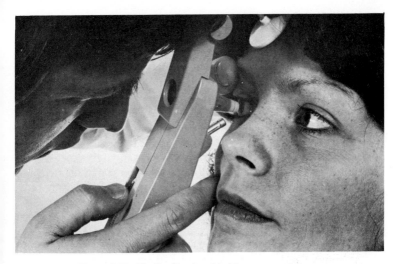

Figure 6.11. *The Perkins hand held tonometer in use.*

night. This symptom is produced by the multiprism effect of the corneal epithelial oedema. Such bouts resolve spontaneously when the patient leaves low-light-level conditions outdoors and enters a room with normal lighting. The light stimulates pupil constriction, opening up the drainage angle and breaking the attack.

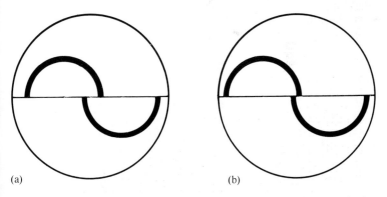

(a)   (b)

Figure 6.12. *The Perkins hand held tonometer in use: observer's view of prism doubled fluorescein-stained tear meniscus. (a) Initial appearance. (b) End point. The pressure reading is taken from the scale when the end point appearance is obtained.*

Chronic open angle glaucoma

In contrast to acute congestive glaucoma, chronic open angle glaucoma (syn. glaucoma simplex, chronic simple glaucoma) is a disease of signs rather than symptoms. It is due to diffuse changes in the ultramicrostructure of the aqueous drainage system. The onset is insidious, slowly progressing over the years. The IOP is usually not grossly raised. There is slowly progressive loss of peripheral vision with encroachment on central vision and eventual blindness. The patient is often unaware of anything other than slight impairment of vision ascribed to advancing years. All too frequently a patient will present with advanced bilateral field loss and the ophthalmoscopic appearance of glaucomatous 'cupping' and atrophy of the optic nerve head (Plate 6.2).

The disease typically appears in the fifth decade. There is a hereditary factor in this type of glaucoma, and in affected families the glaucoma becomes manifest at an earlier age in each succeeding generation. Every effort should be made to detect glaucoma simplex at the earliest stage of reversible field loss, and this can be achieved only by routine annual measurement of IOP in patients aged over 40 years with particular attention to any family history of glaucoma.

The Cover Test

This is a simple diagnostic test used to establish unequivocally the presence or absence of *squint*, which is defined as failure of alignment of the visual axes on the same fixation point. Squint and diplopia are described on page 287.

Ophthalmoscopy (syn. Funduscopy)

The ophthalmoscope is a clinical tool which can be used to examine the entire eye from the cornea back to the retinal plane (syn. fundus oculi). The technique of handling this instrument should be mastered at an early stage in clinical training to become familiar with the normal anatomy of the fundus and its variations, and thereafter to be able to recognise fundus pathology. The fundus oculi offers a unique opportunity to make direct observation of the blood circulation and a portion of central nervous system. The optical principle of the direct ophthalmoscope is simply the observation of returning rays of light from the fundus oculi through the sight hole of a mirror which directs a bright light into the eye.

The retinal image obtained is erect and magnified some fifteen times natural size. Although different makes of ophthalmoscope vary in design and layout of controls, the basic principle is common to all instruments. The most recent instruments give improved illumination from a quartz halogen light source, powered by nickel—cadmium (Hi-power) batteries. The following controls are standard: (1) a combined ON/OFF and sliding rheostat switch to control the brightness of the light beam entering the eye; (2) a ring of focusing lenses ranging in power on either side of a zero setting (no lens) from + 15 in red number, for convex lenses, to −20 in black numerals for concave lenses (the colours are reversed in American and Japanese instruments).

The required lens power is selected by revolving the lens ring, using the thumb or index finger. Convex lenses neutralise the patient's hypermetropia and concave lenses correct for myopia (Figure 6.2). Auxiliary focusing lenses are provided for high degrees of ametropia, although in cases of high myopia a better view is often obtained through the patient's own correcting spectacles, permitting the use of a low-power focusing lens in the ophthalmoscope.

The ametropic examiner has the choice of either wearing his own spectacle correction or racking up the equivalent lens on the ophthalmoscope. Refractive errors in both examiner and subject are corrected by algebraic summation of the ophthalmoscope lens power.

'Major' ophthalmoscopes have a dial to modify the projected light beam giving a choice of a large and a small round aperture for use with large dilated and small undilated pupils. A vertical slit for assessing the degree of convexity or concavity of, for example, the optic disc will also detect the presence of a macular retinal hole from any discontinuity in the beam scanning the macula. A green filter, by absorbing reflected red light (red-free light) increases contrast and enhances resolution of fine blood vessels and haemorrhages, which stand out sharply and are black in colour. Fluorescence funduscopy using the ophthalmoscope with a blue filter and fluorescein angiography using a modified fundus camera are of diagnostic value in defining papilloedema and many other fundus lesions.

Fundus examination through the undilated pupil is possible in a dark room with little or no extraneous light. The small round aperture and low ophthalmoscope illumination minimises pupil constriction. The field of view is limited to the optic disc, however, and a comprehensive examination can be achieved only after full pupil dilatation.

It is very important to be aware of the risk of provoking acute congestive angle closure glaucoma. Before instilling mydriatic drops the following criteria are observed. It is permissible to dilate the pupils of patients *under* 40 years of age, with no previous history of intermittent blurring of vision or coloured haloes associated with ocular discomfort, and after estimating the anterior chamber depth. This is best done using focal illumination and magnification, by shining a hand light obliquely across the cornea and anterior chamber to gauge the distance between peripheral iris and back of cornea. If the anterior chamber appears shallow, and this occurs particularly in middle-aged hypermetropes with early cataract, it is unsafe to use mydriatics. It is also important to remember that patients with recent head injury or undiagnosed acute neurological disorders should not have pupil-dilating drops instilled.

Simple pupil dilation (mydriasis) without paralysis of the ciliary muscle of accommodation (cycloplegia) can best be obtained by instilling a sympathomimetic drop such as phenylephrine hydrochloride 10 per cent. In older patients and diabetic patients who dilate poorly, a stronger mydriatic/cycloplegic is necessary — for example, Tropicamide (0.5 per cent) or longer acting cyclopentolate (0.5 to 1 per cent).

Ophthalmoscopy routine

The following system and handling technique should be put into practice when examining the fundus oculi. The room should be reasonably dark with both patient and examiner seated comfortably. The instrument is switched on and the index finger or thumb placed on the lens adjustment wheel, with the illumination adjusted to a level of brightness comfortable to the patient. The viewing lens wheel is rotated to place a red + 10 lens in the viewing aperture.

The rule is for the observer's right eye and right hand to examine a right eye, and vice versa.

The upper end of the ophthalmoscope is wedged in the angle bounded by nose, brow and cheek. The sight hole is found with the examiner's eye (Figure 6.13). The essential skill is to move and rotate the head and ophthalmoscope as a single unit to aid in the

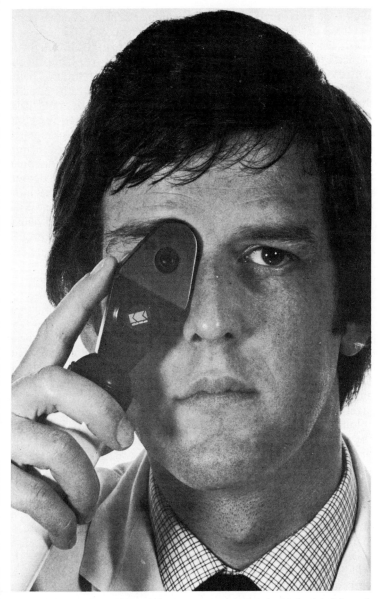

Figure 6.13. *The direct ophthalmoscope: the correct method of holding the instrument.*

alignment with the red reflex. The examiner's fellow eye may either be closed or left open (as in monocular microscopy). The patient is instructed to fix his gaze on a distant object or fixation light to reduce eye movement. The examiner places the free hand on the centre of the patient's brow to elevate the lid of the eye being examined. The centre of the sight hole is aligned with the pupil of the eye. Initial examination is made from a distance of about 10 to 20 cm. The *red reflex*, i.e. light reflected from the blood vessels at the back of the eye, should be clearly seen as a bright orange-red glow. Opacities in the optic media can be seen silhouetted against the red reflex. Peripheral lens opacities have a characteristic radial spoke configuration. Central nuclear cataract appears as an opaque central disc. Diffuse floating opacities suggest intravitreal haemorrhage, which, if severe, causes overall dimming or extinction of the red reflex. A very dark peripheral shadow undulating with ocular movement should be considered a retinal detachment until proved otherwise. The typical funduscopic appearance is seen in Plate 6.4.

Fundus examination

Topographical fundus examination of the eye should be practised following a simple routine to cover the entire fundal territory. The examiner moves forward towards the patient's eye without obscuring the 'fixing' eye (Figure 6.14), turns the viewing lens wheel anticlockwise and progressively reduces the convex lens power so as to focus back towards the retina noting the plane of any opacity on the way. A blood vessel is found and followed back 'against the branches' to the optic disc, the veins being darker in colour than the arterioles. The optic nerve is situated 15° nasal to the mid-eye line, the key orientation feature. After looking at the disc systematically the main branch vessels are followed systematically out to the peripheral quadrants. The extreme periphery is visualised by having the patient turn the eye far outwards in the direction of the peripheral area to be examined.

The macula — the most light-sensitive area — is examined last. When a mydriatic drop has not been instilled a brief glimpse of macula can be obtained using the small round aperture before reflex pupil constriction obscures the view. The central point in the middle of the macular area is the fovea, located temporal to the optic disc by approximately two disc diameters. It is identified as a glistening central point of light coming from the depths of the foveal pit surrounded by a darker macular area. The foveal reflex is sharp and bright in the young fundus, dimming with advancing years.

The overall fundus pigmentation is dependent on the melanin granule content of the retinal pigment epithelial layer, lying between the diaphanous retina and thick blood-filled choroidal vascular coat. Pigment granules are densest beneath the macula and in this area there is an additional yellow pigment (macula lutea) (Plate 6.1). There is also marked ethnic and individual variation in the degree of pigmentation. In Plate 6.1 the overall pigmentation is darker than average. In blondes and redheads pigment is minimal and in the albinoid fundus is almost absent, rendering the labyrinthine choroidal vessel pattern clearly visible (Plate 6.3).

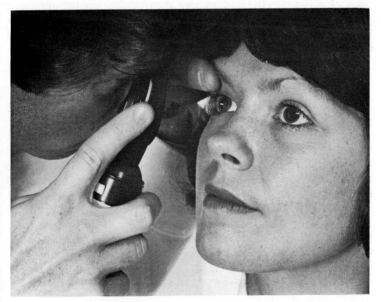

Figure 6.14. *Examining the fundus using a direct ophthalmoscope.*

The retinal vessels

The central retinal artery and vein divide into upper and lower main branches which (each) subdivide into temporal and nasal branch vessels. These major vessels branch and rebranch running towards the retinal periphery in the superficial retinal nerve fibre layer.

Thereafter the vessels run in two planes; a superficial capillary plexus runs in the superficial nerve layer and a deep capillary net lying at the junctional plane between the nuclear layer and outer flexiform layer. There is free communication between the two capillary networks.

The retinal arterioles are surrounded by a capillary-free zone of up to 150 μm, which is the maximum retinal tissue diffusion distance. In the region of the optic nerve head there is a special angio-structure comprising a superficial papillary capillary plexus on the disc surface, giving the normal pearly pink appearance, fed from the central retinal artery, and a deep intrapapillary plexus mainly derived from the posterior ciliary arteries and choroidal circulation. An additional superficial radial peripapillary capillary network surrounds the disc arching above and below the optic disc nerve layer with probable centripetal (venous) flow. In the macular zone the foveal area, which is 0.4 mm in diameter, is completely avascular.

The optic nerve

The region of the optic nerve head deserves special comment, for this region shows wide anatomical variation within the norm.

The optic nerve head is approximately 1.5 mm in diameter; it is formed by converging retinal nerve fibres with supporting glial tissue and intrinsic capillary microcirculation (Plate 6.1). It has the appearance of a vertically elongated disc with a whitish central excavation or cup, through which pass the central retinal vessels. The floor of the cup has a sieve-like appearance (lamina cribrosa) due to penetration of optic nerve fibres through intervening scleral tissue; behind the lamina the optic nerve fibres become myelinated. Myelinated nerve fibres occasionally extend downward through the lamina cribrosa and are seen as opaque nerve fibres (Plate 6.5). The normal physiological cup forms about 30 per cent or less of the overall disc diameter with a distinct unrecessed surrounding rim (Plate 6.1).

Eye diseases

Glaucoma. In glaucoma the cupping extends to the very margin of the disc, giving a sharp temporal edge. The nasal and upper and lower rim remnant is undermined so that the main vessels are obscured until they reappear at the sharp edge to radiate outwards.

Recognition of early glaucomatous cupping is an important observation in the detection of chronic simple glaucoma. Obscuration of the retinal vessels at the superotemporal and inferotemporal disc margins, causing a notched appearance, gives an early clue to the presence of glaucoma. This is confirmed by tonometry and by Goldman perimetry, which demonstrates co-related arcuate visual field defects (Figure 6.5b). As the disease progresses the cup:disc ratio increases ($>1:3$) and there is nasal displacement of the central retinal vessels (Plate 6.2). There are many other causes of optic atrophy but none with the same degree of disc excavation apart from the aftermaths of major incidents of optic disc ischaemia.

Papilloedema. Swelling of the optic nerve head is an important sign of raised cranial pressure. One of the earliest observations is venous distension and loss of spontaneous pulsation even with light digital pressure on the eye. As papilloedema progresses the nerve head swells and elevates with obliteration of the physiological cup and blurring of disc margins. The oedema may extend into peripapillary retina causing concentric light reflexes. The appearance of radial streak haemorrhages from the engorged superficial radial peripapillary plexus is indicative of papilloedema (Plate 6.6). This is of practical value in differentiating from the appearance of pseudo-papilloedema, which often presents in patients with hypermetropia who have small elevated optic discs. The other condition to be considered is hyaline 'colloid' bodies, which, although buried within the optic nerve head, often give the disc margin a scalloped appearance (Plate 6.7). Where there is any doubt, fluorescein angiography should always be carried out to detect extravascular dye leakage into the disc, differentiating between true and pseudo-papilloedema, thereby avoiding unnecessary neurosurgical intervention.

Optic neuritis. Most commonly occurring in multiple sclerosis, this may involve the prelaminar portion of the nerve, causing hyperaemia and florid swelling of the optic disc with superficial microhaemorrhages. In optic neuritis there is always a central scotoma with sometimes profound loss of central vision and impaired pupil reaction, whereas in true papilloedema there is no sustained visual loss, although transient visual blurring may herald acutely progressive papilloedema.

'Pale papilloedema'. This is an acute ischaemic optic neuropathy caused by vascular insufficiency in the optic nerve head (Plate 6.8); in elderly patients with diffuse arteriosclerotic vascular disease or in patients with cranial arteritis, the nerve head is swollen but not hyperaemic, in contradistinction to other forms of papilloedema.

Central retinal vein thrombosis (Plate 6.9). To some extent this simulates papilloedema but is characterised by widespread retinal haemorrhages extending out to the very periphery. Retinal venous thrombosis is usually secondary to immediately adjacent arterial atherosclerosis within the nerve head, causing venous compression, venostasis and eventual thrombotic occlusion. Visual loss is, however, not as marked as in central arterial occlusion and often returns to normal within a few weeks or months. Branch vein occlusions have the same appearance restricted to the upper or lower half of the fundus.

In general, retinal veins are thin walled and distensible as seen in diabetes and the segmental distension of hyperviscosity syndromes (Plate 6.10).

Central retinal artery occlusion. This does not exhibit *disc* swelling but uniform pale oedema of the retina, obscuring the choroidal redness with the exception of the macular area ('cherry red spot') or a wider area from macula to disc if a cilioretinal artery is present (Plate 6.11). It may be caused by local thrombosis over an arteriosclerotic plaque or by embolisation from a remote carotid plaque. The arterioles become thread-like and the disc pale and atrophic. There is sudden irreversible total loss of vision unless a cilioretinal artery is present, when a central island of vision is retained.

Branch arteriolar occlusions are always embolic, and caused by clot impaction, usually at a bifurction (Plate 6.12).

Primary optic atrophy. This implies damage to the nerve behind the eye with usually permanent loss of function. It is caused either by direct pressure on the nerve or after injury. Demyelinating disease selectively affects central retinal nerve fibres forming the temporal disc where pallor is most pronounced. Other uncommon causes are neurosyphilis and hereditary conditions such as Leber's optic atrophy. The appearance of the atrophic disc is 'chalk white' with sharp margins and normal vessels, and there is profound loss of vision or complete blindness (Plate 6.13). In diseases directly affecting the optic nerve head, reactive gliosis gives a yellow pallor with less distinct disc margins. Cavernous atrophy sometimes follows ischaemic neuropathy but is less marked than in advanced glaucoma.

Hypertensive and arteriosclerotic retinopathy. The retinal artery loses its elastic lamina and main muscle coat on entering the eyes so that retinal arterial vessels are really arterioles. The retinal vessel walls are transparent in the normal eye. The appearance is created by the intraluminal blood column with a superimposed central light reflex from the vessel surface. Spontaneous central venous pulsation is often present in the normal eye. The darker veins are wider than the accompanying arterioles in the ratio of approximately 3:2 in diameter. In the younger fundus the vessels show graceful sinuous curves with gentle bifurcations ending in short precapillary arterioles, which immediately form the capillary networks. Arterial sclerosis occurs as a diffuse patchy hyalinisation and fibrosis. Intimal proliferation, sludging and thrombosis can occur. The response to sustained raised blood pressure in this condition is apparent arteriolar attenuation with dilatation of the fibrotic segments. Progressive hypertrophic and fibrotic mural changes result in broader duller reflexes from the vessel wall surface. The reflex colour changes from 'copper' to 'silver' with increasing obscuration of the blood column. Arteriovenous crossing changes occur where the artery crosses the vein and the venous blood column becomes tapered and eventually obscured by further increased arteriolar thickening. It is not surprising that branch vein occlusions occur in these circumstances.

Hypertensive retinopathy in younger patients is initially characterised by diffuse arteriolar narrowing, which is reversible with therapy. In untreated patients the attenuation increases with hypertrophy and some reactive fibrosis producing the appearance of fine variations in the vessel calibre with arteriovenous crossing distortion and nipping (Plate 6.14). The further stages of the retinopathy are seen as scattered haemorrhages, soft exudates and hard exudates in the macular and scattered throughout the fundus. *Soft* (cotton wool) *exudates* are really retinal microinfarcts producing focal axonal swelling; *hard exudates* are fatty transudates through anoxic capillary endothelium (Plate 6.15).

An acute hypertensive crisis is manifested by widespread superficial (streak) haemorrhages from the superficial capillary layer and intraretinal (blot) haemorrhages with many fresh cotton wool exudates and eventually papilloedema with haemorrhages on and around the disc.

Diabetes mellitus. In as many as 90 per cent of diabetics of 20 years' standing there is funduscopic evidence of diabetic retinopathy. Diabetic retinopathy, which can be observed by ophthalmoscopy, represents an angiopathy that is present throughout the entire vascular system. The fundamental initial change is capillary closure which, although undetectable by conventional fundoscopy, is clearly demonstrated in the fluorescein angiogram. Component features of the microangiopathy which can be seen include vascular and extravascular lesions. Capillary microaneurysms are much more evident in a fluorogram (Plate 6.16); venous changes consist of dilation beading and segmented irregularity and are a serious prognostic sign in the young diabetic, being the precursor of rampant neovascularisation.

Extravascular lesions include haemorrhages and exudates. Haemorrhages vary in configuration depending on their location on or within the retina. Very superficial preretinal haemorrhages erupt forward either behind or into the vitreous gel. Hard exudates have a butter-yellow colour, being residual lipid transudates, often forming a ring-like or circinate shape surrounding a focus of gross endothelial incompetence (Plate 6.17). Soft exudates also occur in the younger diabetic and with co-existing hypertension.

Vasoproliferation of abnormal new vessel fans and fronds occurs in front of the optic disc and these are scattered peripherally throughout the retina. Initially these neovascular membranes lie flat on the retina, then sprout forwards into the plane behind the vitreous as mobile vascular fronds (Plate 6.18). Eventually the abnormal endothelium shears, with massive bleeding into the vitreous. The subsequent reactive gliotic traction precipitates retinal detachment (Plate 6.19).

*Sub*retinal new vessels in the macular area of non-diabetic elderly patients are the most frequent cause of permanent blindness in this age group.

A neovascular membrane arising from the choroidal capillaries forms deep to the retinal pigment epithelium giving the appearance of a dirty grey raised mound. Eventually bleeding erupts through into the subretinal space with loss of vision (Plate 6.20). Fluorescein angiography can detect and localise new vessels at an early stage.

Inflammatory processes are most visually disabling when they occur in the macular area. *Toxoplasma gondii, Toxocara canis,* and histoplasmosis are most often implicated in focal retinal and choroidal inflammatory lesions. Toxoplasmosis reactivation adjacent to a healed congenital scar is a not uncommon manifestation (Plate 6.21).

Retinitis pigmentosa, the commonest degenerative retinal disorder, is really a group of conditions with various modes of genetic inheritance. Both eyes are affected, presenting with a history of night blindness and characterised by the appearance of black pigment spicules in the mid-retinal periphery. There is a progressive increase in the pigmentary changes with parallel constriction of the visual field. The final manifestations of the process are dense retinal pigmentation with thread-like vessels, optic atrophy, and grossly constricted or tubular fields. Eventually only a small central island of vision remains (Plate 6.22).

The most frequently occurring neoplastic pigmented lesion seen in the fundus oculi is malignant melanoma of the choroid, characterised by a raised, deeply pigmented mass of several disc diameters at either the posterior pole or periphery (Plate 6.23). Differential diagnosis from a smaller choroidal naevus or choroidal haemorrhage is usually made by fluorescein angiography.

In this section on ophthalmoscopy, selected normal and abnormal conditions of the fundus oculi have been presented and illustrated by colour fundus photographs. It is not intended to give comprehensive coverage of all the ocular manifestations of systemic disease; however, the sooner the technique of funduscopy is mastered the earlier will the clinician be able to observe at first hand the wide variety of disorders of the fundus oculi, which can so often be of diagnostic significance in general medical as well as in primarily ocular disorders.

FURTHER READING

Rosen, E. S. & Savir, H. (1971) *Basic Ophthalmoscopy*. London: Butterworth.
Trevor-Roper, P. D. (1980) *Lecture Notes on Ophthalmology*. 6th edition. Oxford: Blackwell.

7 The Locomotor System

H. L. F. Currey

HISTORY

The cardinal symptoms of joint disease are pain, stiffness, swelling and loss of function. The swelling can readily be accounted for by the pathological changes taking place within the joint, but the mechanism of the pain and stiffness is uncertain. Despite the uncertainties about the mechanism by which joint symptoms arise, the pattern of such symptoms produced by different types of joint disease is often very characteristic, making careful, informed history taking highly rewarding.

Pain

Articular cartilage is insensitive and the synovial lining has a poor nerve supply. Both the fibrous joint capsule and the ligaments are highly sensitive to stretching and presumably to inflammatory changes, and much of the pain of arthritis may arise in these structures. Once joint disease damages nearby bone, pain may arise both from the periosteum and from deep within the bone. Pain may also arise in nearby muscles.

Lay concepts about 'rheumatism' can greatly distort the description by a patient of pains thought to arise in joints. Thus the first objective of the doctor is often to decide whether or not pain actually originates in the joints. Particular hazards in this regard are painful skeletal disorders such as metabolic bone disease and

399

multiple myelomatosis, both of which can produce 'rheumatic' types of pain. In the more peripheral, accessible joints this problem is easier, for joint disease seldom produces pain without providing other clinical evidence of disease, particularly swelling. Trunk or limb girdle pains (arising, for example, from malignant deposits in the spine) present a more difficult problem. Limb joint pain is usually well localised to the joint from which it arises and is provoked by its movement, so the patient is seldom in any doubt about which joint is at fault. An important exception is the hip; pain arising here may be felt only in the knee on that side (referred through the obturator nerve which supplies articular branches to both joints). Shoulder joint pains are usually felt at the point of insertion of the deltoid muscle.

All degrees of severity of joint pain may occur. In early degenerative joint disease (osteoarthrosis) there may be only mild twinges on executing particular movements, especially weight bearing, while at the other extreme, severe, spontaneous and constant pain may arise from a joint affected by septic arthritis, gout or a haemophilic bleed. Most joint pains are increased by activity, but the common painful conditions of the shoulder (capsulitis and frozen shoulder) tend to be worse in bed at night. Neck, limb girdle and trunk pains can be extremely difficult to interpret. Both in the cervical and lumbar regions of the spine, degenerative changes (spondylosis) and intervertebral disc lesions may produce local pain with variable radiation which may be accompanied by pain of nerve root irritation. Both types of pain may be aggravated by movement of the spine, while nerve root pain is characteristically triggered by manoeuvres which raise the intra-spinal pressure, such as sneezing and straining. Inflammatory spinal arthritis, such as ankylosing spondylitis, may produce diffuse aching pain in the back, buttocks and thighs, but (unlike sciatica due to a disc lesion) this seldom extends below the knees. The exact mechanism of much low back pain remains unexplained. Finally, apart from the metabolic and neoplastic bone diseases already mentioned, the pain of certain neurological lesions may mistakenly be ascribed to arthritic conditions. Well-known hazards in this regard are carpal tunnel syndrome (page 429), pre-eruptive herpes zoster (in which the pain has a superficial smarting quality), neuralgic amyotrophy, Bornholm disease and the lightning pains of tabes dorsalis. By contrast, neuropathic (Charcot) joints are characteristically painless, except in the diabetic foot where they may be misleadingly painful.

Stiffness

Stiffness is probably due to a variety of factors. Roughened articular surfaces may increase friction, and muscle resistance ('spasm') may be considerable around an irritable joint. However, the most impressive type of stiffness seen in joint disease — that occurring for example in the early stages of rheumatoid arthritis and typically worst on waking in the morning — is unexplained. Synovitis both within the joint and in the tendon sheaths appears to be the cause of it, but no satisfactory mechanical explanation is available.

Joint stiffness is an imprecise complaint. Many patients find it difficult to separate articular stiffness from pain (understandably, as both may arise from factors such as capsular tension) and the term covers quite different sensations, ranging from slight resistance to all voluntary movements throughout the normal range, to complete blocking of certain movements due to fixed anatomical changes. Thus, careful analysis of this symptom can be most informative. Certain types of stiffness are highly characteristic.

Early morning stiffness occurs in rheumatoid arthritis and other 'inflammatory arthropathies'. The patient awakes with a distressing, painful stiffness of all affected joints which is gradually 'worked off' by activity over a period of half to three hours or longer (to be significant the stiffness must last for at least 30 min). This 'limbering-up time' is a reflection of inflammatory activity and can be used as a measure of the effectiveness of anti-inflammatory drug therapy. A hot bath often provides some relief, but the stiffness may reappear during the day if the patient sits immobile in a chair for a period. Lesser degrees of early morning stiffness may occur in conditions such as systemic lupus erythematosus and rheumatic fever, but in degenerative joint disease (osteoarthrosis) stiffness tends to come on later in the day and after activity. One condition which produces early morning stiffness as severe as that encountered in rheumatoid arthritis is polymyalgia rheumatica.

'Locking' describes intermittent blocking of some part of the normal range of joint movement. It is due to interposition of something between the articulating surfaces and is characteristically seen in meniscal lesions in the knee, producing sudden inability to extend the joint fully. Appropriate manoeuvres may allow full

extension again, but such sudden episodes may be followed by the appearance of effusion. Loose bodies in the knee may produce a similar picture if they get between the articulating surfaces. Both torn menisci and loose bodies may also cause sudden 'giving way' of a knee during weight bearing.

'Trigger finger' results when a thickened segment of a finger flexor tendon has to pass through a narrowed segment of its tendon sheath. It occurs in patients with rheumatoid arthritis and also in otherwise healthy people. Flexion of the affected finger may be noticed to require more effort than usual, and when extension is attempted this proceeds up to a certain point, at which it sticks until greater force is exerted, when the digit suddenly snaps into full extension.

Loss of Function

In order to appreciate the impact of a rheumatological disease on the life of a patient it is necessary to make enquiries about the ability to perform normal activities at home, at work and when travelling. For purposes of crude stratification, overall disability is classified as follows:

Functional capacity
Grade 1: Completely independent without any adaptations at home or at work.
Grade 2: Independent with some adaptations, (e.g. aids and appliances).
Grade 3: Partially dependent (e.g. help needed for dressing or bathing, etc.).
Grade 4: Confined to bed/wheelchair.

Creaking and Cracking

Damaged articular surfaces produce *crepitus* when moved (see below under Examination). When coarse, this may be appreciated by the patient as grating and, in a badly damaged weight-bearing joint, may be clearly audible as an alarming creak or 'klunk'. However, similar sounds arising during shoulder or scapular movements do not necessarily indicate disease.

Joint 'cracking' — the snapping sound arising from a knee during full flexion under load or from a metacarpophalangeal joint during passive hyperextension — is quite different and of no pathological significance. It represents the phenomenon of 'cavitation' in which a bubble of gas forms within the joint.

Pattern of Joint Involvement

The anatomical distribution of joint disease can be highly characteristic. Most familiar is the predilection for *gout* to affect the first metatarsophalangeal joint (podagra). In general, gouty arthritis is centrifugal, affecting mainly peripheral joints and only rarely the hips, shoulders or spine. In this it differs from the other two metabolic deposition arthropathies: pyrophosphate arthritis (pseudogout) involves mainly the larger limb joints, ochronosis the spine. *Rheumatoid arthritis* may affect almost any joint (including oddities such as cricoarytenoid arthritis causing hoarseness and interossicular involvement leading to deafness) but the classical presentation is a peripheral, symmetrical, small joint polyarthritis. By contrast, the *seronegative arthropathies* tend to be less symmetrical and may involve the spine and sacroiliac joints. *Reiter's disease* tends to affect the lower rather than the upper limbs. Finally, it is worth remembering that *primary osteoarthrosis* of the wrist joint is rare. The pattern of joint involvement is discussed further below under Examination.

Extra-articular Complaints in Rheumatic Diseases

History taking in a case of suspected rheumatic disorder clearly must include interrogation about other systems. However, particular attention should be paid to certain features which have high diagnostic significance. An example is *eye inflammation*: a history of conjunctivitis (in Reiter's disease), iritis (in ankylosing spondylitis), dry eye (in Sjögren's syndrome), or scleritis (in rheumatoid arthritis) may provide an important diagnostic lead. *Raynaud's phenomenon* (episodes of white, numb digits, usually provoked by cold) when it appears for the first time in an adult often heralds progressive systemic sclerosis, rheumatoid arthritis or another of the systemic connective tissue disorders. *A skin eruption* can provide the essential clue in the diagnosis of arthritis: psoriasis, erythema nodosum and the 'butterfly' facial erythema of systemic lupus erythematosus are typical examples. There are many others. Enquiry should always be made regarding *genital symptoms*. A history of urethritis, whether gonococcal or 'nonspecific', may be highly relevant, as may a history of painful scrotal ulcers (Behçet's syndrome) or penile psoriasis or circinate balanitis (Reiter's disease). Recurrent painful *mouth ulcers* may indicate Behçet's syndrome and there is an association of ankylosing spondylitis and Reiter's disease with inflammatory bowel disorders.

Family History

Almost all articular diseases show some tendency to familial clustering, making the careful taking of a family history mandatory. Genetic factors are of particular relevance in arthropathies associated with haemophilia, ochronosis (alkaptonuria), hypermobility, familial Mediterranean fever and osteogenesis imperfecta, and can be an important pointer in diseases such as gout, ankylosing spondylitis and psoriatic arthritis. The familial type of osteoarthrosis is expressed, particularly in females, as degenerative changes in the terminal interphalangeal joints of the fingers (Heberden's nodes) and first metacarpophalangeal joint of the thumb, but otherwise in osteoarthrosis and in rheumatoid arthritis the family history is seldom particularly helpful.

Other Factors in the History

Other points which need to be covered include trauma and exposure to, or actual infections (rubella, hepatitis, streptococcal pharyngitis, dysentery, tuberculosis, gonorrhoea and nonspecific urethritis). In addition, diseases of other systems and a drug history, particularly the taking of corticosteroid agents, can be highly relevant.

PHYSICAL EXAMINATION: GENERAL ASSESSMENT

The patient suspected of suffering from a rheumatological complaint requires a systematic examination as outlined in the other chapters. However, certain extra-articular manifestations of rheumatic diseases are so important diagnostically that they require to be sought specifically.

Nodules and tophi

Particularly significant is the *rheumatoid subcutaneous nodule.* This is firm, non-tender, well demarcated and occurs mainly over pressure points, particularly the olecranon, where small nodules may be missed unless the examiner slides his palpating thumb over the subcutaneous ulna. The *subcutaneous nodule of rheumatic fever*, by contrast, is usually detected over the occipital region of the skull. *Gouty tophi* occur particularly in relationship to cartilage and are thus seen arising from joints (Figure 7.1) and from the helix of the ear (Figure 7.2), a characteristic site where they should always be sought.

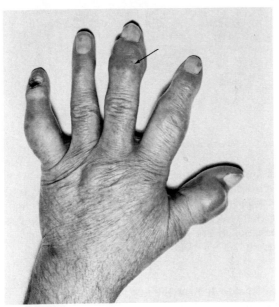

Figure 7.1. *Gouty tophi in the hand. The firm masses of urate arise from the articular cartilage of the finger joints. The scar (arrow) indicates where one tophus has discharged urate.*

Finger nails

Examination of the finger nails may be rewarding. Apart from the clubbing seen in *hypertrophic pulmonary osteoarthropathy*, the characteristic deformity of psoriasis ('thimble pitting', ladder

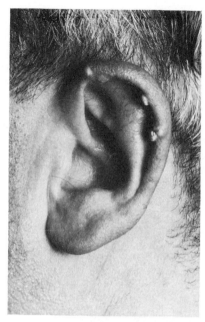

Figure 7.2. *Gouty tophi in the typical position on the helix of the ear.*

pattern, subungual hyperkeratosis, etc.) associated with swelling of the related terminal interphalangeal joint can provide the clue to *psoriatic arthritis*. Rheumatoid arteritis of the digital vessels produces characteristic *nail fold lesions*, i.e. inconspicuous brown dots (cutaneous infarcts) in the nail fold.

Eye

This is a common site for the appearance of extra-articular manifestations of rheumatic diseases. In *Sjögren's syndrome* the dry eyes appear injected and irritable and more detailed inspection reveals the characteristic features of *keratoconjunctivitis sicca* with superficial corneal adhesions ('filamentary keratitis') and punctate conjunctival and corneal staining after instilling a drop of Rose Bengal (indicating the site of death of dry superficial cells). Schirmer's test provides a crude measure of tear secretion: a narrow strip of filter paper is bent over near one end and hooked over the lower eyelid. Normal tear secretion moistens at least

15 mm of the paper in five minutes. The conjunctivitis of *Reiter's disease* is often inconspicuous and may be identified only as injection of the palpebral conjunctiva. Inflammation of the uveal tract *('uveitis')* may range from mild, recurrent *iritis* (anterior uveitis) in patients with ankylosing spondylitis, to *hypopyon* (pus in the anterior chamber) in Behçet's syndrome. Uveitis also occurs in Still's disease and occasionally in Reiter's disease and other systemic connective tissue disorders. The condition must be differentiated from conjunctivitis: there may be deeper pain (as opposed to superficial grittiness), ciliary injection is present in a circumlimbal distribution, and slit lamp inspection reveals the presence of cells in the anterior chamber.

Uveitis is uncommon in adult rheumatoid arthritis, but patients with severe rheumatoid disease (high titres of rheumatoid factor and evidence of arteritis) may develop inflammation of the sclera — *scleritis*. Beginning as an area of scleral injection, it later turns blue-grey as the pigmented layer becomes visible through the thinned sclera (Figure 7.3). The term 'episcleritis' refers to a more superficial lesion. Severe scleritis may actually cause rupture of the eyeball — *scleromalacia perforans*.

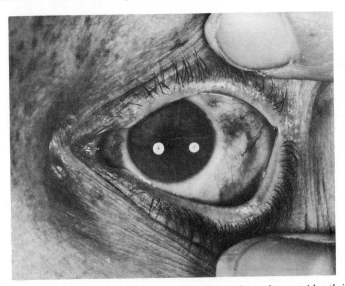

Figure 7.3. *Scleritis of the eye in a patient suffering from rheumatoid arthritis. Inflammatory changes have thinned the sclera so that the underlying pigment is visible.*

Skin

A wide variety of skin lesions may provide the essential clue to the diagnosis of joint disease. *Psoriasis* occurs not only as the typical erythematous plaques with silvery scales (particularly over points of pressure), but as moist lesions in flexures. Sometimes it may present just as 'dandruff' or as nail lesions (see above). *Erythema nodosum*, so often associated with polyarthritis, presents as crops of tender erythematous nodules one to two cm in diameter particularly over the shins. Over the course of a few days these change to the colour of a mild bruise. *Livedo reticularis*, a reticular patterned discoloration of the skin, indicates cutaneous vasculitis and is an important manifestation of polyarteritis nodosa. It must be distinguished from the familiar 'erythema ab igne' caused by repeated irradiation from a heater.

Systemic lupus erythematosus may produce a variety of skin lesions; three of the more important are erythema in a 'butterfly' distribution on the face (cheeks and bridge of the nose), erythema and telangiectasia of the skin at the base of the finger nails, and 'pitting' of the distal finger pulps due to ischaemic loss of tissue. *Reiter's disease* produces characteristic lesions on the soles and palms — 'keratoderma blenorrhagica' or simply 'keratoderma'. These lesions appear first as vesicles, then as pustules (sterile) and thereafter often take on a highly characteristic appearance with circular flaps ('envelopes') of dead skin. Occasionally the skin lesions of Reiter's disease become more generalised as a widespread, erythematous, crusting lesion. On the glans penis there may be, in the circumcised, circular, dry lesions — circinate balanitis — while in the uncircumcised the equivalent lesion is a moist erythematous plaque. *Allergic purpura (Henoch—Schönlein purpura)* produces skin lesions which differ from other types of purpura (e.g. thrombocytopenic) in that the actual purpuric spot may be less conspicuous than the inflammatory papule on which it is situated. These lesions are most common over the buttocks and legs. The skin lesions of *dermatomyositis* tend to be erythematous and scaling. They occur particularly round the eyes and over extensor surfaces. *Scleroderma* (Figure 7.4a, b) is usually recognised in the hands, face and sometimes the anterior chest wall. The skin becomes thickened, hardened (waxy) and bound down ('hidebound') with loss of skin creases and appendages and altered pigmentation (hyper- and/or hypo-). There may also be telangiectases and nodules of subcutaneous calcification.

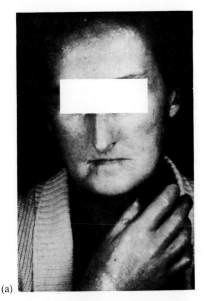

(a)

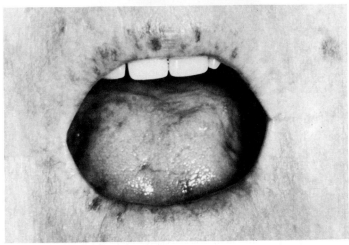

(b)

Figure 7.4. *Systemic sclerosis (scleroderma). a. Face and hand. b. Details of mouth. The skin is sclerotic throughout, with mask-like face. Pigmentary changes can be seen at the wrist, and a subcutaneous deposit of calcium on the thumb. The mouth is contracted and the lips show multiple telangiectasia. Courtesy of Dr R. L. F. Nienhuis, Groningen.*

PHYSICAL EXAMINATION OF THE JOINTS

The Locomotor System as a Whole

Observation should begin as the patient enters the room. Posture, gait, physique and any deformity may provide important information, as may observation during undressing or getting onto the examination couch. It is particularly important to remember that the examination of a joint in the lower limb is incomplete until it has been studied while weight bearing and during walking. At this stage any differences in limb length or muscle bulk should be noted.

The Individual Joint

Look — Feel — Move — Measure

sums up the sequence of steps in examining an articulation and one should add (where applicable):

Compare with the opposite side

While performing the examination, information will have to be obtained about the following.

Swelling

In joints accessible to examination, swelling is usually apparent on inspection, but palpation will be required to differentiate three types: (1) bony, (2) fluid (effusion), (3) soft tissue.

Bony swelling is the osteophytic outgrowth round osteoarthrotic joints. It imparts a hard, gnarled feel to the joint. An *effusion* may be obvious if it distends the joint into a characteristic contour (Figure 7.5), but smaller effusions can be identified only by eliciting 'cross fluctuation', in which the fluid is forced backwards and forwards between two parts of the joint. In the knee joint special manoeuvres greatly assist the identification of effusions (see under Knee; also Figure 7.29a, b). *'Soft tissue swelling'* represents enlargement of the synovial tissues by a combination of hyperplasia, cellular infiltration and oedema. Like an effusion it feels soft to the examiner, but cross fluctuation cannot be elicited. Considerable experience in palpation is needed to assess the relative contributions of fluid and synovial thickening to 'soft' joint swelling.

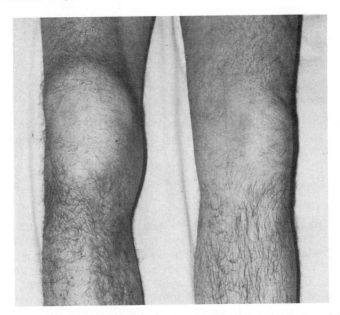

Figure 7.5. *Right knee joint distended with fluid (a bleed in a haemophiliac subject). Note the bulging suprapatellar pouch.*

More localised swellings may also be encountered in the neighbourhood of joints. Around the knee, for example, there may be cystic swellings in the popliteal fossa or distended prepatellar or infrapatellar bursae. These must be differentiated from swelling of the joint proper and the examiner must determine whether fluid can be moved between the cyst and the joint cavity.

Overlying skin

Erythema of the overlying skin is to be expected over a septic or gouty joint; it may occur over joints in rheumatic fever and palindromic rheumatism, but it is uncommon over uncomplicated rheumatoid joints and should not occur in osteoarthrosis. A rise in skin temperature, however, is a much more sensitive index of joint vascularity and is a surprisingly definite physical sign. It is detected by placing, for example, the backs of the fingers against the same part of the joint on each side of the body. The skin temperature over even an osteoarthrotic joint may be appreciably raised if an effusion is present. Over the most acutely inflamed joints (e.g. septic arthritis or gout) there may be actual oedema of the skin, and in the case of gout the skin is often noticeably dry, in contrast to other acute conditions in which it is moist.

Tenderness

Irritability of a joint is detected as tenderness to pressure over the articulation. An arbitrary grading scheme employs the patient's reaction to firm pressure over the joint:

Grade I   The patient complains of pain.
Grade II   The patient also winces.
Grade III   The patient also withdraws the joint.
Grade IV   The patient does not allow palpation.

Irritability of small joints in the hand and foot is a useful pointer to early rheumatoid arthritis. As a rapid screening test for metatarsophalangeal irritability the pinching (Figure 7.6) and squeezing (Figure 7.7) tests are valuable. With larger joints, tenderness due to arthritis should extend over the whole surface marking of the joint. Localised tenderness raises the possibility that a structure outside the joint is involved. Examples where confusion may arise are pre- or infrapatellar bursitis at the knee, 'tennis' or 'golfer's' elbow

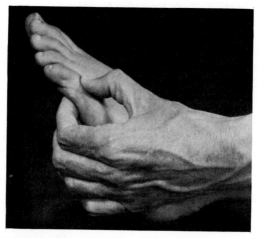

Figure 7.6. *Simultaneously pinching and moving a metatarsophalangeal joint as a test for irritability. Thickening of the joint can also be detected.*

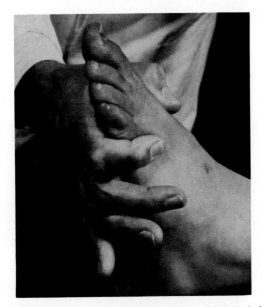

Figure 7.7. *'Squeeze' test for metatarsophalangeal joint irritability.*

(epicondylitis) and De Quervain's syndrome (tenosynovitis) at the wrist. Accurate localisation of the tenderness and demonstration of relatively free and painless movement of the joint establish the correct diagnosis.

Range of movement

Perhaps the most obvious objective in examining a joint is to establish whether it can be put through a full, normal range of movement. If the movement measured is *active* (i.e. performed by the patient) this tests the function of muscles, tendons and nerves, as well as the state of the actual joint and it is for this reason that *passive* movements are more useful for routine examination. In a diseased joint it may be helpful to test both.

When the range of movement is abnormal it must be *measured* and *recorded* (in a manner understandable to others). The most useful measuring instrument is the *goniometer* (Figure 7.8), a protractor with transparent, hinged arms of adequate length.

Modified instruments incorporating spirit levels or plumb lines are useful for special measurements. A tape measure is also needed. The system of recording the range of joint movements is now standardised and is set out in *Joint Motion: Method of Measuring and Recording* by the American Academy of Orthopaedic Surgeons (1966).

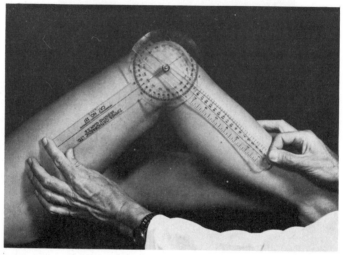

Figure 7.8. *A goniometer is used to measure the range of joint movement.*

According to this, all joint movements are measured from the *zero starting position* in which the body is represented erect with hands by the side and toes, palms and nose pointing straight forwards (except that forearm movements are considered from a zero starting position with the elbow flexed to 90° and thumb pointing straight up). From this zero starting position movements are then recorded as degrees of flexion or extension ('hyperextension' if, as at the knee, extension is abnormal), or supination/ pronation, dorsiflexion/plantar flexion, as the case may be.

Joint mobility is highly variable even amongst patients without any locomotor disease. In general, greater mobility is to be expected in the young, in females and in pigmented races. Apart from the clearly defined genetic diseases such as Ehlers—Danlos, lesser degrees of hypermobility may run in families and may cause joint disease. Such subjects can often extend metacarpophalangeal joints to 90° and touch the forearm with the thumb. Limits of normality for joint movements are difficult to define. When unilateral disease of a paired joint is suspected, much the most useful estimate is a comparison with the opposite side. For the axial joints some elaborate measuring techniques have been developed, but routine assessment depends on the experience of the examiner. While testing the range of movement, note should also be taken of any pain produced by such movement. In an inflamed joint this, like joint tenderness (see above), is a measure of irritability. In acute arthritis pain is produced by movement through any part of the range. When the inflammation is outside the joint (e.g. acute prepatellar bursitis) extremes of movement may be painful (by distorting the nearby soft tissues) but careful examination should reveal a pain-free range within these limits.

Crepitus is a sensation of crunching or grinding transmitted from a moving joint to a palpating hand. The examiner places one hand over the articulation while using the other hand to move the joint passively. Generally crepitus indicates roughening of the articular bearing surfaces and in quality and degree ranges from *fine* in the case of early rheumatoid arthritis to *coarse* in the case of advanced osteoarthrosis (irregular bone ends grinding together). Charcot joints provide the most extreme examples of the latter. Crepitus indicates pathology, except in the case of the shoulder, where crepitus can arise from periarticular structures. The subjective sensation of crepitus and more gross sounds arising from weight-bearing joints are discussed above under Symptoms. Occasionally crepitus may be produced by the movement of tendons through their sheaths. In the forearm this may be a sign of scleroderma.

Deformity

This term, confusingly, is used to describe three joint abnormalities: inability to move through some part of the normal range (e.g. *flexion deformity*), the presence of abnormal alignment of the bones (e.g. *varus deformity* of the knee) and altered relationships of the bearing surfaces (*subluxation* or *dislocation*). The first of these is considered above under Range of movement. Malalignment must be sought in diseased joints, particularly the weight-bearing joints, and it is important to determine the *effect of weight-bearing* on, for example, a varus or valgus knee deformity. By convention, deviation of the distal bone towards the midline is referred to as *varus*, and away from the midline as *valgus*; thus 'bow leg' is genu varum and a 'bunion' is hallux valgus. Such a deformity should be measured, with a goniometer and, if applicable, while weight-bearing, and the examiner must determine the extent to which it can be corrected. Correctable deformities indicate *instability* (see below).

When the opposite bearing surfaces of a joint are partly displaced, the term *subluxation* is used. *Dislocation* describes displacement so gross that the bearing surfaces are no longer in contact.

Stability

Abnormalities of bearing surfaces or ligaments may allow joint movements outside the normal range (e.g. valgus or varus movement in a knee). Such *instability* should be sought, particularly in weight-bearing joints, by passive movements designed to test integrity of the various ligaments (as an example see under Knee joint).

Muscles

Stability tested by passive movements is not the same as stability of a joint in active use. In the latter case the pull of muscles across the articulation plays an important stabilising role. Joint disease leads to wasting and weakness of nearby muscles; thus the assessment of the state of the muscles is an important aspect of examining a joint. Hand or shoulder joint disease may produce muscle wasting so marked as to suggest a neurological lesion, and gross muscle wasting round an articulation may produce a spurious appearance of joint swelling. Knee joint disease produces in particular quadriceps muscle wasting, best documented as thigh circumference at a measured distance above a bony landmark at the knee. However, a rough estimate of quadriceps function may be obtained by palpating these muscles while getting the supine patient to 'press the knee onto the examination couch'.

Neurological examination

The articular system should never be considered in isolation and, in the extremities, it is particularly important to exclude neurological lesions. Not only may arthritis cause neurological lesions (entrapment neuropathies such as carpal tunnel syndrome and ulnar neuropathy) and vice versa (e.g. Charcot joints), but the execution of active joint movements requires the participation of an intact neurological system.

Special tests

Descriptions of special tests applicable only to one particular joint are included in the appropriate sections below.

Functional tests

Integrated functions have to be assessed as well as individual movements of joints. In the hand this involves consideration of matters such as *grip* (see Figure 7.21) and in the lower limbs, *gait*. More elaborate functional assessments are usually carried out in appropriately equipped departments of occupational therapy where all *activities of daily living* can be studied.

PHYSICAL EXAMINATION OF INDIVIDUAL JOINTS

The individual joints are discussed below, beginning with the unpaired, axial joints, followed by the upper limb, then the lower limb joints. As the general principles of examining a joint have already been described, attention will here be focused on the manner in which these techniques are applied in particular anatomical situations. For each articulation the range of normal movements indicated represents an approximate mean normal for an adult based on various authorities (American Academy of Orthopaedic Surgeons, 1966).

Clearly not all patients need to have every joint examined fully. In a routine examination, when joint disease is not suspected, it is usually sufficient to exclude joint swelling or deformity and abnormalities of gait and posture by inspection of the patient's extremities and observation of him in the clinic. To the trained eye this provides important information, not only about the joints, but about the state of the muscles, skin, nails, etc. Inspection of the limbs should include putting the joints through their range of movements passively (again, this is not an isolated exercise to test the joints but provides information about muscle tone and tenderness of bones or soft tissues, etc.). There are, however, two joint movements that should always be tested in a routine examination: the one is *lumbar spine flexion*, the other *hip joint movement*. Experience has shown that it is possible to overlook a rigid lumbar spine or grossly restricted hip joint unless these are specifically sought. When joint disease is suspected then the more detailed examination described below is appropriate.

The Spine

The relative inaccessibility of both the anterior and posterior (facetal or apophyseal) intervertebral joints prevents detailed examination of individual articulations. Nevertheless a carefully performed examination can be highly informative. This demands correct technique, experience of the normal range of mobility and, above all, adequate exposure (a bikini-type examination garment for females is useful).

When spinal disease is suspected the examiner will need to seek evidence, not only of 'rheumatological' lesions such as spondylosis, ankylosing spondylitis and intervertebral disc derangements, but also of infective lesions, metabolic bone disease and neoplasia (e.g. myelomatosis or secondary carcinomatous deposits). For this reason it is particularly important to study the overall shape of the spine with the patient erect (increased flexion is designated *kyphosis*, extension *lordosis* and lateral bending *scoliosis*). Particularly significant is a localised angulation or prominence *(gibbus)*. The posterior spinous processes provide useful surface marks, but their deviation from the midline in scoliosis is minimised by concomitant rotation of the vertebrae. Firm pressure or percussion over the spinous processes may elicit localised tenderness indicative of an abscess, a secondary deposit or an osteoporotic vertebral collapse, while widespread osteoporotic collapse may produce distinct shortening of stature.

Cervical spine

The cervical spine is mobile throughout its length, although the 'nodding' component of flexion/extension takes place mainly at the atlanto-occipital articulation and rotation at the atlanto-axial level. Some degree of degenerative change — spondylosis — is invariable in older patients and affects particularly the C5 to C7 area. Pain or paraesthesiae in the arm reproduced by neck movements is suggestive of nerve root involvement from this cause ('brachial neuralgia') and no examination of the cervical spine is complete without checking the arms for any neurological deficit. When rheumatoid arthritis involves the cervical spine it affects mainly the upper region and occasionally produces serious, even fatal, myelopathy. Care is therefore necessary in examining the rheumatoid neck.

Movements are tested with the patient either standing or sitting upright. The patient is requested to carry out the various movements actively.

Rotation: (75°) 'Look over your shoulder to the right (or left).'

Flexion: (45°) 'Look down — chin on your chest.'

Extension: (45°) 'Look up and tilt your head right back.'

Lateral bending: (45°) 'Bend your head sideways, ear towards your shoulder.'

Thoracolumbar spine

The thoracic region allows more rotation than the lumbar, while bending movements are greater in the lumbar region. Ankylosing spondylitis, which usually starts in the lower spine and spreads gradually up to the occiput, restricts movements in all directions, while disc disorders produce limitation mainly of lumbar flexion. These movements are estimated by careful observation by eye. Adequate exposure is essential.

Flexion (Figure 7.9). The standing patient attempts to touch her toes, without bending her knees, while the observer views the lumbar region from the side. Sufficiently mobile hips may allow the fingers to reach the toes even when the spine is rigid, so it is the observed movement of the lumbar region which is important. Separation of the spinous processes during flexion may be confirmed by placing the finger tips of one hand over them during this manoeuvre, or by actual measurement with a tape measure.

Extension (Figure 7.10). The standing patient bends over backwards, supported behind by the examiner.

Lateral bending (Figure 7.11). The standing patient slides a hand as far as possible down the outside of her leg without allowing her trunk to move forwards. Movement is estimated from behind.

Rotation (Figure 7.12). The patient is seated to fix the pelvis and rotates the shoulders round as far as possible. The examiner observes from above.

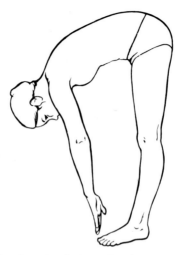

Figure 7.9. *Lumbar spine flexion: adequate exposure is essential.*

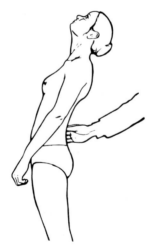

Figure 7.10. *Lumbar spine extension. The examiner's hand supports the patient from behind.*

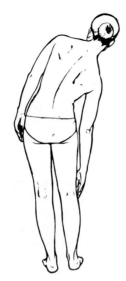

Figure 7.11. *Lateral bending of the lumbar spine: 'Slide your hand down your leg so as to bend sideways, not forwards'.*

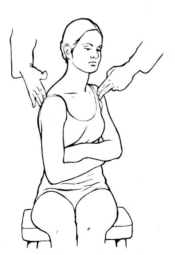

Figure 7.12. *Rotation of the thoracic spine. The patient sits to anchor the pelvis.*

Chest expansion. This useful indication of costovertebral joint mobility is determined by tape measure. A significant reduction (below about five cm, depending on build) characteristically occurs early in the course of ankylosing spondylitis.

In patients with lumbar intervertebral disc lesions there may be pressure on nerve roots, giving leg pain ('sciatica') or other neurological symptoms. Complete examination of the lumbar spine should therefore include a neurological examination of the lower limbs. When a lumbar disc lesion is suspected, *Lasègue's test* (straight leg raising) should be performed. The patient lies flat on her back and the examiner first establishes that hip flexion (with the knee on the same side also flexed) is free and painless (as in Figure 7.26). If it is, the leg (with the knee now straight) is raised passively by the examiner as far as it will go without producing pain. Normally 90° should be possible. This manoeuvre puts the sciatic nerve on the stretch and in the presence of root irritation it may be markedly restricted. Care is necessary to avoid producing excessive pain in patients with acute disc lesions. A corresponding manoeuvre, the *femoral stretch test*, may be positive when there is irritation of nerve roots making up the femoral nerve. With the patient prone the examiner first flexes the knee and then extends the hip on the same side.

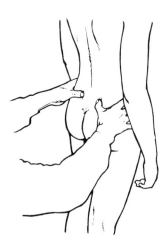

Figure 7.13. *The position of the sacroiliac joints is indicated by a pair of skin dimples. Firm pressure with the thumbs may elicit tenderness.*

Sacroiliac joints

Firm pressure with the thumbs over these joints (the position of which is indicated by two dimples low in the lumbar region) may indicate sacroiliac irritability (Figure 7.13). A more reliable test is that illustrated in Figure 7.14 in which the examiner exerts firm downward pressure over the sacrum with the patient prone. This produces pain in the sacroiliac joints when these are irritable.

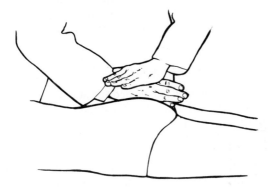

Figure 7.14. *A test for sacroiliac joint irritability. Firm pressure is exerted downwards over the sacrum.*

Sacrococcygeal joint

This joint can be examined adequately only by palpation between an index finger within the rectum and a thumb on the overlying skin. Rheumatological complaints of this articulation are rarely recognised.

Mandibular Joints

A palpating finger placed just in front of the tragus of the ear will feel the condyle of the mandible sliding forward as the jaw is opened. Tenderness, crepitus and clicking may be elicited, and the range of movement is recorded as the distance to which the upper and lower incisors can be separated. These joints also allow protrusion—retraction and side-to-side movements of the jaw.

Shoulder Girdle and Upper Limb

Sternoclavicular and acromioclavicular joints

Both of these articulations are readily accessible for inspection and palpation. Their movements are studied by asking the patient to 'shrug the shoulders'. Degenerative changes and even subluxation of the sternoclavicular joints may make them prominent (although usually painless) in elderly subjects.

In passing, it should be noted that the *manubriosternal* joint may occasionally become painful in ankylosing spondylitis, and that in *Tietze's disease* painful swelling of the upper costal cartilages occurs.

The shoulder (glenohumeral joint)

Exposure of the upper chest is needed for adequate examination of either shoulder. The examiner should stand back and compare the two sides both with the patient standing relaxed and during active abduction of the arms to straight above the head. Muscle wasting is best observed from behind.

Because it is covered by the deltoid muscle, synovial swelling and effusions (which may involve the often-communicating sub-acromial bursa) may not be detected unless gross. Nevertheless the bony landmarks of the joint can be palpated through the deltoid and at the same time the acromioclavicular joint should be tested for tenderness (disorders of this articulation may mimic gleno-humeral pathology).

True arthritis of the shoulder joint is less common than a group of ill-understood disorders (probably not primarily articular) in which pain and/or stiffness are the cardinal features. The patho-genesis of these conditions is less well understood than their titles imply: 'tendinitis' describes a disorder in which passive movements are well retained but in which one particular movement produces pain when executed actively against resistance; the interpretation being that the tendon(s) subserving this movement are at fault. Thus in *supraspinatus tendinitis*, the commonest type, there is a full range of passive movement, but resisted abduction produces pain. Supraspinatus tendinitis also produces a characteristic 'painful arc' on active abduction (Figure 7.15). This is thought to be due to the abnormal tendon impinging on the acromion above and it is abolished by externally rotating the arm. When the signs of tendinitis spread to involve a number of tendons in the rotator cuff the term *capsulitis* is applied. There is uncertainty about the extent to which *subacromial bursitis* represents a separate entity which can be identified clinically. When all shoulder joint movements are markedly limited the condition is called *frozen shoulder*. Predictably, rupture of a tendon leads to loss of the active, but retention of the passive, movement subserved.

Most shoulder movements are a combination of ball-and-socket motion at the glenohumeral articulation combined with sliding of the scapula over the thoracic cage. To test pure glenohumeral movements it is necessary to anchor the scapula by some technique such as that illustrated in Figure 7.16. Apparent crepitus is sometimes elicited in otherwise seemingly normal shoulder joints and, unlike other sites, does not necessarily denote arthritis. Shoulder movements are tested with the patient standing or sitting upright.

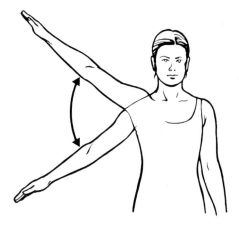

Figure 7.15. *The 'painful arc' of supraspinatus tendinitis. Pain is experienced as the arm moves through the middle range of abduction (indicated by the arrow).*

Abduction: (glenohumeral 90°, total 180°). Figure 7.16 illustrates a method of assessment of passive glenohumeral abduction. Total abduction is usually tested actively. Note that paralysis or rupture of supraspinatus prevents *initiation* of abduction (the deltoid muscle can complete the movement). The 'painful arc' (Figure 7.15) encountered in supraspinatus tendinitis has been mentioned above.

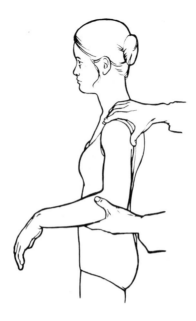

Figure 7.16. *In order to test pure glenohumeral joint movements it is necessary to eliminate scapular movement. Here the examiner tests abduction while anchoring the scapula.*

Adduction: (50°) The arm is carried medially across the front of the chest.

Flexion: (90°) The arm is swung forwards as in marching.

Extension: (65°) The arm is swung backwards as in marching.

Internal rotation: (90°) Rotation can be tested with the arm in various positions of flexion/extension and adduction/abduction. In practice internal rotation is conveniently documented as the height up the back which can be reached with the thumb (Figure 7.17) — a combined glenohumeral and scapular movement.

External rotation: (60°) This is a pure glenohumeral movement (Figure 7.18).

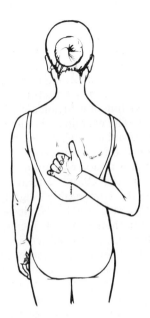

Figure 7.17. *A convenient method of testing total internal rotation (a combined glenohumeral and scapular movement).*

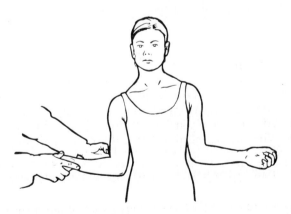

Figure 7.18. *External rotation: a pure glenohumeral movement.*

Elbow

If the patient fully flexes both elbows and points them towards the examiner this allows identification of three bony landmarks forming a triangle (medial and lateral humeral epicondyles and the tip of the olecranon) and allows a useful comparison between the two sides. Synovial swelling or effusion appears as a bulge on either side of the olecranon. The examiner should slide the thumb down the subcutaneous proximal ulna when seeking rheumatoid nodules. This is a common site also for an olecranon bursa or gouty tophus. Two extremely common minor conditions must be differentiated from true arthritis of the elbow: lateral humeral epicondylitis ('tennis elbow') and the comparable, slightly less common condition on the medial side ('golfer's elbow'). In each, elbow movements are full, but there is sharply localised tenderness, which may be difficult to locate, over the affected humeral epicondyle. In addition, extending the wrist against resistance reproduces the pain of tennis elbow; flexing it against resistance reproduces the pain of golfer's elbow. The ulnar nerve can be palpated behind the medial humeral epicondyle. This is a common site for *entrapment neuropathy* due to arthritis. Simple hinge movements take place at the elbow.

Flexion: (150°) The forearm is pressed against the biceps muscle.

Hyperextension: (0°) The arm is straightened and, if possible, carried beyond the zero starting position.

Forearm

A thumb placed about two cm distal to the lateral epicondyle of the humerus will clearly feel the radial head rotating within the annular ligament during passive supination/pronation of the forearm (Figure 7.19). The zero starting position is that in which the elbow is by the side and flexed to 90° with the thumb upright.

Pronation: (80°) The wrist is rotated so that the palm faces the feet.

Supination: (90°) The wrist is rotated so that the palm faces the head.

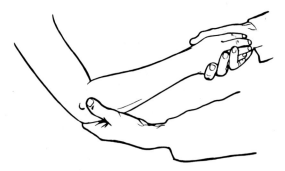

Figure 7.19. *The examiner's left thumb is locating the head of the radius rotating within the annular ligament while his right hand passively supinates and pronates the patient's forearm. The prominence of the lateral humeral epicondyle (the tender site in 'tennis elbow') is just proximal to the examiner's thumb.*

Wrist

Primary degenerative disease of this compound joint is rare, so that the presence of wrist arthritis strongly suggests inflammatory arthropathy, particularly rheumatoid arthritis. However, one must not be misled by conditions which may mimic true carpal synovitis: recent or old ununited fractures of the scaphoid bone, De Quervain's (abductor pollicis longus) tenosynovitis and osteo-arthrosis of the thumb carpometacarpal joint (see below). Cystic synovial swellings (protrusions arising from the carpal joints, occasionally from the tendon sheaths) are common over the dorsum of the wrist in rheumatoid arthritis, while flexor tendon crepitus may be elicited in progressive systemic sclerosis. Finally, anything which increases the volume of carpal tunnel contents may produce compression of the median nerve leading to the extremely common entrapment neuropathy — *carpal tunnel syndrome.*

Flexion/extension movements are readily compared on the two sides by getting the patient to carry out the manoeuvres illustrated in Figure 7.20.

Flexion: (75°) The palm is bent down ventrally.

Extension: (70°) The hand is bent back dorsally.

Radial deviation: (20°) The hand is moved in the plane of the palm towards the thumb.

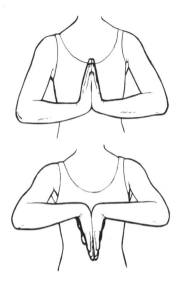

Figure 7.20. *Comparison of the range of wrist movement on the two sides.*

Ulnar deviation: (30°) The hand is moved in the plane of the palm towards the little finger.

Hand

In rheumatic disorders the hand can provide a wealth of useful information and it deserves meticulous attention. This part of the examination is perhaps best carried out with the patient seated by the examiner's desk and it requires a good light. The range of movement of the individual joints requires little comment; most are simple hinges. An exception is the thumb carpometacarpal ('saddle') articulation, at which a range of complex movement is possible: *opposition* brings the tip of the thumb to touch the tip of the little finger, while *abduction* is tested by getting the patient to place the back of his hand flat on the table and raise the thumb straight upwards, starting from a position beside the palm. The small muscles mediating these two movements (opponens pollicis and abductor pollicis brevis) are innervated by the median nerve and hence the importance of testing them when the carpal tunnel syndrome is suspected (similarly, in suspected ulnar entrapment neuropathy, abductor digiti minimi is tested). Clearly, disordered function in the hand may be due to neurological or tendon lesions, even in patients with obvious arthritis, and exclusion of entrapment neuropathy, tendon rupture etc. forms part of the examination of the arthritic hand. In addition to testing movements of individual joints it is necessary to consider the functional integrity of the hand as a whole. The ability, for example, to use a typewriter or hold a walking aid may be critical. A variety of hand grips is shown in Figure 7.21.

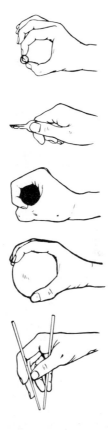

Figure 7.21. *Different types of grip.*

When seeking evidence of early arthritis in the hand, a convenient screening routine is to inspect the two hands side by side for any evidence of joint swelling, then to get the patient to clench and straighten out the fingers (as a rough test of movement), and finally to pinch each finger joint in turn while moving it passively (as in the foot — see Figure 7.6) as a test of joint irritability.

Established arthritis in the hand often produces a characteristic pattern of joint involvement, sometimes in association with typical extra-articular features. *Osteoarthrosis* (Figure 7.22) is recognised by Heberden's nodes at the terminal interphalangeal (TIP) joints

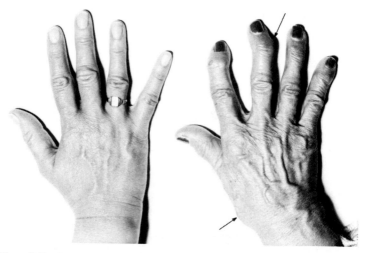

Figure 7.22. *Osteoarthrosis (degenerative joint disease) affecting the hand. Patient's hand on right: normal hand on left for comparison. Note the Heberden's nodes (split-pea sized osteophytes arising from the base of the terminal phalanx) (arrow) and arthritis of the thumb carpometacarpal joint (arrow) producing the 'square hand' appearance. The altered shape of the hand is due to (1) bony swelling of the thumb metacarpophalangeal joint, (2) adduction of the thumb metacarpal and (3) wasting of the associated small muscles.*

and a 'square hand' due to involvement of the thumb carpometacarpal (saddle) joint. *Rheumatoid arthritis* produces symmetrical fusiform swelling of the proximal interphalangeal (PIP) joints and soft tissue swelling of the metacarpophalangeal (MCP) joints. More advanced disease may produce a variety of deformities: ulnar deviation and palmar subluxation at the MCP joints (Figure 7.23), 'button' or 'swan neck' finger deformities and there may be palmar erythema and evidence of digital arteritis in the form of 'nail fold lesions'. Tendon sheath involvement may produce a 'trigger finger' (see above) or a recognisable swelling along the course of a tendon sheath. *Psoriatic arthritis* characteristically produces an asymmetrical pattern of arthritis with TIP joint swelling and psoriatic changes in the nail on the same digit. *Gout* also produces an asymmetrical pattern with tophaceous swellings in relationship to peripheral joints (Figure 7.1). *Progressive systemic sclerosis* may be associated with a mild, small joint polyarthritis in the early stages; the skin changes have been discussed above. The cause of an otherwise obscure polyarthritis may sometimes be explained by the association of finger clubbing and nicotine staining with carcinoma of the lung producing *hypertrophic pulmonary osteoarthropathy*, while the clue to *dermatomyositis* may be erythema and scaling ('collodion patch' lesions) over the knuckles. *Dupuytren's contracture* leads to shortening and puckering of the palmar fascia which characteristically tethers the skin.

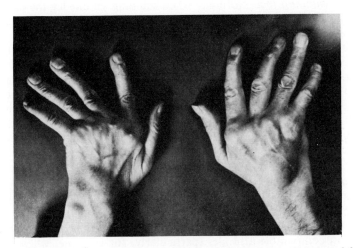

Figure 7.23. *Late rheumatoid arthritis of the hands showing ulnar deviation of the fingers. Note also the wasting of small muscles, the synovial thickening at the wrist joints (with a cystic synovial protrusion on the right), two rheumatoid subcutaneous nodules (over the knuckles on the left), and palmar subluxation of the bases of some proximal phalanges.*

Lower Limb

Hip

Apart from adequate exposure (a bikini-type garment is helpful), examination of the hip joint requires a couch away from the wall and, in the case of the elderly or infirm, the help of an assistant.

As with all lower limb joints, posture and gait may provide important clues about the hip. The depth of the joint from the surface means that it is normally impossible to detect an effusion clinically and testing for joint tenderness, by deep palpation over the centre of the inguinal ligament, is an imprecise observation. Signs of hip joint disease may be mimicked by bone disorders and other nearby lesions. Hip joint disease may lead to fixed flexion and/or adduction deformity and, with destructive changes, to actual shortening of the limb. Partly owing to the depth of the joint from the surface, and the tendency for the patient to compensate by pelvic tilting, these changes may not easily be detected. Because of these difficulties certain special tests are performed when hip joint disease is suspected.

Trendelenberg test. Normally when standing on one leg the pelvis is tilted upwards on the non-weight bearing side to readjust body weight transmission and balance. By contrast, when attempting to stand on a leg in which the hip joint is diseased, the pelvis is liable to sag downwards on the opposite side. This phenomenon is exploited in the Trendelenberg test, which is useful for detecting a hip joint abnormality. It is also positive when muscle weakness prevents normal pelvic tilting. The test is performed by observing the position of the pelvis from behind while the patient raises each foot off the floor in turn. Palpation of the iliac crests may be used to confirm what is usually obvious on inspection (Figure 7.24 a, b).

Leg length measurements. True leg length is measured as the distance between two bony landmarks, for example the anterior superior iliac spine and the tip of the medial malleolus. When measuring this distance care must be taken that the two hip joints are in comparable attitudes (particularly, for example, when one hip has a flexion/adduction deformity). Reduction of true leg length may result from destructive changes in the hip joint.

Apparent leg length is measured from the midline (umbilicus) to the medial malleolus. 'Apparent leg shortening' recorded in this manner (in the absence of true leg shortening) is thus an indication of pelvic tilting; hip adduction producing apparent leg shortening, abduction producing apparent leg lengthening.

Concealed hip flexion deformity. When a patient with a fixed flexion deformity of the hip lies supine on the examination couch she will often instinctively and unconsciously tilt her pelvis by arching her lumbar spine into excessive lordosis and thus allow the leg on the affected side to lie flat on the couch, concealing the hip flexion deformity. The examiner may have been alerted to the presence of such a deformity by noting an abnormal gait or posture

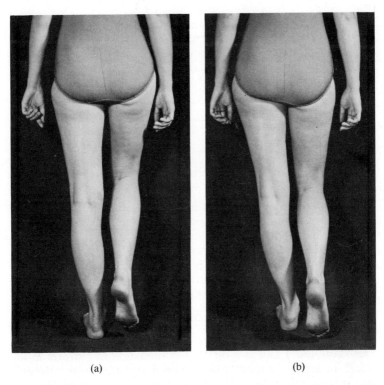

(a)   (b)

Figure 7.24. *Trendelenberg test. Normally when a foot is lifted off the ground the pelvis tilts upwards on that side* (a). *However, when the weight-bearing hip is diseased (or there is weakness of the muscles on that side), the pelvis sags downwards* (b).

(buttocks thrust out posteriorly) or he may detect the excessive lumbar lordosis which allows a hand to slide between the lumbar spine and the couch. In any case this deformity can be revealed by the manoeuvre illustrated in Figure 7.25. The opposite hip is forcibly flexed as far as it will go, thus abolishing the lumbar lordosis (confirmed by the examiner's hand under the lumbar spine), when the leg on the affected side will immediately move into a position of hip flexion. This test is particularly useful in the examination of children.

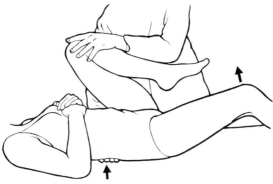

Figure 7.25. *Method of revealing a flexion deformity of the hip joint. Forced flexion by the examiner of the opposite hip abolishes lumbar lordosis (confirmed by a hand placed under back —* arrow) *and the knee on the affected side moves upwards* (arrow) *to reveal the flexion deformity of the hip on that side.*

The ball-and-socket articulation is deeper than in the shoulder, so that the range of each movement is less in the hip. As in the shoulder, ball-and-socket movement has to be differentiated from girdle movement. Thus the examiner must satisfy himself that presumed hip joint movement is not being achieved by tilting the pelvis. This requires observation of pelvic bony landmarks, by the examiner or assistant, while testing hip joint movements.

Flexion: (115°) The thigh is forced down onto the abdomen (as in Figure 7.26).

Extension: (30°) This is a difficult examination to perform in the elderly or arthritic patient, in which instance an assistant is needed. The patient lies on the opposite side while the examiner uses one hand to extend the hip and the other to monitor the position of the pelvis (Figure 7.27). Actual hip joint extension is the angle beyond which any further movement is achieved by tilting the pelvis.

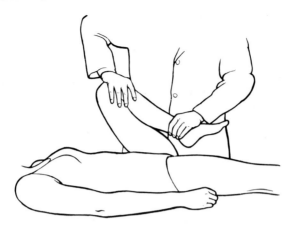

Figure 7.26. *Hip flexion.*

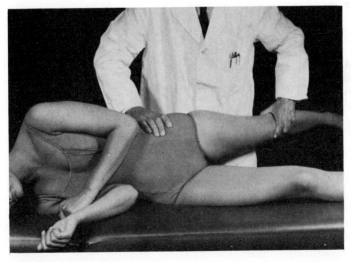

Figure 7.27. *Hip extension. The examiner's right hand is being used to detect tilting of the pelvis.*

Abduction: (50°) With the patient lying supine the leg is carried outwards until further movement tilts the pelvis (detected by the examiner's other hand on the opposite iliac crest).

Adduction: (45°) The leg is carried medially, across the opposite limb, otherwise the technique is the same as for testing abduction.

Rotation: (internal 45°, external 45°) This may be tested with the hip joint in any position of flexion/extension or adduction/ abduction (rolling the leg from side to side on the couch effectively tests rotation in the zero starting position). In practice these measurements are probably most conveniently made with the hip flexed to 90° as shown in Figure 7.28.

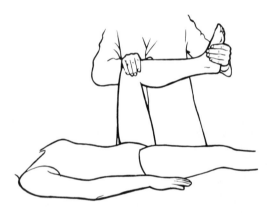

Figure 7.28. *Hip rotation: tested here with the hip flexed to 90°.*

Knee

The knee joint is more accessible for examination than the hip. The outline of the patella is easily palpated and distension of the joint with an effusion produces a characteristic horseshoe-shaped swelling round the patella, with filling of the large suprapatellar synovial pouch (see Figure 7.5). Effectively the knee consists of two compartments: the patellofemoral and the main tibiofemoral articulation. Try to determine the relative contribution of these two compartments to signs such as crepitus and irritability. Move the patella sideways across the femoral condyles and try to palpate its articular surface. The main joint line is opposite the middle of the patellar ligament and the head of the fibula is easily located. The positions of the two collateral ligaments can thus be deduced and these structures can often be palpated by rolling them under the finger tips. Careful palpation of the anterolateral and anteromedial aspect of the join line during flexion and extension may identify a torn or cystic meniscus.

Knee joint disease produces wasting particularly of the quadriceps muscles. This should be recorded as thigh circumference at a set distance above the patella. Palpation of the quadriceps while the supine patient presses the knee downwards onto the couch allows comparison of the state of this muscle group on the two sides.

Very large synovial effusions may be self-evident on inspection (see Figure 7.5) and can be confirmed by eliciting cross-fluctuation between different parts of the joint. Smaller effusions require careful differentiation from synovial (soft tissue) swelling. The fluid nature of an effusion may be established by two techniques: the *patellar tap* (Figure 7.29a) and the *bulge sign* (Figure 7.29b). The latter is particularly useful in detecting small effusions. Remember to examine the back of the knee. Cystic swellings in the popliteal fossa are common in rheumatoid arthritis and are an important cause of pain. Occasionally cystic swellings lower in the calf may represent the late result of synovial ruptures. Anteriorly, pre- and infrapatellar bursitis must be differentiated from arthritis of the knee.

Destructive arthritis of the knee may lead to deformity with altered alignment which is particularly serious in a weight-bearing joint. This should be recorded as the actual number of degrees of varus (medial) or valgus (lateral) angulation of the tibia; and it is important to observe the effect of weight bearing on any such deformity. Destructive lesions tend also to produce laxity of the joint ligaments with instability. Manoeuvres designed to test for laxity of the cruciate and collateral ligaments are illustrated in Figure 7.30.

Flexion: (135°) The calf is pressed against the thigh.

Hyperextension: (5°) The leg is straightened to, and if possible beyond, the zero starting position. Hyperextension is characteristically increased in hypermobile patients — *genu recurvatum.*

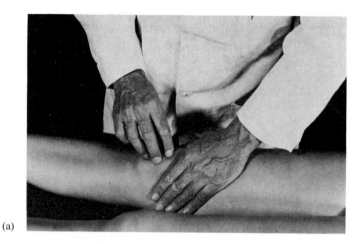

(a)

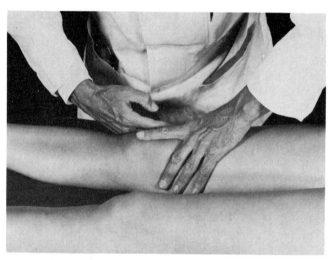

(b)

Figure 7.29. *Two tests for the presence of fluid in the knee joint:* a. *'Patellar tap'. The left hand forces fluid out of the suprapatellar pouch while the fingers of the right hand push the patella sharply downwards. If fluid is present there is a palpable tap as the patella meets the underlying femoral condyles.* b. *'Bulge sign'. The left hand empties the suprapatellar pouch and also, with the index finger, steadies the patella. The fingers of the right hand are drawn alternately along the two sides of the patella, forcing any fluid across the joint to produce a visible bulge on the opposite side.*

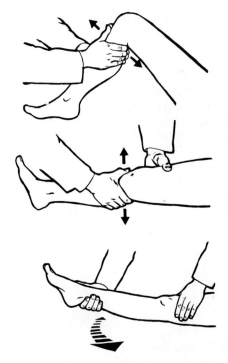

Figure 7.30. *Knee joint stability. Tests for cruciate and collateral ligament laxity.*

Ankle

Arthritis of the ankle joint has to be differentiated from ligamentous strains and sprains, and also from tenosynovitis of related tendon sheaths. For this reason it is particularly important to localise accurately any tenderness or swelling and to determine which movements produce pain. Usually this will establish whether the articulation as a whole is involved. In passing, note whether there is tenderness or swelling at the point of insertion of the Achilles tendon. Tendinitis at this site (with or without bursitis) may occur in patients with spondylitis. The mortise arrangement of the articulation allows only hinge-type movements. These should be tested with the knee flexed.

Dorsiflexion: (20°) The foot is bent upward, toward the shin.

FURTHER INVESTIGATIONS

Many of the investigations used in the diagnosis of joint disease have general application in other systems and these will not be considered here. The discussion which follows is limited to a few selected investigations particularly relevant to rheumatological disorders.

Rheumatoid Factors (Stage and Mannik, 1973)

The serum of about 85 per cent of rheumatoid patients contains detectable autoantibodies directed against immunoglobulin G (IgG). These 'rheumatoid factors' have specificity for antigenic determinants on the Fc fragment of IgG and represent a particular example of antiglobulin formation, a widespread phenomenon of which the biological significance is not understood. Routine laboratory tests for rheumatoid factors detect mainly IgM anti-globulins, and 'seropositivity' is based on these tests. However, more elaborate tests show that rheumatoid factor antiglobulins exist also in other immunoglobulin classes, particularly IgG, and the sera of many patients with 'seronegative' inflammatory arthropathies do actually contain IgG rheumatoid factors not detected by the standard latex and sheep cell tests. Nevertheless the standard tests for rheumatoid factors remain of outstanding value in the diagnosis of rheumatoid arthritis and high titre positivity correlates with a somewhat worse prognosis and with the presence of extra-articular lesions. The test usually becomes positive during the first few months of the disease, but some 15 per cent of otherwise typical rheumatoid patients remain seronegative by the standard tests throughout their illness. Positive tests may be obtained in about four per cent of normal subjects and particularly amongst patients with other systemic connective tissue disorders, with chronic infections and bacterial endocarditis, with liver disease and amongst the elderly.

Antinuclear Antibodies (Reichlin and Mallioli, 1974)

Autoantibodies directed against constituents of cell nuclei are consistently found in the sera of patients suffering from systemic lupus erythematosus (SLE). They are not specific, occurring in other systemic connective tissue disorders and various other diseases; nevertheless they provide the keystone for the diagnosis of SLE. These autoantibodies are mainly in the IgG class. Like rheumatoid factors, the stimulus to their production remains a matter for speculation, but there is evidence that they may play a pathogenic role as constituents of immune complexes. Three tests are used routinely.

LE-cell test

The LE-cell phenomenon occurs when peripheral blood leucocytes (buffy coat cells) from a patient with SLE are incubated after the cells have been processed in a manner which damages some of the cell membranes (thus allowing antinuclear antibodies access to the nuclei). A stained smear is examined for the characteristic LE-cells: polymorphonuclear leucocytes which have phagocytosed masses of nuclear material to such an extent that their own nuclei are pushed to one side. The test is positive in about 80 per cent of patients with SLE. Positive tests may sometimes be obtained in patients with active chronic hepatitis and other systemic connective tissue disorders. The drawback of this test is that it requires a careful and time-consuming search of the stained smear. For this reason it has been largely replaced by the two tests described below.

Fluorescent antinuclear antibody test (ANA test)

Sections of normal animal tissue (e.g. rat liver) are exposed to the patient's serum, when any antinuclear antibody will attach to the liver cell nuclei. After washing, the section is then exposed to antihuman IgG antibody (prepared, for example, in a goat) conjugated to fluorescein. This conjugate attaches wherever there is human IgG on the section and, after further washing, it can be identified by ultraviolet light microscopy. A positive test thus reveals fluorescent staining of the rat liver cell nuclei.

The ANA test is much less demanding on the laboratory than the LE-cell test. It is also more sensitive (all patients with active SLE have positive tests), but less specific. It is thus a useful screening test.

Anti-DNA antibodies (Hughes, 1971)

Amongst the various serum autoantibodies directed against cell nuclei it appears that the presence of those directed against native (double-stranded) DNA correlates best with active SLE. Such antibodies are detected by exposing the test serum to radioisotope labelled DNA (obtained from bacteria). The specific immune complexes so formed are then precipitated using ammonium sulphate and the washed precipitate measured for radioactivity. This gives a measure of 'DNA binding'. In most laboratories a figure of over 25 per cent is positive. Figures of up to 100 per cent may be obtained in active, untreated SLE. This test is the most specific available and the degree of positivity correlates with disease activity.

Synovial Fluid Examination

Bacteriology

The most urgent indication for joint fluid examination is to establish whether or not a joint is infected. When infection is a possibility fluid must always be obtained before starting antibiotic therapy. Examination of stained smears and culture of the fluid is along standard bacteriological lines.

Crystals

The synovitis of gout and pyrophosphate arthropathy (pseudogout) are most accurately diagnosed by identifying the responsible crystals (urate or pyrophosphate) in the synovial fluid. Both types of crystal, being anisotropic, are readily identified employing polarised light microscopy. Clotted specimens are suitable (Currey, 1968).

Cells

The cell content of synovial fluid does not establish the cause of arthritis, unless it be blood in the case of trauma, haemophilia or villonodular synovitis. Most fluids contain cells roughly in proportion to the acuteness of the arthritis and the more acute the arthritis, the higher the proportion of polymorphonuclear leucocytes (Table 7.1). Specimens for cell counts should be mixed immediately with EDTA as anticoagulant.

Table 7.1. *Comparison of cell and protein content in synovial fluid obtained from rheumatoid and osteoarthrotic joints. Approximate range of values to be expected.*

	Osteoarthrosis	Rheumatoid arthritis
Total leucocyte count/μl	0—1000	2000—12 000
Polymorphonuclear leucocytes (%)	10—50	60—95
Total protein content (g/100 ml)	2—4	5—7

Other tests

The protein content of the synovial fluid reflects the acuteness of the arthritis (Table 7.1). The *mucin test* is performed by adding acetic acid to a final concentration of one per cent. Fluid from an acutely inflamed joint gives a scanty clot, while the more nearly normal the fluid is, the firmer the clot. *Rheumatoid factor* tests may occasionally be positive in the synovial fluid at a stage when the serum gives a negative result. Complement component levels tend to fall in active rheumatoid arthritis and SLE.

Tissue Typing (Leading Article, Lancet, 1973)

The tissue antigen HLA-B27 occurs in about seven per cent of the normal population but is possessed by over 95 per cent of patients suffering from ankylosing spondylitis. A relatively high incidence is found also amongst patients suffering from Reiter's disease, psoriatic arthritis of the spondylitic type, sacroiliitis and anterior uveitis. The manner in which this genetic factor operates is not yet understood but already tissue typing has some value in the diagnosis of seronegative arthritis. At present this test is expensive, time-consuming and requires antisera in short supply.

Serum Complement

Determination of serum complement levels may be of value in patients suffering from SLE. Lowered levels occur during active phases of the disease, particularly during the development of lupus nephritis. In rheumatoid arthritis serum levels tend to be normal except when extra-articular disease is active, when they may be reduced.

Antistreptolysin'O' (ASO)Titre

The ability of streptolysin 'O' to haemolyse sheep erythrocytes is inhibited if serum containing ASO is added to the system. This is the basis of the ASO test. A high titre (over 1/800), or a rising titre, is evidence of a recent streptococcal infeetion. The test is thus of some value when rheumatic fever is suspected.

Synovial Biopsy

Material for histology may be obtained at open arthrotomy, by closed (needle) biopsy or at the time of endoscopic examination using an arthroscope.

Radiology

It is important to be selective in ordering x-rays. If unilateral disease is suspected it is usually advisable to x-ray both sides for comparison. In patients with polyarthritis (such as rheumatoid arthritis) three standard films are useful for establishing the diagnosis and following progress: one showing both hands and wrists, one showing both feet and one showing the pelvis (including the hips and sacroiliac joints). Other films should be taken only when required to provide specific information. The diagnostic reward from unselective joint surveys is negligible.

No attempt can be made here to do more than draw attention to some of the more important x-ray changes seen in selected examples of joint disease.

Osteoarthrosis (Figure 7.33)

The diagnosis of degenerative joint disease depends to a large extent on radiology. The involved bone ends show thickening, sclerosis and the outgrowth of bony protuberances (osteophytes). Cystic spaces appear within the periarticular bone and, with cartilage damage, there is progressive narrowing of the normal 'joint space' (representing the space occupied by the radiolucent articular cartilage).

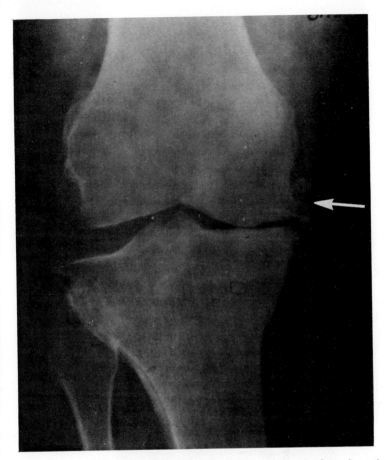

Figure 7.33. *Osteoarthrosis of the knee. Sclerotic bones with osteophytes (arrow) and loss of cartilage ('joint space') on the medial side.*

Rheumatoid arthritis (Figure 7.34)

In the early stages there may be only soft tissue swelling and some thinning of the related bone (periarticular osteoporosis). Later the characteristic erosions appear as bony defects under a breach in the cortex, often starting at the margin of the articular surface. These erosions are highly significant diagnostically; they are the hallmark of the inflammatory arthropathies (rheumatoid arthritis, psoriatic

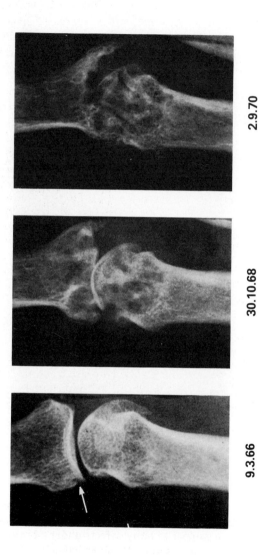

9.3.66   30.10.68   2.9.70

Figure 7.34. *Rheumatoid arthritis in a metacarpophalangeal joint. 1966: one small erosion (arrow). 1968 and 1970: progressive destructive changes and periarticular osteoporosis with loss of cartilage ('joint space').*

arthritis, etc.). The erosions may extend to destroy the whole joint surface. Cartilage damage is indicated by reduction in the 'joint space'. Occasionally, especially in children, the shaft of a bone in the hand or foot may show perosteal new bone formation near an inflamed joint. In Still's disease inflammation near growing epiphyses may result in under- or overgrowth of bones. Finally, damaged rheumatoid joints may develop secondary degenerative changes.

Ankylosing spondylitis (AS) (Figure 7.35)

Characteristic changes are seen first in the sacroiliac joints, with irregularity of the joint space, marginal sclerosis and erosion formation. Later there is fusion. These changes require considerable experience to interpret and are unreliable in patients under 20 years of age. The vertebral changes spread upwards from the sacrum, producing bridging between the vertebrae with syndesmophytes (vertical outgrowths, unlike the more horizontal osteophytes of spondylosis). Finally the whole spine may be converted into a solid bamboo-like tube. Other changes include osteoporosis and erosive changes at the vertebral margins. Facetal (apophyseal) joints are also affected and tend to fuse, as do any affected limb joints.

Other spinal lesions

Early intervertebral disc protrusions may show no changes. Later there is narrowing of the disc space, sclerosis of the adjacent vertebral bodies and local osteophyte formation. Similar changes are seen with increasing frequency in the spines of older patients and are then regarded as indicating degenerative (spondylotic) changes. There is however poor correlation with back complaints. The vertebral osteophytes of spondylosis tend to grow horizontally.

Gout (Figure 7.36)

Because urate is radiolucent, tophi appear as soft tissue swellings or punched-out areas in bone (advanced lesions may calcify). Although sometimes suggestive of rheumatoid erosions, confusion should not arise because such lesions do not appear until the patient already has clinical tophi. Thus, unlike rheumatoid arthritis, x-rays do not aid in establishing the early diagnosis of gout.

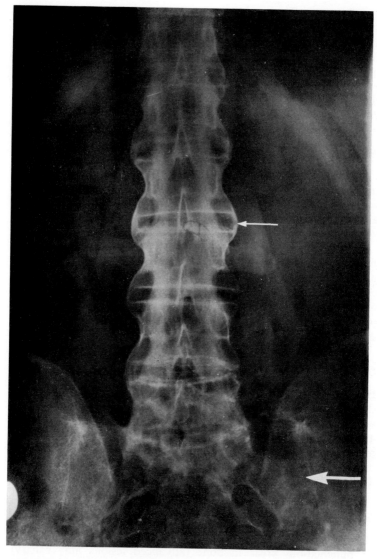

Figure 7.35. *Ankylosing spondylitis. Fusion of sacroiliac joints (large arrow) and bridging between vertebrae with syndesmophytes (small arrow), to form 'bamboo spine'.*

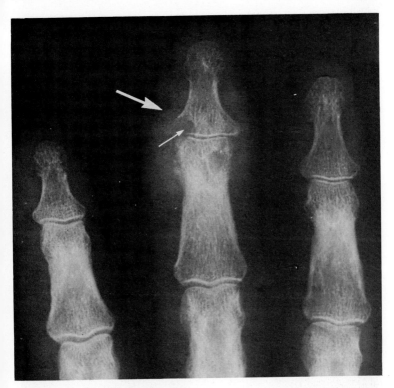

Figure 7.36. *Gout. Soft tissue swelling (large arrow) indicates site of radiolucent tophus. 'Erosion' (small arrow) indicates urate deposit in bone. See text for discussion about the diagnostic value of this sign.*

Pyrophosphate arthropathy (Figure 7.37)

The hallmark of pyrophosphate arthropathy is calcification of joint cartilage ('chondrocalcinosis') best seen in the knee menisci and triangular ligament of the wrist.

Infective arthritis

Pyogenic and tuberculous joint infections produce marked local osteoporosis, going on to a fuzzy bone outline and actual

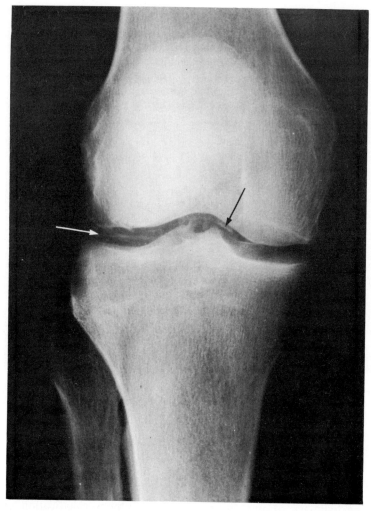

Figure 7.37. *Chondrocalcinosis of the knee. Calcium pyrophosphate dihydrate deposits in menisci (white arrow) and in hyaline articular cartilage of femur (black arrow).*

disappearance of bone. Chronic infections lead to considerable new bone formation. In the spine it is useful to remember that infections destroy the intervertebral discs, while they are preserved in secondary neoplastic lesions.

FURTHER READING

American Academy of Orthopaedic Surgeons (1966) *Joint Motion: Method of Measuring and Recording.* Edinburgh: Churchill-Livingstone.

Currey, H. L. F. (1968) Examination of joint fluids for crystals. *Proceedings of the Royal Society of Medicine,* **61,** 969-972.

Hughes, G. R. V. (1971) Significance of anti-DNA antibodies in systemic lupus erythematosus. *Lancet,* **ii,** 861-863.

Jayson, M. I. V. (1976) Diagnosis and assessment. *Clinics in Rheumatic Diseases,* **2,** 1-297.

Kelley, W. N., Harris, E. D. Jr, Ruddy, S. & Sledge, C. B. (1980) *Textbook of Rheumatology.* Philadelphia, London: W. B. Saunders.

Leading Article (1973) Ankylosing spondylitis and the HL-A antigen, W27. *Lancet,* **i,** 921-922.

Reichlin, M. & Mallioli, M. (1974) Antigens and antibodies characteristic of systemic lupus erythematosus. *Bulletin on the Rheumatic Diseases,* **24,** 756-760.

Stage, D. E. & Mannik, M. (1973) Rheumatoid factors in rheumatoid arthritis. *Bulletin on the Rheumatic Diseases,* **23,** 720-725.

8 The Skin

W. Frain-Bell

Normal skin varies between one person and the next but usually not to a great extent unless, for example, the individual is atopic, when the skin may well be generally dry and scaly. The skin normally becomes drier with age. Some individuals have a more greasy skin than others, particularly those who are seborrhoeic. In most people, however, the skin is neither abnormally dry nor greasy and any variation which might indicate systemic disease is usually easily recognised, although subjective observations need not necessarily have a somatic origin. Human skin also varies in colour, for ethnic and climatic reasons, with the fair-complexioned Celt at one extreme and the pigmented African at the other. Although the colour of the skin changes in response to a variety of exogenous and endogenous stimuli, this is infrequently the result of treatable systemic disease.

HAIR

The distribution, colour and type of hair and the various patterns of constitutional baldness will vary within any group of normal people, and in particular between the sexes and those of different ethnic origin. Loss of hair is probably noted or complained of more often than increased growth. Usually there is a reduction in the amount of scalp hair with ageing, which will follow either the male or female patterns of constitutional baldness. A sudden progressive loss of scalp hair may indicate alopecia areata or, less often, a response to systemic disease (see below).

In the neonatal period, scalp hair follicle growth is synchronous, in that 80 per cent of follicles are in the growing phase at the same time, but from then on growth becomes and remains asynchronous unless this pattern is disturbed for pathological or physiological reasons. The hair growth cycle consists of a growing phase (anagen), a short involution phase (catagen), and a resting phase (telogen), at the end of which the hair is shed, being pushed out by the new, growing hair. Certain diseases and physiological states, such as pregnancy, cause scalp hair growth to become synchronous so that all the hairs reach the resting phase at the same time, leading ultimately to sudden diffuse hair loss (telogen effluvium). The hair then starts to grow again with the arrival of the anagen phase, although sometimes regrowth is incomplete, especially in those for whom the trigger factor was pregnancy or the stage of hair fall was prolonged.

In *constitutional female pattern baldness* there is usually a history of a slow, progressive, diffuse loss of scalp hair, particularly over the vertex, without the temporal recession seen with the male pattern. Other female members of the family are often similarly affected and they tend to have fine rather than thick hair. There may also be a history of episodes of increased hair fall of the telogen effluvium type in which subsequent regrowth is incomplete. In the later stages there may be some reduction in the number of follicles.

The commonest reasons for loss of scalp hair are probably either constitutional baldness, alopecia areata or telogen effluvium. The diagnosis of *alopecia areata* is usually straightforward when there are multiple patches of hair with the characteristic exclamation mark (!) appearance (Figure 8.1), but difficulties can arise when, as sometimes happens, the loss is of the diffuse, non-patchy type.

Misuse of certain hairdressing techniques may cause fracture of the hair. Hair styles which result in traction, for example the pony tail, and the habit of twisting or pulling the hair more commonly seen in the younger age groups (trichotillomania) may disturb scalp hair growth and require consideration in differential diagnosis.

Amongst the features of certain developmental abnormalities is an effect on the hair follicle which is recognisable under the microscope, for example the beaded hair of monilethrix.

X-ray, cytostatic and anticoagulant treatment may lead to hair

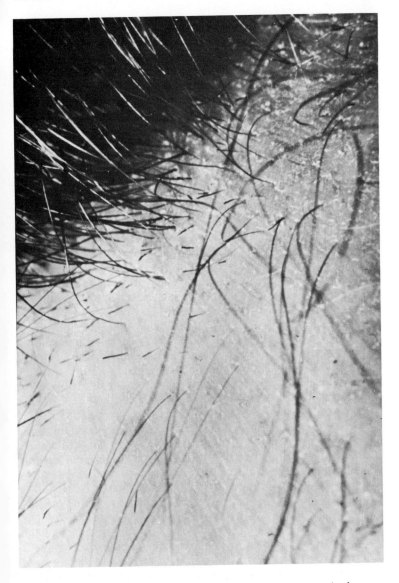

Figure 8.1. *Allopecia areata. Exclamation mark (!) hairs are present in the upper spreading edge of the patch of baldness.*

fall; the hair usually regrows unless the follicles have been destroyed. Disturbance of hair growth can occur in association with diseases affecting most systems.

Sometimes the scalp will be found to be scarred with a permanent loss of follicles. In this instance hair loss may be due to a variety of conditions, such as bacterial or fungal infection, lupus erythematosus and some forms of lichen planus. Confirmation of the cause suspected on clinical grounds will depend on appropriate histological, mycological and other investigations.

NAILS

Variation in the colour, shape and form of the nails is common and most often has a simple explanation: it is attributable to systemic disease in only a minority of instances. Thickening, irregularity and discoloration are usually due to local factors such as trauma (Figure 8.2) or infection (Figure 8.14), or arise in association with benign dermatoses such as dermatitis and psoriasis (Figure 8.10b) — particularly if only some of the digits are affected. Certain nail dystrophies are recognised to be classically associated with systemic disease, such as koilonychia (iron deficiency anaemia), brittleness and ridging (ischaemia), dilated nail fold capillaries with or without haemorrhages (collagen vascular disease), pallor which is more marked proximally (hypoalbuminaemia, hepatic and renal disease), splinter haemorrhages (trauma, vasculitis, endocarditis), and the temporary cessation or alteration in rate of growth due to episodes of illness which produce the transverse ridging or Beau's lines.

In *chronic debilitating disease* there is usually some thinning and loss of elasticity of the skin, along with a fine dry scaling of the skin surface, a waxy pallor and sometimes an Addisonian type of pigmentation of the skin (i.e. at pressure areas and on the palms) and the mucous membrane. Fine lanugo hair may appear over the body and the scalp hair may become lank and sparse and the nails brittle.

On examination of any skin a variety of small lesions and skin *growths* can be demonstrated, the majority tending to be one or other of the melanocytic naevi, papillomata and keratoses of seborrhoeic type, angiomata, and, less commonly, solar keratoses and basal cell epitheliomata. Rarely, otherwise benign lesions such as papillomata or angiomata may suddenly increase in number and, in such situations, systemic disease must be considered.

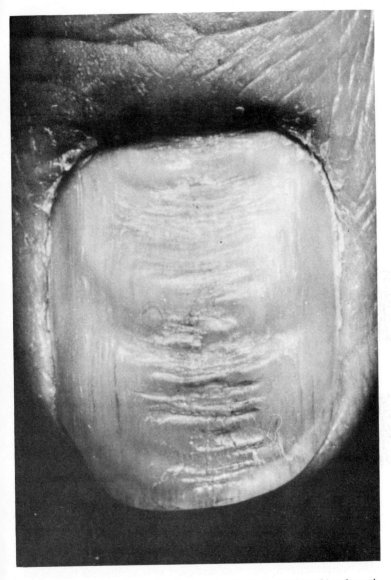

Figure 8.2. *A common form of nail dystrophy due to trauma, resulting from the habit of rubbing the nail fold with the index finger.*

The skin can be affected as a manifestation of non-organic disease and the absence of any visible abnormality probably enables this diagnosis to be made more readily in the skin than with other systems. Examples of this are subjective complaints of severe burning and itching without visible abnormal changes, parasitophobia, fear of loss and/or increase of hair, neurotic excoriations, and dermatitis artefacta. The diagnosis of a non-somatic disorder is justifiable only after the exclusion of organic disease, an example being porphyria, as in erythropoietic protoporphyria (acute discomfort with minimal signs) and hepatic porphyria (increased skin fragility).

HISTORY

Most of the common skin diseases are unrelated to detectable abnormalities of other systems. Thus, the taking of a *personal history* in a patient with a skin eruption or growth will differ in certain ways from that used in general medical history taking. The patient and clinician are both usually able to see what is complained of without support from specialised techniques. In addition, the symptoms will be few — such as pruritus and, less often, discomfort or pain. The clinician is therefore concerned with morphology and with the visible changes that have occurred throughout the natural history of the eruption, with the site or sites of onset and the subsequent distribution, and with how these features have varied in response to treatment and other measures. In this way a provisional clinical diagnosis or differential diagnosis is arrived at, and may be confirmed subsequently, where necessary, by the use of techniques such as biopsy, skin testing, phototesting and mycology, in addition to the usual range of biochemical and other investigations.

It is preferable to take a full history prior to the examination and the desire to have a quick look should be resisted. It is important to know whether the *primary site* was on covered or exposed skin and to determine the relationship of this site to possible contact allergens or irritants and to the known distribution of the various dermatoses. Whether the primary site is no longer affected must also be ascertained; this would suggest that additional factors may have become involved — for example, an initial contact dermatitis may have triggered off a constitutional atopic or a seborrhoeic reaction; alternatively, allergic sensitivity to an ingredient of a medicament used for initial treatment could have accounted for a change in emphasis away from the primary site. The subsequent *distribution* of the eruption will often point towards the diagnosis: the presternal and interscapular presentation in seborrhoeic dermatitis with or without flexural involvement; the limb flexure lichenification in atopic dermatitis; the affection of the shins in erythema nodosum.

Information should be obtained on whether the reaction is episodic with periods of complete or partial freedom, whether this occurs as a result of, or is independent of, treatment, and whether it is persistent with fluctuations in severity as in chronic psoriasis; whether there have been other attacks of the same or other forms of skin disease, and whether there is any response to treatment. It is necessary to record domestic and occupational factors in relation to contact allergy or irritation. A personal history of atopy (asthma, eczema, hay fever) or of known allergies may be obtained. A record should be kept of present and past illnesses and their treatment, this being of particular importance in the assessment of possible drug eruptions and cutaneous markers of systemic disease.

A *family history* is important but less so than the personal details. Guidance can be obtained as to the presence or otherwise of constitutional skin diseases such as atopic dermatitis or of general illness such as diabetes (cutaneous moniliasis, vasculitis), rheumatoid arthritis (psoriasis), and autoimmune diseases — for example pernicious anaemia or thyroiditis (vitiligo and alopecia areata) — and on whether there is any familial skin infection or infestations.

DIAGNOSIS

Fortunately, the skin is limited in its ability to produce morphological changes and the recognition of one or more of the following, along with the history, will usually lead to a reasonably accurate provisional clinical diagnosis:

1. *Surface change:* scaling, crusting, thickened/lichenified, excoriated, follicular involvement, exudation, ulceration, bleeding
2. *Colour*
3. *Erythema:* monomorphic or polymorphic (macules, papules, target lesions, nodules) with or without oedema
4. *Urticaria:* wheal, papule, angio-oedema
5. *Blister:* vesicle, bullae, haemorrhagic, scald-like
6. *Haemorrhage:* petechiae/purpura, ecchymosis

Examination of the buccal mucosa is important because it may provide supporting evidence for a diagnosis suspected from the examination of the skin.

In the differential diagnosis of skin tumours and growths, note should be made of the following:

(a) Distribution: single or multiple
(b) Development: sudden or gradual
(c) Situation: within the skin (dermal and/or epidermal), subcutaneous or deeper
(d) Change in appearance: size, shape (peripheral spread, satellites), colour, surface (altered horn formation, nodulation/ulceration/haemorrhage), consistency (induration)
(e) Symptoms: itch/pain

As with abnormality in many other systems, the skin is affected by a relatively small number of common conditions or reactions. It is necessary, therefore, to be able to recognise dermatitis (eczema), psoriasis, the erythematosquamous eruptions, the common infections, certain changes in hair and nail growth, the common benign and malignant tumours, and to know which of the reactions of the skin to systemic disease are common and which are specific to a disease. In so doing, reactions and growths outside these common problems will be noted to be unusual and atypical, and specialised guidance and help can then be sought.

The two main 'constitutional' reactions of the skin — eczema/dermatitis and psoriasis — obviously must start some time and the clinician may therefore on occasion observe the first appearance of such reactions, but usually there is the history of a relatively long duration with periods of prolonged activity. The erythematosquamous eruptions, on the other hand, tend to be episodic and often, although not always, limited to a single attack or to a number of attacks over a period of months or years. Nail changes as part of a constitutional dermatosis such as psoriasis, due to persistent trauma or to ringworm infection, are all long term. Common growths in the skin usually appear at various stages of life and often increase relatively slowly in size and number with any morphological changes in the individual lesion being gradual. Sudden appearance and relatively rapid increase in size or number suggest an infective origin such as virus warts or, less likely, more serious disease. Therefore, variations from the common patterns of behaviour of skin changes, progressive morphological changes in individual lesions or the sudden appearance of multiple growths are warning signs requiring assessment and appropriate action. A

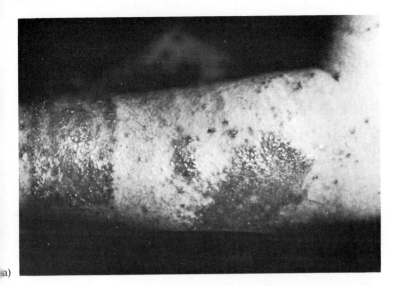

a)

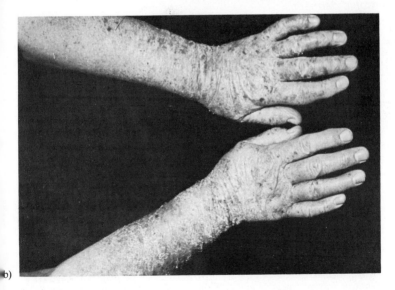

b)

Figure 8.3. *Dermatitis (eczema). (a) Acute — multiple vesicles and papules on an oedematous erythematous background. (b) Chronic — scaly thickened erythematous skin.*

confident recognition of what is common is the basis for the appreciation of atypical features and happenings. This is particularly so with cutaneous disease, where the diagnostic problem is constantly apparent.

COMMON DERMATOSES

Eczema/Dermatitis

The morphological features of eczema/dermatitis are illustrated in Figure 8.3. Various constitutional forms or patterns can be recognised and classified by associating parts of this spectrum of morphological changes with the distribution (Figure 8.4), history and other features. These different forms are: atopic, seborrhoeic, varicose/stasis, discoid (nummular), contact, and exfoliative (universal). There are important practical advantages to be gained from the correct recognition of these separate forms of dermatitis.

Atopic dermatitis.

Although morphologically a dermatitis, particularly so in the younger subject, atopic dermatitis often presents in the adolescent and the adult with extensive thickening (lichenification) and dusky discoloration of the skin, which is especially prominent in the bends of the elbows and knees (Figure 8.5), on the face, neck and upper third of the trunk, and on the hands and wrists (Figure 8.6). Usually activity is manifested by episodes of severe pruritus leading to extensive excoriation and further thickening of the skin rather than to morphological eczema. Commonly, although not always, appearing first in early childhood, it can persist with variable

---

Figure 8.4. *Distribution of the various forms of dermatitis. (a) Atopic dermatitis. Commonly affects the bends of the elbows and the knees, the face, neck, upper third of trunk, and the hands and wrists. (b) Seborrhoeic dermatitis. Affects particularly the scalp, facial creases, presternal and intrascapular areas of the trunk, and the flexures. (c) Contact irritant dermatitis. Finger web distribution resulting from exposure to water and physicochemical irritants. (d) Contact allergic dermatitis. Due to dyes used in tights, appearing at sites of maximum absorption of the allergen as a result of friction, sweating and occlusion. (e) Contact allergic dermatitis. Due to footwear factors such as rubber adhesives, most commonly affecting the sides of the feet, particularly the heel, and spreading on to the dorsum of the big toe and the neighbouring skin.*

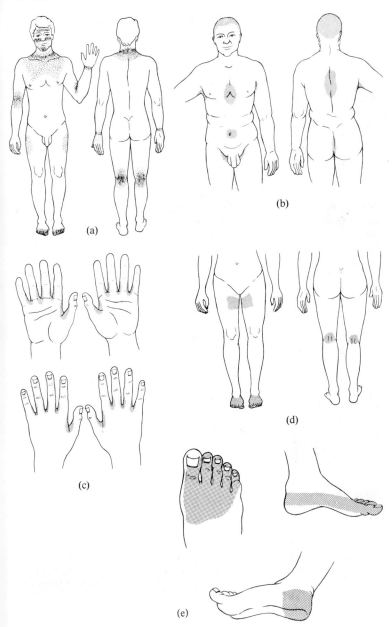

(a)

(b)

(c)

(d)

(e)

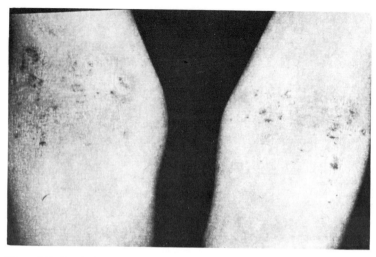

Figure 8.5. *Atopic dermatitis. Excoriated lichenified dermatitis of the elbow bends.*

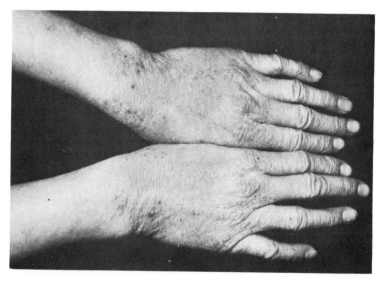

Figure 8.6. *Chronic lichenified atopic dermatitis, affecting the backs of the hands and the wrists.*

severity well on into late adult life. Inflammatory reactions of the skin are common in infancy and only a relatively small number are examples of atopic eczema. It is therefore not possible on the basis of clinical features alone to make a diagnosis of atopic eczema in the infant, other than to suspect it if there is positive evidence of atopy (i.e. eczema, asthma, hay fever) in close relatives.

Individuals with atopic eczema are particularly prone to deal inadequately with certain virus infections such as those of herpes simplex and vaccinia, on account of which appropriate protective and avoidance measures are required, especially in the younger subject. A tendency to develop cell-mediated contact allergic dermatitis is probably not much greater than that for the non-atopic subject. On the other hand, the dryness of the skin, which is a prominent feature in most atopics, leads to occupational problems if there is exposure of the skin of the hands to degreasing agents or other physicochemical irritants.

Seborrhoeic dermatitis

Seborrhoeic dermatitis is different and has few, if any, features in common with atopic dermatitis. This allows for ease of diagnosis. Certain difficulties, however, arise in assessing the infant, in the diagnostic relevance of intertrigo and, on occasions, in differentiation from psoriasis, particularly when the reaction is prominent in the scalp.

The skin of a patient with seborrhoea is often greasy, particularly on the face, but not necessarily so. Patients are liable to suffer from dandruff (pityriasis capitis), which may lead to a dermatitis reponse in the scalp either spontaneously or as a result of scratching. Scratching may result in secondary infection although sometimes infection follows over-zealous treatment including excessive shampooing. Commonly dandruff is the first stage of seborrhoeic dermatitis and in many individuals the skin reaction remains confined to the scalp, with perhaps minimal affection of eyebrows, facial creases and behind the ears. There is a tendency to develop chronic external otitis. It is important to appreciate that dermatitis of the scalp, face and ears is only sometimes indicative of seborrhoeic dermatitis and more commonly occurs as a manifestation of contact dermatitis. However, an initial allergic or irritant contact dermatitis may trigger off a constitutional seborrhoeic dermatitis reaction which then becomes chronic. The only manifestation of seborrhoeic dermatitis may be patches of scaly erythema of the presternal and/or interscapular skin. Reactions of the skin similar to those seen on the scalp and face may occur in the body flexures, umbilicus and pubic skin. Intertrigo is particularly liable to occur in the seborrhoeic individual, especially if he or she is overweight and if secondary cutaneous moniliasis has been encouraged by injudicious use of topical steroid preparations without additional measures to deal with yeast infection.

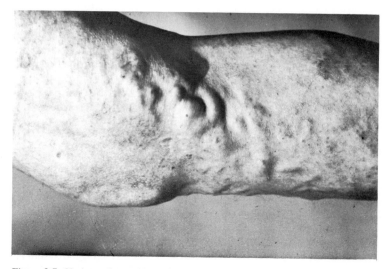

Figure 8.7. *Varicose dermatitis. Dilated varicose veins in association with a patchy eczematous reaction.*

Varicose/stasis dermatitis

Varicosity of the veins of the lower limbs is common. In time the skin of the leg below the knee becomes irritable, patchy eczema appears and the condition is labelled *varicose dermatitis* (Figure 8.7). The mechanism for this reaction is little understood but the same sequence of events can occur in the absence of demonstrable varicose veins, particularly in late middle-aged and elderly males. The condition is often self-limiting, requiring minimal treatment, but in some patients the process increases in severity and may disseminate to the skin of the upper limbs, face and elsewhere.

Stasis dermatitis, on the other hand, refers to a different sequence of events following initial deep venous thrombosis, leading to chronic oedema and induration of the skin of the distal third of the leg, often with episodes of superficial phlebitis and eventual ulceration. The dermatitis element affects the distal half of the leg below the knee and is subsequently episodic, becoming more persistent with the passage of time.

Discoid (nummular) eczema

The importance of this not uncommon variety of eczema lies in the fact that, although it represents a constitutional response of the skin, and is likely to occur only in certain predisposed individuals, it is frequently caused by exogenous irritant factors, when it affects the skin of the fingers and hands, and, as such, is then a manifestation of contact dermatitis. The name 'discoid' (or 'nummular') refers to the appearance of multiple discrete coin-shaped patches of eczema. In addition to the affection of the skin of the back of the hands (Figure 8.8a) and fingers it is often distributed symmetrically over the skin of the upper (Figure 8.8b) and lower limbs and parts of the trunk.

Contact dermatitis

Contact dermatitis is a common skin disorder. An initial contact reaction may aggravate or trigger off one of the constitutional responses and, therefore, in the same individual it is possible to make a diagnosis of, for example, both contact dermatitis and atopic dermatitis. This is a dermatitis occurring at a contact site and certain distribution patterns are of assistance in arriving at this diagnosis (Figure 8.4).

Contact dermatitis usually occurs because the skin reacts to physicochemical factors and, less commonly, to contact allergens acting through cell-mediated immunological mechanisms. The technique of skin testing used to confirm the presence of contact allergy is simple but important (see page 519).

Rarely a dermatitis response is morphologically atypical, or the various features do not fit into one or other of the patterns of reaction already described. Such a situation arises, for example, in the early stages of the cutaneous reticulosis and in particular in mycosis fungoides (Figure 8.9). On occasion, also, the dermatitis may become universal, when the term *exfoliative dermatitis* or erythroderma is used. Such atypical patterns of response are thus more likely to be cutaneous markers of systemic disease.

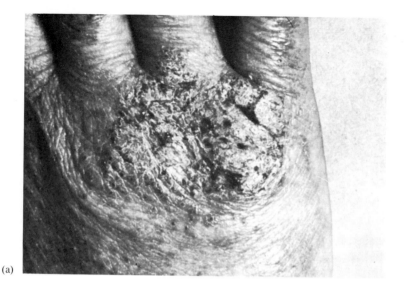

(a)

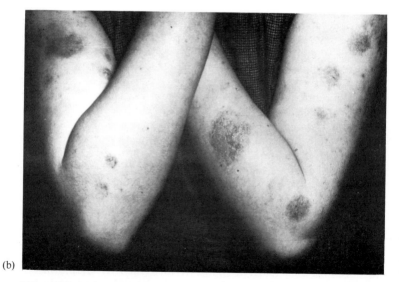

(b)

Figure 8.8. *Discoid (nummular) eczema. Discrete coin-shaped patches of scaly erythema (a); similar reaction produced by exposure to physicochemical irritants (b).*

Pompholyx

'Pompholyx' is a widely used term which requires recognition since this disorder will appear for different reasons, some of which are more important than others. Blisters, usually small vesicles, are a common lesion on the skin of the fingers, palms and soles of the feet. They usually occur as a dyshidrotic manifestation secondary to partial blockage of sweat pores in circumstances which have resulted in increased sweating. An attack of this form of dyshidrotic pompholyx can range from extensive vesicle formation over the palm and sides of the fingers to relatively mild localised scaling without visible vesicle formation.

Another manifestation of pompholyx is that of pompholyx eczema. The intra-epidermal vesicular formation as part of the eczematous process is modified by the thicker surface keratin layer found on the palms and fingers, as a result of which an eruption develops which is closely similar to that of dyshidrotic pompholyx.

The reaction of the skin to the presence of a fungus infection of the feet can lead to a similar pompholyx response on both hands and feet.

Psoriasis

Psoriasis affects one to two per cent of the population and occurs at all ages and in both sexes. A family history of psoriasis is common and the inheritance is probably autosomal dominant with incomplete penetrance. This genetic predisposition results in the development of the cutaneous condition only in those individuals who are in addition exposed to other, unknown factors, which may include certain infections.

As a result of increased epidermal cell proliferation the cutaneous lesions develop, which consist of variable-sized well-demarcated erythematous papules and plaques with surface silvery scaling (Figure 8.10a). The individual lesions may be small as in *guttate psoriasis* (Plate 8.1), but commonly appear as large plaques classically distributed on the elbows, knees and scalp, although any part of the body skin can be affected. Pruritus is uncommon except in the elderly. Affection of the body flexures may occur in the elderly and in those who, as a result of obesity, are liable to develop flexural intertrigo. A dystrophy of both finger and toe nails is common (Figure 8.10b). Psoriasis can be a disabling and distressing condition, both for the patient and for the family, but is usually not

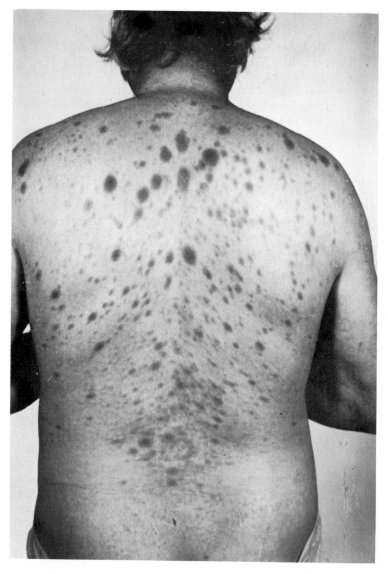

Figure 8.9. *Leukaemia cutis. Dusky violaceous nodules and papules.*

serious or life-threatening except in the acute pustular or universal erythrodermic forms, both of which may be precipitated by the use and subsequent withdrawal of systemic corticosteroid drugs. The patient with the universal erythrodermic form of reaction may demonstrate systemic changes such as cardiovascular insufficiency, impaired temperature regulation, protein and water loss, and malabsorption as a result of the shunting of blood from the gut to the erupting skin.

There is an association with arthritis of rheumatoid type. The psoriatic arthritis may be restricted to a relatively mild involvement of the distal joints of the fingers and toes or be severely disabling with affection of the spine and sarcoiliac joints. In both these forms the rheumatoid factor is absent.

Acne Vulgaris

This disease affects the majority of adolescents to a variable degree at some time during their developing years, and continues into adult life in approximately 5 per cent of those affected; it may trouble a few in middle age. Persistence of the condition for many years is seen particularly with the severe form of cystic acne conglobata.

Acne vulgaris first occurs with the onset of puberty, at which time androgen production is increased in both sexes. As a result the sebaceous glands are stimulated to secrete sebum, thereby allowing the growth within the follicle of bacteria such as *Propionibacterium acnes*, which produce enzymes that convert the triglycerides of sebum to free fatty acids. These are comedogenic and become involved in the subsequent inflammatory reaction and alteration in the follicular epithelium. From the early comedone formation, the inflammatory reaction leads to the production of the papule, pustule and nodule of the classical acne morphology.

It is known also that subjects with inflammatory acne develop an immune response to *P. acnes* and that there is an association between the severity of the condition and the antibody titres to *P. acnes.*

Acne conglobata is a severe destructive form of the disease. There is scarring which may be hypertrophic and, characteristically, nodulocytic lesions, sinuses and double comedones are present. It is sometimes associated with hidradenitis suppurativa and pilonidal cysts.

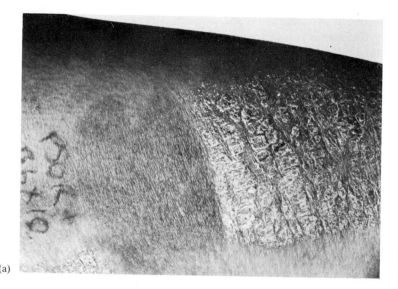

(a)

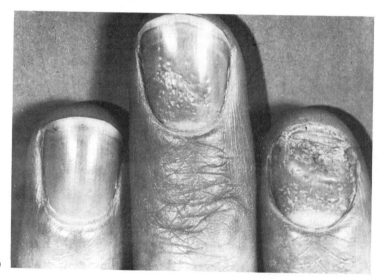

(b)

Figure 8.10. *Psoriasis. (a) An erythematous well-defined plaque with superficial silvery scaling. The left half of the plaque has been successfully treated by the combination of 8-methoxypsoralen and UVR. (b) Nail dystrophy. Pitting, discoloration and thickening of the nails.*

Certain environmental factors will affect the acne process, such as exposure to oils, halogenated hydrocarbons, occlusive cosmetics and localised friction. Acne may also be a feature of certain endocrine disorders, as in Cushing's syndrome and adrenal virilism, and of liver disease, and may be caused or aggravated by drugs such as corticosteroids, phenytoin, rifampicin, lithium and chlorpromazine.

INFESTATIONS AND INFECTIONS

Pruritus

Widespread or localised pruritus is common but it is rare for this symptom to have any serious significance. If there is a pruritic eruption, and not simply pruritus, the commonest cause is a reaction of the skin to the bite of an ectoparasite such as the human or animal scabies mite or the ordinary animal flea. Such reactions involve immunological mechanisms, which may be modified by systemic diseases such as the reticuloses or by therapy which inhibits the immune responses. Thus, the clinical presentation of, for example, cutaneous reactions to ectoparasites and also to fungus infections can be modified and the diagnosis missed. The term 'tinea incognito' has been coined for a fungus infection modified by injudicious treatment with topical steroid preparations.

The variation of the incubation period in human scabies accounts for the apparent absence of similar eruptions in near relatives and friends at the time when the patient is first seen. The treatment, also, of single members of a family group instead of the whole group regardless of apparent affection helps to confuse the contact history and of course the subsequent efficacy of treatment. If the source of the mite is an animal such as a dog, then other members of the family may escape affection and prophylactic treatment has to be directed towards the animal source. Not enough use is made of the simple procedure of standing the offending animal on a newspaper so as to facilitate the collection of 'brushings', which are then passed to a veterinary surgeon for examination.

The elderly may suffer from scabies or from pediculosis but this is less often the cause of irritation in the older age groups than the more common problem of 'senile pruritus'. A satisfactory explanation has still to be found for this condition, in which the irritation can be widespread. Senile pruritus often appears to be precipitated by temperature changes and is particularly troublesome at bedtime. It is made worse by the drying action of bathing. Scratching, perhaps combined with intolerance to a local application, will lead to secondary eczematisation.

Children not infrequently react to flea bites with the usually itchy, but short-lived, immediate urticarial wheal with or without central blister formation. The lesions are often grouped and localised at clothing constriction sites. In some children the eruption persists with the development of pruriginous nodules at the sites of the original wheals, presenting a mixed morphological picture of *papular urticaria*.

Widespread pruritus may be due to systemic disease, for example impaired hepatic or renal function, malignancy and other illnesses, but these are all very rare causes of pruritus with or without a primary eruption.

Impetigo

Impetigo due to infection of the skin with the staphylococcus or streptococcus is relatively rare in the adult, although so-called impetiginised dermatitis as a secondary phenomenon in a primary eruption does occur. Impetigo usually presents in the younger age groups and may be bullous with the epidermal cleavage situated subcorneally so that the blister roof soon ruptures to give a raw, red, crusted eruption with occasional scattered, flaccid, peripheral bullae (Figure 8.11). It is important that the presence or absence of a nephritogenic streptococcus is determined and appropriate systemic antibiotic treatment instituted.

Infection of pilosebaceous follicles varies and the depth and type of response of the host skin can lead to either *folliculitis* of superficial or deep type or to *furuncles, carbuncles* and *cellulitis.* Although infection of this type necessitates the exclusion of metabolic disease such as diabetes, it is more likely to be due to a chronic primary dermatosis such as a dermatitis which may have been treated with antibiotics in association with topical steroid preparations, whereupon the skin has been colonised by staphlococci.

Viral Infections

Of these the most common is the human *wart* virus, producing a range of benign tumours, usually multiple, which vary in appearance, being often filiform or digitate on the face and neck, raised

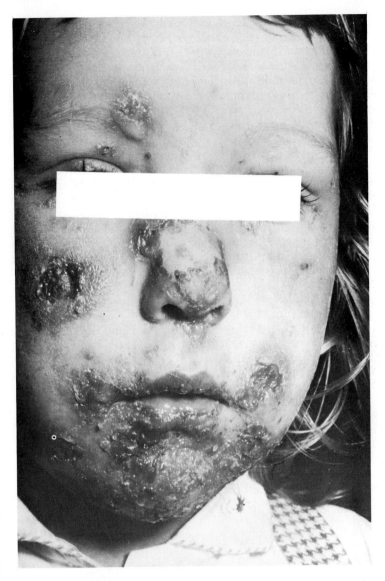

Figure 8.11. *Impetigo. Oedematous erythema with crusting and blistering of the skin.*

and 'verrucous' on the fingers and hands, depressed into the skin of the sole (plantar verruca), and sometimes small and flat with a brownish colour (plane warts) or as a plaque consisting of tightly packed small warts (mosaic warts). Diagnostic difficulties usually only arise in the adult with a single warty tumour or with a plantar callosity, which, in the adult, is much more common than a plantar verruca. In the verruca, scraping of the lesion will demonstrate the interruption of the epidermal ridge pattern and the presence of capillary bleeding points.

The *herpes simplex virus* (Type I in non-genital and Type II in genital herpes) infection commonly presents as recurrent, mild reactions, particularly on the face, in the form of grouped vesicles on a swollen erythematous base with subsequent crusting; occasionally there is adenitis or erythema multiforme. The affection may present with linear lesions particularly in the lower thoracic or lumbar region (zosteriform herpes simplex), which require differentiation from herpes zoster. The primary infection may present in early childhood as a severe herpetic gingivostomatitis with pyrexia and systemic upset. A severe widespread disseminated vesicular eruption is occasionally seen in the atopic eczema herpeticum.

In *herpes zoster* ('shingles') the virus remains dormant after a primary or subclinical attack of chicken pox, being reactivated by a subsequent, unknown stimulus. The herpes zoster eruption is preceded by three or four days of localised discomfort with paraesthesia or pain over the involved neural segment. The eruption is usually in the form of a unilateral and segmental collection of vesicles on an erythematous base which become pustular and are associated with a systemic upset and lymphadenitis. Widespread lesions may develop (disseminated zoster) and indicate a possible lymphoreticular disorder such as a malignant reticulosis. Persistent pain (postherpetic neuralgia) may occur after the eruption has healed, particularly in the elderly subject. The possibility of pressure by a tumour on the posterior root ganglia needs also to be considered.

Fungal Infections

Of the superficial fungal infections, that which affects the skin of the feet (tinea pedis, 'athlete's foot') is common. Affection of hands is uncommon, when the fungus is usually *Trichophyton rubrum*; the feet, toe nails and finger nails are all then likely to be

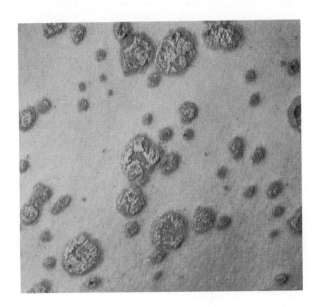

Plate 8.1

Guttate lesions of psoriasis.

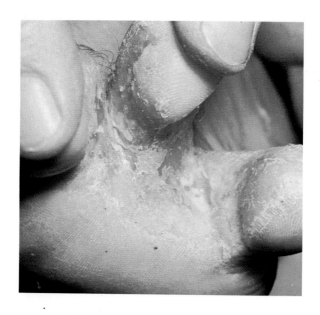

Plate 8.2

Tinea pedis. Macerated interdigital intertrigo often maximally involving the fourth and fifth and third and fourth toe webs.

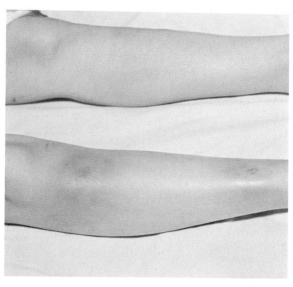

Plate 8.3

Erythema nodosum. Inflamed nodules and plaques most commonly seen on the anterior legs.

Plate 8.4

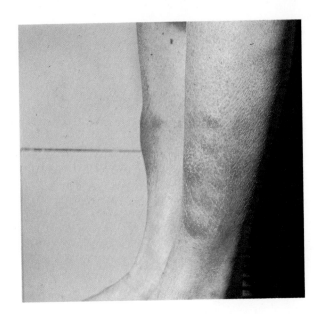

Pretibial myxoedema.

Plate 8.5

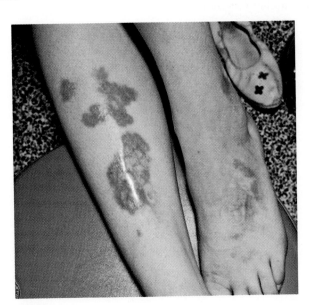

Necrobiosis lipoidica.

chronically affected. Chronic *T. rubrum* infection of the hands can present as a unilateral dry scaly palm, a somewhat bizarre reaction which can be confirmed by appropriate mycological studies.

The severity of the reaction in *tinea pedis* varies depending on the interaction between the mycelium in the skin and the patient's immune response, and on physical factors such as sweating and heat. The clinical presentation ranges from a low-grade mild interdigital scaling (Plate 8.2), which may or may not be itchy, to an acute vesiculo-bullous response affecting the whole foot, perhaps spreading up the leg with secondary eruptions on the skin elsewhere, especially on the hands. A similar interplay between the fungus and the skin occurs when the source of the fungus is farm animals such as cattle, leading to *tinea circinata* (Figure 8.12), with relatively mild low-grade reaction at one extreme and, at the other, a more acute bogy tumour formation labelled a *kerion* (Figure 8.13), which is usually seen on the scalp or beard area. Confirmation of the clinical diagnosis is obtained by microscopical examination of scrapings of the skin and, if necessary, culture studies.

Scalp ringworm in children is uncommon but should always be considered in any young person presenting with a scaly, partially bald patch or patches in the scalp. Examination of the area under Wood's lamp may indicate a *Microsporun* infection by fluorescence.

Tinea versicolor may be confused with vitiligo in that it presents as chronic, multiple, depigmented, lightly scaly, yellowish-brown patches most commonly on the skin of the trunk. Failure of these patches to tan following exposure to sun in the summer accentuates the appearance of the eruption and facilitates the clinical diagnosis, which can be confirmed by the demonstration of the responsible fungus on microscopical examination of surface scales.

Yeast infection, particularly with *Candida albicans*, is common, partly because of the widespread use of topical steroid preparations in the treatment of inflammatory reactions of the body flexures. Monilial intertrigo manifests as red raw, often painful, itchy skin with peripheral scaling and sometimes outlying small pustules. It is likely to be due to the injudicious use of such steroid preparations in an overweight subject who has developed a primary inflammation of the skin folds of, for example, the groin and axillae. Inflammation is likely to occur in such situations from sweating and friction as a response to seasonal or occupational alterations in temperature or following enforced restriction of movement in the elderly and in those temporarily confined to bed.

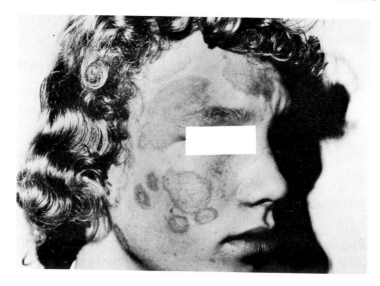

Figure 8.12. *Tinea circinata.*

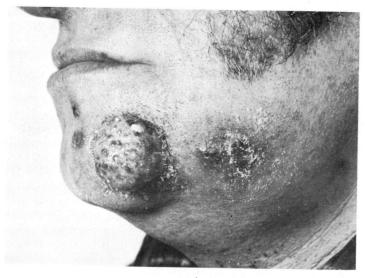

Figure 8.13. *Kerion. A bogy pustular swelling of the hair-bearing area of the chin.*

Candida albicans is also a major factor in the persistence of a chronic paronychia (Figure 8.14) which has developed upon a wet environment after minor trauma to the skin of the nail folds; it is also responsible for thrush infection of the mucous membranes of the mouth and vagina and for balanitis.

Although diabetes should be looked for in all cases of cutaneous moniliasis, it will rarely be found. The presence of chronic mucocutaneous moniliasis may be associated with abnormalities of immune mechanisms.

THE ERYTHEMATA

Apart from the eczematous reactions and certain specific common dermatoses such as psoriasis, the next most frequently observed group of skin disorders is the erythemata or erythematosquamous eruptions. The erythemata result from a reaction of the small cutaneous blood vessels leading to a range of morphological changes such as macules and papules, with a background of

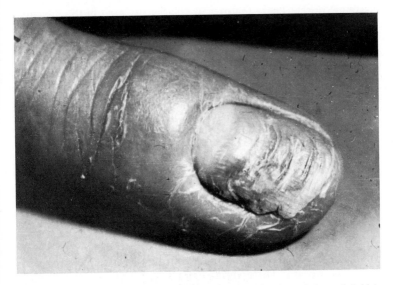

Figure 8.14. *Chronic monilial paronychia. Tender bolstering of the nail fold in association with dystrophic growth of the nail.*

oedematous erythema. When the reaction is more acute, vesicles or larger bullae may appear in association with a variable amount of destruction of the epidermis, best seen in the more acute forms of erythema multiforme and in toxic epidermal necrolysis (Lyell's disease). Purpura and other evidence of blood vessel wall damage such as haemorrhagic bullae may also be seen. In the erythemata, therefore, the morphological changes, and thus the descriptive labels applied, will depend on the severity of the reaction and on the effect on the different layers of the skin. With the exception of erythema marginatum, said to be specifically associated with acute rheumatism, many of the forms are linked with infection, drug administration or systemic disease or are regarded as idiopathic.

Erythema multiforme, in its mildest and most commonly seen form, presents as a bilateral, symmetrically distributed eruption consisting of macules, papules and iris (target) lesions, with a background of erythema and oedema distributed over the limbs, especially the extensor aspects, the face and, to a variable extent, on to the trunk. In the acute form the reaction of the skin is more widespread with bullae which are often haemorrhagic. There is loss of epidermis, affection of the mucous membranes, particularly the buccal mucosae and the lips, and symptoms and signs of a general systemic upset. These features are classically seen in the Stevens—Johnson syndrome (Figure 8.15).

Erythema nodosum presents as erythematous nodules 2.5 to 5.0 cm in diameter which are painful as well as being tender to touch. They are commonly seen on the anterior aspects of the shins (Plate 8.3) and less frequently on the skin of the thighs and upper limbs. An associated systemic reaction is variable and may be absent. The erythematous nodules vary in number and may continue to appear over a period of a number of days, the whole reaction, however, often being present for no longer than three to four weeks and usually less if the patient is confined to bed during the first week or two. As individual lesions clear they present colour changes similar to a resolving bruise.

Erythema induratum is uncommon as the incidence of tuberculosis infection has dropped. It presents with indurated nodules and plaques on the back of the calves of the legs leading to a varying amount of tissue destruction and scarring. There is often an abnormal reaction to cold as demonstrated by livedo reticularis or cutis marmorata. Differential diagnosis is from other forms of nodose erythema and is based on histological evidence of a tuberculous granuloma.

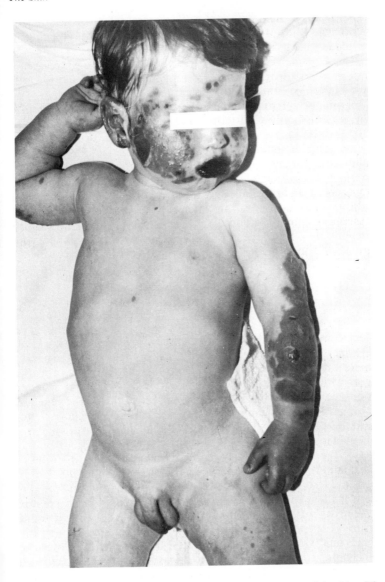

Figure 8.15. *Stevens—Johnson syndrome. Oedematous erythema of the skin of the face and limbs (bullae), also involving the buccal mucosa.*

Toxic epidermal necrolysis (Lyell's disease) resembles scalding of the skin with the development of widespread areas of erythema and raw tender patches.

Of the remaining relatively rare erythemata, e.g. erythema gyratum repens (Figure 8.35), investigations are directed towards the exclusion or otherwise of systemic disease.

It is important to define and recognise these erythemata since they are commonly used terms, and, although they may occur in different persons for different reasons (infection, drugs, systemic disease, or idiopathic), certain aetiological factors are more commonly present in some erythemata than in others, e.g. recurrent herpes simplex infection in erythemata multiforme; streptococcal and tuberculous infection and sarcoidosis in erythema nodosum; and tuberculosis in classical erythema induratum but not in the more common nodose erythemata, in which the underlying vasculitis may be found, for example, to be in association with periarteritis nodosa.

URTICARIA

The lesion seen in urticaria is a localised swelling of the skin from oedema of the dermis. It presents as an itching erythematous papule which rapidly enlarges to form the characteristic urticarial wheal with central pallor and surrounded by erythema; separate lesions may coalesce to form rings with central clearing. There may be an associated, usually asymmetrical, localised swelling of, for example, part of the face (angio-oedema) and, less often, large subcutaneous swellings (giant urticaria) which may occur on any part of the body. It is likely that histamine is responsible for the wheal in most cases of chronic urticaria, although other substances, such as serotonin, kinins, prostaglandins, anaphylatoxin and acetylcholine, will produce a similar form of cutaneous response.

Acute urticaria, as seen for example in penicillin allergy and in serum sickness, is of sudden onset with widespread urticarial wheals and lasts for a number of days; on occasion it may lead on to chronic urticaria. The majority of cases of chronic urticaria are idiopathic and may last with fluctuating severity for months or even years; the remainder are examples of physical urticaria (i.e. due to pressure, heat, cold or light) and, more rarely, cholinergic urticaria.

Chronic idiopathic urticaria is more commonly, but not exclusively, seen in the atopic and in the female. A specific responsible allergen is rare. Aspirin will aggravate the condition in about one third of the cases, possibly by inhibition of prostaglandin synthesis. It is not yet known whether this common form of urticaria is mediated by pharmacological or immunological mechanisms.

In the *physical urticarias* a relatively small group occur as a result of exposure to heat or to cold, the latter presenting in a number of different forms. In *hereditary cold urticaria* the inheritance is autosomal dominant. It starts soon after birth and lasts throughout life, being precipitated by a cold environment. *Symptomatic cold urticaria* occurs in paroxysmal cold haemoglobinuria or in association with cold agglutinins or cryglobulinaemia, for example in myeloma or systemic lupus erythematosus. In *idiopathic cold urticaria* the onset is usually in early adult life, the urticaria developing as a result of direct contact with cold substances.

Urticaria following exposure of the skin to sunshine *(solar urticaria)* is rare although an urticarial wheal is not an uncommon feature of the response of the skin to light in polymorphic light eruption, the commonest of the photodermatoses to affect females. It can indicate the presence of a photoactive substance in the skin, for example the accumulation of a metabolic product such as porphyrin in erythropoietic protoporphyria, or of a therapeutically administered photoactive substance.

In *cholinergic urticaria* there is the sudden development of multiple small urticarial wheals following exercise, heat or emotional disturbance. This is caused by the liberation of acetylcholine subsequent to activity of the sweat glands.

In *hereditary angio-oedema* there is a dominantly inherited absence of C_1 esterase inhibitor, as a result of which kinins and other vasoactive peptides are formed which induce gross oedema following minor trauma. The resultant subcutaneous swellings last for a number of days, producing intestinal colic from bowel involvement and asphyxia from upper respiratory tract involvement. In vitro chemical tests are available for the confirmation of the diagnosis.

DRUG ERUPTIONS

The possibility that a reaction of the skin may be due to a substance administered as part of the treatment or investigation of a disease requires consideration. It is unfortunate, therefore, that, other than for the urticarial response in penicillin sensitivity, there are still no reliable laboratory tests for the diagnosis of a drug eruption suspected on clinical grounds.

Certain drugs are recognised as being capable of producing specific cutaneous responses: for example the lupus erythematosus syndrome from hydrallazine, isoniazid, penicillamine and procainamide; a fixed drug eruption from phenolphthalein; and pigmentation and photosensitivity from chlorpromazine and other phenothiazines. Usually, however, the diagnostic problem is the occurrence of a widespread symmetrical eruption in a patient under treatment. A drug eruption usually develops fairly rapidly, perhaps preceded for a day or two by pruritus. The rash is bilateral and symmetrical, and commonly consists of an admixture of erythema, oedema and morbiliform lesions. More severely affected patients have blisters, purpura and other evidence of skin vessel damage. The rash usually spreads rapidly and is often associated with an increase in symptoms of a systemic disturbance. The skin is limited in its pattern of reaction and therefore an eruption may be common to a number of drugs, although, as mentioned above, certain drugs have a tendency to produce specific skin lesions. Continued administration of a drug responsible for a skin reaction may result in universal affection of the skin — for example exfoliative dermatitis or erythroderma. Systems other than the skin may be affected.

CUTANEOUS VASCULITIS

A number of conditions with both cutaneous and systemic involvement are due to inflammatory reactions of the blood vessels; reference has already been made to examples of these, such as Henoch—Schönlein purpura, erythema multiforme, erythema nodosum, and erythema induratum. Periarteritis nodosa, granulomatous vasculitis in the form of Wegener's granulomatosis, and temporal arteritis all may have extensive involvement in other systems in addition to the changes seen in the skin. The inability to determine specific causal factors makes classification of 'vasculitis' difficult.

Lupus erythematosus, dermatomyositis and scleroderma can be grouped together as collagen—vascular disorders. In *lupus erythematosus* the reaction may be confined to the skin (Figure

8.16), but in the acute systemic form there is involvement of many of the body systems. In *scleroderma* there is a cutaneous form, morphoea, as well as systemic scleroderma. The latter often presents as Raynaud's phenomenon, which may be the only manifestation for some years, to be followed by the sclero-dermatous tightening and atrophy of the skin of the fingers and hands. Characteristically, the changes are noticeable on the face, particularly around the mouth, with tightness and puckering of the lips, and occasionally the development of numerous spider

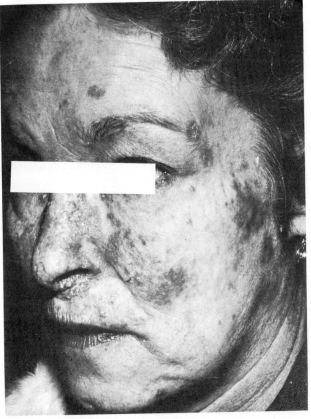

Figure 8.16. *Cutaneous lupus erythematosus. Fixed erythematous patches with follicular plugging and some degree of scarring over the butterfly area of the face.*

angiomata. Involvement of the oesophagus leads to dysphagia. Additional symptoms arise depending on the severity of the affection of other systems.

Blisters (vesicles/bullae) occur in a variety of dermatoses but there are three conditions in which their formation is an important and major diagnostic feature, namely, pemphigus, pemphigoid and dermatitis herpetiformis. *Pemphigus* affects the middle-aged, presenting as a blistering eruption in which the blister soon ruptures to leave extensive raw tender areas. A shearing strain-type of pressure on uninvolved skin can result in the production of a blister (Nikolsky's sign). The appearance of the eruption varies with the situation of the blister at the different levels of the epidermis and, when very superficial, it closely simulates exfoliation (pemphigus foliaceous). The mucous membranes are often involved. *Pemphigoid*, on the other hand, affects an older age group with an eruption consisting of intact tense blisters (sometimes haemorrhagic) on a background of oedematous erythema (Figure 8.17), the mucous membranes being rarely affected. In *dermatitis herpetiformis* (Figure 4.5) the eruption is itchy and affects particularly the extensor aspects of the limbs (especially knees and elbows) and the buttocks, with mixed features of eczema, oedematous erythema, urticaria and small blisters. The rapidity of response to dapsone (diaminodiphenyl sulphone) is such that the administration of the drug can be used both diagnostically and therapeutically. There is an association with coeliac disease.

In addition to confirmation of the clinical diagnosis by routine histological studies of biopsy material, immunofluorescent staining techniques can provide important additional information for differential diagnosis. In pemphigus vulgaris, IgG antibody reacts with an antigen in the intercellular membrane resulting in an intra-epidermal blister, whereas, in pemphigoid, the IgG reacts with the basement membrane leading to a subepidermal blister. In dermatitis herpetiformis IgA is directed against the epidermal basement membrane.

THE REACTION OF THE SKIN TO 'LIGHT'

The ultraviolet (UV) component of the solar spectrum (Figure 8.18) can damage living cells; the structure of DNA is such that it will absorb ultraviolet radiation (UVR), and the resulting damage has to be repaired quickly otherwise the cell dies or survives with

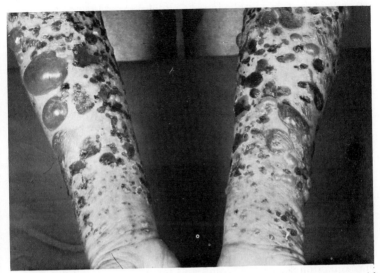

Figure 8.17. *Pemphigoid. Tense intact bullae, some of which are haemorrhagic with background erythema.*

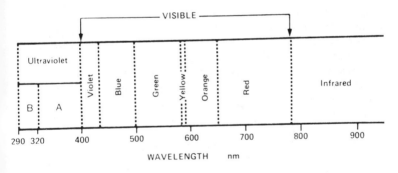

Figure 8.18. *The solar spectrum.*

altered function. It is this altered functioning cell which leads in time to the development of a localised malignant change seen in an early stage in actinic keratosis (Figure 8.30). In addition to cell repair the skin will, in response to exposure to UVR, thicken and increase melanin pigmentation, the potential for the latter depending on genetic, racial and environmental factors. At one extreme is the fair-complexioned Celt who responds to exposure to sunshine with erythema and freckling, and at the other extreme the dark-skinned African. The former is at risk of developing premalignant and malignant skin changes if he should reside for any length of time in parts of the world where the amount of UVR is greater than that to which he is genetically adapted. Degenerative changes in the collagen framework of the dermis will lead in time to loss of elasticity, manifested by wrinkling of the exposed skin (Figure 8.30). Similar degeneration will affect the lower lip, resulting in actinic cheilitis, and in some leads on to squamous cell carcinoma, which is a serious lesion with a greater potential to metastasise than when arising from exposed skin. In certain rare developmental abnormalities there is an inability to repair UV-damaged cellular DNA because of impaired enzyme function. Thus, in xeroderma pigmentosum the process of UV-induced malignant change is speeded up leading to the production in the skin of all the features of premalignant (dryness, wrinkling, freckling, keratoses, keratoacanthoma) and malignant (basal cell and squamous cell epithelioma and malignant melanoma) change (Figure 8.19).

The skin will also react to light if photoactive substances are present. These substances may be derived from a number of different sources — drugs such as phenothiazines and sulphonamides, or a metabolic byproduct as in certain types of porphyria. Depending on their structure, they will absorb different wavelengths throughout the solar spectrum; thus, porphyrin absorbs and reacts to visible light between 400 and 700 nm, whereas chlorpromazine and other phenothiazines react to the UV wavelengths below 400 nm. The subsequent reactions make use of either *phototoxic* or *photoallergic* mechanisms (Figure 8.20). In porphyria there is increased skin fragility and blister formation and alterations in pigmentation and hair growth, whereas a similar phototoxic reaction following parenteral administration of chlorpromazine leads to dusky erythema and pigmentation of the exposed skin. Absorption of certain photoactive substances directly into the skin from external contact and their subsequent combination with UVR commonly leads to a photoallergic response involving cell-mediated immune mechanisms.

The clinical diagnosis of cutaneous photosensitivity is simple when there is a history of a skin reaction on exposed sites only, when the disorder is confined to the sunshine months, and when the severity of the response is directly related to the amount of

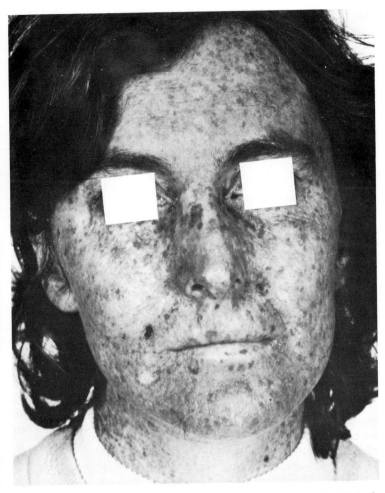

Figure 8.19. *Xeroderma pigmentosum. Premalignant and malignant changes in the skin with dryness, keratoses, freckling and scarring from previous kerato-acanthomata, basal cell epithelioma and cheilitis.*

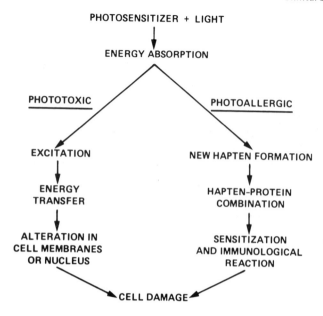

Figure 8.20. *Phototoxic and photoallergic mechanisms.*

exposure. Sometimes, however, the wavelengths of light to which an individual has become 'sensitive' may be present all the year round (e.g. visible light) and in this instance the seasonal history is lost or at least modified. If the changes in the skin seen by the patient are not simply sunburn erythema or a red rash but comprise increased fragility and blisters, then an association with sun exposure is likely to be missed. Certain of the photodermatoses also owe their chronicity to factors other than photosensitivity, such as contact allergic sensitivity.

It is necessary therefore to have access to the technique of phototesting, which will determine whether the response of the skin differs from normal and, if so, will define the wavelengths of UVR and/or light responsible for the abnormal reaction, i.e. the action spectrum of the eruption (Figure 8.39). In addition, a modified skin patch test, called a photopatch test (see below), is used to demonstrate the presence or otherwise of photocontact allergic sensitivity (Figure 8.38).

TUMOURS

Although the skin can be affected by many tumours, those which are common are relatively few in number (see Table 8.1).

Table 8.1. *Common skin tumours*

Melanocytic naevi and malignant melanoma
Seborrhoeic keratoses, skin tags and squamous papilloma
Histiocytoma
Neurofibroma
Angioma: capillary, cavernous, spider telangiectasis, granuloma telangiectaticum (pyogenic granuloma) and Campbell de Morgan's spots
Solar keratosis
Epithelioma: basal cell, squamous cell and intra-epidermal
Keratoacanthoma
Epidermal/epithelial naevi

Melanocytic Naevi ('Mole')

The *lentigo* is a common brown or dark-brown macule, usually first seen in childhood. It is permanent, although sometimes it fades with age. The majority do not show transition towards a junctional melanocytic naevus but this can occur in childhood. The *melanocytic naevus* is also common, often seen first in childhood and increasing in number throughout life with a reduction in old age. It appears in a variety of forms (Figure 8.21a), the term 'junctional' being used when the proliferation of naevus cells is confined to the epidermal/dermal junction. This is in contrast to the 'dermal' form, where collections of cells are seen only in the dermis, and the 'compound' variety, when both sites are involved. These are benign lesions although malignant melanoma may rarely develop, particularly in the junctional form. The *congenital pigmented naevus*, which is present at birth (Figure 8.21b), may affect extensive areas of the skin and has a greater potential for malignant change.

Malignant lentigo (lentigo maligna) most commonly affects the skin of the face of middle-aged and elderly subjects. It presents as a flat, brown to dark-brown patch which may be slightly raised with some colour variation at different parts and an irregular margin (Figure 8.22). Untreated, it may change to a more invasive tumour when pigmentary changes and eventually localised nodule formation develop (Figure 8.23).

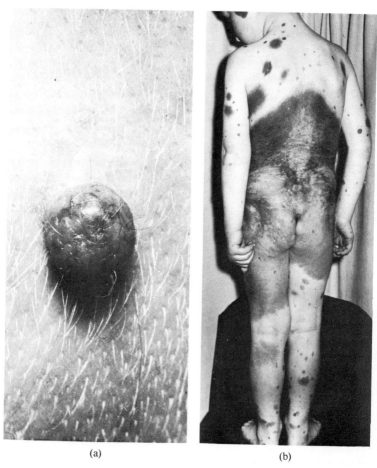

(a)   (b)

Figure 8.21. *Melanocytic naevi. (a) Melanocytic naevus. (b) Congenital pigmented naevus.*

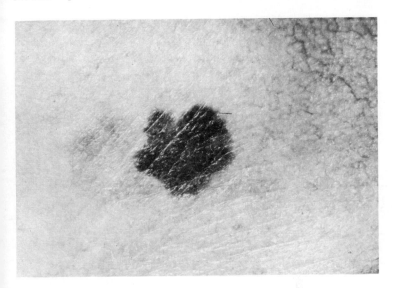

Figure 8.22. *Lentigo maligna. Pigmented patch on the cheek showing variations in the depth of pigmentation and irregularity of peripheral growth.*

Malignant melanoma usually presents in one of two forms. A superficial spreading melanoma is commonly encountered in the fourth or fifth decade. It is a pigmented lesion (Figure 8.24) which has been growing slowly over a number of months or years and which may then cause mild itching or discomfort. There may be a deepening in pigmentation and an inflammatory reaction related to the advancing edge. Depigmentation may be present elsewhere in the lesion. The nodular melanoma variety does not stem from a pre-existing pigmented lesion but as a nodule in the skin, which is usually, but not necessarily, heavily pigmented (Figure 8.25). It has a tendency to early invasion of the dermis and the prognosis is worse than with the superficial spreading variety.

Seborrhoeic Keratoses (Skin Tags)

Considered to be dominantly inherited, seborrhoeic keratoses affect both sexes equally frequently, are commonly numerous, and increase in number from middle age onwards. They range in size

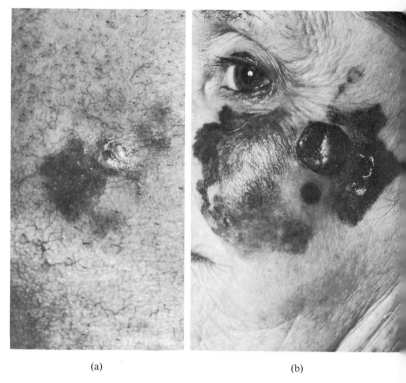

(a)   (b)

Figure 8.23. *Lentigo malign melanoma. Showing within the pigmented patch a dark-black nodule, indicating malignant melanoma (a). The development of melanoma in a lentigo maligna (b).*

from a few millimetres to two to three centimetres, and from small flat yellowish spots to large warty plaques which appear stuck on to the skin (Figure 8.26). Some may be smooth-surfaced and domed with follicular orifices which contain keratin plugs (Figure 8.27). They are commonly seen on sites containing sebaceous glands and tend to be pedunculated, not keratotic, when present round the eyes or in the body flexures. Skin tags are related to seborrhoeic keratoses and are commonly seen on the skin of the neck and trunk, particularly in middle-aged women. A profuse eruption of seborrhoeic keratosis may follow a dermatosis such as dermatitis and may rarely be a cutaneous manifestation of systemic malignancy.

Histiocytoma (Dermatofibroma)

This is a common benign tumour usually affecting the skin of the limbs and is particularly common in the female. It is a small firm nodule usually single, but occasionally multiple, which is attached to the epidermis. The tumour is freely movable over the underlying tissues and has a colour range from pink or red to brown and ivory-white when of long duration. A histiocytoma is thought to follow insect bites or other forms of minor trauma.

Neurofibroma

A neurofibroma may be solitary but when multiple (neurofibromatosis, von Recklinghausen's disease) is dominantly inherited and associated with cafe-au-lait spots. The single lesion is usually first seen in adult life, while multiple neurofibromatosis occurs in later childhood or in early adolescence. Tumours arise from peripheral nerves and their supporting structures and may be associated with renal, endocrinal and skeletal abnormalities.

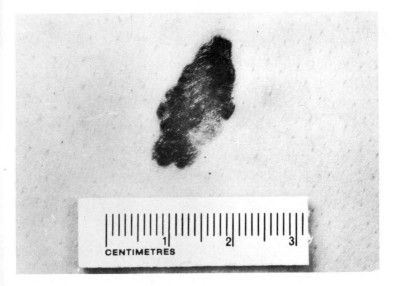

Figure 8.24. *Superficial spreading malignant melanoma. Showing variation in depth of pigmentation with irregular peripheral spread and an area of hypopigmentation.*

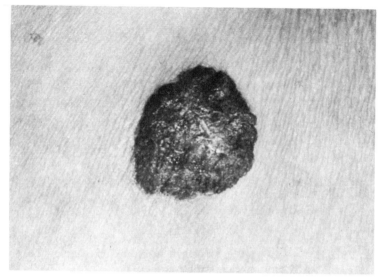

Figure 8.25. *Nodular melanoma.*

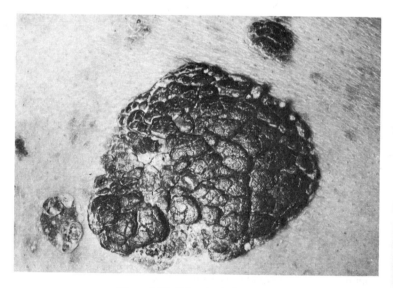

Figure 8.26. *Seborrhoeic keratoses.*

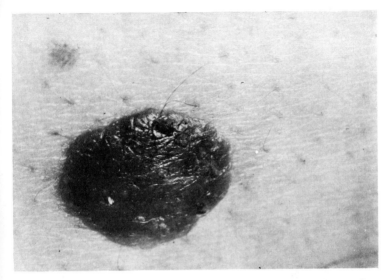

Figure 8.27. *Seborrhoeic keratosis. This form of seborrhoeic keratosis is sometimes called basal cell papilloma in view of the absence of superficial horn formation and the appearance of a smooth-surfaced dome-shaped lesion with keratin plugging of the follicular orifices.*

Cutaneous Haemangioma

These hamartomatous lesions include the *capillary angioma* (port-wine stain) — the commonest birth mark — and the *cavernous angioma* (strawberry mark). The latter may be present at birth but usually does not appear until a few weeks later, first as a small red macule which slowly increases in size to reach the final strawberry appearance at about six months of age (Figure 8.28). It usually affects females and normally remains unchanged, perhaps increasing in size with the growth of the child, before resolving spontaneously with the appearance of pale areas and increasing flaccidity. Sixty per cent disappear by the third year and most of the remainder by six or seven years of age.

Granuloma telangiectaticum (pyogenic granuloma) is a commonly seen red nodule comprising proliferating capillaries. It often follows trauma and is usually rapidly growing. Granuloma telangiectaticum occurs in both sexes, at any age, and ulcerates and bleeds easily. It may be pedunculated, being situated most often on

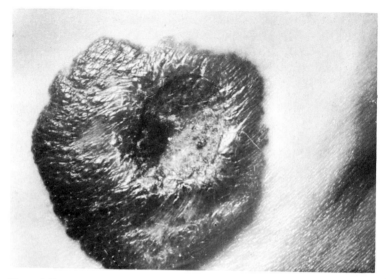

Figure 8.28. *Cavernous haemangioma (strawberry mark). Well-circumscribed raised red lesion with central necrosis.*

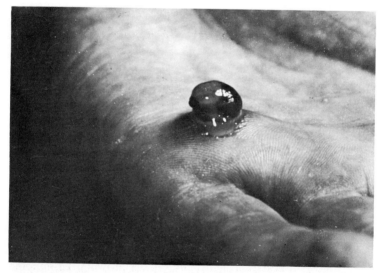

Figure 8.29. *Pyogenic granuloma. Rounded brownish-red nodule with a collar of acanthotic epidermis.*

the skin of the hands and feet and particularly on the fingers or toes (Figure 8.29). It does not usually disappear spontaneously.

Spider telangiectasis consists of a central arteriole with fine radiating vessels. The lesions are present in 15 per cent of normal individuals; they are commonly seen in children but can be associated with pregnancy, liver disease and scleroderma (systemic sclerosis), where they are found only on the face. In *hereditary haemorrhagic telangiectasis* (Rendu-Osler-Weber syndrome) the lesions are punctate or linear rather than spider-like, occurring most frequently on the upper half of the body, e.g. face, lips, ears, conjunctivae and, invariably, on the mucous membranes of the nose, mouth, nasopharynx and gastrointestinal tract, with the danger of haemorrhage from any of these sites.

Campbell de Morgan's spots (cherry angiomata) are small, raised, bright-red angiomata which usually occur on the skin of the trunk in middle-aged and elderly individuals. They are common and have no clinical significance.

Solar Keratosis

The skin ages on exposed sites mainly as a result of the accumulated effect of UVR, leading eventually to premalignant changes in the

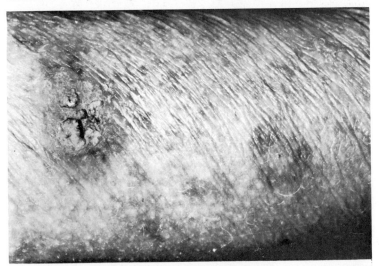

Figure 8.30. *Premalignant skin. Senile purpura with wrinkling of the skin, variable pigmentation and a solar (actinic) keratosis.*

form of dryness, loss of elasticity, patchy hypopigmentation and hyperpigmentation, haemorrhages (senile purpura), and ultimately localised areas of abnormal keratin formation (early solar keratosis) (Figure 8.30). The solar keratosis is thus seen on exposed skin such as the backs of the hands, the rims of the ears and the face, and in the older age groups. In those with fair complexion and of Celtic origin the lesion appears earlier in life, especially if the individual has been exposed to sunshine for any length of time. It is an irregular crusted lesion which may be flat or raised, with variable horn formation. On the face it may appear as rough, yellow or dirty-brown scaly plaques. It is potentially malignant but frequently fails to progress towards squamous cell carcinoma in the lifetime of the subject. Similar UV ageing of the lips, especially the lower lip, is much more likely to lead to squamous cell carcinoma. Carcinogens additional to UVR such as tar, inorganic arsenic, ionising radiation and radiant heat may all lead eventually to malignant change, as may chronic skin ulceration.

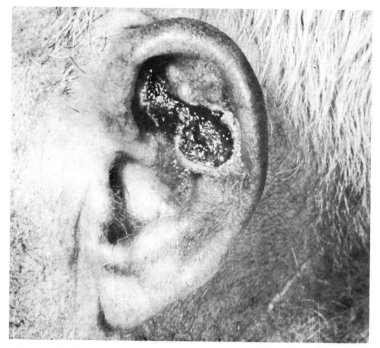

Figure 8.31. *Squamous cell epithelioma. Chronic indurated ulcer of the pinna.*

Epithelioma

The development of *squamous cell carcinoma* should be suspected when the lesion becomes indurated and feels firm on palpation with the induration appearing to extend beyond the visual margin of the lesion. In time the central keratotic crust is shed to produce either ulceration or an otherwise eroded indurated margin with perhaps a purulent exudate in the base (Figure 8.31).

Intra-epidermal epithelioma (carcinoma) as seen in Bowen's disease forms scaly, sometimes erythematous, plaques, most commonly appearing on the skin of the trunk. The lesions are often multiple, slow growing and their slightly raised margin is sharply demarcated from the neighbouring normal skin (Figure 8.32).

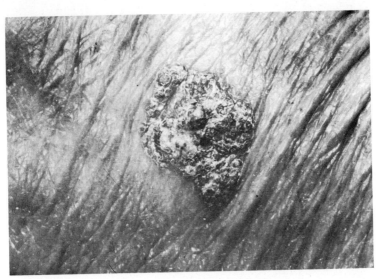

Figure 8.32. *Intra-epidermal epithelioma. Scaly erythematous well-circumscribed persistent plaque on the skin of the back of the hand.*

Developing from the basal cells, *basal cell carcinoma* is the commonest malignant tumour of the skin. It is locally destructive but rarely metastases. Basal cell carcinoma is more common in males above the age of 40 years and occurs predominantly on the upper and central parts of the face. Exposure to ultraviolet light

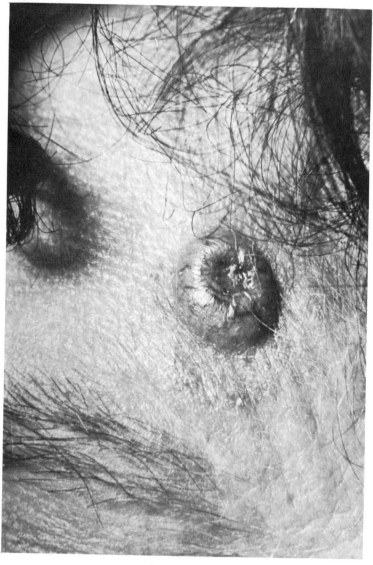

(a)

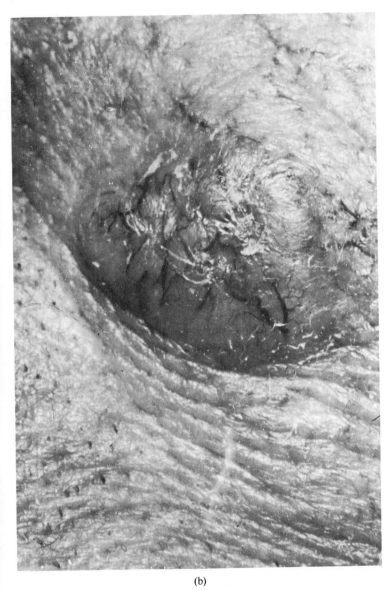

(b)

Figure 8.33. *Basal cell epithelioma. (a) Nodulo-ulcerative form, showing pearly border with telangiectasis and central ulceration. (b) Cystic form.*

and/or some modifications of the cells of an adnexal structure are considered to play a part in the development of this type of tumour. Basal cell carcinoma may be solitary or multiple. It usually starts as a small translucent papule and develops into a number of different forms. The nodulo-ulcerative form is the commonest (Figure 8.33a), but the lesion may be pigmented, cystic (Figure 8.33b), superficial or morphoeic.

Keratoacanthoma

This is a relatively common benign tumour of the exposed skin. Middle-aged and elderly males are particularly affected. It seems likely that cutaneous carcinogens such as UVR and tar can be aetiological factors, as may also infection in association with minor skin injuries.

It originates from pilosebaceous follicles and starts as a skin-coloured or reddish papule which soon enlarges rapidly to reach its maximum at about four weeks, when it presents as a fleshy smooth nodule, usually one to two cm diameter, with some telangiectasis and a central keratin-filled crater. Thereafter spontaneous resolution takes place, usually over the next three months, by a gradual increase in the central keratin plug in parallel with flattening of the surrounding fleshy circumference, leaving a puckered crenated scar. This natural history may vary, with the total duration being many months or with recurrence after curettage, excision or apparent resolution (Figure 8.34).

A number of less common growths arise from epidermal and adnexal structures and these are called epidermal or epithelial naevi, examples of which are sebaceous naevus and nevo syringocystadenoma papilliferum. Similar less common growths arise from adnexal structures, for example the syringoma from eccrine sweat glands.

THE RETICULOSES

The reticuloses may affect the skin, presenting non-specific changes such as purpura, haemorrhage, erythemata and atypical eruptions which may mimic either dermatitis or psoriasis; specific infiltrations and nodules may also be seen (Figure 8.9). In mycosis fungoides, which is considered to be a T-cell lymphoma, the condition may remain confined to the skin throughout life, but

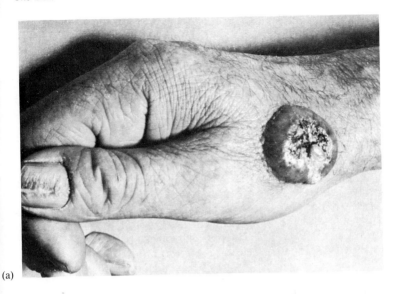

(a)

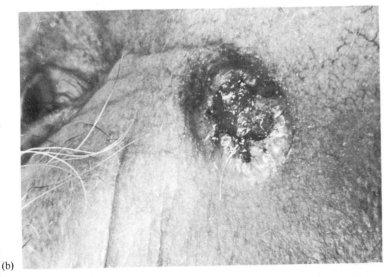

(b)

Figure 8.34. *Keratoacanthoma. (a) A firm round nodule with central horn formation. (b) The central horny plug has been shed and the overhanging epidermal edge is now receding.*

occasionally a reticulosis will eventually involve internal organs. Two stages of eruption can often be demonstrated, with, initially, a widespread formation of scaly, usually irritable plaques, perhaps with somewhat bizarre shapes, suggestive of an atypical dermatosis such as dermatitis or psoriasis or a mixture of the two. In the later stage nodules appear, which in time will ulcerate.

CUTANEOUS MANIFESTATIONS OF MALIGNANCY

Certain cutaneous signs and symptoms suggest the possibility of underlying malignant disease. Direct invasion by malignant cells, as in Paget's disease, or secondary cutaneous metastases from a distant primary cancer are encountered. Skin haemorrhage in the form of purpura, petechiae and ecchymosis may occur in leukaemia and the dysproteinaemias. Systemic malignancy must always be excluded when there is generalised pruritus or a chronic widespread idiopathic pruritic eruption, although in the majority of instances this will be found to be a benign symptom unconnected with any systemic disease. Persistent severe infection of the skin, to which the leukaemia patient is particularly prone, may be due to viral infection (herpes simplex, herpes zoster), chronic candidiasis, systemic fungal infection, or chronic boils. Increased viscosity may be present as Raynaud's phenomenon or erythromelalgia.

In addition there are a number of more specific skin conditions ('skin markers') which are suggestive of systemic malignancy. These include:

Acanthosis nigricans
Dermatomyositis
Acquired ichthyosis
Acquired hypertrichosis
  lanuginosa (malignant down)
Pachydermoperiostosis
Exfoliative dermatitis/
  erythroderma
Bowen's disease
Erythemata: erythema gyratum
  repens

Arsenical keratosis/
  pigmentation/basal cell
  epithelioma
Reticulohistiocytoma
Carcinoid
Palmoplantar keratoderma
  (Howell—Evans syndrome)
Gardner's syndrome
Peutz—Jeghers syndrome

A number of these conditions are extremely rare, such as acanthosis nigricans, acquired hypertrichosis lanuginosa, pachy-dermoperiostosis, arsenical keratosis/pigmentation, reticulohistio-cytoma, and palmoplantar keratoderma.

Dermatomyositis

This is an inflammatory condition of the skin and the muscles and is associated with malignancy in 30 per cent or more of affected subjects. The myositis element may be minimal or undetectable but when present consists of aching and weakness of the muscles leading to difficulty in sitting up in bed or climbing stairs. There is often erythema and oedema of the face, particularly around the eyes, with a purplish-red heliotrope colour. Elsewhere there is an affection particularly of light-exposed areas with erythema, telangiectasis and atrophy. On the hands there is often periungual telangiectasis with scaly lesions over the knuckles.

Acquired Ichthyosis

Dryness of the skin (mild ichthyosis, xeroderma) is common and not infrequently associated with atopy and, as such, is benign and remains throughout life. Also, in certain elderly subjects the skin becomes dry and itchy with advancing years. Very rarely, however, an adult will suddenly develop widespread dry scaling of the skin, often with an element of increased pigmentation which may be associated with a reticulosis, particularly Hodgkin's disease.

Exfoliative Dermatitis/Erythroderma

Universal skin changes either in the form of dermatitis or persistent scaly erythema and oedema (erythroderma) may be due to a reticulosis, which should be suspected once the more common causes such as contact allergic sensitivity and drug-induced reaction have been excluded.

Bowen's Disease

When this form of intra-epidermal epithelioma appears on exposed skin it is probably due to long-term UVR exposure. If it develops on covered areas, and particularly if multiple, then previous ingestion of inorganic arsenic is a possibility. There may also be an associated tendency to develop malignancy of one or more systems and particularly the respiratory, gastrointestinal or genito-urinary systems.

Erythemata

The relationship between the erythemata and systemic disease has already been referred to. In erythema gyratum repens, the erythematous reaction moves slowly over the body surface, producing a pattern resembling the grain of wood (Figure 8.35). It is particularly associated with malignant disease of the breast and lung.

Carcinoid Syndrome

In this disorder there is recurrent facial flushing with eventual permanent dilatation of the capillaries.

Gardner's Syndrome

In this syndrome there is an association between multiple sebaceous cysts, polyposis of the colon, dental abnormalities, osteomas of the facial bones and skin fibromata, with a tendency for malignant change to develop in the intestinal polyp.

Peutz—Jeghers Syndrome (see Figure 4.7)

Multiple, small, brown-pigmented spots around the mouth and on the lips and neighbouring buccal mucosa are associated with intestinal polyps and, less commonly, polyps in the stomach or colon.

CUTANEOUS CHANGES IN GASTROINTESTINAL DISEASE

Reference has been made to changes in the skin which raise the possibility of malignancy within the gastrointestinal tract. There remain a number of other skin conditions which are associated with gastrointestinal disease:

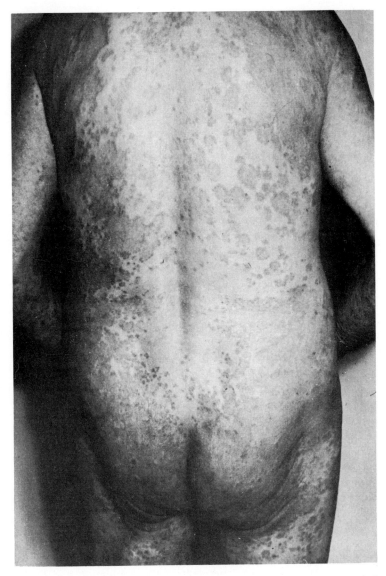

Figure 8.35. *Erythema gyratum. Fluctuating, bizarre, bilateral, symmetrical, widespread gyrate erythema.*

Aphthous ulcers
Benign mucosal pemphigoid
Vitiligo
Pyoderma gangrenosum
Dermatitis herpetiformis
Acrodermatitis enteropathica
Behçet's syndrome

Hereditary haemorrhagic
   telangiectasia
Blue rubber bleb naevi
Malignant papulosis
Henoch—Schönlein purpura
Kaposi's sarcoma
Pseudoxanthoma elasticum
Ehlers—Danlos syndrome

Some of these conditions are extremely rare, particularly blue rubber bled naevi, malignant papulosis, Kaposi's sarcoma, pseudo-xanthoma elasticum, and Ehlers—Danlos syndrome.

Aphthous ulcers (see Figure 4.4)

This type is common and consists of one or more ulcers of the buccal mucosa which are shallow and painful with a white base and a margin of erythema.

Recurrent oral ulceration is seen in ulcerative colitis, Crohn's disease, coeliac disease, and in Behçet's syndrome.

Benign Mucosal Pemphigoid (Cicatricial Pemphigoid)

The vesiculobullous element is a common feature of many cutaneous reactions but in two specific conditions this blister element predominates, those of pemphigus and pemphigoid (see page 490). The level of blister formation differs in that, in the former, it is intraepidermally situated and, in the latter, sub-epidermal. A variant, which is called benign mucosal pemphigoid, develops mucosal lesions in addition to the bullous lesions on the skin. Involvement of the eyes and the mucous membrane of the mouth leads to scarring. The reaction may spread down to involve the lining of the oesophagus.

Vitiligo

In vitiligo, areas of depigmentation occur at various sites because of destruction of the pigment-forming melanocytes. It is a common condition affecting 1 to 2 per cent of the population and has an association with autoimmune conditions such as pernicious anaemia, atrophic gastritis, hyperhydroidism, thyroiditis, adrenal insufficiency, some forms of uveitis and sympathetic ophthalmia.

Pyoderma Gangrenosum

This can occur on any skin site in approximately 10 per cent of patients with ulcerative colitis. It presents as erythematous swellings, followed by pustulation and the development of indurated plaques with undermined edges and areas of ulceration.

Acrodermatitis Enteropathica

This is a recessively inherited disorder which presents in infancy as an erythematous eruption with vesicles, pustules and crusting. Secondary *Candida* infection affects particularly the skin around the mouth and anogenital region, fingers and scalp. Diarrhoea and alopecia occur. The disease is due to zinc deficiency probably as a result of a defect of gastrointestinal zinc absorption, although an abnormality yet to be defined may be common to both the bowel and the skin.

Behçet's Syndrome

In this condition recurrent ulcers appear on both the buccal mucosa and the genitalia and may be associated with cutaneous lesions resembling erythema nodosum and superficial migratory thrombophlebitis. There may be involvement of the respiratory and central nervous systems and gastrointestinal ulceration may occur.

Hereditary Haemorrhagic Telangiectasia (Rendu-Osler-Weber Disease)

See page 503.

Henoch—Schönlein Syndrome (Anaphylactoid Purpura)

This is a manifestation of leucocytoclastic vasculitis. It affects children and young adults as a purpuric eruption which may be initially an urticarial erythema. The lesions occur particularly on the skin of the lower extremities and buttocks but may also affect the trunk, arms and face. There is frequently joint pain and renal and abdominal complications, the latter being associated with colic, haemorrhage and intussusception.

ENDOCRINE DISEASE AND THE SKIN

Pituitary

In acromegaly the skin is coarse, greasy, pigmented and thickened, along with hypertrichosis; in hypopituitarism there is hypopigmentation and thinning of the skin and loss of sexual hair. In addition, there are the characteristic and diagnostic cutaneous features of Cushing's syndrome with striae (Figure 9.14), hirsuties, pigmentation, acne, purpura, and a tendency to develop chronic fungal infection *(Trichophyton rubrum* or *Pityrosporon orbiculare)*.

Thyroid

In hyperthyroidism the skin is warm and sweating and there may be a complaint of irritation. There is an increased incidence of alopecia areata and vitiligo and a tendency to scalp hair fall of the telogen effluvium type. Pigmentary changes are variable. Pretibial myxoedema (Plate 8.4) occurs in association with thyrotoxicosis, usually following treatment. The lesions are situated over the anterior aspect of the lower legs in the form of thickened waxy plaques with prominent hair follicles and resulting from the accumulation of acid mucopolysaccharide in the dermis. In hypothyroidism the skin is dry, pale, coarse and swollen, with loss of scalp and, occasionally, eyebrow hair.

Adrenals

In addition to the pigmentation of Addison's disease, which is widespread but often accentuated on exposed skin and at sites of friction, there are the changes of adrenal virilism (Figures 9.5 and 9.6) to be considered such as hirsuties, acne and male pattern baldness.

Diabetes Mellitus

Skin conditions associated with the development of diabetes include infection, particularly with *Candida*, and ischaemic changes. Other skin disorders encountered include vitiligo, xanthomatosis (page 519), necrobiosis lipoidica and diabetic dermopathy.

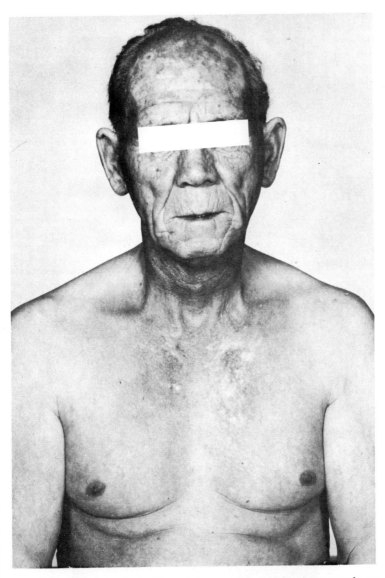

Figure 8.36. *Hepatic porphyria. Pigmentation, scarring and sclerodermatous change affecting the exposed skin of the face and neck.*

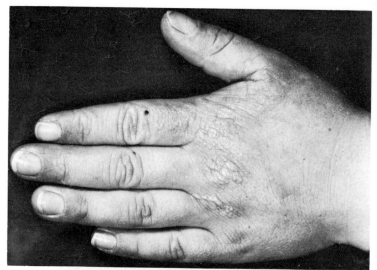

(a)

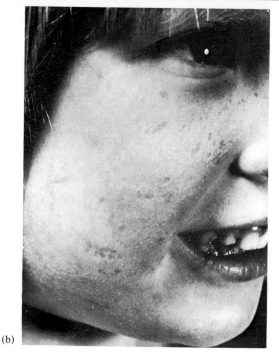

(b)

In *necrobiosis lipoidica* a thickened plaque develops which is yellowish in colour at the centre and violaceous at the periphery, gradually becoming atrophic with telangiectases and a tendency to ulcerate. It is usually seen on the shins but can appear on other parts of the legs and in the skin elsewhere (Plate 8.5). In *diabetic dermopathy* red papules or small nodules develop on the skin of the lower legs which may ulcerate to leave small depressed scars and pigmentation.

METABOLIC ABNORMALITIES AND THE SKIN

Porphyria

In hepatic porphyria, porphyria variegata, congenital erythropoietic porphyria and erythropoietic protoporphyria, abnormal amounts of porphyrins accumulate in the skin which then combine with light to produce characteristic cutaneous changes. In *hepatic porphyria* there is increased skin fragility with blisters, scarring and hyperpigmentation, increased growth of hair and, in more severe cases, sclerodermatous changes (Figure 8.36). In the rare *congenital erythropoietic porphyria* the destruction of tissue is that much greater. In *erythropoietic protoporphyria*, particularly as it presents in the United Kingdom, the symptoms are often more prominent than the signs. There is a complaint of severe discomfort, often pain, in the exposed skin associated with swelling. This swelling may be minimal and can result in thickening of the skin, particularly over the knuckles, with accentuated skin lines and fine linear scarring on the face (Figure 8.37).

Hyperlipidaemia

In disturbances of lipid metabolism various forms of xanthoma may be seen in the skin. Plane xanthomata, as xanthelasma, occur on the eyelids, in the palmar creases and on the sides of the neck or

Figure 8.37. *Erythropoietic protoporphyria. (a) Characteristic thickening of the skin over the knuckles with accentuation of the skin lines and a fine linear scarring of the face (b).*

trunk, and are to be found in association with Types II, III and IV hyperlipidaemia. The tuberous xanthomata appear as raised nodules over the extensor aspects of joints and on the buttocks and are associated with Types II and III hyperlipidaemia. They may show a particular predilection for extensor tendons (tendinous xanthomata) such as those over the knuckles and round the elbows, and in this instance are associated with Types II and III hyperlipidaemia. In the eruptive xanthomata there is a sudden rapid development of smaller yellow papules, usually in association with diabetes mellitus and Types I, II, III and IV hyperlipidaemia.

INVESTIGATIVE TECHNIQUES

Patch and Photopatch Testing (Figure 8.38)

The allergens suspected of being responsible for the contact dermatitis are applied to the centre of a series of patches (Figure 8.38a), using a concentration which is known to be non-irritant for normal skin. These patches are then applied to the skin of the back (Figure 8.38b) and removed 48 hours later. The production of a localised eczematous reaction indicates the presence of allergic sensitivity (Figure 8.38c). The allergens listed are those most commonly found to produce contact allergic sensitivity and, as such, can be used for screening purposes.

The technique of photopatch testing is similar to that of patch testing except that the area is subsequently irradiated with measured amounts of selected wavebands of UVR or light.

Phototesting (Figure 8.39)

The technique of phototesting consists of irradiating the skin with increasing amounts of energy at special selected wavebands with a view to determining the minimal erythema dose (Figure 8.39a). The table lists the dose in mJ/cm^2 required to produce a minimal reaction of the skin in relationship to the dose at which no reaction could be detected, e.g. at the 295 nm peak the minimal response dose is 2.7 mJ/cm^2 and the no-response level is at 2.2 mJ/cm^2 (Figure 8.39b). These data allow the action spectrum to be plotted as illustrated in Figure 8.39c, the bars recording the range between the minimal response and no-response levels. The action spectrum

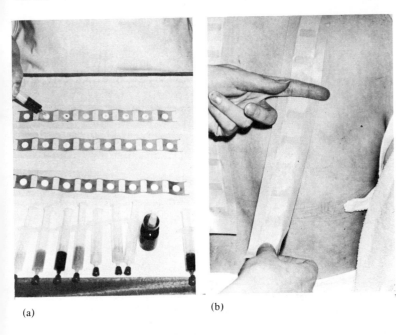

(a)　　　　　　　　　　　　(b)

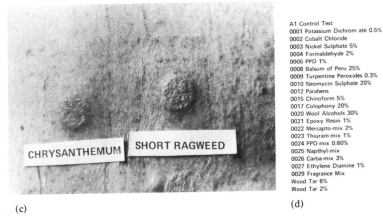

CHRYSANTHEMUM　　SHORT RAGWEED

A1 Control Test
0001 Potassium Dichrom ate 0.5%
0002 Cobalt Chloride
0003 Nickel Sulphate 5%
0004 Formaldehyde 2%
0005 PPD 1%
0008 Balsum of Peru 25%
0009 Turpentine Peroxides 0.3%
0010 Neomycin Sulphate 20%
0012 Parabens
0015 Chinoform 5%
0017 Colophony 20%
0020 Wool Alcohols 30%
0021 Epoxy Resin 1%
0022 Mercapto-mix 2%
0023 Thiuram-mix 1%
0024 PPD-mix 0.60%
0025 Napthyl-mix
0026 Carba-mix 3%
0027 Ethylene Diamine 1%
0029 Fragrance Mix
Wood Tar 6%
Wood Tar 2%

(c)　　　　　　　　　　　　(d)

Figure 8.38. *Technique of patch testing. The syringes contain the various materials (a) which are applied in measured amounts to the line of discs which are backed with non-irritant non-allergic adhesive materials which are then applied to the skin of the back (b) and a positive reaction is indicated by an eczematous response (c) present 48 to 72 hours later. The list of allergens used for screening purposes can be seen in (d).*

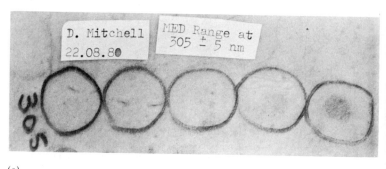

(a)

SCREENING PROCEDURE

5 nm   ½BW
Day 1

Wavelength nm	Dose mJcm⁻²				
254	1.5,	4.7,	15,	33	
295	2.7,	6.8,	18,	47	
300	1.5,	4.7,	15,	33	
305	2.7,	6.8,	18,	47	
310	1.5,	4.7,	15,	33	
315	1.5,	4.7,	15,	33	
320	10,	22,	33,	82,	270
325	100,	330,	820		
330	270,	680,	1200		
335	1200				
340	1200				

Day 2

Six separate doses (20% difference)
between the no response level and the
MED

(b)

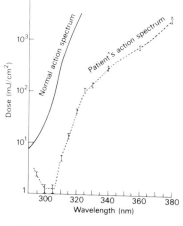

(c)

Figure 8.39. *Technique of photopatch testing. The skin is irradiated at a series of wavelengths, e.g. from 254 to 340 nm as in (b) with increasing doses, with a view to defining the minimal response dose, which can be seen as the fourth dose (a) at a wavelength peak of 305 nm. This minimal response dose defined for a series of wavelengths allows for the determination of the patient's action spectrum (c).*

for the individual patient is compared to that found in a group of normal subjects using the same technique (normal action spectrum).

FURTHER READING

Fitzpatrick, T. B., Eisen, A. Z., Wolff, K., Freedberg, I. M. & Austen, K. F. (Ed.) (1979) *Dermatology in General Medicine.* 2nd Edition. New York: McGraw-Hill.

Rook, A., Wilkinson, D. S. & Ebling, F. J. G. (Ed.) (1979) *Textbook of Dermatology.* 3rd Edition. Oxford: Blackwell Scientific Publications.

Shuster, S. (1978) *Dermatology in Internal Medicine.* London: Oxford Medical Publications.

9 The Endocrine System

C. W. H. Havard

HISTORY

The hormones of the endocrine system control the rate of growth, rate of metabolism of the body, the physical development and gonadal function, the response to stress, the proper distribution of water and electrolytes between intracellular and extracellular tissues, and the metabolism of calcium. It is small wonder, therefore, that the manifestations of endocrine disease are protean. Symptoms as different as loss of weight, sweating or pigmentation may be features of endocrine disorders. When taking a medical history questions relating to all body systems must be asked in a routine manner. The clinical approach will differ depending upon how the problem presents. Thus if a patient presents with shortness of stature, the symptoms and signs of pituitary or thyroid deficiency should be sought with special interest and vigour because these are the two most important glands concerned with growth. Alternatively, if a patient has a goitre special interest will be taken in the symptoms and signs of thyroid dysfunction. It is therefore useful to discuss in general some of the more important endocrine symptoms and signs, realising, however, that many of these may also be manifestations of disease in other systems.

Growth

Skeletal growth does not proceed at a uniform rate but rather in cycles. It is most rapid in infancy, slowing thereafter until puberty is reached when there is a secondary spurt. In boys this occurs between the ages of 13 and 15 and in girls between the ages of 11 and 13. The ultimate height depends on both genetic and environmental influences.

Certain individuals wish to be tall and they or their parents may complain of shortness of stature because they have not attained their desired height. When considering the possibility of a disorder of growth it is important to know the height of siblings and of parents and also the age at which the puberty growth spurt occurred in other members of the family. Charts relating height to age have been devised and give an indication of the normal rate of growth. The wide variation in normal children is immediately apparent on studying such charts (Figures 9.1, 9.2). Deviations from the mean of this wide range are called percentiles. Centile or percentile charts describe the distribution of a characteristic in a population. They are obtained by measuring a specific characteristic in a large population of at least 1000 of each sex at each age. For each age there will be a height above and below which 50 per cent of the population lie and this is called the 50th centile. The 50th centile indicates the mean height at a particular age. Such tables are less reliable around the age of puberty because of variation in the age of onset. Minor variations from the mean do not warrant investigation, but if the height of an individual falls below the third centile (three per cent of normal children have a height which falls below the third centile) or above the 97th centile, investigation is required. Changes in the rate of growth are also important and skeletal proportions may provide useful information. There are many children who are normal but are small in relation to their parents. The problem is merely one of growth delay; these children take rather longer to reach maturity and there is also a proportional delay in their skeletal maturation.

The actual height must always be assessed in relation to maturity. The change in skeletal proportions is one manifestation of maturity but other features include the maturing of facial features (with the growth of the nose and jaw) and dental development. Maturity of bone can readily be measured by the radiological bone age. Although smallness of stature and immaturity of the skeleton are features of hypopituitarism, in this disorder the velocity of growth is also impaired.

Measurement of height

The routine examination should include the measurement of the height and weight, not only for their immediate value but also for future reference. The height should not be measured by marks on the kitchen or consulting room door but by the correct instrument. The basic requirements are a firm horizontal platform on which the child stands, a moving horizontal platform which rests on the head, and a rigid surface on which he can hold himself vertical. The child should be encouraged to stretch to his full height to limit any observer error. The relative contribution of the limbs and the trunk to the total height may provide useful clinical information. It is therefore important to measure the distance of the symphysis pubis to the ground as this is essentially the contribution of the lower limb to the total height. A similar assessment of limb growth is provided by the span which is obtained by measuring the distance between the extremities of the middle finger when the arms are fully outstretched. In the normal adult the span equals the height. At birth the ratio of the trunk to the limb length is 1.7 to 1.0. The legs grow more rapidly than the trunk so by the time a child is ten years of age the segments are of equal length and remain so. Limb growth is hormonally determined. In eunuchoidism the span exceeds the height. Hypothyroid dwarfs retain their infantile proportions but in hypopituitarism an adult pattern occurs.

Bone growth is influenced by many hormones, of which growth hormone is the most important. Excess production leads to marked increase in epiphyseal cartilage growth rate and a deficiency leads to a marked reduction in the growth rate. Although deficient growth hormone production is called hypopituitarism, the primary defect is not infrequently in the hypothalamus and is due to a deficiency of the growth hormone releasing factor. Excess thyroxine leads to a slight increase in growth rate and a deficiency, as in hypothyroidism, causes a marked reduction. Much of this effect is due primarily to a deficiency of thyroid hormone but in hypothyroidism all endocrine functions are reduced including that of the pituitary. Androgens and oestrogens lead to an increase in the growth rate of epiphyseal cartilage and are responsible for the puberty growth spurt, though deficiencies of these hormones have no effect on the rate of growth. Excess production of these hormones accelerates skeletal maturation more than linear growth so that the ultimate height is reduced by their excess. Excess corticosteroid hormones reduce the growth rate but deficiencies have little effect on growth.

(a)

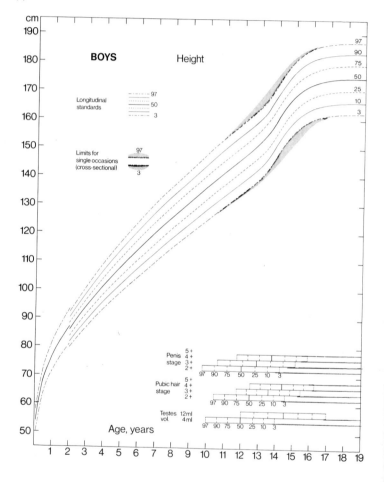

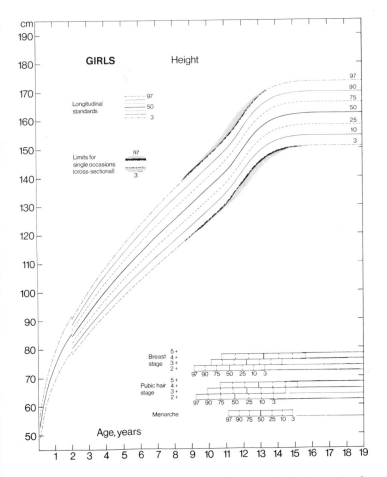

Figure 9.1. *Centile charts for height. Courtesy of Professor J. M. Tanner, London.*

(a)

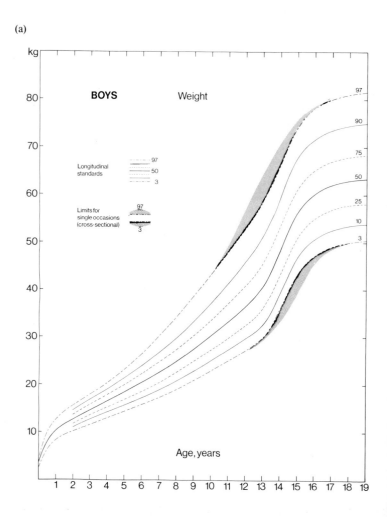

(b)

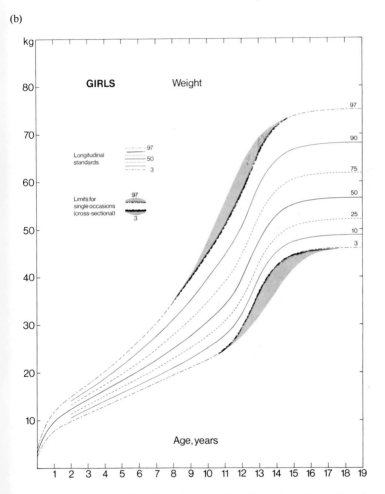

Figure 9.2. *Centile charts for weight. Courtesy of Professor J. M. Tanner, London.*

Shortness of stature

Most patients with shortness of stature do not suffer from endocrine disease. The majority are in fact perfectly normal and are the three per cent of normal children whose height lies below the third centile. The problem is to distinguish these children from those who are short because of disease. The commonest reason for being short and normal is to be the child of short parents and charts are available which relate height to age, taking into account parental height; but in this situation common sense is as good a guide as statistics. Deficiencies in protein and oxygen are more common than endocrine disease, and the cessation or slowing of linear growth and a failure to gain weight are the first effects of deficient protein or calorie intake. In the underdeveloped countries there are large numbers of children who are underheight and underweight as a result of a diet inadequate in protein or calories without other clinical evidence of disease. Malnutrition also occurs in malabsorption. Oxygen is necessary for the growth of tissue and it is therefore not surprising to find shortness of stature a typical feature of cyanotic heart disease and chronic respiratory disease. Children need love as well as food and disturbed family relationships can lead to failure of growth. Many of the syndromes associated with chromosome abnormalities may be associated with disorders of skeletal development and *Turner's syndrome* and *Down's syndrome* are examples of chromosome anomalies associated with shortness of stature. These children usually look abnormal. Clinical features such as webbing of the neck suggest ovarian infantilism, and short metacarpals suggest *pseudohypoparathyroidism*. Dwarfism due to deficiency of growth hormone is rare and hypothyroidism is more common. *Cushing's syndrome* in children is always associated with retardation of growth. Inherited bone disorders such as achondroplasia or osteogenesis imperfecta and acquired bone diseases such as rickets are common causes of short limbed dwarfism.

Having established that the patient has a disorder of growth there are many causes of shortness of stature that must be considered when seeking the relevant symptoms and signs which will lead to the correct aetiological diagnosis.

The main causes are shown in Table 9.1.

Tallness of stature

Tallness is usually constitutional in origin and the normal body proportions are maintained. Thyroxine increases the growth of

Table 9.1. *Causes of short stature.*

1. Constitutional delay in growth
2. Genetic
3. Nutritional
   a. Deficient intake
   b. Intestinal malabsorption
   c. Chronic renal disease
   d. Chronic infection
   e. Protein-losing disorders
4. Hypoxia
   a. Cyanotic heart disease
   b. Chronic pulmonary disease
5. Chromosome abnormalities
   a. Turner's syndrome
   b. Down's syndrome
6. Skeletal diseases
   a. Achondroplasia
   b. Hurler's syndrome
7. Endocrine diseases
   a. Hypopituitarism
   b. Hypothyroidism
   c. Cushing's disease

epiphyseal cartilage and rapid growth is seen in children with *thyrotoxicosis*. Androgens and oestrogens in excess stimulate skeletal growth but they have an even greater effect on skeletal maturation so that although a child with one of these disorders may be initially tall for its age the ultimate height will be shortened. Tallness of stature is a feature of *eunuchoidism* and of *Klinefelter's syndrome* and also of individuals with XYY chromosome constitution. It is also a feature of a few rare congenital syndromes such as *Marfan's syndrome* and *generalised lipodystrophy*. True *gigantism* results from excessive growth hormone secretion by a pituitary adenoma occurring before the epiphyses have fused (Figure 9.3) with the period of rapid growth occurring in late childhood and early puberty. The clinical features of *acromegaly*, though not apparent at first, usually appear during adolescence. When excessive production of growth hormone appears after the epiphyses have fused it is no longer possible for any increase in height to occur. Growth hormone does, however, stimulate the growth of other tissues apart from epiphyseal cartilage and overgrowth of the soft tissues occurs including the connective tissues of the skin and subcutaneous tissues. This gives rise to the coarsening

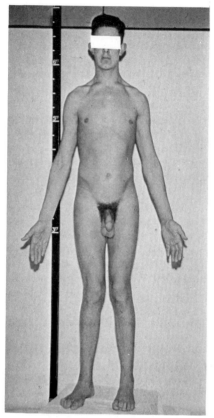

Figure 9.3. *Gigantism.*

of the features and the increase in the size of the hands and feet that are so typical of acromegaly (Figure 9.4). Ligaments and synovial membranes are affected and acroparaesthesiae or a carpal tunnel syndrome may occur. Cartilage is affected and the overgrowth of nasal and aural cartilage causes enlargement of the nose and ears. There is overgrowth of the maxillary bone and lengthening of the face, while overgrowth of the ramus of the mandible gives rise to prognathos.

Body Weight

Various tables relating weight to height and age have been published. There is a wide variation in normal children and even in the adult it is not easy to relate weight to height as there is considerable variation in bone structure and lean body mass. The mesomorph is often mistakenly diagnosed as obese because of a large skeletal and muscle mass. Body fat can be estimated clinically by measuring the skin fold thickness over the scapular or triceps areas with callipers.

Loss of weight

Loss of weight is commonly due to deficient food intake or intestinal malabsorption and is infrequently the result of endocrine disease. When loss of weight is not associated with any impairment of appetite a metabolic disorder is probable and thyrotoxicosis is the most common cause. Diabetes mellitus is another disease in which loss of weight may occur without any impairment of appetite. Adrenal insufficiency is constantly associated with loss of weight and is usually accompanied by anorexia. Anorexia nervosa results in extreme loss of weight and also amenorrhoea; it is a psychiatric disease and not primarily an endocrine problem.

Gain in weight

Obesity is usually the result of over-eating and lack of physical exercise, but genetic factors are important and emotional disturbances often lead to altered feeding habits. Excess fat is stored in the subcutaneous tissues, especially those of the breasts, buttocks and thighs. Satiety gives comfort to the depressed patient.

Endocrine diseases are uncommon causes of obesity and indeed they are sometimes the result, for diabetes mellitus is often a consequence of obesity. Nevertheless, certain endocrine disorders do cause obesity. Hypothyroidism reduces the rate of body metabolism and is associated with a gain in weight. Corticosteroids induce a characteristic distribution of obesity with a deposition of fat over the trunk and proximal parts of the limbs and this is a frequent feature of Cushing's syndrome. If plethora and hypertension are associated with obesity the clinical suspicion of Cushing's syndrome should be aroused. Hyperinsulinism may increase appetite and lead to a gain in weight and this may be a

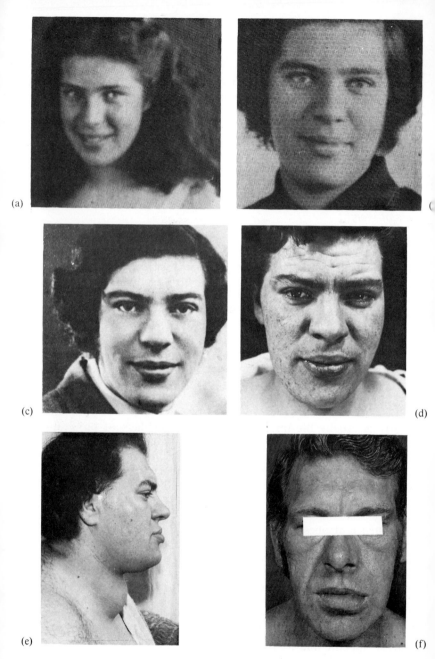

Figure 9.4.

feature of insulin-secreting tumours of the islets of Langerhans. Excessive weight is frequently gained in pregnancy and may not be subsequently lost. Babies of diabetic mothers are overweight. Hypogonadism in the male after puberty is associated with obesity. The polycystic ovary syndrome (Stein—Leventhal syndrome) should be suspected when a gain in weight is associated with oligomenorrhoea and hirsutism. Patients with obesity are often assumed to have some disturbance of endocrine function but in the majority of obese patients there is no detectable endocrine disease. Nonetheless it is wise to keep in mind the possibilities of hypothyroidism, Cushing's syndrome and insulinoma.

Hair

There are three types of hair: (1) lanugo hair; (2) vellus hair; (3) terminal hair. *Lanugo hair* is fine silky hair which covers the fetus and is normally shed in utero. It is seen over the backs of adults who have anorexia nervosa. *Vellus hair* is also fine, rarely exceeding three cm in length and covers the body surface with the exception of the scalp, eyelashes and eyebrows. *Terminal hair* is coarser and is derived from vellus hair by a thickening of the vellus shaft. It is produced on the scalp in childhood, appearing in the pubic area and axilla at puberty and later over the limbs and, in the male, over the chest and shoulders. The growth of hair is cyclical and no new hair follicles appear after birth. Anagen is the term given to the active growth phase of the cycle and this is followed by a period of rest. Anagen may be shortened by any systemic disease, protein deficiency and shock, while the cycle can be interfered with by drugs, especially cytotoxic agents and sometimes anticoagulants. Disturbances of the growth cycle produce the sparse, coarse hair characteristic of hypothyroidism (see page 56).

Loss of hair

Baldness in the male is common and is due to a combination of heredity, ageing and androgenic stimulation which is particularly important. Eunuchs do not lose their scalp hair and temporal

Figure 9.4. *Acromegaly.* a to e, *The stages of development in a woman.* f, *Acromegaly in a man.*

recession of scalp hair in women with virilisation is common. However, the urinary oxosteroid excretion is not unduly high in bald men. Loss of scalp hair is almost a constant finding in the disease of dystrophia myotonica. *Alopecia areata* is the most common local disease of scalp hair in which the hair becomes brittle and breaks off near the scalp. Lice and fungus infections also lead to loss of scalp hair. Scantiness of the outer third of the eyebrow is often quoted as evidence of hypothyroidism but it occurs too frequently in normal individuals to be of any diagnostic relevance.

The absence of facial hair in the male is a feature of hypogonadism whereas in hypopituitarism the loss of body hair is more complete because adrenal androgen production is also lost. Loss of axillary hair in the female occurs in adrenal insufficiency but not in the male because of the additional source of androgen from the testis.

Hirsutism

Hirsutism means an increased growth of body and facial hair and is one of the commonest problems in endocrinology. Much clinically useful information can be obtained from the examination of the distribution of body hair. Whilst hirsutism may be a feature of virilisation it does not necessarily mean increased androgen production particularly when it is confined to the face. When hirsutism is accompanied by other features of virilisation, such as amenorrhoea, atrophy of the breasts, acne, deepening of the voice, temporal scalp recession, clitoral hypertrophy and the appearance of a masculine body contour, it is always an indication of endocrine disease and of a need for investigation (Figure 9.5). In disorders of virilisation the distribution of hair changes towards that of the male. Hirsutism of beard and moustache areas (Figure 9.6) first appears and this is followed by an extension of pubic hair up to the umbilicus. Hair may then increase on the limbs and appear on the chest.

There is a wide range of facial and body hair growth in both normal men and women. Mediterranean women have more body hair than Nordic races but the Japanese and Chinese have little body hair, even in the male. Genetic factors are also important but their inheritance is complex and little understood. Increased hairiness in women asserts itself in many normal situations,

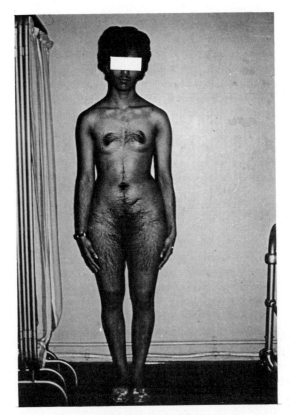

Figure 9.5. *Virilisation.*

especially at puberty, during pregnancy and after the menopause and can be induced by many drugs, particularly phenytoin, diazoxide and corticosteroids. Virilisation may be induced by drugs and especially important are the anabolic hormones, all of which have some androgenic activity and some of the progestogens have androgenic effects.

The endocrine control of hair growth is mediated through the secretion of androgens, the most potent being testosterone. However, the ability to respond to androgens is an intrinsic quality of the hair follicle itself and the ability to metabolise androgens by the skin is variable. Androgens are derived from the adrenal cortex, the testis and, to a lesser extent, from the ovary. Most androgens

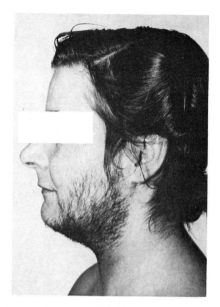

Figure 9.6. *Facial hirsutism.*

are excreted in the urine as 17-oxosteroids. In males the production of testosterone contributes as little as three mg per day to the urinary excretion of 17-oxosteroids. Thus it is possible for a virilising tumour of the ovary, such as arrhenoblastoma, to increase testosterone production from the female level of one mg per day to the male rate of seven mg per day and cause severe virilisation and yet for the urinary oxosteroid level to increase by only three mg per day.

When a woman develops hirsutism of endocrine origin the two major sources of increased androgen production are the adrenal and the ovary. If the adrenal gland is the source of androgens the oxosteroid excretion is usually high, but when the ovary is the source of androgen it is likely to be testosterone and the oxosteroid excretion may be little raised. The ovarian disorders which may produce hirsutism are the polycystic ovary syndrome or ovarian tumours, and the commonest adrenal disorders are adrenal tumours, Cushing's syndrome and congenital adrenal hyperplasia. The polycystic ovary is often palpable on vaginal examination and some ovarian tumours are often large enough to be felt. Adrenal tumours are rarely palpable.

Appetite

The appetite may be increased, decreased or perverted.

Increase in appetite

Increased appetite is a feature of several endocrine diseases. In thyrotoxicosis the increase in appetite is commonly associated with a loss of weight due to the enhanced rate of metabolism. This association of loss of weight and increased appetite is useful clinical information for it is limited to few disorders, thyrotoxicosis being the most familiar, but it may also occur in diabetes mellitus. Pancreatic steatorrhoea is another disorder with this association whilst in most other disorders of intestinal malabsorption the appetite is reduced. Increased appetite is a feature of Cushing's syndrome due to the excess production of cortisol but in this endocrine disorder there is a gain in weight. Patients with insulinoma frequently discover that the other symptoms of hypoglycaemia such as paraesthesiae, sweating and mental confusion can be rapidly corrected by the intake of sugar or sweets so that they learn to carry around on their person a supply of carbohydrate to combat symptoms of hypoglycaemia as they arise. This may lead to weight gain.

In rare hypothalamic disorders patients may lose their sense of fullness after food, resulting in excessive intake and consequent weight gain.

Diminution in appetite

Anorexia is usually a feature of gastrointestinal disease or malignant disease and only rarely is it seen as a manifestation of endocrine disorders. Indeed, in hypothyroidism when decreased physical and mental activity might be expected to lead to loss of appetite this does not usually occur and as a result patients with hypothyroidism gain weight. Eating is so often a habit rather than a physiological response to calorie requirement that disorders reducing energy requirements are frequently associated with no reduction in intake. One endocrine disorder which usually presents with anorexia and loss of weight is adrenocortical insufficiency or Addison's disease. Anorexia nervosa is a psychiatric disorder with an associated endocrine dysfunction in which there is a revulsion against food and the patient loses weight.

Perverted appetite

Perverted appetite is a manifestation of psychiatric rather than endocrine disease.

Gastrointestinal Symptoms

There are two endocrine diseases which present more commonly to the gastroenterologist than the endocrinologist because the predominant symptoms are gastrointestinal. The first is adrenocortical insufficiency in which loss of weight is constant and is associated with anorexia, nausea and diarrhoea. The second is hyperparathyroidism where anorexia, nausea, vomiting and constipation all result from hypercalcaemia. Diarrhoea is often a feature of hyperthyroidism and constipation is the rule in myxoedema and hyperparathyroidism.

Sweating

Sweating is often a useful diagnostic symptom in endocrine disease. There are two types of sweat glands. *Eccrine glands* are found over the entire skin, are supplied by cholinergic sympathetic nerve fibres and secrete a clear watery fluid. *Apocrine glands* occur in the axilla and anogenital region, are larger than eccrine glands and are associated with hair follicles into which they open. They are not innervated and secrete a turbid fluid which on bacterial decomposition gives rise to the typical body odour.

There are two varieties of sweating. The eccrine glands are responsible for emotional sweating; sweating of the hands and feet and axillary sweating are usually due to anxiety and the limbs are cold. It has been postulated that the teleological basis was to permit a firmer grip with well-lubricated palms under conditions of stress, and is surely an advance on the South American monkey that urinates on its hands and feet when frightened. Diffuse sweating over the whole body counters the rise in body temperature which may occur in a hot climate, after exercise or in conditions such as thyrotoxicosis when the metabolic rate is increased. In these situations the limbs are warm.

The differentiation between anxiety states and hyperthyroidism is often difficult and the difference in the temperature of the extremities is one of the most useful physical signs; cold in anxiety states and warm in hyperthyroidism. Paroxysmal profuse sweating may be a feature of phaeochromocytoma due to the pharmacological effects of enhanced catecholamine production and here the sweating is usually episodic and associated with pallor. Episodes of sweating are a feature of menopausal flushing and hypoglycaemia. Enhanced greasy sweating of apocrine glands is a symptom of activity in acromegaly and during the active phase of the disease patients complain of excess sweating with the greasy sweat causing some to have an unpleasant odour.

Excessive or inappropriate sweating of eccrine glands is a distressing complaint due to enhanced sensitivity of the sweat glands of palms, soles and axillae to autonomic stimulation: primary hyperhidrosis. The symptoms may be as bad in winter as in summer, are often precipitated by emotional or mental stress and sweat may literally drip off the hands, feet and from the axillae.

Pigmentation

The major pigments that colour the normal skin are haemoglobin, melanin and bilirubin. In disease states these and other pigments may be responsible for abnormal pigmentation of the skin. For example, bile pigments give the yellow discoloration of jaundice, carotene the orange discoloration of *myxoedema*, chromogens the sallow tint of *renal failure* and melanin the darkening of the skin in *Addison's disease.* Increased pigmentation due to melanin is also seen in *Cushing's syndrome, pregnancy, acromegaly* and malnutrition. In *haemochromatosis* and haemosiderosis the skin becomes a slatey brown colour due to a combination of increased melanin and deposits of iron. Prolonged ingestion of *heavy metals* such as silver, arsenic and mercury will colour the skin, and *drugs* such as mepacrine may cause marked pigmentation.

Pigmentation of the skin is a feature of primary *adrenal insufficiency.* The pigment is melanin and its enhanced production is due to raised levels of ACTH. Pigmentation of the skin similar to that found in *Addison's disease* is a feature of *Cushing's syndrome* due to bilateral adrenal hyperplasia. If pigmentation is marked it is suggestive of a *pituitary tumour* secreting ACTH or of an oat-cell carcinoma of lung producing an ACTH-like polypeptide. Minor degrees of pigmentation occur in classical Cushing's syndrome when it is due to excess ACTH production. Conversely in hypopituitarism the lack of ACTH leads to a decrease in skin melanin, depigmentation of the areolae of the breasts and a loss of the capacity to tan after exposure to the sun.

Vitiligo is a localised depigmentation of the skin due to loss of the functional activity of melanocytes. It is most common in dark-skinned individuals and may cause great cosmetic embarrassment. The patches of depigmentation may coalesce to form large areas of depigmentation. If the melanocytes of the hair follicles are affected patches of white hair will appear. The cause is unknown but there is a definite association with certain endocrine disorders — especially hyperthyroidism and Addison's disease.

Skin

Normal skin has a fine texture and a slightly moist surface. In hypothyroidism (Figure 9.7) it becomes coarse, pale and dry and there is often a distinct yellow tint due to carotinaemia. There may be associated peripheral cyanosis due to sluggish peripheral circulation. The subcutaneous tissue becomes thickened giving the doughy appearance of non-pitting oedema from which the name myxoedema was derived and it is particularly obvious around the eyes. This may sometimes give the appearance of a nephrotic syndrome and the patient with myxoedema in Figure 9.7c was referred to hospital as a case of nephrotic oedema.

Soft tissue overgrowth is the characteristic feature of acromegaly and this is particularly striking in the face, hands and feet giving rise to the coarse features. The skin appears leathery and there is exaggeration of the skin pores and markings. The increase in subcutaneous tissue can be assessed objectively by measuring the thickness of the heel pad by x-ray and this is a useful diagnostic investigation for acromegaly. There is excessive sweating and the skin becomes oily due to increased sebaceous gland activity.

The skin becomes finer and more like that of the female in male hypogonadism and also in hypopituitarism where excessive wrinkling of the skin may be a feature. In hypoparathyroidism the skin is dry and scaly and the nails are often brittle and ridged.

Flushing of the skin of the face and neck is the most classical feature of the carcinoid syndrome. Four types of rash have been described: (1) a brief diffuse erythematous flush affecting face, neck and anterior chest; (2) a violaceous flush associated with conjunctival suffusion, lacrimation and telangiectasia; (3) flushes

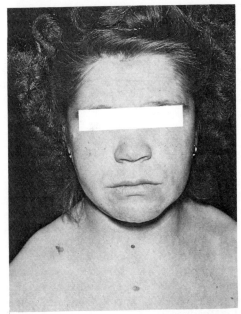

Figure 9.7a. *Primary myxoedema. Courtesy of Dr M. Wilkinson, Dundee.*

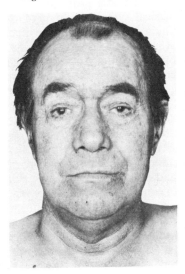

Figure 9.7b. *Primary myxoedema.*

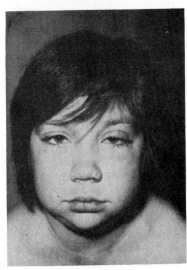

Figure 9.7c. *Child of 16 with myxoedema.*

lasting two to three days, associated with lacrimation, salivary gland swelling, facial oedema and hypotension, and usually found with bronchial tumours; (4) bright red patchy flushing in patients with gastric carcinoid tumours who produce histamine. The vasomotor effect is due to the escape from the tumour into the circulation of 5-hydroxytryptamine, bradykinin, histamine and other vasoactive peptides which dilate the small blood vessels of the face.

Menstruation

The menstrual history must include the age of onset of menstruation, which is called the menarche, and the details of the menstrual cycle. The regularity of the menses, the length of the period and the amount of blood loss are all relevant. Any history of intermenstrual bleeding should be sought. The discussion of the menstrual cycle should lead to enquiry about pain during sexual intercourse (dyspareunia), and whether orgasm is experienced. These subjects are unlikely to be discussed by the patient unless a direct enquiry is made and as they may be caused by, or result in, psychological difficulties it is important that patients are given the opportunity to discuss them. Patients with these problems often present to the doctor with other physical symptoms of psychosomatic disease and it is only by taking a full medical history that these problems are likely to be discovered and resolved.

Primary amenorrhoea is a pathological failure to commence menstruation. There is enormous variation in the age of onset of menstruation and in Britain the mean age is 13 years with a range of 10 to 16 years. Menstruation occurs approximately every four weeks and lasts from three to seven days. Precocious menarche may be diagnosed if there is vaginal bleeding before the age of 10 years. The onset of the menarche is preceded by the earlier manifestations of puberty which include the appearance of breast tissue and by the growth of vulval and pubic hair. Breast growth usually begins between the ages of nine and 13 years and is the first sign of secondary sex development to appear. The time from the beginning of breast development to the menarche may be anything from six months to five years but the average is 2.3 years. As puberty approaches there is a spurt in growth due to ovarian production of oestrogens and the adrenal production of androgens.

The menstrual cycle begins when bleeding commences and ends

on the day before bleeding. The cycle is commonly recorded as a fraction, the numerator being the number of days menstruation lasts and the denominator the length of the cycle. A cycle of 4/28 indicates that a woman with a cycle of 28 days menstruates for 4 days. As some women cannot be absolutely precise about dates it may be helpful to give an indication of the range of the bleeding, e.g. $4\pm1/28\pm3$. The menstrual loss is composed of endometrial cells from the breakdown of endometrium following the fall in oestrogen and progesterone production, together with secretions and blood. The amount of blood lost with each normal period varies from 20 to 80 ml and a woman normally uses three to four pads daily. Oestrogens are produced by the graafian follicle, oestrogens and progesterone by the corpus luteum and these hormones prepare the endometrium for implantation should an ovum become fertilised during that cycle. In the absence of fertilisation the corpus luteum degenerates, the plasma levels of oestrogen and progesterone fall and this results in the breakdown of the endometrium. Infrequent periods are described as oligomenorrhoea and when menstruation is too frequent it is called polymenorrhoea. Pain associated with menstruation is called dysmenorrhoea.

Disorders of menstruation may be indicative of gynaecological or endocrine disease and are best considered under the following symptoms:
1. Amenorrhoea.
2. Menorrhagia.
3. Bleeding unrelated to menstruation, which may be prepubertal, intermenstrual or postmenopausal.
4. Dysmenorrhoea.

Amenorrhoea

The most important point to ascertain in the patient with amenorrhoea is whether this is primary or secondary as the aetiology is likely to differ. Primary amenorrhoea is diagnosed if the patient has not started menstruating by the age of 17. Secondary amenorrhoea is present if vaginal bleeding ceases before the age of 40 years, there having been an intervening period of normal menstruation. It is essential to ascertain whether the amenorrhoea is apparent or real. Apparent amenorrhoea may be due to the fact that a normal menstrual flow is unable to escape because there is obstruction in a part of the genital canal such as an imperforate hymen or congenital defects of absence of vagina or uterus. This should be considered seriously when primary amenorrhoea persists several years after development of the breasts and pubic hair. It is likely to be associated with pelvic pain, and the diagnosis can usually be made by physical examination which must be directed towards finding out whether the essential organs, namely the uterus and ovaries, are present and normal.

Primary amenorrhoea. True primary amenorrhoea may be due to ovarian failure or to deficient production of the trophic hormones by the hypothalamus or pituitary. If the cause is ovarian there is no production of oestrogen and progesterone so there will be no breast development or pubic hair. The patient may be tall due to failure of epiphyseal closure. More commonly, however, primary ovarian failure is genetic in origin due to chromosome anomalies affecting the X chromosome; these patients are commonly short in stature and may have the other skeletal stigmata such as webbing of the neck, cubitus valgus, and widely spaced nipples as in Turner's syndrome (Figure 9.8).

Primary amenorrhoea also follows a failure of production of gonadotrophins as a result of pituitary or hypothalamic disease. Pituitary tumours including chromophobe adenomas and cranio-pharyngiomas may be responsible, or vascular causes such as a haemorrhage, or trauma to the base of the skull. In many of these patients no obvious cause can be found and the defect is due to a congenital failure of the hypothalamus to secrete the releasing hormone that controls pituitary gonadotrophin production.

Other causes of primary amenorrhoea include disorders that produce excessive androgens for these suppress pituitary gonado-trophin production; but these patients will have evidence of virilisation. Generalised systemic diseases may suppress gonado-trophin production and these include malnutrition, malabsorption, chronic renal failure and obesity.

Secondary amenorrhoea. Secondary amenorrhoea is usually defined as the cessation of menses for six months or longer. If menstruation has once been established there cannot be any serious congenital anomaly of the genital tract and the uterus and ovaries must have been functioning. The commonest cause of secondary amenorrhoea is pregnancy and this must be excluded before further investigation is undertaken. The menopause is the commonest manifestation of primary ovarian failure but it is rare before the

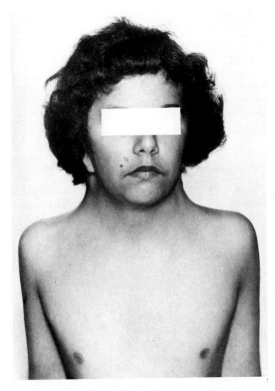

Figure 9.8. *Girl of 16 with Turner's syndrome.*

age of 40. The polycystic ovary syndrome causes secondary amenorrhoea which is usually associated with obesity, hirsutism and infertility. Secondary amenorrhoea is frequently the result of disturbances of hypothalamic—pituitary function. Whilst this disturbance may be the result of pituitary tumours or infarction it is more usually associated with chronic debilitating diseases, or protein malnutrition, or is functional in origin. Stress and psychiatric problems are common causes of secondary amenorrhoea. Virilising syndromes are associated with amenorrhoea as the raised level of androgen suppresses pituitary gonadotrophin production. Secondary amenorrhoea may occur in women who have been taking oral contraceptives, especially if there were menstrual irregularities before going on the pill. Amenorrhoea also occurs with excessive pituitary production of prolactin which may or may not be associated with galactorrhoea. Although pituitary production of gonadotrophins is not usually impaired in this situation the raised levels of prolactin antagonise the effects of gonadotrophins on the ovary.

Oligomenorrhoea refers to the situation where the menstrual cycle is lengthened to six or eight weeks. Ovulation may occur. It may be caused by an abortion or pregnancy and is due to deficient gonadotrophin production by the pituitary.

Menorrhagia

Menorrhagia is defined as excessive menstrual bleeding. It is frequently the result of uterine disorders such as fibroids, uterine malignancy or a bleeding diathesis that interferes with endometrial haemostasis. It may also be due to a failure to ovulate; if there is no ovulation no progesterone is produced and the endometrium shows the characteristic hyperplasia of prolonged oestrogen stimulation and this gives rise to excessive and prolonged bleeding. Prolonged oestrogen therapy may similarly lead to marked endometrial hyperplasia. Other sources of excess oestrogen may be from an ovarian tumour, or as a manifestation of an incomplete abortion. Menorrhagia is a common feature of hypothyroidism. *Dysfunctional uterine haemorrhage* is a term used to describe menorrhagia when it is not associated with any pelvic or haematological abnormality.

Bleeding unrelated to menstruation

Bleeding unrelated to the menses is usually of gynaecological rather than endocrine origin and it is important to exclude carcinomas of the cervix and genital tract. Ovulation bleeding may occur two weeks before menstruation; this is usually transient and scanty and can always be suppressed with drugs that suppress ovulation, such as the contraceptive pill. Postmenopausal bleeding may be the result of atrophic vaginitis or carcinoma of the uterus or vagina and a gynaecological examination is mandatory. Oestrogens given for menopausal symptoms may cause postmenopausal bleeding and oestrogen-producing tumours of the ovary are occasionally responsible.

Menstruation before the age of 10 is not usually due to gynaecological disorders. It is most frequently the result of precocious puberty when the hypothalamus stimulates the pituitary to produce adult levels of gonadotrophin prematurely. In children with precocious puberty it is important to exclude pituitary and pineal tumours.

Dysmenorrhoea

Painful menstrual periods are associated with ovulatory cycles but the aetiology is obscure. Dysmenorrhoea may be secondary to pelvic inflammatory disease, endometriosis, to fibroids or to retroversion of the uterus. In the majority of patients there is no obvious cause and the condition can be relieved by suppressing ovulation with the contraceptive pill.

Impotence

This is a persistent inability to attain or sustain erection of the penis for sufficient time to obtain satisfactory coitus. Temporary impotence is extremely common. The majority of cases of impotence are functional in origin and secondary to emotional problems. It often occurs in anxiety and is a not infrequent occurrence in young men during such stresses as examinations. Honeymoon impotence is a transient situation that occurs in sensitive individuals but a more insidious onset may occur later in life with the irreconcilable problems of failing attraction of the wife and a guilt-ridden desire for extramarital experience.

The parasympathetic nerves, S2,3,4, through the nervi erigentes, produce erection and ejaculation and the sympathetic nerves through L2 and 3 are responsible for emission of semen into the urethra. These nerve pathways are also involved in micturition and if impotence is associated with urinary symptoms, it is very likely to be the result of *autonomic neuropathy*, especially secondary to diabetes mellitus or chronic alcoholism. Tabes dorsalis may also be responsible. Perineal prostatectomy may be followed by impotence if there has been damage to the prostatic nerve plexus. Disorders of the lateral spinothalamic tract may also cause impotence as they carry the afferent fibres from the nervi erigentes to the thalamus and this is why impotence may be a feature of disseminated sclerosis, Friedreich's ataxia or spinal injuries. The degeneration of the central processes of the posterior root ganglion cells with interruption of afferent impulses causes impotence in tabes dorsalis. Impotence may also be a feature of hypogonadism whether this is primary or secondary to hypopituitarism and the clinical evidence of hypogonadism such as deficient secondary sex characteristics usually make this cause obvious. Impotence, like amenorrhoea in the female, can be an early symptom of Cushing's syndrome or a pituitary tumour. It may also occur as a result of hyperprolactinaemia, whether this is drug induced or secondary to a microadenoma of the pituitary. Impotence may be due to testicular atrophy secondary to haemochromatosis, dystrophia myotonica or deficient pituitary gonadotrophin production accompanying malnutrition or malabsorption.

PHYSICAL EXAMINATION

Thyroid Gland

The thyroid gland is shaped like a butterfly and consists of two lobes closely related to either side of the trachea and joined by an isthmus which is a thin band of thyroid tissue in front of the trachea at the level of the second ring. It is the largest endocrine gland and weighs about 30 grams. Accessory thyroid tissue is occasionally found at the base of the tongue: a lingual thyroid.

The normal thyroid gland cannot be seen or felt unless the neck is unusually thin, so a palpable gland should be regarded as enlarged. Enlargement of the thyroid gland is called a goitre (Figure 9.9).

The thyroid gland should be examined with the patient in the sitting position and with the neck moderately extended making the thyroid more prominent to both inspection and palpation. The gland should be inspected from in front but palpated from behind the patient. A feature that distinguishes the thyroid from other masses in the neck is its movement on swallowing, because the gland is intimately connected with the larynx. Thus the patient should be asked to swallow when the thyroid gland is being inspected or palpated and to facilitate this he should be asked to drink a glass of water. This sign alone is often sufficient to establish the diagnosis of an enlarged thyroid. Rarely a thyroid swelling may not move on swallowing if it is due to a malignant growth of the gland that has infiltrated other structures but this is usually obvious on physical examination. The clinical features for any mass should then be sought, in particular the size, shape, position, consistency and mobility.

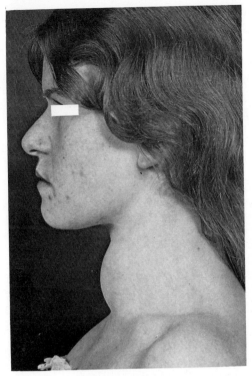

Figure 9.9. *Goitre.*

If the thyroid is enlarged it is important to decide whether there is any retrosternal extension of the goitre and this is probable if it is not possible to feel below the lower border of the gland. The thyroid in the neck may occasionally be of normal size in the presence of retrosternal enlargement. X-ray examination of the thoracic inlet is the most useful way to demonstrate retrosternal extension. Pain or tenderness indicate acute inflammation and acute thyroiditis may occur as a result of a virus infection or rarely bacterial inflammation. The shape of the gland must be assessed. Commonly both lobes are enlarged but asymmetrical enlargement also occurs. The consistency of the gland is important as this may give a lead to the aetiology of the goitre. Hard glands are usually due to chronic thyroiditis or malignancy, soft glands are usually colloid goitres of iodine deficiency. Auscultation of the gland is helpful and the presence of a bruit indicates increased vascularity which suggests that the glandular enlargement is that of a toxic goitre producing hyperthyroidism. The blood flow through the normal thyroid is about 150 ml per minute but in a toxic goitre may exceed one litre per minute which gives rise to an audible and even palpable bruit. This increased blood flow has important functional consequences for the increased cardiac output necessary to maintain the blood flow may precipitate heart failure in the elderly or in patients with underlying heart disease.

The examination of a goitre is not complete until the neck has been examined for enlarged lymph nodes; the presence of lymphadenopathy will suggest that carcinoma of the thyroid is the likely aetiology of the goitre.

It is important to know the common causes of thyroid enlargement so that examination of the gland can be directed towards an attempt to establish the likely aetiology. A goitre may be: (1) simple colloid goitre; (2) lymphadenoid goitre; (3) toxic goitre; (4) subacute thyroiditis; (5) carcinoma; (6) Riedel's goitre.

The *simple colloid goitre* is a result of iodine deficiency and is in effect a compensatory hypertrophy of the gland to cope with iodine deficiency or a defect in hormone synthesis. This type of goitre commonly appears in childhood particularly around puberty when the increased demands of thyroid hormone are made, and during pregnancy. The thyroid swelling is soft, diffuse and symmetrical. Over a period of years waxing and waning of gland activity with the associated hyperplasia and involution may lead to a nodular consistency.

The *lymphadenoid goitre* of chronic or autoimmune thyroiditis (Hashimoto's disease) is a uniform or hard goitre due to the chronic inflammatory cell infiltration and subsequent fibrosis. It is often associated with hypothyroidism.

The consistency of a *toxic goitre* in the younger age group is usually soft and the gland is vascular so that a bruit may be audible. In older patients the toxic gland may be nodular. The characteristics of a toxic goitre are, however, the associated symptoms and signs of hyperthyroidism.

Subacute thyroiditis is usually obvious because of the tenderness of the gland and the characteristic distribution of the associated pain.

Undifferentiated *carcinoma of the thyroid* is usually distinguishable from chronic thyroiditis by its asymmetry but the differentiated carcinomas of the thyroid appear as single nodules in the thyroid gland and cannot be distinguished clinically from small areas of haemorrhage or focal areas of thyroiditis or hyperplasia. Thus if a thyroid gland contains a single palpable nodule this must be regarded as malignant until proved otherwise, and the only certain way to establish the diagnosis is by biopsy. Any single nodule in the thyroid should be investigated by a radioactive scan of the gland. If the nodule takes up the radioactive iodine it is unlikely to be malignant. If the nodule is cold, that is, it does not take up the radioactive tracer, malignancy is a real possibility and the nodule should be explored and removed.

Riedel's goitre or woody thyroiditis is remarkable because of its hardness and even more remarkable because of its rarity.

The finding of an enlarged thyroid prompts an immediate clinical assessment of the thyroid function. The important symptoms of thyrotoxicosis have already been discussed and are summarised in Table 9.2. The most useful physical signs of hyperthyroidism are as follows.

Table 9.2. *Main symptoms of thyrotoxicosis.*

Weight loss
Increased appetite
Diarrhoea
Tiredness
Palpitations
Exertional dyspnoea
Nervousness
Excessive sweating
Heat intolerance
Muscle weakness
Amenorrhoea

Persistent tachycardia. The normal pulse frequency is 70 to 80 per minute. It is increased in conditions of cardiac and respiratory failure but other signs of these disorders will usually make the correct diagnosis apparent. The pulse frequency is also increased in anxiety states and it is this condition that is most likely to give rise to confusion in diagnosing hyperthyroidism. It may be possible to relax and reassure the anxious patient so that after five or ten minutes the pulse frequency falls. If the patient is in hospital a sleeping pulse rate is a useful physical sign to differentiate the anxiety state from hyperthyroidism as the tachycardia of hyper-thyroidism continues throughout sleep and a sleeping pulse rate of more than 80 per minute makes the diagnosis of hyperthyroidism highly probable. It must, however, be remembered that many thyrotoxic patients will have sleeping pulse rates of less than 80 per minute.

Excess thyroxine causes vasodilatation, and an increased cardiac output. This results in the full volume collapsing pulse that is characteristic of thyrotoxicosis.

Hot moist extremities. As a result of vasodilatation the extremities in hyperthyroidism are warm and moist. This contrasts with cold moist extremities of the patient with an anxiety state.

Hyperkinesia and tremor. One of the effects of the increased metabolic activity of the nervous system is the restless hyperactive state called hyperkinesia. This is commonly associated with a fine tremor of the extended hands.

Thyroid bruit. In many patients with a toxic goitre auscultation over the thyroid will reveal a vascular bruit due to the increased vascularity of the gland. Whilst many thyrotoxic patients do not have a bruit over the gland, its presence is almost pathognomonic of a toxic goitre.

Examination of the eyes in thyrotoxicosis

The two major eye manifestations of thyroid disease are exophthalmos and lid retraction. *Lid retraction* is due to the increased adrenergic stimulation that is characteristic of hyperthyroidism. It is therefore related to the degree of hyperthyroidism and improves when the thyrotoxicosis is controlled. *Exophthalmos* or proptosis refers to a forward displacement of the eyeball due to the increased content of retro-orbital tissue (Figure 9.10). Although this is one of the immunological features of Graves' disease it is in no way related to the degree of hyperthyroidism and is not directly affected by the control of the thyrotoxicosis. It must be distinguished from retraction of the eyelids which causes an illusion of exophthalmos. Normally the upper eyelid lies between the border of the iris and the limbus of the cornea. When there is lid retraction the white of the sclera is visible between the border of the iris and the upper eyelid. This is commonly associated with lid lag which is due to the asynchronous movements of the upper lid and eyeball. This sign is elicited by asking the patient to follow the movement of the examiner's finger in a vertical direction first upwards then downwards. The patient's head should be stationary and the examiner's finger should be moved slowly.

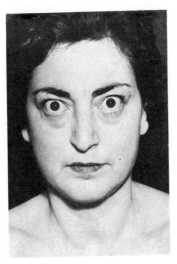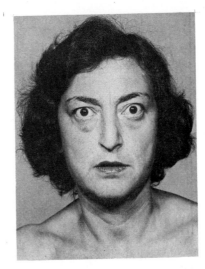

Figure 9.10. *Exophthalmos in a patient with hyperthyroidism; at presentation (left) and eight years later (right), showing some improvement.*

In exophthalmos the white of the sclera is visible above and below the iris. The acute angle between the upper lid and the roof of the orbit is lost and there is frequently periorbital oedema. The proptosis can be assessed by examination of the eye from above or, better still, from the side where the bony lateral margin of the orbit provides a baseline from which the degree of forward protrusion can be gauged. The only way to be sure of the presence of exophthalmos is to measure it. A simple perspex scale that can be rested into the lateral margin of the orbit is all that is required and the distance between the margin and the anterior surface of the cornea is measured. Readings with such a simple exophthalmometer usually show a forward protrusion of more than 18 mm in exophthalmos.

Although exophthalmos may be a feature of any retro-orbital space-occupying lesion, if it is bilateral or if it is associated with lid retraction it is essentially a feature of thyroid disease. It commonly starts shortly after the development of hyperthyroidism but it may arise months or even years after thyrotoxicosis has been treated successfully. Conjunctival oedema or chemosis may also occur due to the impaired venous drainage precipitated by the increased retro-orbital pressure. Exophthalmoplegia is commonly associated, giving rise to diplopia. The extraocular muscles become oedematous and infiltrated with mucopolysaccharide and consequently there is impairment of muscle function. Involvement of the inferior rectus muscle is most common and causes reduction in upward gaze. The eye movements controlled by the inferior oblique are also frequently affected and upward and inward ocular movements are reduced. The severity of the ophthalmoplegia is not directly related to the magnitude of ocular protrusion and it appears to bear an inverse relation to the degree of thyrotoxicosis.

Clinical features of thyroid myopathy

A proximal myopathy is common in hyperthyroidism. Physical examination reveals evidence of muscle weakness in 80 per cent of patients with thyrotoxicosis and electromyographic evidence of myopathy is even more common. The muscle weakness can be demonstrated most simply by an inability to raise both legs off the bed for a period of 15 seconds which is normally easily done. Obvious wasting of the pectoral and pelvis girdle muscles and the muscles of the thighs is often apparent and the muscles particularly affected are the deltoid, supraspinatus and quadriceps (Figure 9.11). The muscular wasting tends to be symmetrical. Winging of the scapulae from weakness of serratus anterior is not infrequent and wasting of the gluteal muscles is apparent in many male patients. Occasionally the muscle weakness and wasting may be severe and may even be the presenting feature of thyrotoxicosis. The cause of the myopathy is uncertain but it always resolves when the hyperthyroidism is controlled. The catabolic effects of thyroid hormones on protein metabolism may be associated with some reduction in muscle bulk and power but it has no effect on the electrical changes during contraction and is therefore not the cause of the myopathy. The rapidity with which myopathy may develop in thyrotoxicosis, the absence of obvious structural change in the muscle fibres and the constant recovery which follows control of the hyperthyroidism support a biochemical abnormality as the cause.

Examination of the muscles in hypothyroidism is less rewarding. The striking neuromuscular sign in myxoedema is the delay in relaxation of the ankle jerk which is a most useful physical sign of hypothyroidism.

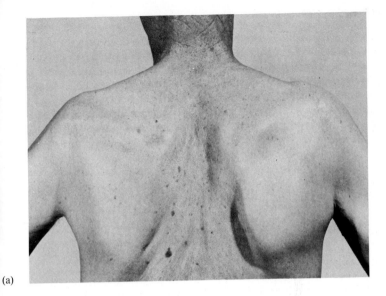

(a)

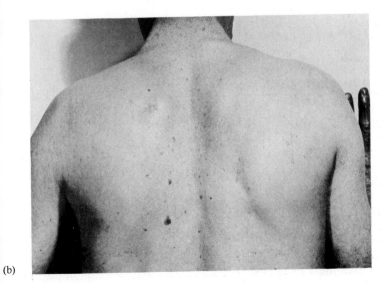

(b)

Figure 9.11. *Thyrotoxic myopathy before* (a) *and after* (b) *treatment of hyper-thyroidism.*

Hypothyroidism

If the patient has a simple colloid goitre or the generalised firm enlargement of chronic thyroiditis the possibility of hypothyroidism must be considered. The most useful physical signs of hypothyroidism are: (1) The skin is dry and coarse. (2) The pulse frequency is slow. (3) The physical and mental activity of the individual is retarded. (4) The voice may be hoarse, and the hair coarse. (5) The ankle jerk shows a delay in the phase of relaxation, which is often readily detectable by the eye.

A summary of investigation of thyroid function is given in Table 9.3.

Table 9.3. *Investigation of thyroid function.*

Screening test
  Serum thyroxine (immunoassay or competitive protein binding)
  T3 uptake
  T3 binding index

Further investigation of possible hyperthyroidism
  Serum T3 (immunoassay)
  TRH test

Further investigation of hypothyroidism
  Serum TSH (immunoassay)

Investigation of chronic thyroiditis
  a. Serum antibodies to thyroglobulin
  b. Serum antibodies to thyroid microsomal antigen

Parathyroid Gland

The parathyroid gland is not amenable to physical examination and even tumours of the parathyroid are rarely palpable. The symptoms and signs of parathyroid disease are dependent on the alteration in the serum concentration of calcium which is controlled by the hormone of the parathyroid glands — parathyroid hormone. It acts on bone, the kidney and the gut, inhibiting bone formation and mobilising calcium and phosphate and increasing their absorption from the small intestine. It promotes the renal excretion of phosphate, potassium and sodium and the retention of calcium, magnesium and hydrogen ions. A lack of parathyroid hormone leads to hypocalcaemia which causes the symptoms and signs of hypoparathyroidism. Increased neuromuscular excitability is the hallmark of hypocalcaemia. On the motor side this is manifest by muscular cramps, twitching, dysarthria and carpopedal spasms. In children laryngeal stridor is common. On the sensory side hypocalcaemia results in paraesthesiae in arms and legs and occasionally in the area around the mouth. In younger individuals epilepsy may be a manifestation of hypocalcaemia and in older persons amnesia or even frank psychosis may occur. Prolonged hypocalcaemia leads to changes in the ectodermal tissues: the skin becomes dry and scaly, the nails become brittle and deformed, body hair becomes sparse, the teeth become hypoplastic and lenticular cataracts may develop.

There are two useful physical signs to detect latent tetany and they carry the names of the physicians who first described them. Chvostek described the muscular twitching that occurs in the facial muscles, especially those of the upper lip, when a sharp tap with the finger is applied over the facial nerve in front of the ear. Although it is a manifestation of the neuromuscular excitability of hypocalcaemia it does occur in some normal people. Trousseau described the production of carpopedal spasm by reducing the circulation in the arm with a sphygmomanometer. The cuff should be inflated to a pressure exceeding the systolic blood pressure and maintained for three minutes. In hypocalcaemic states a carpal spasm is provoked and the hand adopts the position described as 'main d'accoucheur' in which there is flexion of the metacarpophalangeal joints, extension of the interphalangeal joints and opposition of the thumb (Figure 9.12). This physical sign is rarely positive in normal individuals.

These symptoms and signs are due to the neuromuscular excitability of hypocalcaemia. They are not specific for hypoparathyroidism, and are also seen in the hypocalcaemia of osteomalacia or intestinal malabsorption.

Excess production of parathyroid hormone is usually due to an adenoma of one or more of the parathyroid glands. These tumours do not usually exceed the size of two cm, and are commonly much smaller. They are therefore not palpable. The clinical features of hyperparathyroidism may be divided into four groups.

1. *Clinical features due to hypercalcaemia and hypercalcuria* are common to all hypercalcaemic states and consist of generalised muscular weakness and lassitude, anorexia, nausea, vomiting and constipation. Mental changes such as depression, confusion and even delusions may appear. Polydipsia and polyuria occur, in part

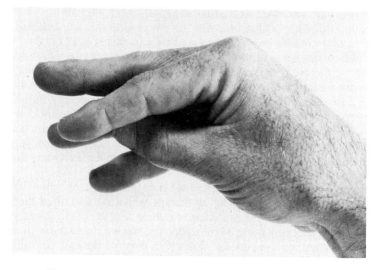

Figure 9.12. *Hand of a patient with positive Trousseau's sign.*

due to the osmotic diuretic effect of the hypercalcuria but more importantly to resistance to the effects of antidiuretic hormone on the distal renal tubule that develops in states of hypercalcaemia. The symptoms of hypercalcaemia are dependent on the level of the serum calcium and the acuteness of onset of the hypercalcaemic state. Lesser degrees of hypercalcaemia are asymptomatic. Moderate degrees of hypercalcaemia present as described above. In cases where there is a rapid onset of severe hypercalcaemia (serum calcium 4.0 mmol/l or 16 mg/100 ml) abdominal pain may be severe, and the patient usually develops severe muscular hypotonia and vomiting and may pass into a coma.

2. *Clinical symptoms of visceral calcification* secondary to the hypercalcaemia. Calcification is especially common in the kidney and this gives rise to renal stones which frequently present with haematuria and renal colic. The majority of patients with renal stones, however, have idiopathic hypercalcuria without hypercalcaemia but some five per cent of patients who present with renal stones do have primary hyperparathyroidism. Looked at from another angle, renal stone is the mode of presentation for 60 per cent of patients with hyperparathyroidism.

The other organ particularly susceptible to visceral calcification is the eye, so that conjunctival and eyelid deposits occur and more commonly deposits affect the cornea causing a band keratitis. The corneal calcification tends to occur near the corneal scleral junction and is present in 25 per cent of patients with hyperparathyroidism (Figure 9.13).

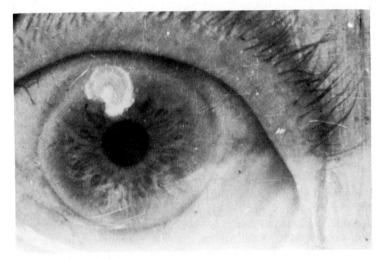

Figure 9.13. *Corneal calcification in primary hyperparathyroidism and hypercalcaemia. Courtesy of Dr C. Paterson, Dundee.*

3. *Effects of parathyroid hormone on bone.* This leads to a generalised resorption of bone, which is sometimes replaced by a highly cellular fibrous tissue giving rise to osteitis fibrosa which is a pathological rather than a clinical entity. The bones are soft and break easily so that bone pain and pathological fractures occur. The skeletal pains may be vague and ascribed to rheumatism. When they are more severe they are frequently diagnosed as arthritis or neuritis.

4. *Features due to diseases commonly associated with hyperparathyroidism.* The two most important of these are peptic ulcer and pancreatitis. Twenty-five per cent of patients with hyperparathyroidism have duodenal ulcers. Conversely 1.3 per cent of patients with duodenal ulcer have hyperparathyroidism. This is much higher than would be expected by chance as a recent survey of all ambulatory patients attending a hospital outpatient clinic

revealed that one in every 1000 patients had hyperparathyroidism. There is also an increased incidence of acute pancreatitis in patients with hyperparathyroidism and occasionally this is the mode of presentation.

A summary of the investigation of parathyroid function is given in Table 9.4.

Table 9.4. *Investigation of parathyroid function.*

Serum calcium
Serum inorganic phosphate
Urinary calcium
Serum parathyroid hormone (immunoassay)
Radiological investigation of skeleton for:
  subperiosteal erosions
  osteitis fibrosa

Adrenal Cortex

The adrenal gland itself is not amenable to physical examination and even tumours of the gland are rarely large enough to be palpable. The gland secretes three hormones: (1) cortisol; (2) aldosterone; and (3) androgens, the most important of which is androstenedione. Of these three hormones cortisol is essential to life. Clinical symptoms and physical signs are of great importance to the diagnosis of adrenal disorders, although definitive diagnosis depends ultimately on the demonstration by chemical means of excessive or inadequate secretion of one or more of the adrenal hormones.

Hypoadrenalism (Addison's disease)

A deficiency of cortisol is associated with anorexia, nausea and often diarrhoea. Loss of weight is constant. Symptoms may also arise as a result of hypoglycaemia which is a consequence of deficient gluconeogenesis. The symptoms of hypoglycaemia may be subdivided into those due to the lack of cerebral glucose such as mental confusion, dysarthria and ataxia, and those due to the increased secretion of catecholamines, the homeostatic response to promote the mobilisation of liver glycogen, when sweating, palpitations and often nausea occur. Cortisol is necessary to excrete water so that nocturia is a common symptom of adrenal insufficiency and represents the delayed excretion of the day's water intake. When the blood levels of cortisol fall the hypothalamus stimulates the pituitary production of ACTH. ACTH is similar in structure to MSH and has some MSH-like action so that in primary adrenal insufficiency the patient becomes pigmented, especially the flexor surfaces and palmar creases. In diseases that destroy the adrenal gland aldosterone production will be impaired and this gives rise to sodium depletion and hypotension. The symptoms that result from hypotension are lightheadedness and syncope, especially when standing erect. Deficiencies of adrenal androgens will not give rise to symptoms in the male because of the alternative source of androgens from the testis but in the female the adrenal androgens are the important source of anabolic steroid and muscular weakness, lack of vigour and loss of axillary hair will result from this deficiency. The main symptoms of primary adrenal insufficiency are summarised in Table 9.5.

Table 9.5. *Symptoms of primary adrenal insufficiency.*

Tiredness
Loss of weight
Gastrointestinal symptoms:
  anorexia
  nausea
  diarrhoea
Hypotension
Hypoglycaemia
Pigmentation of skin and buccal mucosa
Nocturia
Mental changes

Hyperadrenalism (Cushing's syndrome)

In some diseases adrenal hormones are produced in excess giving rise to characteristic clinical pictures depending on which hormone is in excess. When cortisol production is increased (or when patients are given large doses of cortisol as part of their treatment) a classical clinical syndrome develops which bears the name of the man who originally described it — Cushing's syndrome. The individual gains weight and the obesity often has a characteristic distribution over the face (Figure 9.14a, b) shoulders and neck, and distal parts of the limbs are spared. Indeed, because of catabolic action of cortisone there is marked wasting of muscle and the limbs may show a strikingly wasted appearance in contrast to the large amount of fat laid down proximally. The catabolic effect of excess cortisol induces a weakening of the vascular supporting tissue and a thinning of the skin. This gives rise to the purple striae which are characteristic of Cushing's syndrome and which result from the stretching of the skin due to the increase in adipose tissue and extravasation of blood from the weakened capillary supporting matrix. The striae appear over the shoulders, thighs and abdomen (Figure 9.15). Excess cortisol produces hypertension because of sodium retention while osteoporosis results from excessive calcium loss. The increased weight adds a great strain to the softened vertebral column and back pain and even pathological fractures occur. Cortisol also increases cerebral excitability and may even lead to frank psychosis. The main diagnostic features of Cushing's syndrome are summarised in Table 9.6.

Table 9.6. *Diagnostic features of Cushing's syndrome.*

Obesity
Hypertension
Purple striae
Easy bruising
Symptoms of osteoporosis
Symptoms of diabetes mellitus
Psychosis

The increased production of adrenal androgens leads to features of virilisation in the female (page 538). The excess androgen may be the result of bilateral hyperplasia due to excess ACTH production or secondary to an autonomous adenoma secreting androgens.

Aldosteronism

The increased production of aldosterone will lead to sodium retention and potassium loss. Aldosterone acts on the distal renal tubule at the cation exchange site where sodium is reabsorbed in exchange for potassium. Sodium retention produces hypertension but patients with primary aldosteronism usually present with the symptoms of potassium loss which are muscular weakness or even paralysis. Hypokalaemia also reduces the sensitivity of the renal tubule to antidiuretic hormone and many of the patients have polyuria. Oedema is not a feature of primary aldosteronism because after some 300 to 400 mmol of excess sodium has been retained, which is a quantity sufficient to expand the extracellular

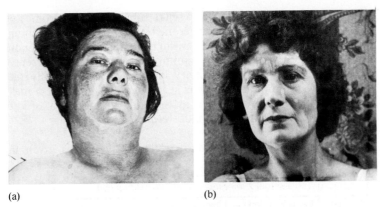

(a)   (b)

Figure 9.14. *Patient with Cushing's syndrome before treatment* (a) *and after treatment* (b).

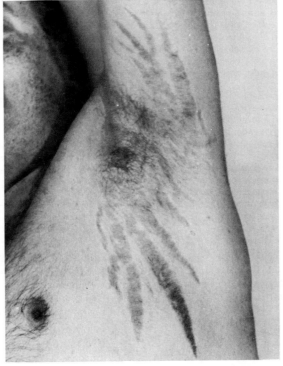

Figure 9.15. *Purple striae of Cushing's syndrome.*

volume two to three litres, the renal tubule escapes from the sodium-retaining effects of aldosterone by reabsorbing less sodium in the proximal tubule. The mechanism of this escape phenomenon is not fully understood but it is tempting to postulate the presence of a natriuretic hormone. Primary aldosteronism is usually the result of an autonomous adenoma secreting aldosterone or it may be due to areas of hyperplasia in the zona glomerulosa of the adrenal cortex secreting excess aldosterone.

A summary of investigation of adrenal function is given in Table 9.7.

Table 9.7. *Investigation of adrenal function.*

1. a. Plasma cortisol at 0900 and 2400 hours
   b. Urinary oxogenic steroids
   c. Urinary free cortisol

2. *Tests of adrenal reserve when adrenal insufficiency is suspected*
   a. Synacthen test: The plasma cortisol is measured before and 60 minutes after 250 μg of synthetic ACTH (Synacthen)
   b. Plasma cortisol response to insulin-induced hypoglycaemia

3. *Tests of autonomy of adrenal glands in suspected cases of adrenal hyperfunction*
   Dexamethazone suppression test: The plasma cortisol and urinary oxogenic excretion are measured before and after:
   0.5 mg dexamethazone six-hourly
   2 mg dexamethazone six-hourly
   Normal subjects will suppress after the small dose of dexamethazone. Cushing's syndrome due to adrenal hyperplasia will not suppress after a small dose but will suppress after the large dose of dexamethazone. Patients with Cushing's syndrome due to adrenal tumours will not suppress on either dose of dexamethazone.

Adrenal Medulla

The adrenal medulla secretes adrenaline and noradrenaline. *Hypofunction* of the adrenal medulla does not give rise to symptoms or signs because there are alternative sources of these catecholamines at the neuromuscular junctions. Indeed, after bilateral adrenalectomy the excretion of noradrenaline remains unchanged. Excess production of one or both of these hormones occurs as a result of a metabolically active tumour of the adrenal medulla: *phaeochromocytoma*. These tumours, which account for less than one per cent of patients with hypertension, are usually small and rarely palpable. Pressure on the abdomen will, however, often produce a rise in blood pressure or an increase in sweating. The diagnosis is therefore made on the clinical history or from the presence of hypertension, and is confirmed by the biochemical measurement of the urinary concentrations of adrenaline, noradrenaline, dopamine or their breakdown products. Noradrenaline is the catecholamine most consistently produced in excess and is the physiological stimulator of alpha-adrenergic receptors, giving rise to vasoconstriction of the skin, splanchnic and coronary vessels, pupil dilatation and gut relaxation. Adrenaline stimulates both alpha and beta adrenergic receptors causing an increase in the rate and force of cardiac contraction. The symptoms which result from excess of these catecholamines are paroxysmal palpitations, sweating and feelings of anxiety. The most useful physical signs are pallor and hypertension during an attack. The hypertension may be intermittent but is usually persistent when the secretion of catecholamine is sustained.

Pancreas

The endocrine aspects of the pancreas are either those of excess production of insulin by tumours of the beta cells or those resulting from a relative deficiency of beta-cell function and insulin production resulting in diabetes mellitus. In neither situation is the physical examination of the pancreas itself helpful. Endocrine tumours of the pancreas are too small to be palpable on clinical examination of the patient and the clinical diagnosis of insulinoma is made on the history of episodes of hypoglycaemia (page 535), and confirmed by the biochemical determination of the blood glucose level and serum insulin concentration.

Deficiencies of beta-cell function are manifest by the symptoms and signs of *diabetes mellitus*. This disease occurs in all parts of the world and the sexes are equally affected. It occurs at all ages though nearly 80 per cent of all diabetes cases occur in elderly obese patients and most of the remainder in young thin persons. Ketosis is much more common in younger patients and is indicative of more severe depletion of insulin. The most common presenting symptoms are polyuria, polydipsia and loss of weight. Glycosuria often leads to balanitis in men and pruritus vulvae in two thirds of all women who present with diabetes, this being associated with an inflammation of the vulvae. The polyuria is due to the osmotic diuretic effect of the sugar in the urine. In younger patients the hyperglycaemia is usually associated with ketosis and when this is severe there may be drowsiness and coma. On the other hand older patients with diabetes mellitus are frequently non-ketotic but drowsiness and coma may occur when the blood sugar is very high ($>$900 mg per 100 ml, 55 mmol/l) as a result of cellular dehydration. This is the consequence of increased extravascular osmotic pressure caused by the glucose which draws water out of the cells, and the cells of the central nervous system are the most sensitive to dehydration. The reason why some patients develop ketosis and others do not is uncertain but it seems probable that circulating levels of insulin in the non-ketotic disease are sufficient to prevent the accelerated release of free fatty acids and their subsequent degradation to ketones. The loss of weight is the consequence of mobilisation of the fat stores and gluconeogenesis from protein, and also the loss of sugar in the urine which may often exceed 100 grams per day. Ketoacidosis may itself give rise to symptoms such as anorexia, nausea, vomiting and abdominal pain.

There are no abnormal physical signs in uncomplicated diabetes mellitus. In severe cases there is wasting and dehydration and the smell of acetone can usually be detected in the breath. If ketosis is severe there is often air hunger characterised by deep breathing, and clinical evidence of dehydration with sunken eyes, a dry cool inelastic skin and a rapid thready pulse. Drowsiness is the rule and may proceed to coma.

Complications

Diabetes mellitus not infrequently presents with one of its complications and complete physical examination must be undertaken to seek evidence of these. The most important complications are vascular disease, peripheral neuropathy, cataracts and renal disease. *Vascular disease* is most commonly detected by the examination of the optic fundus where capillary microaneurysms can often be seen and also small dot-like haemorrhages. The hyperlipidaemia associated with diabetes leads to scattered hard waxy exudates. More rare and much more serious is the proliferative retinitis which may accompany diabetes mellitus; in this new blood vessels proliferate causing retinal detachment and haemorrhage with severe scarring and loss of vision.

Atherosclerosis develops at an earlier age and in a more severe form in the individual with diabetes affecting the coronary arteries and especially the arteries of the lower limbs. Evidence of peripheral ischaemia should be sought. The peripheral pulses should be examined and the volume of popliteal, dorsalis pedis and posterior tibial arteries assessed and the status of the arterial wall determined. Evidence of impaired tissue perfusion may be seen in the form of coldness of the limbs, and tissue necrosis which is especially probable around pressure points such as the heel, and over the first metatarsal head where tight shoes readily produce ischaemia in the diabetic. The larger blood vessels should be auscultated for bruits which are especially probable over the abdominal aorta, renal arteries, iliac and femoral vessels.

The symptoms and signs of *peripheral neuropathy* are considered on page 305. In diabetes mellitus the common form of peripheral neuropathy is a sensory neuropathy. The urine should always be tested for protein as well as sugar and ketones as part of the routine examination of the diabetic because proteinuria may be a manifestation of either urinary tract infection, a common complication of diabetes, or the more serious renal disorder of diabetic glomerular sclerosis. This nodular lesion in the glomerulus, first described by Kimmelstiel and Wilson, is a diffuse capillary disorder similar to the microaneurysms of the retina and indeed the lesions of kidney and retina are clinically associated. The skin should be examined for xanthomas which are small hard yellow nodules: they are a manifestation of the hyperlipidaemia of diabetes and are usually associated with vascular disease.

Pituitary Gland

The pituitary gland lies in the sella turcica, a depression of the sphenoid bone, and it is covered by a layer of dura mater, called the diaphragma sellae, through which the pituitary stalk passes. The gland comprises an anterior and a posterior lobe, each of which have separate origins and independent function. The pituitary gland is not amenable to physical examination and the physical evidence of pituitary disease depends either upon detecting the symptoms and signs of excess or deficiency of one or more of the pituitary hormones, or on the detection of damage to the optic chiasma or cranial nerves which may occur when a pituitary tumour extends out of the pituitary fossa. The functioning of the anterior pituitary gland is controlled by the hypothalamus which secretes regulatory hormones into the portal venous system which flows from the median eminence to the anterior lobe.

Anterior pituitary

The anterior pituitary secretes six hormones.

Growth hormone (GH) stimulates the growth of epiphyseal cartilage and is essentially anabolic in action.

Follicle-stimulating hormone (FSH) stimulates the growth of the ovarian follicle and hence controls oestrogen production in the female and stimulates the growth of the seminiferous tubules and spermatogenesis in the male.

Luteinising hormone (LH) is essential for ovulation and the formation of the corpus luteum. In the male it stimulates the development of the Leydig cells of the testis and hence the production of testosterone.

Adrenocorticotrophin (ACTH) regulates the adrenal secretion of cortisol and androgens having in addition a direct action on the melanocytes of the skin leading to skin pigmentation.

Thyrotrophin (TSH) regulates the production of thyroxine and tri-iodothyronine by the thyroid gland.

Prolactin stimulates the growth and development of the ducts and alveoli of the breast in concert with other hormones and is the major factor concerned with milk secretion.

All these anterior pituitary hormones are under the control of regulatory hormones from the hypothalamus.

Hypothalamic regulating hormones. Hypothalamic regulating hormones which affect the release of each of the six anterior pituitary hormones have been identified. Their blood levels are only one thousandth of those of the pituitary trophic hormones. Release of thyrotrophin, adrenocorticotrophin, growth hormone, follicle-stimulating hormone and luteinising hormone is stimulated by hypothalamic hormones whilst release of prolactin is inhibited. The prolactin release inhibiting hormone is dopamine. The structure of the releasing hormones for TSH, FSH—LH, and GH is now known and these releasing factors have all been synthesised. Thyrotrophin releasing hormone (TRH) is already in clinical use as a diagnostic test of thyroid function but has no therapeutic application. FSH—LH releasing hormone provides a useful diagnostic test of gonadotrophin reserve in patients with pituitary disease and has potential for the treatment of infertility and amenorrhoea in patients with functional hypothalamic disturbance. The therapeutic use of GH releasing hormone has yet to be established. Most cases of congenital deficiency of GH, FSH, LH and ACTH are due to defects in the hypothalamic production of releasing hormone and are not due to a primary pituitary disorder, so that the therapeutic implication of the recently synthesised group of releasing hormones is considerable. Galactorrhoea is frequently due to raised levels of circulating prolactin resulting from impairment of the tonic inhibition exerted on the pituitary by the hypothalamus and treatment with prolactin-release inhibiting hormone may be of therapeutic value.

Disorders of the anterior pituitary are associated with oversecretion or with a deficiency of one or more of these trophic hormones.

Hypofunction of the anterior pituitary. Deficiencies of trophic hormone production lead to gonadal failure, adrenocortical insufficiency, hypothyroidism and, in children, dwarfism. Isolated failure of a single pituitary hormone is uncommon and when it occurs it is usually a genetic deficiency of the relevant hypothalamic releasing factor and hence is apparent early in life. When the pituitary suffers any generalised disease, either as a result of pituitary tumours, granulomas such as sarcoidosis, syphilis or eosinophilic granuloma, or from a vascular disorder such as postpartum necrosis, there is usually a sequential failure of hormone production. Growth hormone and gonadotrophin hormone fail first while ACTH failure tends to occur late and TSH failure is intermediate. Growth hormone deficiency in the child is associated with shortness of stature and immature facies. *Gonadotrophin deficiency* in the male causes impotence, loss of libido, and loss of body hair whilst in women amenorrhoea and infertility occur. *ACTH deficiency* gives rise to the symptoms of cortisol deficiency: anorexia, weakness, nausea and vomiting. Lack of ACTH is responsible for the lack of pigmentation of the skin and nipples in patients with hypopituitarism. *Pituitary TSH deficiency* is responsible for the symptoms of hypothyroidism. However the swelling of the skin and subcutaneous tissue so characteristic of myxoedema is unusual when thyroid failure is secondary to pituitary disease. Hypopituitarism in adolescence leads to infantilism (Figure 9.16).

The local glandular lesion is of clinical importance and of diagnostic value in the case of pituitary tumours when the patient presents with headaches or visual defects. The headache may be bitemporal, frontal or vertical and the visual defect is usually a bitemporal hemianopia due to impingement of the tumour on the optic chiasma. Optic atrophy may occasionally occur. The patient

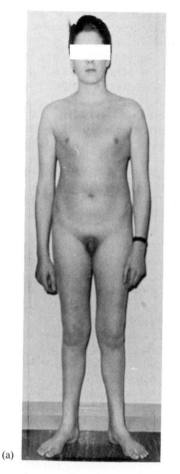

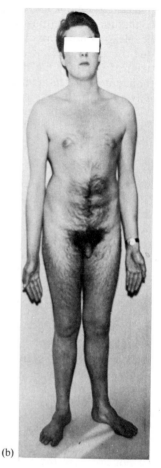

(a)　　　　　　　　　　　　　　　　(b)

Figure 9.16. *Man of 22 with hypopituitarism before* (a) *and after* (b) *treatment.*

often mentions that he walks into people because he has failed to see them coming up on one side and examination of the visual fields is therefore of great importance. Less common is a third nerve palsy from lateral extension of the tumour. In patients in whom the hypopituitarism is the result of damage to the hypothalamus the presentation may be one of hypothalamic disturbance in which the sleep rhythm is disturbed with somnolence by day and insomnia at night, appetite is increased, there is a gain in weight, defects in temperature regulation lead to hypothermia or less frequently hyperthermia, and diabetes insipidus with intense polydipsia and polyuria may occur.

Hyperfunction of anterior pituitary. Hyperfunction of the anterior pituitary is usually confined to a single hormone and is nearly always the result of a pituitary tumour. An eosinophilic adenoma results in excess growth hormone production and will produce gigantism in adolescence or acromegaly in the adult.

Gigantism. This is due to excess growth hormone production in adolescence and is a rare disease. There is a generalised overgrowth of the skeleton and soft tissues. It requires to be distinguished from eunuchoidism, Klinefelter's syndrome and XYY chromosomal constitution.

Acromegaly. Acromegaly occurs in one in 10 000 of the population, usually in the third and fourth decades. The symptoms and signs of acromegaly are due to: (1) the excess growth hormone production; and (2) the presence of an intrasellar tumour. Both sexes are equally affected. It is an insidious disease in which the hands and feet enlarge, the nose broadens and the lower jaw protrudes. Because of the gradual progression the patient is frequently unaware of the changes which are most often noticed by relatives or the doctor who have not seen the patient for some time (see Figure 9.4). Once the epiphyses have fused excess growth hormone cannot produce any further increase in height but it can stimulate the growth of the connective tissues such as ligaments, capsules and synovia causing the carpal tunnel syndrome and acroparaesthesiae. The effect of growth hormone on the skin and soft tissues give rise to the coarsening of the features: nasal and aural cartilage overgrowth produces enlargement of the nose and ears while bone overgrowth of the maxilla lengthens the face and that of the ramus of the mandible is responsible for prognathos.

Proliferation of deep layers of joint cartilage results in thinning of articular cartilage which eventually causes premature osteoarthrosis. Viscera such as the tongue, liver, adrenal and thyroid enlarge. The heart is also affected but the increase in cardiac size is not associated with increase in performance and, indeed, the increased growth may lead to fibrosis of cardiac muscle and cardiomyopathy. Hypertension is commonly associated with acromegaly. Because growth hormone is an antagonist of insulin there is a decrease in carbohydrate tolerance and frank diabetes mellitus occurs in 20 per cent of cases.

In addition to these clinical manifestations of excess growth hormone production the symptoms and signs referable to the pituitary tumour itself may occur. In particular headache is a feature of 90 per cent of patients with acromegaly. Suprasellar extension is unusual so that bitemporal hemianopia is uncommon.

Cushing's syndrome. Excess ACTH production will result in bilateral hyperplasia of the adrenal glands and increased production of cortisol to produce Cushing's syndrome which has already been considered under the adrenal gland disorders. Pituitary tumours may cause Cushing's syndrome, but the main defect in this disorder when it is associated with bilateral adrenal hyperplasia is in the hypothalamus where the receptors which normally respond to rising levels of circulating cortisol by reducing corticotrophin releasing hormone production become less sensitive, so that higher levels of cortisol are required before production of corticotrophin releasing factor is reduced.

Precocious puberty. This disorder results from the premature production of adult levels of gonadotrophins and is more common in girls. The young female will develop secondary sex characteristics and menstruate at an early age (three to eight years) and the young boy will develop puberty early and the testes approach adult size. Such children are tall for their age as their growth velocity is consistent with the normal puberty growth spurt, but their mental and bone age is consistent with their chronological age. Tumours of gonadotrophin-producing cells of the pituitary do not occur though gonadotrophin production is a regular feature of choriocarcinomas and some teratomas. Premature puberty or precocious puberty arises because the puberty spurt of gonadotrophin occurs prematurely. The mechanism controlling the release of gonadotrophins is not fully understood. A common releasing hormone from the hypothalamus stimulates both FSH and LH release.

It is important to distinguish between true precocious puberty and sexual precocity. In male sexual precocity, which is usually due to excessive production of androgens by the testis or adrenal, the testes are small, there is azoospermia and the gonadotrophin levels are low. Testicular causes are tumours whilst adrenal causes may be hyperplasia or tumour, with excessive adrenal androgen production. If it is due to the less common cause of a testicular tumour producing androgens, this is obvious on clinical examination of the testes. In the female sexual precocity is usually due to an oestrogen-secreting ovarian tumour which is palpable per rectum by the time the syndrome presents.

Galactorrhoea. Abnormal galactorrhoea is the inappropriate secretion of milk in a patient who is not nor has recently been pregnant. It is due to the increased production of prolactin by the anterior pituitary. Only a small proportion of patients with hyperprolactinaemia have galactorrhoea. A number of other hormones, such as oestrogens, progesterone, thyroxine and cortisone, are necessary for the full development of the breast before prolactin can induce lactation. Hyperprolactinaemia causes infertility due to anovulation and amenorrhoea more frequently than it causes galactorrhoea and this is due to the impaired response of the ovary to gonadatrophins in the presence of increased circulating levels of prolactin. Hyperprolactinaemia is an important cause of infertility and amenorrhoea. Prolactin is the only pituitary hormone that is under the control of hypothalamic inhibition. The other pituitary trophic hormones are under the control of hypothalamic releasing hormones. Dopamine is the hypothalamic hormone that inhibits the release of prolactin.

Drugs such as reserpine and methyldopa which deplete the brain stores of dopamine will cause the increased pituitary production of prolactin. Drugs that block the effects of dopamine have a similar effect and these include phenothiazines, the butyrophenones, and metoclopramide, all of which are in common usage. Drugs which act at the hypothalamic level, such as the oral contraceptives, may suppress the prolactin inhibiting hormone and cause enhanced prolactin secretion. Damage to the pituitary stalk will also suppress prolactin inhibiting hormone. TRH causes the release of prolactin as well as TSH, so that hyperprolactinaemia may be associated with primary hypothyroidism. Pituitary tumours may secrete prolactin and 50 per cent of patients with chromophobe adenomas have hyperprolactinaemia; the resulting amenorrhoea is commonly due to the raised prolactin levels rather than damage to gonadatrophin producing cells. These tumours are often small and may not cause enlargement of the pituitary fossa. Growth hormone is structurally similar to prolactin and many patients with acromegaly have hyperprolactinaemia.

Hyperprolactinaemia in men causes impotence and galactorrhoea is rarely seen. Gynaecomastia without galactorrhoea is much more common in men and prolactin plays no part in uncomplicated gynaecomastia. Simple gynaecomastia is associated with oestrogen concentrations which are in excess of effective androgen activity.

Thyroid stimulating hormone. Excess TSH production by the

pituitary is rare. It may cause hyperthyroidism but this is usually due to stimulation of the thyroid by an antibody called the thyroid stimulating antibody, or is a result of excess thyroid hormone production by an autonomous adenoma of the thyroid gland.

A summary of investigation of anterior pituitary function is given in Table 9.8.

Table 9.8. *Investigation of anterior pituitary function.*

1. *Measurement of growth hormone*
   a. *When deficiency of growth hormone is suspected:*
      The serum growth hormone is measured at 30-minute intervals for 2½ hours following insulin-induced hypoglycaemia. Hypoglycaemia is a stimulus to growth hormone production
   b. *When excess growth hormone production is suspected:*
      The serum growth hormone levels are measured in response to hyper-glycaemia induced by a glucose tolerance test. Hyperglycaemia suppresses normal growth hormone production

2. *Measurement of gonadotrophic hormone*
   LH—RH test
   In this test serum LH and FSH are measured before and 20 and 60 minutes after the intravenous injection of 100 µg of the hypothalamic hormone LH—RH

3. *Measurement of adrenocorticotrophic hormone*
   This is indirectly measured by determining the plasma cortisol levels at half-hourly intervals for 2½ hours following insulin-induced hypoglycaemia. Hypoglycaemia is a stress that normally stimulates ACTH production

4. *Measurement of thyroid stimulating hormone*
   TRH test
   In this test the serum TSH is measured before and 20 and 60 minutes after the intravenous injection of 200 mg of the hypothalamic releasing hormone TRH

5. *Measurement of prolactin*
   Serum prolactin levels (immunoassay)

6. *Radiological investigation of pituitary function*
   a. Skull x-ray for size of pituitary fossa
   b. X-ray of hands for bone age

Posterior pituitary

The posterior pituitary stores the hormones vasopressin and oxytocin which are produced by the hypothalamic neurosecretory cells. Hyperfunction of the posterior pituitary does not occur. When *inappropriate secretion of the antidiuretic hormone* does arise it is usually due to ectopic production of arginine vasopressin-like polypeptides by an oat-cell carcinoma of the bronchus. Extra-cellular hyponatraemia is associated with over-hydration of the brain and this results in confusion, convulsions and even coma. Inappropriate ADH secretion may also be associated with infections of the lungs and central nervous system; in such patients the urine is often more concentrated than plasma so that, in a sense, there is an inappropriate secretion of ADH if one considers the plasma osmolality as the only stimulus to ADH production. There are, however, other stimuli such as volume depletion, hypotension and pain.

Deficient production of antidiuretic hormone causes *diabetes insipidus*. It may be the result of a primary or secondary tumour in the area or from infiltration by chronic granulomatous tissue as in sarcoidosis or syphilis. These days the cause is frequently trauma to the base of the skull following a road traffic accident. Not infrequently diabetes insipidus is idiopathic. The symptoms are those of intense thirst, polydipsia and polyuria, and the only physical sign directly related to the lack of vasopressin is the large volume of almost colourless dilute urine which commonly reaches a figure of 8 to 12 litres per day.

There are a number of other disorders causing polyuria and polydipsia which must be considered. The more important are diabetes mellitus, chronic renal failure, psychogenic polydipsia and hypercalcaemia. The basic disturbances which may give rise to polyuria are: (1) inadequate secretion of vasopressin; (2) inability of the kidney to elaborate a concentrated urine despite adequate vasopressin; (3) the persistent excessive intake of water.

Both hypercalcaemia and hypokalaemia impair the ability of the renal tubule to respond to the effects of vasopressin and in hyper-calcaemia there is in addition the osmotic diuretic effect of the increased calcium in the urine. Structural and functional damage to the loop of Henlé causes polyuria since it is in this area that the countercurrent system of sodium reabsorption renders the renal medulla hyperosmotic to plasma permitting water to be absorbed from the collecting ducts along an osmotic gradient. Damage may occur both to the loop of Henlé and to the collecting tubules themselves in chronic renal disease but the polyuria rarely exceeds three litres and the presence of albuminuria will enable clear differentiation from diabetes insipidus. In diabetes mellitus the osmotic effect of the glucose in the urine prevents the reabsorption of adequate water despite the presence of vasopressin. In psychogenic polydipsia there is a compulsion to drink water although there is no dehydration and no primary defect in urinary water reabsorption. When water is restricted these patients can produce concentrated urine.

Breasts

Female breast tissue consists of glandular, fibrous and adipose tissue. It is subject to alterations in size and consistency as a result of physiological changes which occur during menstruation, pregnancy and lactation whilst some degree of atrophy commonly follows the menopause. The female breast is composed of about 20 lobes each in turn consisting of several lobules. The lobules are constructed of glandular tissue which opens into a small ductule and is surrounded by loose connective tissue. The lobules are separated by dense fibrous tissue and fat. Each lobe is drained by a duct and the ducts converge beneath the nipple to open onto the surface. The development of the duct system is stimulated by oestrogens and that of the glandular tissue by progesterone. There is thus a constant hyperplasia and involution taking place during the fluctuating levels of ovarian hormones during the menstrual cycle. The changes during pregnancy are even more striking and the release of the pituitary hormone prolactin is necessary for the secretion of milk.

There is considerable variation in the size of the normal breast because of varying tissue sensitivity to ovarian hormones. Women frequently complain of a failure of the breast to develop to what they consider a desirable size but this is usually not due to any hormonal deficiency if menstruation is normal and no increase in size can be anticipated from the administration of ovarian hormones. Less commonly there is a failure of the development of one breast in which there is a deficiency in tissue sensitivity to hormonal influences. An occasional patient is troubled by extremely large breasts and this is due to an increased tissue responsiveness to normal hormonal influences.

Tenderness of the breasts is a frequent symptom especially during the premenstrual period and results from fluid retention secondary to the relative excess of oestrogen to progesterone. An accentuation of the process leads to the development of small cysts in the ducts which may be palpated as multiple nodules in the breast.

The breasts are the most frequent sites of carcinoma in women so that no physical examination in a woman is complete until both breasts have been palpated. For the purpose of clinical examination the breast is traditionally divided into the nipple, the areola and the upper, lower, inner and outer quadrants. Examination of these areas must then be followed by palpation of the regional lymph nodes that drain the breast in the axillae and supraclavicular fossae. Inspection of the breasts should be undertaken with the patient stripped to the waist. The symmetry and contour of the breasts are noted and the situation, prominence and inclination of the nipples assessed. With the patient lying down the breasts are palpated and evidence of local enlargement, palpable masses, discoloration and venous dilatation sought by inspection and palpation. It is often useful to ask the patient to raise her arms above her head and this may produce evidence of dimpling of the skin when there is carcinomatous attachment.

The breasts should be palpated with the flat of the hand, thereby making the mass of a tumour much more obvious and lessening the effect of the diffuse nodularity of cystic mastitis. Palpation of the breasts is best performed with the patient lying on her back and each quadrant is systematically felt. The chief object of the examination is to detect a hard, fixed mass hidden in the glandular tissues. If a mass is palpated it is then felt with the finger tips to define its characteristics (page 25). Carcinomas tend to be attached to superficial and deep structures and if a lump is attached in this way it is almost certainly a carcinoma. If it is not, a carcinoma cannot be excluded and palpable lumps must therefore be biopsied before a diagnosis can be made. The nipples and areolae must be examined and any discharge sought. Inversion of the nipple, discharge from the breast or ulceration are the important features sought in examination of the nipples.

Breast tissue in the male is rudimentary but at puberty transient gynaecomastia is normal. Otherwise gynaecomastia is usually a feature of Klinefelter's syndrome or the result of drugs such as oestrogens, spironolactone or phenothiazines (Figure 9.17). Carcinoma of the male breast occurs rarely.

Female Genitalia

Before examining the female genitalia it is important that the patient is in the correct position, the bladder empty and the light

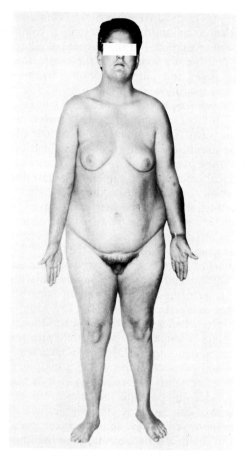

Figure 9.17. *Gynaecomastia.*

adequate. The correct position is for the patient to be on her back with the legs drawn up, the soles of the feet together and the legs rotated externally so that the knees are wide apart.

Vulva

The vulva is first inspected, noting in particular the condition of the skin and any atrophic changes in the labia. The labia are parted using two fingers and the patient asked to strain down which demonstrates any weakness of the vaginal walls, the presence of a cystocele and in more severe degrees of prolapse descent of the vault enabling the cervix to become visible. Atrophic changes in the vagina are indications of deficient oestrogen production. Infection of the vagina produces erythema and a discharge, the quality and quantity of which should be noted.

Digital examination

Digital examination is performed to assess the state of the uterus which is a midline structure and to examine the laterally placed ovaries. The glove is lubricated with a non-irritant jelly and the index and middle fingers of the right hand gently introduced into the vagina, pressing the vaginal wall backwards. At the same time the left hand is placed above the symphysis pubis so that both hands can be manoeuvred to assess the size, position and mobility of the pelvic organs. The cervix is felt first and attention should be given to whether it points backwards or forwards in relation to the long axis of the vagina. If the uterus is anteverted the cervix points backwards and if the uterus is retroverted the cervix points forwards, if the body of the uterus can be felt through the anterior fornix it is anteverted, if it is felt through the posterior fornix it is retroverted.

The normal uterus is seven to eight cm long, five cm across and three cm thick. The walls are smooth and it is fully mobile in the anterior and posterior direction. Restricted mobility is abnormal and infection or endometriosis often causes a fixed retroversion. Irregularity of the uterine outline suggests fibroids.

Adnexa

The adnexa are felt through the lateral fornices. Normal fallopian tubes are not palpable. The right ovary is easier to feel than the left as the latter is often obscured by a loaded bowel. The normal ovary is hard, smooth, mobile and tender on pressure. It measures about 4 cm by 1.5 cm but the presence of a corpus luteum causes slight enlargement. Ovarian swellings may be so adherent to the uterus that differentiation from uterine swellings may be impossible on vaginal examination.

Speculum examination

A bivalve speculum can be passed with the patient in the dorsal position. It is passed upside-down so that the screw or rachet is uppermost. If the purpose of the examination is to look at the cervix and take a smear this position will suffice. More information is, however, gained by placing the patient in the left lateral position with the buttocks to the edge of the couch and the right leg flexed more at the hip than the left and the right shoulder forwards in relation to the left.

The normal appearance of a well-oestrogenised vagina is a rugose epithelial surface with a pearly white discharge formed from desquamated epithelial cells. The atrophic vagina is flat, shiny and bleeds easily on touch by a spatula. Infection produces erythema and purulent discharge. The cervix is usually covered by squamous, stratified epithelium. It is smoother than the vaginal wall but the epithelium is of similar quality. Childbirth often splits the cervix and exposes the cervical canal which is lined with mucous membrane. This is really an ectropion of the cervix but does not require treatment unless responsible for symptoms of excessive discharge or dyspareunia. The cervix should be examined for the presence of an erosion which is overgrowth of the cervical squamous epithelium by columnar epithelium. Annular erosions of less than one cm in diameter are usually of no significance.

Pelvic examination should be completed by rectal examination as the supporting ligaments of the uterus are best felt by rectal examination. These may be thickened by endometriosis when nodules are usually palpable and by infection when the ligament is indurated and thick.

Testes and External Genitalia

Testes

The testes should be examined both in the recumbent position and with the patient standing. The patient is more relaxed when lying down and it is easier to palpate the testes, but the patient should also be examined standing or a varicocele, which is dilatation of the veins of the pampiniform plexus, may be missed. In the normal male the left testis hangs lower than the right. The testes are palpated gently to determine their size and contour and consistency. An estimate should be made of their size, but it is only after palpation of many hundreds of testes that a clear idea can be obtained of the normal range. The mean size of the testis is 4.5 cm in length and 2.5 cm in width, and it is normally sensitive to even gentle pressure. If one testis is small it suggests previous infection or injury. Mumps and syphilis are the common infections which affect the testes.

The epididymis and spermatic cord are also examined. The epididymis lies posterolateral to the testis to which it is closely attached. The spermatic cord can be examined between the thumb and forefinger and is normally smooth and even. Many infections affect the epididymis, including *Escherichia coli*, staphylococci and gonococci, and tuberculosis usually produces a characteristic nodular change in the epididymis with thickening of the cord. The presence of fluid around the testis *(hydrocele)* should be sought and if this is thought to be present confirmation should be obtained by transilluminating the area with a pocket torch pressed against the area. An empty scrotum on one or both sides must lead to a search for undescended or ectopic testes. The undescended testis can commonly be palpated in the inguinal canal.

If a testis is larger than normal a tumour should be suspected, especially if it is irregular. Testicular tumours are usually painless and not tender.

Swellings within the scrotum should be examined in the same way as other swellings (page 25). They commonly contain fluid and this can be confirmed by transillumination. Hydroceles, spermatoceles and cysts of the epididymis are the main possibilities and they can be diagnosed by their anatomical relationship to the testes.

The external genitalia must also be examined. The phallus should be inspected. If foreskin is present it should be retracted and the urethral orifice examined. The glans penis is inspected for scars or ulceration, chancres and urethral discharge sought and the inguinal lymph glands palpated. The commonest anomaly of the external genitalia is hypospadias in which there is malposition of the urethral orifice and this may occur in 1 in 300 boys. Phimosis is a condition in which contracture of the prepuce prevents its retraction over the glans. It predisposes to balanitis and may be sufficiently severe as to cause obstruction to the flow of urine.

Cryptorchidism. In undescended testes the testes are either within the abdomen or the inguinal canal. The testes are undescended in 10 per cent of males at birth, in two per cent at one year of age but after puberty unilateral or bilateral cryptorchidism is found in only 0.3 per cent. Undescended testes must be distinguished from ectopic testes where the testis has strayed from the normal path of descent. Common sites for ectopic descent are in the perineum, femoral and superficial inguinal areas. It is important to diagnose cryptorchidism at an early age as undescended testes are a significant cause of infertility and have an increased risk of malignancy. Up to the age of five years undescended testes may show normal maturation of the seminiferous tubules but between six and 10 years only eight per cent are normal and by 11 years of age all are abnormal.

If both testes are small hypogonadism is suggested which may be primary or secondary to pituitary gonadotrophin failure. The commonest cause of primary testicular failure is Klinefelter's syndrome. In this disorder there is atrophy of the seminiferous tubules with consequent azoospermia, whilst Leydig cells are commonly spared and hence androgen production is unaffected. This syndrome is frequently associated with gynaecomastia and the breasts should therefore be examined carefully with this in view. If an individual has small testes the physical features of eunuchoidism should be sought which are: span exceeding height, female hair distribution, high-pitched voice, infantile genitalia, and female body contour.

A summary of investigation of gonadal function is given in Table 9.9.

Table 9.9. *Investigation of gonadal function*

1. *Testicular function*
    Sperm count
    Serum testosterone
    Urinary oxosteroid excretion
    Urinary oestrogen excretion
    Response of serum testosterone to injection of human chorionic gonadotrophin
    Chromosome karyotype or buccal smear
    Serum FSH and LH
    Skull x-ray for pituitary fossa

2. *Investigation of ovarian function*
    Urinary oestrogen excretion
    Vaginal cytology
    Serum prolactin
    Response of urinary oestrogen to follicle stimulating hormone
    Clomiphene stimulation test
    Gynaecography or laparoscopy
    Chromosome karyotype or buccal smear
    Serum FSH and LH
    Skull x-ray for pituitary fossa

FURTHER READING

Bayliss, R. I. S. (1974) Investigations of endocrine disorders. *Clinics in Endocrinology and Metabolism*, Vol. 3, No. 1. London: W. B. Saunders.

Hall, R. Anderson, J., Smart, G. A. & Besser, M. (1980) *Fundamentals of Clinical Endocrinology*. 3rd edition. London: Pitman Medical.

Williams, R. H. (1981) *Textbook of Endocrinology*. Philadelphia: W. B. Saunders.

Wills, M. R., Havard, C. W. H. & Roylance, P. J. (1979) *Laboratory Investigation of Endocrine Disorders*. London: Butterworth.

10 Haematology

J. E. Pettit and A. V. Hoffbrand

In patients with blood disorders, the diagnosis of the type of abnormality and where necessary the underlying disease is often made on the basis of laboratory investigations. The clinical history may be unrewarding and physical examination may show few or no signs. The most important organs or tissues to be affected by the blood dyscrasia are the skin, mucous membranes, liver, spleen, lymph nodes and central nervous system. Blood and bone marrow are readily accessible, and a wide range of haematological investigations is now possible so that an accurate diagnosis can be made in virtually all patients once a blood abnormality is suspected. Full diagnosis will depend on recognising the exact type of haematological abnormality and, where necessary, on detecting an underlying disease outside the haemopoietic system that is causing the abnormality in the particular patient. Nevertheless, the clinical history and physical examination are of great importance in suggesting that a blood disease may be present and the correct line of investigation, in grading the severity and overall effects of the disease in the particular patient and in deciding on the best management. Moreover, since many blood abnormalities are familial or drug-induced, these aspects of the clinical history are of particular importance in patients with blood diseases.

Diseases of the bone marrow often result in anaemia, neutropenia or thrombocytopenia either alone or in combination (i.e. pancytopenia). In a minority of patients, excess numbers of red cells, white cells or platelets are produced. In this chapter, the possible clinical signs and symptoms of the patient with anaemia, neutropenia or thrombocytopenia are described, as well as the features of patients with excess production of these elements and of those with other defects of bone marrow, reticuloendothelial or coagulation systems which are conveniently considered with them.

ANAEMIA

Anaemia is one of the most common signs of illness in clinical medical practice. It is usually defined as a haemoglobin in adult males of less than 13.5 g/dl and in females of less than 11.5 g/dl, though a few laboratories have slightly different criteria. In children before puberty, the normal is above 11.0 g/dl. Although for practical purposes anaemia is defined on the basis of the haemoglobin concentration in a given volume of blood, it must be remembered that this concentration depends both on the total circulating red cell mass and on the total plasma volume. In most patients with a decreased red cell mass, the plasma volume is increased to maintain the blood volume constant and thus anaemia occurs. In acute blood loss, red cell mass and plasma volume are both reduced and symptoms are related to the reduction in total blood volume, rather than to anaemia. They manifest as progressively severe degrees of shock. 'Spurious' anaemia due to haemodilution may occur in pregnancy, overhydration, renal failure, liver diseases and in conditions where there is gross splenomegaly, whereas 'spurious' polycythaemia due to a relative decrease in plasma volume may occur in dehydration, and also in an ill-understood disorder known as 'stress polycythaemia'.

Clinical Features

The presence and severity of symptoms depends on the speed of onset of anaemia, the age of the patient, whether or not cardiac or pulmonary disease is present and on the type of anaemia present. When anaemia develops rapidly, particularly in old people, symptoms are more severe than those of slowly progressive anaemia in the young who may develop a haemoglobin of 8 g/dl or less before seeking medical attention. Children are particularly well able to adapt to anaemia of insidious onset.

The symptoms of anaemia also depend on the nature of the anaemia. In general, in *chronic anaemia* there is an adaptation in the oxygen dissociation curve of haemoglobin by which it gives up oxygen more readily to tissues ('a shift to the right in the curve'). This is brought about by an increase in red cell 2,3-DPG (2,3-diphosphoglyceric acid), a compound which competes with oxygen for binding haemoglobin. Because of the sigmoid shape of the haemoglobin oxygen dissociation curve, uptake of oxygen at the lungs is barely, if at all, impaired by increased red cell 2,3-DPG. On the other hand, at tissue oxygen tensions, release of oxygen to the tissues is considerably enhanced because of the increase in red cell 2,3-DPG. This shift is exaggerated in some haemoglobin-opathies, e.g. sickle cell anaemia, and in some metabolic abnormalities, e.g. pyruvate kinase deficiency. In these conditions, patients may be remarkably well and have a good exercise tolerance despite very low haemoglobin levels.

Symptoms and signs also depend on the *type of anaemia* since there may be associated features, e.g. unconjugated hyperbilirubin-aemia in haemolytic and megaloblastic anaemias, haemoglobinuria with intravascular haemolysis, and glossitis in megaloblastic anaemia or iron deficiency. Symptoms of a myeloneuropathy may occur in vitamin B_{12} deficiency. In many bone marrow disorders leucopenia and thrombocytopenia lead to infections and haemor-rhage as well as to anaemia. There may also be features of a disease such as carcinoma of the stomach or a peptic ulcer which lead to iron deficiency. Finally, in many general medical disorders such as renal failure, liver disease, chronic inflammations or malignancy, anaemia may be just one manifestation when those of the primary disease dominate the clinical picture.

The main clinical features are due to changes in the *circulation and respiratory systems* which are marked only if the anaemia is severe. Shortness of breath, dizziness or faintness may develop during exercise or excitement. Fatigue, lassitude and generalised muscular weakness may also be prominent symptoms. In older subjects, congestive heart failure, angina pectoris or intermittent claudication may be the main features.

On examination, there may be a rapid bounding pulse, the cardiac output being increased in nearly all subjects with a haemoglobin less than 7 g/dl. In adults, this is largely due to an increase in stroke volume rather than to tachycardia, but in children, tachycardia is relatively more marked. Decreased peripheral vascular resistance, decreased blood viscosity and increased cardiac output account for the bounding pulse and may also result in systolic bruits over the carotid and cranial arteries. Cardiac murmurs, usually systolic and maximum at the apex or pulmonary areas, are common in severe anaemia when not only increased turbulence and blood flow but actual dilatation of the heart with mitral and tricuspid incompetence may occur.

The *skin* may be pale in anaemia but this depends more on the state of the skin circulation than on the haemoglobin level. Pallor of the skin may also result from fluid retention in the subcutaneous tissues as in myxoedema or renal disease. The conjunctivae, mucous membranes of mouth, lips and pharynx and the nail-beds give a better indication of anaemia than the skin. The skin and appendages may show other changes in particular types of anaemia. Jaundice of the conjunctiva and skin suggests haemolysis. Bilirubin above 70 mmol/l is unusual unless there is cholestatic jaundice due to gallstones (which are common in some chronic haemolytic anaemias) obstructing the common bile duct. Of course, all the other causes of jaundice may occur incidentally in the anaemic patient. Jaundice occurs in patients with large internal haematomas and also in megaloblastic anaemia due to excessive breakdown of haemoglobin in the bone marrow ('intra-medullary haemolysis'). In some cases of vitamin B_{12} or folate deficiency, widespread skin pigmentation with melanin, reversible by B_{12} or folate therapy, develops.

A greenish hue to the skin, 'chlorosis', has been described in young women with iron deficiency but is only rarely seen nowadays. Chronic leg ulcers occur in sickle cell anaemia, hereditary spherocytosis and rarely in other haemolytic anaemias. They probably occur because of blockage of the microcirculation with consequent tissue anoxia, exaggerated by the lowered oxygen delivery due to anaemia.

In cold antibody haemolytic syndromes, anaemia is worse in cold weather and may be associated with Raynaud's phenomenon. There may be discoloration and cyanosis of exposed parts, particularly tips of the fingers, toes, nose and ear-lobes.

The *nails* in some patients with chronic iron deficiency become concave (koilonychia) (Figure 10.1). More commonly, they become brittle. Loss of lustre and thinning of the *hair* may also be seen. In some patients with pernicious anaemia, early greying of the hair is a feature but is of genetic origin rather than due to vitamin B_{12} deficiency, which it may precede by many years. Vitiligo is also associated with pernicious anaemia.

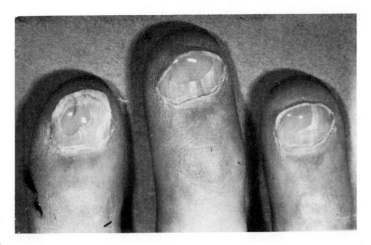

Figure 10.1. *Koilonychia in a 60-year-old woman with iron-deficiency anaemia. The nails are concave and can hold water, as shown.*

Alimentary manifestations are mainly seen with specific types of anaemia. Glossitis occurs in megaloblastic anaemia and, less commonly, in iron deficiency which may also cause angular cheilosis and dysphagia, rarely with pharyngeal webs. An altered appetite ('pica') with demands for unusual foods, e.g. ice, chalk or dirt, also occurs in some patients with iron deficiency.

An enlarged *spleen* from whatever cause may reduce appetite and cause discomfort after a large meal. If it is extremely large, a dragging sensation in the left hypochondrium may be a prominent symptom. The spleen may enlarge in any severe anaemia when the red cell life is shortened and the spleen undergoes 'work hypertrophy'. Repeated blood transfusion also leads to splenic enlargement due to iron overload. A spleen more than a few centimetres enlarged suggests that an underlying disease itself may be causing splenomegaly, even in the absence of anaemia or when anaemia has been corrected, e.g. liver disease with portal hypertension, a myeloproliferative disease or a lymphoma.

In nutritional anaemias, symptoms or signs of a disease of the gastrointestinal tract which causes the deficiency may also be present, e.g. a neoplasm or 'piles' in iron deficiency, coeliac disease or tropical sprue in folate deficiency, intestinal stagnant loop in vitamin B_{12} deficiency. As chronic haemorrhage is one of the most frequent causes of anaemia it is most important to make enquiry about blood loss from the alimentary tract.

Excessive blood loss from the female reproductive tract is one of the most frequent causes of anaemia. As pregnancy is often associated with a negative iron balance details of past obstetric history should be obtained from all women patients.

Urinary features are uncommon in anaemic patients. Mild proteinuria may be caused by extreme anaemia, while dark urine occurs when there is intravascular haemolysis with haemoglobinuria. Haemosiderinuria also occurs but is only detected by staining a centrifuged deposit for iron released from desquamated renal tubular epithelial cells. Haematuria occurs in bleeding disorders as well as with local lesions of the renal tract, and if chronic, may lead to moderate iron deficiency. Microscopic haematuria is found in sickle cell disease or trait.

Common symptoms of anaemia involve the *nervous system.* Headache, tinnitus, vertigo, lack of concentration are all frequent features. Symptoms and signs of a peripheral neuropathy or of posterior or lateral column damage may occur in severe vitamin B_{12} deficiency. In general, these are symmetrical and affect the legs more than the arms. In some cases, an optic neuropathy or dementia are the main features.

The *optic fundus* may show abnormalities in any severely anaemic patient, particularly when anaemia develops rapidly and retinal anoxia occurs because there is inadequate time for circulatory compensation to the anaemia. Papilloedema is rare but flame-shaped or punctate haemorrhages are more frequent.

Some anaemic patients are *febrile.* A fever of up to 38° to 38.5°C may occur in severe megaloblastic anaemia and less frequently in other very severe anaemias. An associated infection, particularly if the patient is severely neutropenic, must always be excluded.

Family History

This is particularly important in patients suspected of congenital haemolytic anaemias. Inheritance is dominant in hereditary spherocytosis and elliptocytosis; anaemia, jaundice, gallstones or splenectomy have usually occurred in a parent, sibling, grandparent, uncle or aunt. Inheritance is autosomal recessive in sickle cell anaemia and thalassaemia and there may have been no symptoms of the disease in family members who carry the trait.

Inheritance is sex-linked in the common types of glucose-6-phosphate dehydrogenase (G-6-PD) deficiency and in the rare disease, congenital sideroblastic anaemia, and in these conditions males show the most severe manifestations though occasional females do show mild clinical abnormalities. The rare congenital aplastic anaemia known as Fanconi's anaemia which is associated with defects of other organs, e.g. absent radii, other skeletal deformations or renal abnormalities, is inherited as an autosomal recessive. A family history is also often obtained in some of the acquired anaemias, particularly in pernicious anaemia in which close relatives may have had the same disease or may have shown thyroid abnormalities or other autoimmune disorders which also occur more commonly in pernicious anaemia patients.

Drug History

A knowledge of the occupational status and previous drug therapy is important in any patient with anaemia. There is almost no haematological abnormality that cannot be reproduced by drugs. The more common include a history of aspirin ingestion in patients with iron deficiency; anticonvulsant therapy related to folate deficiency; chloramphenicol or phenylbutazone therapy associated with patients with aplastic anaemia; sulphonamide, phenacetin or antimalarial drugs precipitating a haemolytic episode in patients with underlying G-6-PD deficiency; methyldopa therapy as a cause of autoimmune haemolytic anaemia; immunosuppressive and cytotoxic drug therapy for patients with anaemia associated with neutropenia and thrombocytopenia due to bone marrow damage. In certain occupations, subjects are exposed to chemicals which may cause bone marrow aplasia or hypoplasia. This applies particularly to patients who are exposed to insecticides, organic solvents, benzene derivatives or to lead. Hair dyes and deodorants may also cause marrow hypoplasia rarely.

Social History

Poverty and mental abnormalities may lead to a poor dietary intake with consequent nutritional deficiencies; the most frequent manifestation being folate deficiency. Vegans tend to become vitamin B_{12} deficient. Alcohol is a direct toxin to the marrow and patients who drink spirits without taking a good diet tend to develop anaemia which, in some cases, is associated with megaloblastic change due to folate deficiency or sideroblastic anaemia due to a disturbance of pyridoxine metabolism but in other cases appears to be due to the direct toxic effect of alcohol on the bone marrow. In chronic alcoholics anaemia of liver disease may also be present. Residence in certain tropical areas (e.g. India, Singapore, Puerto Rico), may lead to tropical sprue with consequent folate or vitamin B_{12} deficiency, while iron deficiency anaemia due to infestation with ankylostoma is one of the most common causes of anaemia in the tropical areas. Malaria may also cause anaemia in the tropics but is usually diagnosed because of other features.

Racial Origins

Sickle cell anaemia and trait are found in Negro individuals, whether from Africa or from other parts of the world, but sickle cell anaemia also occurs in subjects of other ethnic groups, particularly in the Middle East and in India. Beta-thalassaemia occurs in subjects of Mediterranean origin, particularly from Greece, Cyprus, Turkey and Middle Eastern countries but also occurs in other areas of the world with less frequency. Alpha-thalassaemia syndromes are more common in the Far East. G-6-PD deficiency in which anaemia occurs mainly after drugs or eating the broad bean (favism) occurs in the Mediterranean, while in Negro individuals and other racial groups G-6-PD deficiency is more particularly associated with drug sensitivity. Pernicious anaemia occurs more commonly in subjects of Northern European origin than in other racial groups, while megaloblastic anaemia due to coeliac disease is also particularly common in residents in some countries, e.g. Ireland.

Particular Features of Anaemia in Children

Children do not usually develop symptoms or signs of anaemia until this is quite severe. They often present with an intercurrent infection or diarrhoea and vomiting and anaemia is only diagnosed after a blood examination. In general, tachycardia is a more prominent sign than a bounding pulse. In congenital haemolytic anaemias there may be an expansion of the marrow cavity which affects the shape and size of several of the bones. This is particularly common in thalassaemia major when so-called 'bossing' of the skull and widening of the bones of the face may cause a typical facies. Radiographs of the skull show the classical 'hair-on-end' appearance (Figure 10.2) which results from such expansion of the marrow cavity. This is less commonly seen in other severe congenital haemolytic anaemias, e.g. spherocytosis or pyruvate kinase deficiency. In sickle cell anaemia the history is usually dominated by crises of abdominal pain, back pain or bone pain due to infarction of tissues. In some patients, haemolytic or aplastic crises may also lead to a rapidly increasing severity of anaemia with increasing symptoms. Repeated bone infarcts may lead to alteration in appearance of the patients, who are typically slender and may show shortening of digits.

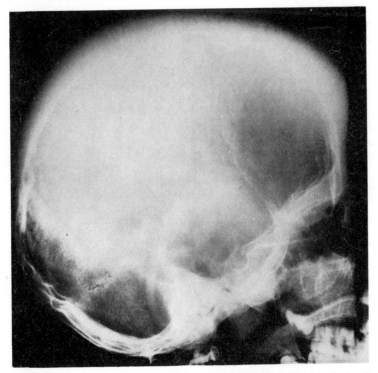

Figure 10.2. *The skull x-ray of a 6-year-old boy with homozygous beta-thalassaemia showing thickening of the vault of the skull and the 'hair-on-end' appearance.*

The Blood Count and Film Examination

The initial haematological investigations comprise a blood count and the examination of a stained blood film. With modern automated electronic counters accurate computed red cell indices (MCV, MCH, MCHC) readily indicate what morphological class of anaemia, e.g. hypochromic microcytic, macrocytic or normo-cytic, the patient is likely to be suffering from. Examination of the blood film, the cornerstone of haematology, provides an essential check on these indices and the rest of the blood count and in many patients identifies the type of anaemia present. Figures 10.3 and 10.4 illustrate the features of iron deficiency and megaloblastic anaemias; spherocytosis and polychromasia would point to a haemolytic anaemia and so on. No definite pattern of red cell indices is found in combined deficiency of iron and folate or with many important anaemias associated with red cell anisocytosis, poikilocytosis and fragmentation; examination of the blood film is essential for the recognition of such abnormalities. The reticulocyte count, a valuable index of erythropoietic response to anaemia, is also of great value in the initial definition of anaemia.

The additional presence of severe thrombocytopenia and neutro-penia may reflect generalised bone marrow failure rather than a selective abnormality of erythropoiesis and suggests aplastic anaemia, leukaemia or marrow infiltration. Often the exact diagnosis is only made after the examination of aspirated bone marrow and other detailed laboratory studies have been performed.

BLEEDING DISORDERS

The normal haemostatic mechanism involves the complex inter-action of a number of factors. Primary arrest of haemorrhage results from vasoconstriction and elastic recoil of severed blood vessels together with the formation of platelet plugs. Activation of blood coagulation converts the fluid column of blood in the vessel into an insoluble fibrin clot which reinforces the sealing effect of the vascular and platelet components of haemostasis. Bleeding disorders thus result from deficiency or qualitative defects of platelets, from structural abnormalities of blood vessels or from deficiencies of the blood coagulation factors. It is often possible to distinguish which of these abnormalities is most likely to be present during the initial clinical evaluation of the patient with a bleeding

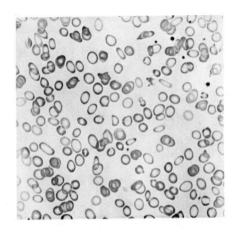

Figure 10.3. *Peripheral blood film in severe iron deficiency anaemia (haemoglobin 5.5 g/dl, MCH 17 pg, MCV 59 fl) showing red cell hypochromia, microcytosis and poikilocytosis. (May—Grunwald—Giemsa × 350.)*

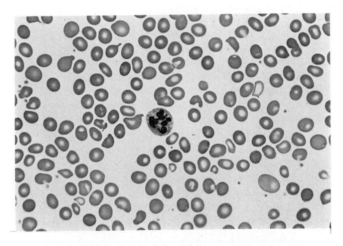

Figure 10.4. *Peripheral blood film in untreated pernicious anaemia (haemoglobin 4.6 g/dl, MCH 40 pg, MCV 122 fl). The red cells show oval macrocytosis, aniso-cytosis and poikilocytosis and the neutrophil present is hypersegmented. (May—Grunwald—Giemsa × 350.)*

disorder. Disorders of platelets and small blood vessels classically present as 'purpuras' with prominent cutaneous and mucosal bleeding. On the other hand, repeated haemarthroses and deep dissecting haematomas dominate the clinical course of patients with hereditary coagulation disorders.

Clinical Features

Petechiae and ecchymoses

Multiple skin petechiae and ecchymoses are collectively referred to as *purpura*. Petechiae are 'crops' of small capillary haemorrhages which vary from pinpoint size to a few millimetres in diameter (Figures 10.5, 10.6). Although they are most visible in the skin, mucous membranes and the retina, the internal organs of the body are not spared from this type of haemorrhage. Petechiae are most frequently the result of *thrombocytopenia*. The small blood vessels of the skin and mucous membranes are subjected to constant

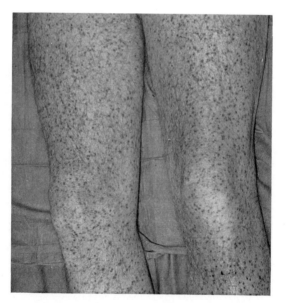

Figure 10.5. *Petechial haemorrhages in a 61-year-old man with severe thrombocytopenia (platelets 10 × 10^9/l) due to acute myeloblastic leukaemia.*

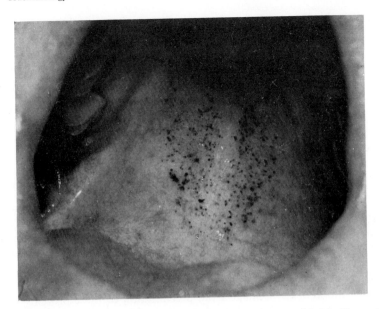

Figure 10.6. *Petechial haemorrhages on the palate of a 16-year-old girl with severe thrombocytopenia (platelets 20 × 10⁹/l) due to infectious mononucleosis.*

shearing and it is likely that minor breaches of vascular integrity are normally sealed by platelet aggregation. The spontaneous development of petechiae is usually associated with platelet counts of less than $20 \times 10^9/l$. Although they may occur anywhere on the skin thrombocytopenic petechiae tend to be more conspicuous in sites subjected to pressure or venous constriction, e.g. on the legs in the ambulant or adjacent to garters or girdles. When the thrombocytopenia is very severe and has been rapid in development, e.g. in immune drug-induced thrombocytopenia, the petechiae may be confluent and in the mouth they are frequently accompanied by haemorrhagic vesicles or bullae.

Ecchymoses (small bruises) result from the confluence of petechiae or from haemorrhage from vessels larger than capillaries. In the thrombocytopenic patient they may appear spontaneously or surround venepuncture sites. Although multiple ecchymoses characterise the bleeding disorders, it should be remembered that isolated ecchymoses are normal findings, especially in women and small children.

Petechiae are a feature of *scurvy*. The earliest 'crops' are usually seen around hair follicles on the medial surfaces of the thighs and buttocks (the so-called 'saddle area'). Some defect in the micro-vascular supporting tissue (ground substance or collagen) is the probable reason for the haemorrhagic tendency in this condition. Rather indolent purple ecchymoses measuring up to five cm in diameter may be found in the elderly. This *senile purpura* is most often seen on skin areas exposed to sunlight, e.g. on the backs of the hands and neck, and on the extensor surfaces of the forearm. Atrophy of dermal collagen and elastin and loss of subcutaneous fat in the elderly weakens the supporting tissue of the dermal microcirculation which becomes more susceptible to shearing strain.

Petechiae and ecchymoses are seen in some patients with *paraproteinaemias*, e.g. myelomatosis, Waldenström's macro-globulinaemia, benign monoclonal gammopathy, cryoglobulin-aemia or cryofibrinogenaemia. Some of these proteins interfere with platelet function and fibrin formation and small vessel haemorrhages may also result from hyperviscosity of the blood or from blood vessel damage from precipitation of these proteins in the cooler parts of the skin. Deposition of amyloid in the micro-circulation may also produce purpura in patients with *amyloidosis*.

In the *allergic purpuras* the skin lesions are more variable. The petechiae and ecchymoses associated with the Henoch—Schönlein syndromes or with drug-induced vascular purpuras may be accom-panied by itching, tingling sensations, erythema and urticarial swelling. In occasional patients the small vascular lesions may either be associated with herpetic-like vesicles or become necrotic with superficial ulceration. The lesions of allergic purpura may be generalised or have a symmetrical proximal distribution. The thighs and buttocks are often the most severely affected regions.

The frequently fatal but fortunately rare condition known as *purpura fulminans* is characterised by the widespread development of large, painful, confluent and necrotic ecchymoses. Almost any area of skin may be affected. The extremities, face, buttocks and lower back are often the worst affected areas and some patients develop symmetrical peripheral gangrene. The condition is usually seen in children who are recovering from scarlet fever, varicella or other infections. In most cases, there has been evidence of associated disseminated intravascular coagulation with thrombocytopenia and coagulation factor deficiencies. The cause of this catastrophic syndrome is unknown. It has been suggested that antigen—antibody complexes may trigger the vascular damage and intravascular coagulation. A similar condition occurs rarely in patients with meningococcal septicaemia.

In the coagulation disorders ecchymoses are usually large and the skin discoloration is often the result of subcutaneous spread of haemorrhage from haematomas in deeper tissues.

The tiny vascular malformations which are the essential lesion of *hereditary haemorrhagic telangiectasia* may be confused with petechiae. These permanent bright red or purple spots are most noticeable on the face, ears, tongue, lips, plantar and palmar surfaces. Although they are the same size as petechiae they characteristically blanch on pressure. The lesions do not appear until adult life and they become more numerous with advancing age. Bleeding from the telangiectasia of the gastrointestinal mucosa produces a state of chronic severe iron deficiency. Purpuric areas should also be distinguished from Campbell de Morgan spots.

Haemarthroses

Major joint haemorrhage is the main clinical problem in patients with severe classical haemophilia (haemophilia A or factor VIII deficiency) and Christmas disease (haemophilia B or factor IX deficiency). Although a history of minor joint trauma may be obtained, bleeding from the synovial vessels is usually spontaneous. The knees, elbows, ankles and wrists are the most frequently and severely affected joints; other joints, e.g. shoulder, hip, temporomandibular, small joints of hands and feet are occasionally involved. The patient complains of severe pain, the affected joint is tender, warm and may be grossly distended. There is limitation of movement and often accompanying muscular spasm and the joint may be held in a position of flexion. With initial haemarthroses haemorrhage into the periarticular tissue may result in tracking of blood to the skin over the joint. However, in joints subjected to many haemorrhages, thickening of the joint capsule tends to prevent further external bruising. After repeated haemarthroses retained blood induces a state of chronic inflammation in the affected joint. The synovial membrane thickens, develops villi and becomes highly vascular, and a weakening of the joint supporting tissues occurs. These changes, together with atrophy of muscle groups related to the joint, e.g. quadriceps and hamstrings if the knee is involved, only serve to increase the susceptibility of the damaged joint to further injury and haemorrhage. Chronic joint haemorrhage results in degenerative joint changes and mechanical derangement of articular surfaces. Disuse demineralisation, loss of articular cartilage, bone 'lipping' and osteophyte formation produces deformity and crippling. The end result is often permanent fixation of the affected joint by bony or fibrous ankylosis.

Patients with inherited or acquired defects of coagulation factors other than VIII or IX often show easy bruising and spontaneous and excessive post-traumatic bleeding. Spontaneous haemarthroses are, however, most unusual. Joint haemorrhage is also rare in patients with thrombocytopenia. Swollen tender joints may develop in some patients with allergic purpura due to periarticular inflammation and oedema. These changes are not associated with haemorrhage into the joint cavity.

Soft tissue haematomas

The spontaneous development of soft tissue haemorrhage is another feature of severe haemophilia and Christmas disease. Dissecting haematomas may involve large areas of muscle or deep fascial layers. The patient complains of pain and is often febrile. Spontaneous bleeding into the tongue, throat or neck is particularly dangerous as airway strangulation sometimes occurs. Haemorrhage into the retroperitoneal fascial spaces or into the psoas muscle produces considerable problems in differential diagnosis. Associated pain, tenderness and fever may mimic almost any cause of the 'acute abdomen'. Right-sided haematomas may be confused with appendicitis even to the extent of their producing a positive 'psoas' sign (right thigh held in flexion and the accentuation of pain by hyperextension of the right hip joint). Ischaemic contractures may follow extensive haemorrhage into limb muscles, e.g. Volkmann's contracture of the forearm.

Other spontaneous haemorrhage

Epistaxis, haematemesis, melaena, rectal bleeding or *haematuria* may accompany any haemorrhagic disorder. Haemoptysis is very rare. *Gum bleeding* occurs frequently in patients with thrombocytopenia or scurvy. Continuous small vessel gastrointestinal haemorrhage is characteristically seen in hereditary haemorrhagic telangiectasia but is also seen in patients with severe thrombocytopenia or the myeloproliferative disorder, essential thrombocythaemia. *Menorrhagia* is often the principal clinical problem of women with severe thrombocytopenia or von Willebrand's disease. Other rare coagulation disorders with autosomal inheritance and the hereditary platelet function disorder known as thrombasthenia (Glanzmann's disease) may also be associated with excessive menstrual blood loss. Although spontaneous central nervous system bleeding is not common in patients with haemorrhagic diatheses, cerebral haemorrhage is a prominent cause of death in severely thrombocytopenic patients.

Excessive post-traumatic bleeding

Prolonged *bleeding from superficial cuts and abrasions* is a feature of thrombocytopenia. Although this superficial haemorrhage from small blood vessels may occur in patients with von Willebrand's disease because of their functional platelet abnormality it does not usually occur in haemophilia or other hereditary disorders of blood coagulation. This type of post-traumatic haemorrhage is immediate and frequently may be controlled by local pressure. The onset of *post-traumatic bleeding* in patients with haemophilia and other coagulation disorders may be delayed for several hours as early haemostasis may be accomplished by vascular reaction and platelet plugging. The typical prolonged and excessive bleeding associated with these disorders is not stopped by local pressure and is frequently life-threatening.

The response to trauma provides an excellent screening procedure for a haemostatic defect and a previous history of surgery or traumatic injury without bleeding complications virtually rules out a hereditary disorder of blood coagulation. In severe haemophiliacs, although there is an absence of factor VIII in the blood at birth, serious haemorrhage is rare at the time of delivery or during the first few months of life. Serious bleeding from the umbilical stump is most unusual and large cephalohaematomas are infrequent. Early circumcision may or may not be associated with excessive haemorrhage. The loss of deciduous teeth may cause few problems but the extraction of permanent teeth in haemophiliacs is associated with excessive bleeding. Following a tooth extraction in a normal adult, moderate haemorrhage may continue from the tooth socket for up to two hours and minor oozing of blood generally persists for up to two days. In the haemophiliac profuse socket haemorrhage may continue for several days.

Relation of severity of disorder to clinical features

The severity and frequency of abnormal bleeding episodes in patients with hereditary coagulation disorders are related to the degree of deficiency of the involved coagulation factor. This is well illustrated in haemophilia. The most severely affected patients with factor VIII levels of less than one to two per cent suffer from recurrent spontaneous and crippling haemarthroses and soft tissue haemorrhage. In patients with one to five per cent level of factor VIII, spontaneous bleeding episodes are less frequent and less severe and there is seldom permanent orthopaedic deformity. However, like the most severe haemophiliacs, this group of patients may suffer from exsanguinating haemorrhage after trivial injury. Patients with 5 to 25 per cent level of factor VIII do not have spontaneous haemorrhage but excessive bleeding accompanies minor surgery, trauma and dental extractions. Patients with the mildest form of haemophilia with factor VIII levels between 25 and 50 per cent are often undiagnosed. Excessive bleeding occurs in these patients only after a serious accident or following major surgery.

Although it is more difficult to relate clinical manifestations directly to platelet levels in patients with thrombocytopenia, spontaneous bleeding and purpura are usually associated with platelet counts of less than $20 \times 10^9/l$. Patients with idiopathic thrombocytopenic purpura and other causes of excessive peripheral platelet destruction often show less haemorrhage than patients with similar degrees of thrombocytopenia resulting from marrow failure, e.g. aplastic anaemia or leukaemia. This has been attributed to a predominantly young functionally superior platelet population in idiopathic thrombocytopenic purpura and other conditions in which the platelet life-span is short. The platelet count is normal in bleeding disorders related to abnormalities of platelet function, e.g. hereditary thrombasthenia or aspirin-induced thrombopathy. Paradoxically, spontaneous gastrointestinal haemorrhage occurs in patients suffering from essential thrombocythaemia and platelet counts consistently above $1000 \times 10^9/l$. This may result from occlusion and necrosis of small vessels with subsequent rupture. Thrombosis may also be a feature of the clinical course in patients with high platelet counts.

Family History

In all patients with a history of easy bruising or haemorrhage, it is important to establish whether this has been life-long and whether there is a family history of bleeding. The inheritance of the most common disorders of blood coagulation, haemophilia and Christmas disease, is sex-linked. In suspected patients, enquiry should be made about evidence of the disease in male siblings and maternal uncles. One-third of haemophiliacs have no family history of the disease. In the rare coagulation disorders characterised by autosomal recessive inheritance, a positive family history is often difficult to obtain but in some patients there is history of consanguinity. Hereditary haemorrhagic telangiectasia and von Willebrand's disease are inherited as autosomal dominant conditions and a positive family history frequently spans several generations.

Drug History

In many patients with bleeding disorders enquiry into recent drug or chemical exposure is important. Drug-induced thrombocytopenia may occur as a result of generalised toxic bone marrow depression (aplastic anaemia), from selective megakaryocyte depression or as a result of drug-induced immune destruction of circulating platelets. Aspirin is an occasional cause of purpura due to its damaging effect on platelet function and several drugs have been implicated in causing vascular purpura. Patients taking coumarin or indanedione anticoagulants may bleed because of overdosage or because some other drug interferes with the plasma binding or metabolism of the anticoagulant.

Haemostasis Screening Tests

Although attention to the patient's history and a thorough clinical examination are most important in the evaluation of a bleeding disorder, the definitive diagnosis is usually made only after laboratory assessment.

The bleeding time and platelet count are used to detect quantitative and qualitative platelet defects. The prothrombin time is sensitive to deficiencies of coagulation factors II, V, VII and X and is typically prolonged in liver disease, vitamin K deficiency and during oral anticoagulation. The activated partial thromboplastin time is sensitive to deficiencies of factors V, VIII, IX and X and thus is able to detect the most important hereditary coagulation disorders, haemophilia (deficiency of factor VIII) and Christmas disease (deficiency of factor IX). This latter test is also sensitive to the presence of heparin. In disseminated intravascular coagulation, low fibrinogen levels and the presence of fibrin degradation products can be detected by the fibrinogen titre, a prolonged thrombin time and one of the screening tests for fibrin degradation products. Thrombocytopenia should be confirmed by platelet counting. Prolongation of the prothrombin time and activated thromboplastin time indicates reduced levels of coagulation factors. The whole blood coagulation time is prolonged in severe haemophilia and during heparin therapy. The observation of clot retraction after one hour's incubation provides a guide to platelet function and smaller than normal clots indicate fibrinogen deficiency. The results of haemostasis screening tests in patients with the rather ill-defined vascular purpuras are usually normal.

More definitive tests needed for diagnosis include bone marrow examination, platelet function and survival studies and coagulation factor assays.

GRANULOCYTE DISORDERS

The dominant clinical features of patients with defective neutrophil function or numbers are bacterial infections. These usually occur when the neutrophil count falls to less than $0.5 \times 10^9/1$ and are particularly frequent when the count is $0.2 \times 10^9/1$ or less. The incidence may be related partly to the functional efficiency of the neutrophils which varies widely according to the cause of the neutropenia. Patients with acute agranulocytosis are most frequently seen after therapy with a drug which causes an immune or 'toxic' neutropenia. They present with *sore throat* and *fever* which becomes rapidly more severe with prostration, dehydration, shock and possible early death. There may be severe necrotic *ulceration* of the mouth and pharynx. With lesser degrees of neutropenia the most common features are recurring *infections*, particularly of the mouth and pharynx, other mucocutaneous junctions and of the skin. Because of neutropenia, pus is not formed and bacteraemia may occur without features of localised infection. In rare patients with normal numbers of neutrophils which are functionally defective, chronic granulomas may develop. These patients often give a history of recurring pneumonia, tonsillitis and other local infections and may ultimately succumb to an overwhelming infection.

Excess numbers of granulocytes only lead to clinical features in malignant and myeloproliferative diseases which are discussed in the next section.

LEUKAEMIAS, LYMPHOMAS AND MYELOPROLIFERATIVE DISEASES

The clinical features of these disorders are protean. In the leukaemias the features depend largely on whether the disease is of the chronic or acute variety and on the nature of the main cell type involved, lymphocyte or granulocyte. Moreover, in some patients the course of the disease changes from one to another of these syndromes, e.g. from chronic granulocytic to acute myeloblastic leukaemia or from polycythaemia vera to myelosclerosis. The symptoms and signs of the malignant lymphomas are so varied that it is impossible to mention any but the main features here.

Clinical Features

The symptoms of many of these patients, especially when the disease is advanced, are due to anaemia, neutropenia and thrombocytopenia caused by bone marrow failure. These are particularly frequent in patients with acute leukaemia or myeloma in which early presenting features are of malaise, general ill-health, fatigue, recurring or persistent sore throats and purpura or haemorrhage. Immunoglobulin deficiencies in myeloma, lymphatic leukaemias and poor granulocyte function in myeloid leukaemias may all aggravate the tendency to infection (Figure 10.7). *Excessive bleeding* resulting from thrombocytopenia may be exaggerated because of lack of clotting factors in acute promyelocytic leukaemia when disseminated intravascular coagulation is a feature. In the chronic leukaemias and myelosclerosis, similar symptoms may occur but often the patient's complaints are related to the grossly enlarged spleen or to a raised metabolic rate which causes sweating, heat intolerance and loss of weight. The *spleen* may cause heaviness or a dragging pain in the left hypochondrium. Splenic infarction may produce acute abdominal pain, and there may be difficulty in

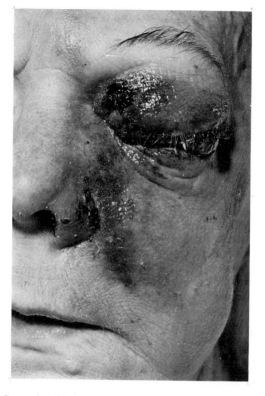

Figure 10.7. *Severe facial infection in a 55-year-old woman with acute myelomonocytic leukaemia.*

taking a full meal or frequency of micturition due to pressure of the enlarged spleen on adjacent organs.

Common presenting symptoms of patients with a lymphoma are a *lump* due to lymphadenopathy most frequently in the cervical region, general feelings of ill-health, fever, and loss of weight. The *fever* in Hodgkin's disease in a minority of patients is of the intermittent type. Generalised *pruritus* and pain after alcohol ingestion occur, particularly in Hodgkin's disease. In patients with a localised lymphoma outside the reticuloendothelial system, as with carcinoma, almost any clinical syndrome may develop, depending on the size of the mass, its rate of growth and where it is situated, e.g. brain or spinal cord, gastrointestinal tract, skin, lungs. In Burkitt's lymphoma tumours occur frequently in the jaw.

Pain in the joints due to gout caused by the increased cell and purine turnover may be a feature of all these disorders, particularly in chronic granulocytic leukaemia and myeloproliferative diseases. *Bone pain* is a characteristic feature of myeloma but also occurs in acute leukaemia and myelosclerosis. Among these disorders, however, spontaneous fractures are virtually confined to myeloma.

The symptoms of polycythaemia vera are somewhat different. A ruddy complexion, headaches, dizziness, visual disturbances, and symptoms related to peripheral vascular obstruction or haemorrhage, are common features. Pruritus, particularly after bathing, is characteristic, and may be due to histamine release from excess numbers of basophils. Despite the possible variety of symptoms, it is important to recognise that a proportion of patients with all these conditions, particularly with chronic lymphocytic leukaemia, have no symptoms at all when they are first diagnosed because an incidental blood count is performed.

Physical examination of a patient suspected of one or other of these disorders is helpful both in diagnosis and staging the disease.

Features of anaemia, neutropenia or thrombocytopenia are common. *Skin* may show pallor, petechiae or ecchymoses and jaundice which may be due to haemolysis or to cholestasis if there is a tumour mass obstructing the common bile duct. In polycythaemia vera, the skin typically shows a ruddy cyanosis; excoriation due to pruritus is common in this condition and in Hodgkin's disease. There is an increased incidence of herpes zoster in patients with lymphomas and chronic lymphocytic leukaemia. Infiltrations of the skin with leukaemic or lymphomatous cells may cause a variety of widespread eruptions, the best recognised being 'mycoses fungoides'. Patients with macroglobulinaemia and myeloma may show purpura due to blockage of capillaries with abnormal plasma protein and in some patients with myeloma or lymphoma cutaneous vascular lesions may occur in cold weather due to blockage of small vessels in the extremities, face and ears.

Wasting, most marked in the extremities, may be due to the combination of anorexia and raised metabolic rate due to excess turnover of cells and to growth of tumour tissue in the marrow, spleen, lymph nodes and elsewhere.

Changes in the *mucous membranes* occur principally in the patient with acute leukaemia. Oral ulceration and bacterial or fungal infections are common. *Gum hypertrophy* is seen typically in acute monoblastic leukaemia (Figure 10.8). Ulceration and infection of other mucous membranes and mucocutaneous junctions are also common problems.

Sternal tenderness is elicited by pressure over the manubrium sternae. It is an indication of expansion of the bone marrow and the physical sign is not confined to the leukaemias and myeloproliferative disorders but may be found in any severe anaemia.

The *eyes* may show important changes. There may be pallor of the conjunctivae or jaundice of the sclerae. Suffusion and a bloodshot appearance of the conjunctivae and engorgement of the fundal vessels are seen in severe polycythaemia. Fundal haemorrhages and exudates are more characteristic of acute leukaemia or hyperviscosity. Papilloedema suggests meningeal infiltration by leukaemia or lymphoma.

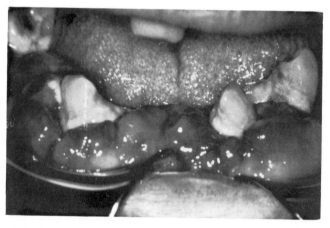

Figure 10.8. *Gum infiltration and hypertrophy in a 38-year-old female with acute monoblastic leukaemia.*

Lymph Nodes

In the malignant lymphomas, chronic lymphocytic leukaemia and acute lymphoblastic leukaemia, almost any group of lymph nodes may show enlargement. Nodes in the anterior or posterior cervical triangles, supraclavicular, axillary, epitrochlear or inguinal regions may be detected by the patient or by the clinician during the initial physical examination. Grossly enlarged nodes may produce visible swellings. Occasionally patients notice 'lumps' under the skin during daily activity, e.g. shaving or washing, while others become aware of neck thickening. The enlarged nodes are detected by the careful and systematic palpation of superficial lymph node areas. During the examination the patient should be positioned so that the overlying skin is freely mobile and the underlying muscles are relaxed. The initial palpation should be gentle and most physicians search with a circular motion of the fingertips, steadily increasing the pressure applied as the search area deepens. Sometimes the cervical nodes are palpated more easily when the patient performs the Valsalva manoeuvre.

In the malignant lymphomas and particularly in Hodgkin's disease, enlargement of one or other group of superficial lymph nodes is usually the presenting manifestation of the disease (Figure 10.9). The cervical nodes are involved in over 60 per cent of patients with Hodgkin's disease. The next most frequent sites of involvement, in decreasing order, are axillary, mediastinal and inguinal. The nodes vary in size but may reach several centimetres in diameter. They are usually of rubbery consistency, smooth, firm and non-tender. In many patients individual nodes remain discrete but with the most aggressive types of lymphoma, extracapsular extension of the malignant cells may result in fusion of adjacent involved nodes and fixation to surrounding tissues. In acute and chronic lymphatic leukaemia, lymph node enlargement tends to be generalised or present in more than one region. The nodes are firm, discrete and usually not tender.

In myeloid leukaemias, lymph node enlargement is usually not a feature.

Differentiation of leukaemic and lymphomatous node enlargement from other causes of lymphadenopathy is often difficult. Anterior cervical nodes frequently enlarge in response to infections of the mouth or pharynx. When lymphadenopathy follows acute infection, the nodes are classically soft and tender and the overlying skin may show erythema and oedema. With widespread antibiotic usage suppuration of nodes is now rare. As a result of repeated upper respiratory tract infections the palpation of discrete nodes of less than one centimetre in diameter in the cervical region is considered a normal finding in children. It is not unusual to find isolated small nodes in the inguinal region of adults but lymphadenopathy in other areas must be considered abnormal. The lymph node enlargement associated with infectious mononucleosis is usually bilateral and more frequently involves node groups deep

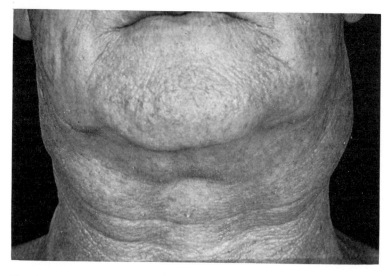

Figure 10.9. *Cervical lymphadenopathy in a 67-year-old man with non-Hodgkin's lymphoma.*

and posterior to the sternomastoid muscle than those of the anterior cervical, axillary and inguinal regions. Involvement of the posterior auricular nodes suggests rubella infection. While sinus formation and radiological evidence of calcification are characteristic of tuberculous nodal involvement, nodes involved by metastatic cancer are classically fixed, irregular and stone-like in consistency. In many chronic inflammatory conditions the lymph nodes are firm and there is a tendency towards fusion and matting; the clinical distinction from lymphoma may be impossible. Microscopy and bacteriological studies on an excision biopsy is the only certain way to define the aetiology of chronic superficial lymphadenopathy.

In the leukaemias and lymphomas, there is frequently involvement of internal lymph nodes. Chest x-ray may reveal the presence of mediastinal lymphadenopathy. Occasionally massive enlargement of mediastinal nodes may be detected by percussion or suspected by tracheal displacement. Enlarged nodes in the thoracic inlet may produce signs of superior mediastinal obstruction. Retroperitoneal lymph node enlargement may cause abdominal symptoms through pressure or infiltration of surrounding structures and very occasionally the abdominal nodes may be large enough to become palpable. Their recognition has been greatly facilitated by the recent development of abdominal lymphangiography.

The principal features in the *abdomen* are likely to be hepatic and splenic enlargement. The largest spleens, which may extend beyond the umbilicus and reach the pelvis, occur in chronic granulocytic leukaemia and myelosclerosis, though in occasional patients with these diseases the spleen may be only slightly enlarged and perhaps impalpable. The spleen is firm, the notch may be palpable and the surface is smooth. If an infarct has occurred recently, a friction noise may be heard on auscultation over the area of perisplenitis. Lesser degrees of splenomegaly, rarely extending beyond the umbilicus, are found in chronic lymphocytic leukaemias, Hodgkin's disease and other lymphomas and in about three-quarters of patients with polycythaemia vera. In acute leukaemias and myeloma, the spleen is often impalpable, but some degree of splenomegaly may be found, particularly in acute lymphoblastic and monoblastic forms.

Examination of the urine is most valuable in multiple myeloma when Bence Jones proteinuria (excretion of immunoglobulin light chains) occurs in about 60 per cent of cases. Non-specific proteinuria may also occur in this disorder while Bence Jones proteinuria occurs occasionally in patients with a non-Hodgkin's lymphoma.

Neurological signs occur in a proportion of patients. They may be due to infiltration of the central nervous system by leukaemia or lymphoma. Meningeal leukaemia causes neck stiffness, photophobia, papilloedema and in some cases localising neurological signs. Lymphomatous involvement of the brain or spinal cord may lead to signs of a space-occupying lesion in these tissues. Cerebral thrombosis or haemorrhage is a serious complication of polycythaemia vera and also of the thrombocytopenia that may occur in many of these disorders.

Whatever the clinical features, the diagnosis of leukaemia is made by careful examination of the blood (Figure 10.10) and bone marrow, while a lymphoma is diagnosed by histological examination of tumour tissue, usually an excised lymph node. Additional essential information is often obtained by special appropriate investigations such as cytogenetic and cytochemical studies, analysis of serum and urine proteins, lumbar puncture, bone marrow trephine, radiological studies including lymphangiography (Figure 10.11), ultrasonography, computerised whole body tomography and, in some cases, laparatomy and splenectomy.

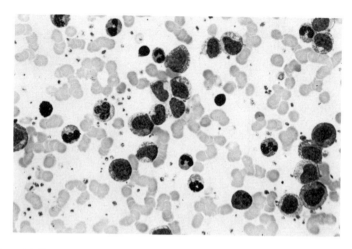

Figure 10.10. *Peripheral blood film in chronic granulocytic leukaemia. (Total white cell count 137 × 10⁹/l.) The dominant white cells seen are myelocytes, metamyelocytes and neutrophils. (May—Grunwald—Giemsa × 350.)*

Polycythaemia vera must be distinguished from 'spurious' and 'secondary' polycythaemia by full blood count, bone marrow, blood volume studies and by other special tests.

FURTHER INVESTIGATIONS FOR BLOOD DISORDERS

Examination of Peripheral Blood

Bone Marrow Examination

This relatively simple and safe procedure provides essential diagnostic information in the majority of patients with diseases of the blood. Marrow may be obtained by aspiration or by trephine biopsy.

Marrow aspiration

The most frequently used sites are the sternum, the posterior or anterior iliac spines and, in infants under two years, the upper and medial surfaces of the tibia. Following the injection of a local

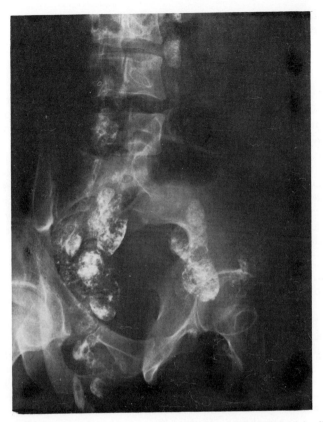

Figure 10.11. *Lymphangiogram in a 40-year-old man with Hodgkin's disease showing enlargement of para-aortic, pelvic and inguinal lymph nodes.*

anaesthetic into the skin and periosteum a special needle with a well-fitting stilette and adjustable guard is employed to penetrate cortical bone and about 0.5 ml of marrow is aspirated. The usual method of study combines the examination of Romanowski stained films made from the aspirated material and an estimation of iron content by staining with potassium ferrocyanide (Perls' reaction). Additional techniques employed in some cases include the examination of 'squashed' marrow fragments and histological sections cut from marrow fragments treated with suitable fixatives.

Special biochemical, immunological, cytogenetic or culture techniques may give useful information in appropriate cases.

Trephine bone biopsy

When marrow aspiration fails to provide adequate samples for examination, e.g. in myelosclerosis and some patients with aplastic anaemia, and in patients suspected of having marrow infiltration by malignant lymphoma, metastatic tumour or granuloma, bone marrow aspiration should be supplemented by histological study of a trephine bone biopsy. In addition to the study of haematoxylin and eosin stained sections silver impregnation techniques are employed to delineate reticulin architecture. An iliac site is preferred by most physicians and the microtrephines currently used for percutaneous bone biopsy are only slightly more traumatic than standard aspiration needles.

Lymphangiography

It is usually not possible to detect enlargement of abdominal and pelvic lymph nodes by clinical examination. Many of these node groups may be delineated by lymphangiography. Following the injection of radiopaque oil into the lymphatic channels on the dorsum of the feet, lymph nodes in the inguinal, pelvic and para-aortic regions can be visualised radiologically (see Figure 10.11). Lymphangiograms are most frequently used to study patients with malignant lymphoma. If this diagnosis has been established by biopsy of accessible nodes or other involved tissues the choice of treatment depends upon knowledge of the anatomical extent or stage of the disease. As the iodised contrast medium is retained in the lymph nodes for several months repeated abdominal x-rays are often used to monitor the effects of treatment on the progression of the lymphoma. Involvement of the abdominal and pelvic nodes by metastatic carcinoma or their enlargement due to other causes, e.g. tuberculosis or other infections, connective tissue disorders, sarcoidosis, may also produce positive lymphangiograms. Although filling defects and node displacement are more often seen in nodal involvement by metastatic carcinoma, in most patients a reliable radiological distinction between the various causes is not possible.

Ultrasonography

This non-invasive technique may be useful in suspected lymphoma for determining whether an abdominal mass is solid or cystic and in detecting enlarged coeliac axis, retroperitoneal or pelvic lymph nodes.

Whole Body Computerised Axial Tomography (CAT Scan)

This is a valuable technique for detecting enlargement of lymph nodes or other organs in the abdominal or thoracic cavity and for monitoring their changes in size with therapy. It is, however, expensive and not widely available.

FURTHER READING

De Gruchy, C. (1978) *Clinical Haematology in Medical Practice* (Ed.) Penington, D., Rush, B. & Castaloli, P. Oxford: Blackwell.

Hardisty, R. M. & Weatherall, D. J. (1974) *Disorders of the Blood.* Oxford: Blackwell.

Hoffbrand, A. V. & Lewis, S. M. (1981) *Postgraduate Haematology.* London: Heinemann.

Williams, W. J., Beutler, E., Erslev, A. J. & Rundles, R. W. (1977) *Hematology.* 2nd edition. New York: McGraw-Hill.

Wintrobe, M. W. (1974) *Clinical Hematology.* 7th edition. Philadelphia: Lea and Febiger.

11 The Psychiatric Assessment

P. G. Campbell and G. F. M. Russell

Psychiatric assessment requires a systematic but flexible approach if it is to be performed confidently and reliably. The primary means of assessment is the *clinical interview*; the interviewer will thereby elicit a *psychiatric history* and examine the patient's *mental state*. An essential part of the skill of interviewing is the ability to establish, if possible, a relationship of *rapport* with the patient so that he can communicate freely. This will help to make the interview more informative and to prepare a sound basis for an alliance in further investigations and treatment should they be needed.

In any medical assessment the psychiatric dimension deserves attention. At the very simplest level this will mean giving every patient some opportunity to express himself openly about his anxieties and his perception of his difficulties. Psychological and social problems may emerge which will affect his capacity to cooperate in investigations or to gain maximum relief from treatment of physical disease. His symptoms may become recognisable, partially or entirely, as expressions of psychiatric disturbance. In Great Britain, conservative estimates suggest that about one in three patients who consult their general practitioners have significant psychological problems. Only about one in 20 of these will be referred to a psychiatrist. Many of them will present not with the major syndromes of psychiatric disorder but with a mixture of bodily and mental symptoms in a setting of personality weaknesses, social difficulties and stressful interpersonal relationships,

Such problems may present to the doctor in any speciality, either in the guise of bodily complaints requiring investigation or as complications of established physical pathology. A mother may present her child for treatment of some trivial complaint when it is really she who needs help with the problems of her daily life.

To be able to recognise and treat the many psychiatric disorders which should not require referral to a specialist, as well as to perform at least the first-line assessment of the rarer gross or complex disorders so that he can organise prompt and appropriate action, the doctor will need a technique of assessment which is readily adaptable to the presenting situation. With increasing experience he will become alert to verbal and non-verbal cues from the patient's behaviour which indicate the possibility of psychiatric disorder and the need for the provision of adequate time for a detailed enquiry. The approach outlined in this chapter is based on the belief that, just as the physical examination is most reliably mastered when learned as a comprehensive routine, so the psychiatric examination can best be learned by acquiring familiarity with a comprehensive structure.

AIMS OF ASSESSMENT

The clinician conducting a psychiatric assessment aims to build up a comprehensive longitudinal and cross-sectional picture of the patient's life and mental functioning. He will then be able to exclude significant abnormality or to formulate a provisional diagnosis in descriptive terms, elucidate possible pathogenetic and aetiological factors and decide on strategies of further investigation, management and treatment.

Each of these two aspects, the longitudinal and cross-sectional, incorporates many inter-related facets of the patient's life which can be listed under three major headings as *psychological, social* and *physical.*

Psychological. Subjective experiences, attitudes, fantasies, wishes. Behaviour.
Psychological functions, conventionally categorised as:
  1. cognitive: e.g. perception, thinking, learning, remembering.
  2. affective: e.g. feeling, emotion.
  3. conative: e.g. motivation, volition.

Intelligence.

Psychological development, formative learning experiences, educational attainment.

Premorbid personality (i.e. before illness).

Unconscious mental mechanisms and psychodynamics.

Social. Immediate social environment (family, occupation marriage, etc.), interactions with the people who compose it and events which affect it.

The wider social culture and subculture to which he belongs.

Physical. Genetic constitution.

Physiological functions and physical health.

Physical interventions with drugs etc. medically prescribed or self-administered.

The physical environment.

Psychological, social and physical factors will all need to be taken into account when any psychiatric problem is assessed.

SOURCES OF INFORMATION

The patient himself will be able to supply only a limited amount of the array of information required. For the assessment to be as comprehensive as possible, therefore, it will be necessary to obtain biographical data and details of the onset of illness from other informants, preferably with the patient's consent. The doctor or social worker may need to interview members of his family, friends or colleagues. Medical records of previous psychiatric or physical illness will need to be reviewed. Information from these sources will be supplemented as appropriate by nursing observations, special investigations including physical and psychological tests, occupational assessment and home-visiting.

Such detailed assessment will not be required in most cases. Usually an initial interview with the patient and perhaps a close relative or other informant and a physical examination will outline significant psychological, social and physical problems and their possible inter-relationships sufficiently clearly to enable a provisional formulation to be made.

The beginner in psychiatric assessment may be tempted to accept the patient's own account over-credulously, but experience will soon show how very misleading an impression may be gained if the information from others is not sought, either directly or with the aid of a social worker. In many cases, too, efforts to enlist the family's active support in treatment will be crucially important. In recent years an increasing interest in the role of family tensions and conflicts in the precipitation or exacerbation of psychiatric disorder in one or more family members has led to the development of techniques of family assessment and therapy, predominantly in child psychiatry.

MAJOR CATEGORIES OF DISORDER

Socially deviant individuals (or simply the people one fears or disapproves of) are often condemned in popular parlance as 'sick' or 'mad', but one should not equate deviations of behaviour from social norms with psychiatric illness. Although dividing lines between normality and psychiatric disorder and between different categories of disorder are at present often difficult to draw precisely, there are several practical guidelines which will prove helpful and which do not demand theoretical assumptions. Adherence to the classification of mental disorders contained in the International Classification of Diseases (ICD 9, 1978) is important for consistency in communication. Details of its application are explained in a glossary, *Mental Disorders: Glossary and Guide to their Classification* (W.H.O., 1978).

Psychiatric illness

Psychiatric illness, in the narrow sense of syndromes of psychosis and neurosis, should only be diagnosed if the patient has undergone a disabling change from his usual self by developing unequivocal signs and symptoms of illness, i.e. if morbid abnormalities of psychological or psychophysiological functions have appeared which cause concern to the patient or others by reason of their distressing effects. They are abnormalities not only in relation to statistical population norms but also *in relation to the patient's own norms of experience and behaviour.* Their form, severity and relative independence of the patient's volition cannot be wholly explained by alterations in his environment. Acute symptoms arising as a rapidly transient response to a situation of exceptional physical or emotional stress have been given a separate ICD classification as *acute reactions to stress.*

Categories of psychosis and neurosis. Illnesses due to recognised physical disease are categorised according to their identifiable organic pathology as the organic *dementias* and other *organic psychoses*. Other *psychoses* (schizophrenia, manic-depressive psychosis, paranoid states, etc.) and *neuroses* (anxiety, hysterical, phobic, obsessive—compulsive, depressive, etc.) are characterised in purely descriptive terms as syndromes according to the predominant symptoms and signs.

Personality disorders

Here the deviation is from statistical norms rather than individual ones. *Personality disorder* is diagnosed if the patient's abnormalities are deeply engrained features of an enduring maladaptive life-style and the degree of deviation is such as to cause suffering to the patient himself or to society at large. The term is preferable to the older and more ambiguous 'psychopathy'. Subcategories of personality disorder are named descriptively according to the predominant traits (cyclothymic, schizoid, obsessive—compulsive, hysterical, paranoid, etc.).

Disordered personalities may develop symptoms of neurosis or psychosis. If these amount to a distinct syndrome of illness, two diagnostic categories may be required, one for the illness and the other for the personality disorder.

Other disorders

Deviations from social norms form the basis for classification of the *sexual deviations* and *behaviour disorders of childhood*. Abnormal indulgence, psychological and physical dependence and harmful effects on the individual characterise *alcoholism* and *drug dependence*. Disorders with associated tissue damage or marked physiological dysfunction which appear to be precipitated, exacerbated or maintained by psychological upheavals constitute the *psychosomatic disorders*.

Mental subnormality

The Mental Health Act of 1959 defines subnormality as '. . . a state of arrested or incomplete development of mind . . . which includes subnormality of intelligence and is of a nature or degree which requires or is susceptible to medical treatment or other special care and training of the patient.' 'Severe subnormality' indicates subnormality of such a degree that the patient is, or will be, incapable of living an independent life or of guarding against serious exploitation.

Four categories of severity of subnormality are listed by ICD 9, differentiated by IQ levels (test unspecified) from 'mild' (IQ 50—70) down to 'profound' (IQ <20).

THE STATUS OF PSYCHIATRIC DIAGNOSIS

Compared with most medical diagnoses, psychiatric diagnoses may seem insubstantial and arbitrary, lacking known aetiological or pathophysiological significance in the individual patient and often limited to the descriptive syndromal level. Some outspoken critics of psychiatry deride the exercise as a misleading imitation of the method of physical medicine. Such criticism is a reminder of the dangers of treating psychiatric diagnoses in a reified way. It can too easily be forgotten that diagnosis is a name for a pattern of illness and not an all-pervading attribute of the ill person.

Clinical experience and research, however, show that psychiatric diagnoses serve a useful purpose to designate common syndromes of disorder with broad implications about likely course over time and responsiveness to different types of treatment. In addition they provide a necessary basis for statistical and research studies.

NEED FOR INDIVIDUAL AND MULTIFACTORIAL APPROACH

While psychiatric diagnosis will be one goal of psychiatric assessment, there are other goals which have equal or greater importance in elucidating what help the patient needs. These will demand close attention to the unique psychological, social and physical circumstances of the individual and his capacities and wishes. It will be necessary to determine exactly what aspects of his functioning are implicated in his difficulties, how these affect his ability to lead a fulfilling life and what opportunities his social situation affords for future assistance and support. The questions of *why* he has these difficulties and how their *meaning* should be interpreted are usually harder to answer and more conjectural. Theories abound, but ignorance and uncertainty have to be tolerated.

Although it is usually possible to identify precipitating, exacerbating or other contributory causes of disorder, explanations in terms of necessary or sufficient causes are seldom possible except perhaps where there is ascertainable physical disease. Psychiatrists adopt a multifactorial approach, recognising that psychiatric disorders may arise from complex interactions of psychological, social and physical factors. In this respect there is a broad consensus of opinion supported by research findings.

Some of these points may be illustrated by a clinical example.

CASE HISTORY A 44-year-old single woman of middle-class background had been working as a secretary before the onset of psychiatric illness. She was admitted to hospital under compulsory order after accosting a policeman in the street and offering him 'rectal sex'. On admission it emerged that she had recently taken up employment attached to a hotel as a call-girl specialising in anal intercourse, advertising herself as follows:

'Ex-model gives French lessons, backward students a speciality.'

When invited to comment after seeing a videotape of an assessment interview with her, a group of novice psychiatric nurses responded by immediately suggesting that her behaviour must be due to 'sexual frustration' or 'overwork'. Psychiatrists who assessed her were, by contrast, struck by the fact that she displayed primary delusions, a complex persecutory delusional system and lack of insight, believing she was the recipient of messages transmitted to her from a long-absent male friend through the medium of newspaper headlines and car number-plates which instructed her to offer rectal sex. In addition she believed that a former landlord was circulating obscene photos and articles about her.

The manner of development of these beliefs and the absence of other significant abnormalities led to agreement that the descriptive diagnosis was paranoid schizophrenia. She had been a rather shy and retiring person with limited social contacts before illness. There was no known family history of psychiatric disorder nor any obvious stresses which might have contributed to the insidious development of her delusions some months previously. Treatment consisted mainly of phenothiazine medication and hospital admission until her symptoms had receded and she was able to find accommodation and a job as a secretary. It was accurately predicted that if medication was maintained by continuing outpatient supervision her delusional beliefs would not seriously interfere with her life by determining her actions.

While it is true that the social unacceptability of this patient's behaviour brought her to medical notice, a diagnosis of psychiatric illness was made not on grounds of social deviance, but by reason of the *form* of the abnormalities of psychological function she displayed, which represented a very marked change from her normal self. Her illness took the form of paranoid delusions; their content was mainly erotic and sexual in nature. Form rather than content is the major basis for diagnosing different syndromes of illness. Content is likely to reflect the individual patient's life experiences. Descriptively the patient's illness was classified as paranoid schizophrenia, but the diagnosis leaves questions of pathogenesis and aetiology unanswered. It could conceivably have been brought about by psychological and environmental factors acting on a personality predisposed by genetic or other constitutional vulnerability. Similar symptoms might, however, have been precipitated by drug abuse, or they could be an atypical presentation of a physical disease such as cerebral neoplasm, an endocrine disorder or other lesions affecting cerebral function. Known physical precipitants such as these could be excluded by appropriate investigations. Further advances in knowledge may possibly demonstrate biochemical lesions or other neuropathological changes as underlying causes for such 'functional' illness.

Too often doctors are inclined to regard a psychiatric and a physical diagnosis as mutually exclusive, asking 'Are these symptoms due to physical or mental disorder?' Such a crudely dualistic approach ignores the fact that all mental events take place in a biological substrate and that mind—body interactions are exceedingly complex and largely obscure. Psychiatric and somatic illness frequently coexist. For example, a syndrome of depressive illness may be diagnosed and treated in a patient with serious or even terminal physical disease:

CASE HISTORY. A man of 56 with severe chronic bronchitis was admitted to hospital for the third time in respiratory and cardiac failure. Ten days after admission he was noted to be persistently tearful, terrified of dying and convinced there was nothing to live for. His physical prognosis did indeed seem very poor, but it was recognised that his mental state of overwhelming despair and terror combined with early morning waking, hopelessness and diurnal variation of mood was consistent with a diagnosis of depressive illness. Treatment with a tricyclic antidepressant was started and two weeks later, although his respiratory function was still grossly impaired, he was cheerful, talkative, eating and sleeping well, and fulsome in his expressions of gratitude for his treatment.

THE INTERVIEW

The Setting of the Interview

The setting in which a psychiatric interview is attempted can do much to determine its fruitfulness. Lack of privacy, noisy and uncongenial surroundings and obvious pressure of time distract the patient and make it harder for him to talk freely or cooperate in tests. It is wise if possible to see him alone initially before other informants are interviewed. Quiet, privacy and comfortable seating are essential requirements. A desk placed between interviewer and patient hinders free communication, so that if a desk is needed it is best to seat the patient at its side. Use of two easy chairs may encourage greater relaxation.

Starting the Interview

The interviewer, if not already known to the patient, should introduce himself and explain the reasons for the interview. The nature of any preliminary information available to him should be outlined briefly in terms that are unambiguous and that will not be unduly upsetting.

In general it may be said that the interviewer should aim to convey sincere interest, calm receptivity and understanding respect for the patient's views. Exaggerated bonhomie, excessive formality or casualness or any hint of disingenuousness will strike a false note, which even seriously ill patients may be quick to detect. It will be helpful to give the patient adequate opportunity to ask questions about the purpose of the interview and later about the interviewer's opinions as to what is wrong and what needs to be done. In this way it may be possible to win the patient's confidence or at least lessen his distrust, a problem which is often especially important when dealing with adolescent patients or those with paranoid disorders.

Directing the Interview

The course and duration of the interview will depend on the circumstances and the interviewer's preferences. It will be essential, however, to keep in mind a structured framework to which history and observations can be related in order to ensure comprehensiveness, ease of recording and communicability of findings.

In many cases it will be best to let the patient tell his own story of his current difficulties and his past life. The interviewer need intervene only to guide him into describing areas of biography he has not mentioned and to ask for clarification of uncertain points or further relevant details. Imposition of too organised a structure from the start will be inhibiting and will prevent the interviewer gaining valuable insights by observing the sequence, relative emphasis and significant omissions from the patient's spontaneous narrative.

Examination of the mental state starts from the moment of first contact with the patient. His speech and behaviour during the interaction with the interviewer will be evaluated in relation to what has been gleaned about his life history including his educational attainment, his personality before illness, his previous health and his present circumstances. More detailed enquiry to review symptoms, systems and mental functions can await the completion of an adequate outline of the history in the earlier stages of the interview.

Questions are often most freely answered if the interviewer proceeds from the general to the particular and from emotionally more neutral, factual and impersonal areas to more sensitive ones. Open-ended questions or suggestions are to be preferred early on to more direct questions which may constrain the patient to give a normalised, socially acceptable answer which he may be reluctant to correct later once he has committed himself to something less than the truth. 'Tell me about your marriage', for instance may evoke a reply quite different from the conventional affirmative elicited by 'Is your marriage happy?' The severely withdrawn and preoccupied patient may answer questions which do not trespass on his inner world of private fantasy, whereas questions about his recent behaviour and state of mind, if asked too soon before any contact has been made, may be met with grudging monosyllables or even total silence and apparent lack of response. Once talking, he may be gently drawn on to more personal matters.

With increasing expertise the interviewer will find it possible to weave his enquiries into a more natural flow of conversation so as to avoid disjointedness or the formality of interrogation. The art of good listening demands more than inert passivity: interjections such as 'mm', 'yes', 'I see', nods of assent or brief statements summarising what the patient has conveyed will communicate interest and encouragement. Tactful but firm control of the interview will be needed if the patient is over-talkative or digresses on irrelevancies.

If the patient is unable to provide a coherent history of his past life and present predicament, or is extremely suspicious or quickly tired, attention should be directed early on to elucidation of his mental state. This may be particularly necessary with elderly patients, for whom the help of another informant is indispensable in compiling a reliable history.

Focus of Observation

If he is to learn as much as possible from his assessment, the interviewer should strive to focus his attention in three major ways during his time with the patient:

The objective focus

He should attempt to gain an objective view of the patient's history and mental state so that his assessment is reliable and without bias. Corroborative evidence from other informants may be needed. Extensive research has shown that psychiatric assessment of the same patient by different trained observers can provide consistent results only if the assessors look for clearly ascertainable evidence and describe their findings in definable and standardised terms.

The empathic focus

He should try to understand the patient empathically as an individual by putting himself in the patient's shoes, so to speak, in order to see past events and current circumstances as the patient sees them. In this way he will encourage rapport and prevent breakdown of the interview and may see more deeply into the patient's experiences, difficulties and needs. The interviewer must, however, acknowledge the limitations of his empathy and not claim to understand more than is justified. It is a common error, for instance, to empathise with a depressed patient to the extent of accepting his view that his mood is warranted by his circumstances, thereby overlooking the likelihood that his current preoccupations may be a product of depression rather than its cause.

The interactional focus

He should try to be alert to the interactional processes between himself and the patient, both to learn more about the patient's mental state and personality, and also to recognise that some of the patient's behaviour may be an artificial and potentially misleading product of the interview or of the context in which it occurs. Development of the interviewer's ability to understand his own emotional responses may help him to see the patient more objectively and not to mistake his own needs for the patient's. If the patient makes him feel helpless and angry, for example, it is important that he understands that his reaction may reflect a lack of confidence in himself rather than a deficiency in the patient.

The importance of these three foci, which should be considered in any assessment, is particularly illustrated where antisocial or violent behaviour is the presenting problem.

CASE HISTORY. A diabetic man of 56 who had had a previous below-knee amputation terrified the nurses on his ward by trying to put his hand up their skirts and by responding even to friendly overtures with outbursts of rage, on one occasion throwing a tray of food at the nurse who had just handed it to him. Psychiatric assessment helped the nurses to accept that he was mentally disabled rather than 'mad' or 'bad'. *Objectively*, he was found to show marked suspiciousness and lability of mood and to be functioning at a moderately subnormal intellectual level. Life-long mild subnormality of intelligence and unsociable, paranoid personality traits had been exacerbated by superimposed cerebral damage due to arteriosclerosis. *Empathically*, one could understand his bewilderment in the hospital setting, his fear of losing his long struggle for independence and his feelings of sexual frustration. *Interactionally*, one could recognise that smiling at him was liable to be misinterpreted as mockery, thus precipitating his violent outbursts. To his demented and disinhibited mind, the proximity of attractive girls was tantamount to a sexual invitation.

THE HISTORY

The aim of the psychiatric history is to elicit information about the development and course of illness and to relate this to the context of the patient's past and present life, his strength and weaknesses of personality and his previous adjustments to stress. Major headings and a brief outline of the scope of each area of enquiry are indicated in the following scheme which forms the basic structure for recording (and recounting) the history.

Reason for referral

Complaints (if any)

As reported in the patient's own words.

Present illness

Problems experienced, severity and effects, mode and timing of development, situational relationships, accompaniments, course, variability, treatment already received. (Present illness may alternatively be recorded at the end of the history so that it can be seen against the background of other historical information.)

Family history

Father, mother and siblings — biographical details. Where brought up and by whom. Family history of mental disorder and psychiatric treatment. Family relationships and atmosphere. Separations, bereavements — dates and reaction.

Personal history

Early development — mother's pregnancy; birth, infancy, milestones.

Childhood health — including behaviour disorders, neurotic symptoms.

Schooling — schools attended, scholastic attainments. Interests. Relations with peers and teachers. Examinations.

Adolescence — changes in attitudes, relationships, behaviour.

Occupations — detailed history, including military service. Reasons for change. Satisfaction. Relationships. Ambitions. Dates and nature of most recent employment.

Sexual history — puberty, menarche, menstruation. Sexual education. Masturbation. Hetero- and homosexual experience, fantasies, inclinations. Sexual relationships. Satisfaction or difficulties. Contraception. Pregnancies.

Marital history — biographical details, occupation and health of spouse. Quality of relationship. Children.

Medical history — serious illnesses, operations, head injuries. Hospital admissions. Treatment.

Previous mental health — details of previous treated or untreated psychiatric disorders. Duration, precipitating factors. Treatment, efficacy and by whom.

Antisocial behaviour — delinquent or criminal behaviour. Convictions.

Drug use and abuse — alcohol, tobacco or other drugs of dependence. Hypnotics, tranquillisers, analgesics.

Current life situation and review of past year — housing, domestic relationships. Financial situation. Job opportunities. Social life. Recent conflicts, disappointments, bereavements or other changes. Recent physical health (system review, if appropriate). Contact and relationship with medical and social welfare agencies.

Personality before illness

1. Capacity for interpersonal relationships — ease, intimacy, social role.
2. Attitudes to self — strengths, weaknesses. Future ambitions.
3. Moral attitudes and standards.
4. Mood and temperament. Stability or variability.
5. Hobbies and leisure interests.
6. Fantasy life, day-dreams, dreams.
7. Reactions to stress, disappointment or frustrations.

Some attention to all areas indicated by the headings above will be required in any comprehensive assessment, but the relative emphasis allotted to each will depend on the nature of the presenting problem. The historian's task is not merely to amass data but is also to engage in an active process of exploration and abstraction, bringing the patient's life into both broad and narrow perspective in order to delineate meaningful patterns of development and change.

Before the history of the present illness is discussed in more detail further aspects of history taking warrant special attention:

Assessment of Premorbid Personality

The patient's premorbid personality is composed of the constellation of attitudinal, behavioural and physical characteristics which constitute his individuality as seen by others and by himself. He will inevitably be limited in his capacity to know or describe this. Illness may have brought about a personality change, or may have altered his perception of his personality before illness, so that information from others is essential. Self-deprecatory feelings resulting from his current mood-state may cause a depressed patient, for example, to describe his past life as being one of repeated failures, inadequacy and unhappiness. When well, his view of himself and his life-circumstances will be quite different, as others can confirm.

Evidence suggestive of abnormal personality or frank personality disorder may emerge from many areas of the history. Probable indicators of disorder include one or more of the following: recurrent failures and conflicts in interpersonal relationships, marked over-dependence on others, frequent changes of employment, repeated brushes with the law or other authorities, recurrent episodes of aggressive or impulsive behaviour, multiple drug abuse, repeated self-injury or overdoses, repeated medical or surgical treatment of unexplained physical symptoms, long-standing instability of mood, marked tendencies of perfectionism or other obsessional traits, excessive introspectiveness and aloofness, recurrent behavioural disorder or minor neurotic symptoms arising in response to the normal stresses of life.

Self-revelation

In contrast to investigation in the realm of somatic disease, where the doctor can expect the patient to tell him accurately where he feels any pain, the elucidation of psychological distress is often obscured by the patient's evasion, distortion or denial. He may hope that the doctor will somehow be able to heal his troubled mind without being told where, mentally, it hurts or what is really distressing him. He may hint at difficulties by offering bodily symptoms or may adopt other kinds of 'illness behaviour' in an attempt to mobilise help from his family or from other important people in his life. Sexual disorder, alcohol or other drug dependence, or other problems whose revelation the patient fears would bring censure and humiliation may remain partially or completely concealed for years. In addition, as is emphasised in psychoanalytic theory, there may be powerful unconscious mechanisms of defence which ward off anxiety and become manifest as 'resistance', the opposition to the uncovering of unconscious processes.

The interviewer, too, will find some topics easier to talk about than others. Practice will be needed before, for instance, he feels comfortable inquiring about details of the sexual history including masturbation and sexual fantasies. As in other areas where intimate personal details are asked about, plain speaking without recourse to vague euphemisms will help the patient to speak frankly and with a minimum of embarrassment, but it may well take time (and more than one interview) before the patient feels sufficiently at ease with the interviewer to talk freely.

The Current Social Situation

One aspect of the patient's life which requires careful assessment in every case is his current social situation, including accommodation, job opportunities and the quality of available social support. These factors may be equally or more important than the nature of his disorder in determining what can or should be done to help. Often, for instance, it is lack of family support, of suitable accommodation or of suitable supportive services in the community rather than the severity of illness which necessitates admission to psychiatric hospital and may hinder early discharge.

Careful charting of the year (or more) before onset of overt symptoms and comparison with previous years will often reveal evidence of premonitory changes in the patient's wellbeing which may be related to specific preceding events. The significance of these events as precipitating factors should not be overlooked.

The statistical relationship between life-events and subsequent psychiatric and physical morbidity is being explored in recent research which shows that liability to many kinds of 'functional' psychiatric disorder and also to physical illness may be increased after stressful events such as bereavement or a rapid accumulation of life-changes. By scoring the latter in terms of their commonly experienced degree of significance, Holmes, Rahe and others have shown that there is a relationship between the total score accruing over a given period and the subsequent liability to illness.

One must, however, recognise that the patient's attribution of causative significance to events which preceded illness may be mistaken. Distressing events such as marital strife may have been the consequence of incipient but as yet unrecognised illness rather than the trigger which helped to bring it on.

HISTORY OF PRESENT ILLNESS

Symptoms

Any psychological symptom, or any bodily complaint which is suspected of being precipitated or aggravated by psychological factors, can be explored systematically. The following outline will serve as a useful structure with the complaint of 'depression' used as an example.

Clarification of the symptom

What is the precise meaning that the patient is trying to convey?

The patient may amplify his complaint by the following statements: 'I feel I am in a dark endless tunnel', 'I weep for no reason or when someone talks to me kindly', 'I feel constantly as if there is a dark cloud over me'. Or he may actually mean something different: e.g. that he feels bored or easily irritated.

Severity of symptoms: effects on his daily life

The severity of the symptom may be assessed from the statements of the patient himself. They should be supplemented by the opinion of a close relative or friend: has his distress been outwardly evident? The effects on his daily life should be ascertained: has his work capacity been reduced? Have his personal relationships been impaired? Has he lost interest in leisure or intellectual activities?

The patient's wife may, for example, report that she has found him weeping, and that he has returned from work feeling exhausted. He may have become quarrelsome and difficult to live with. His hobbies may have been abandoned weeks before.

Time relationships

It is important to establish the date of onset of the psychological complaint, its rapidity of development, its constancy or variability (both during each day and from day to day). Has the symptom ever appeared in the past, and for how long?

A patient complaining of depression may indicate that it began insidiously three months previously, that at first it fluctuated in severity but that during the past month it reached a constant plateau of maximum and unabated severity. A bout of depression of similar or lesser severity might have occurred ten years previously, and lasted for six months with recovery occurring spontaneously over the course of three to four weeks.

Preceding events: current situation

It may be possible to elicit that the symptom in question comes and goes according to events or factors which can therefore be viewed as having some causal significance. Thus it may be found that the onset of the symptom was preceded by important events in the patient's life, a few weeks or days previously. Or its severity may be influenced by his current social situation or the quality of his personal relationships with key persons around him. Other variables — social, psychological, somatic or chemical in nature — may be found to determine the severity of the symptoms. Enquiries should also be made about the results of previous treatments or attempts at self-help.

For example, a patient's morbid depressive symptoms may have become evident a few weeks after the death of his spouse, or after losing his job. In the case of a woman, the depression may at first be evident only during the week preceding the onset of menstruation, to become more constant at a later date. The severity of the symptom may be found to fluctuate with the fortunes of his marriage or with his consumption of alcohol; the patient may say that he has sought relief of his current depression from alcohol. It may be learned that ten years previously, recovery from an earlier depressive episode had been accelerated by treatment with antidepressant drugs or with ECT.

Disturbances likely to be associated with the primary symptom

Knowledge of the nature of psychiatric disorders and increasing experience will lead the clinician to anticipate the likelihood of other symptoms or disturbances being present.

A depressed patient is likely to complain of sleeplessness and loss of appetite. He may lose interest in the future; he may express regret for previous events in his life or even blame himself; he may display an abnormal preoccupation with his bodily functions. These disturbances in various combinations are likely to express themselves in suicidal ideas or acts, which should be enquired into.

The patient's interpretation of symptoms (insight)

The patient's attitude to his symptom should be explored by asking such questions as: How do you explain the onset of the trouble? In what way do you think you may need help?

A depressed patient is likely to ascribe his feeling of sadness to a preceding misfortune; but he may come to his doctor reluctantly adding that the trouble is due to his own fault and that, in any case, he is beyond any help.

THE COURSE OF PSYCHIATRIC DISORDER

Determining the course of the patient's disorder is often helpful in diagnosis. The life-history should be scrutinised for previous episodes of illness, their nature, precipitants (if any), duration, response to treatment and extent of recovery. Alternatively or in addition, personality traits may be detected which have been accentuated from time to time to the extent of becoming trouble-some as symptoms. Sometimes a patient's history from early years will reveal a complicated succession of illnesses and symptoms; it will then be useful to construct a *life-chart*, comprising four columns:

1. The patient's *age*, from the date of birth.
2. All *psychiatric disorders*, with dates of onset, remission and treatment.
3. *Physical illness*, with dates.
4. *Personal events* in the patient's life.

By correlating the four columns one will be able to see at a glance the pattern of illnesses and possible relationships to personal events.

Differences between Personality Disorder and Psychiatric Illness

Reference has already been made to the distinction between psychiatric illness and personality disorder. The former initially reveals itself by the new occurrence of a syndrome with an identifiable onset, which may be acute over hours or days or gradually over weeks or months. The latter represents a virtually life-long abnormality of personality with a propensity to develop symptoms or behavioural disturbance at periods of stress; the disorder appears to have emerged during the patient's early years in childhood and adolescence without identifiable time of onset. There may be a tendency towards amelioration of the disorder with increasing age.

It is difficult to define the distinction in such a way that there is no area of overlap. The pattern of development of symptoms and their apparent relationship with the premorbid personality should be assessed in each individual case. In some patients the presenting problem can be seen clearly as an exaggeration of existing personality traits rather than a syndrome of illness.

CASE HISTORY. A 30-year-old engineer was suspected of suffering from schizo-phrenia because he made unprovoked attacks on his wife during the later stages of her first pregnancy, on one occasion punching her in the stomach. Before the delivery he also attacked a nurse in the obstetric hospital after she had indignantly refused his attempt to bribe her to 'get rid of' the child as soon as it was born. When admitted to a psychiatric hospital he readily disclosed that after learning of his wife's pregnancy he had had fantasies of killing his child, and had entertained visual images of hitting the baby's head with a hammer until blood spurted. On closer study of his early history it became clear that the patient's eccentricities were long-standing and probably related to an unusual and deprived childhood. Both parents had died during his infancy. Brought up by elderly grandparents, he led a lonely, restricted life. In adolescence and after, he would attack his grandmother when he lost his patience with her, for example by knocking away her crutches. He hated uncertainties and was rigidly meticulous and fastidious about cleanliness and orderliness. His wife's pregnancy conjured up for him a world disrupted by a slobbering, vomiting, nappy-soiling infant.

This information enabled his recent disturbances to be seen as severe exaggerations of long-established personality traits. There was no new syndrome of illness and no specific symptoms indicative of schizophrenia. After psychological treatment he came to accept his child and settled back into his previous eccentric personality.

In other patients neurotic symptoms occur which do amount to a named syndrome of illness but which are consistent with previous episodes of symptoms in response to stressful life-events. Each time they may recur in similar or closely related form, for example, as described in the following.

CASE HISTORIES. A young married housewife developed agorophobia: she was unable to leave the house unaccompanied and was terrified of crowded shops and of travelling on buses. She had always been of a rather anxious, dependent personality and at the age of 10 she had had an episode of school-refusal on moving to a new district.

A middle-aged man developed persistent hypochondriacal complaints with great concern about his bowel function and digestion. In adolescence he had had a period of undiagnosed 'indigestion' about the time when his parents were reunited after a brief separation. He had a long-standing interest in athletics and keep-fit activities and seemed to have been unduly concerned with his bodily functions since his 'teens.

A patient's vulnerability to develop recurrent neurotic disorders usually betrays itself early in life. This accounts for the maxim that hysterical symptoms of neurotic origin do not occur for the first time in middle age or beyond: there will have been previous hysterical episodes or anxiety symptoms at times of personal stress. If this is not the case, 'hysterical' symptoms at this age should strongly be suspected of arising from organic disease or depressive illness.

The Time-Course of Psychiatric Illnesses

Limited duration and full recovery

Acute illness. A sudden onset over hours or days, with a profound change in behaviour and mental state followed by complete recovery within one or more weeks is typical of *acute confusional states* due to toxic, infective or metabolic interference with cerebral function. *Acute atypical psychosis*, without ascertainable physical aetiology, is rarer, but may also run a short self-limited course.

More prolonged illnesses. A more insidious onset and a duration of weeks or months is typical of *affective disorder* (depression or mania). Before the introduction of modern treatment methods, accounts of affective illness such as involutional melancholia lasting as long as two to three years were common, but again recovery was complete. Even in the elderly a complete remission is to be expected from depressive illness so long as it is not complicated by physical disease of the brain. The course of most *neuroses* is highly variable, with a tendency towards partial or complete remission, but there may be a chronic or fluctuating course. Psychiatric illnesses which can last as long as three to five (or even more) years but can still be followed by complete recovery include *obsessional neurosis* and *anorexia nervosa*; partial recovery is also common.

Recurrent and cyclical psychiatric illnesses

Affective disorders. Depressive and manic illnesses tend to recur, but with full recovery between each episode. Depression may recur each time or there may be alternation, usually irregular, between depression and mania in the 'bipolar' type of manic-depressive illness. The frequency of recurrence is extremely variable, ranging from decades of intervening good health at one extreme, to rapid alternations of mood state lasting weeks or even only days without intervening stability.

Schizophrenic illnesses. These may recur as acute episodes with or without intervening deterioration, but there is usually likely to be evidence of residual continuing disability in between acute episodes, in contrast to affective disorders. The very rare form, *periodic catatonia*, shows a more or less regular and frequent alternation between states of excitement or stupor and normality.

As already mentioned, *neuroses* may follow an intermittent course with recurrent episodes of disturbance, usually precipitated by physical or emotional stress. Recurrent psychiatric illnesses with acute episodes may also result from persistence of an *underlying organic disease* (e.g. porphyria) or from continuing indulgence in a *toxic substance* (e.g. alcohol, barbiturates, amphetamines or other drugs).

Prolonged illnesses with a deteriorating course

Affecting all mental functions including memory and intellect. A progressive downhill course characterises various *organic dementias*, the rapidity and pattern of dementia depending on the nature of the underlying cerebral disease. The onset of dementia is usually insidious but an acute onset may occur (e.g. following head injury, a subdural haematoma, a cerebrovascular accident or encephalitis). Progression is often slow and relentless, e.g. senile dementia, Alzheimer's disease, Huntington's chorea) or it may show fluctuations, with periods of greater mental clarity or of acute confusion leading to stepwise deterioration (e.g. in cerebral arteriosclerosis), or it may be rapidly fatal (e.g. cerebral tumours). Occasionally a dementia can be arrested through withdrawal of a responsible agent (e.g. alcohol) or as a result of treatment (e.g. for neurosyphilis).

Affecting principally volition, initiative and emotional life. The personality may deteriorate in such a way as to result in withdrawal from social contacts and responsibilities, loss of initiative and drive, shallowness and inappropriateness of emotional response and incoherent thinking. These are features of the gravest forms of *schizophrenia.* Such progression may occur slowly over several years, fostered perhaps by the harmful effects of institutional life, or it may occur following successive episodes of acute illness. With modern treatment and active policies of rehabilitation, however, a severely deteriorating course should be more rarely seen than formerly. The personality changes, too, are not necessarily irreversible.

Prolonged disability without progression or fluctuation

Persistent intellectual impairment or change of personality without ensuing deterioration or fluctuation may follow non-progressive cerebral damage resulting from such causes as trauma, encephalitis, anoxia or chemical intoxication. When damage is congenital or sustained in early life, some degree of mental subnormality is the likely outcome.

THE MENTAL STATE

To examine the mental state, the interviewer explores the patient's current psychological functioning by observing his behaviour in the interview, his spontaneous utterances and his responses to questions and tests.

The areas for assessment and the headings for record-making are outlined in Table 11.1. All areas require at least brief description and comment.

Table 11.1. *Areas for assessment.*

Appearance and general behaviour
  General description. Conscious level. Facial expression. Motor activity. Dress and hygiene. Observations by others.

Speech
  Flow, speed, quantity, spontaneity, coherence and relevance.

Mood (affect)
  Quality, severity, constancy, reactivity, appropriateness. Attitudes to self and to the future. (Vegetative functions: sleep, appetite, libido, excretion.)

Preoccupations and content of thought
  Including: suicidal ideas and intentions, obsessive—compulsive phenomena, hypochondriacal or other morbid ideas, delusions and misinterpretations.

Abnormal perceptions and sensations
  Hallucinations, illusions. Depersonalisation and derealisation.

Cognitive functions
  Consciousness, orientation, attention and concentration, memory, language functions, intelligence.

Insight and appraisal of illness

Observations and Inferences

Examination of the mental state demands a skilful technique, acquired only by practice. In this and other respects it is quite closely analogous to physical examination, for the examiner's aim in both is essentially the same: to elicit by clinical observation reliable and valid evidence of normal or abnormal function, and to be able to make inferences about its significance. But there are, of course, major differences. Evidence of mental dysfunction is primarily verbal and behavioural rather than somatic, and it only rarely has a demonstrable pathophysiological basis which can be elucidated or confirmed by physical investigations. The purely clinical method by which evidence of abnormal function is observed and interpreted is, therefore, of paramount importance.

The procedure can be regarded as consisting of three main stages or *levels*:

Level A (Observation)

Items of evidence are collected by observing behaviour and evaluating the content of speech.

Level B (First-order abstraction)

Symptoms and signs which can be assigned to definable categories (e.g. anxiety, delusions) and their degree of severity or fixity are inferred from the evidence, together with areas of unimpaired function.

Level C (Second-order abstraction)

The pattern of symptoms and signs, their relative diagnostic specificity and their compatibility with named syndromes of disorder are evaluated.

These levels of observation and abstraction can be illustrated by a brief example showing how one aspect of a patient's overt behaviour is assessed.

CASE EXAMPLE. The patient is a 46-year-old accountant. During the interview he frequently breaks off in mid-sentence to comment on noises audible to the interviewer outside the room, a door slamming, a babble of voices, a car back-firing. Questions often have to be repeated because instead of answering them the first time the patient remarks on details such as a picture on the wall, a hole in the interviewer's shoe, the pattern on the carpet. From the observations (Level A) the interviewer concludes that the patient shows marked *distractibility* (Level B) in that his attention appears to be unduly distractible by stimuli irrelevant to the task in hand. Further observations and abstractions are needed before the interviewer can decide at Level C whether the non-specific sign of distractibility is consistent in this patient with a syndrome such as an acute confusional state or other organic psychosis, hypomania or schizophrenia or whether it is of no morbid significance. Other evidence from the interview allows more judgements at Level B to be made: the patient displays pressure of talk, flight of ideas, grossly elevated mood, irritability, grandiose ideas and lack of insight. Orientation and memory appear unimpaired. The interviewer recognises these findings as having varying diagnostic weighting in his overall judgement at Level C that the mental state is suggestive of a manic illness. Additional evidence from the patient's history which shows the time-course of the disorder, together with negative findings on physical examination, need to be taken into account before a diagnosis of a syndrome, in this case a manic episode in a manic-depressive psychosis, is confirmed.

The reason for drawing attention to the logical steps in psychiatric examination is that each stage of abstraction is liable to error. Symptoms have to be carefully evaluated to determine their exact nature. The history has been primarily concerned with the patient's own account of them; the mental state examination is concerned more with the interviewer's detailed review of evidence of recent abnormal experiences and functioning and his opinion of its significance.

An example may be given which illustrates a common source of confusion when the levels of observation and abstraction are inadequately distinguished.

CASE EXAMPLE. A patient says *'I'm depressed'*. The interviewer may or may not accept this item of evidence (Level A) as a reliable datum contributing to an opinion that the patient has a *depressed mood* (Level B). Further observations and review of the history may lead him further to regard the depressed mood as part of a syndrome of *depressive illness*. He may, on the other hand, decide that it is consistent with one of the many other syndromes in which some degree of depressed mood may occur, or he may decide it reflects long-standing personality traits or that it is of no morbid significance. The important point is that the patient's statement alone does not lead inevitably to the conclusion that he has a significantly depressed mood in the psychiatric sense. He may be using the term in a personal way to describe, say, a transient feeling of dissatisfaction or boredom, or he may simply be trying to convey a certain impression. The converse is also important. Not uncommonly patients with depressed mood-states deny feeling depressed. Their depressed mood may be due to depressive illness.

The three levels described can be thought of as steps in a logical hierarchy which can be traversed inductively or deductively. In clinical practice, the interviewer can use his knowledge of symptoms and syndromes as well as the evidence already elicited to direct him into areas where evidence of disorder can be expected or significant discrimination made by the finding of normal function. Screening questions will be useful for excluding the likelihood of disorder or to point the way for more searching enquiry.

Some findings will be of much more specific diagnostic significance than others. If there is clouding of consciousness, organic cerebral dysfunction is strongly suggested and all other symptoms may be attributable to this cause. If cognitive function is intact but there are 'first-rank' symptoms of schizophrenia, all other symptoms may be of subordinate importance. If cognitive function is intact and there are no first-rank symptoms of schizophrenia but there is gross elevation or depression of mood, again all other symptoms may be subordinate and due to affective illness.

Classification

The study of classes of symptoms and signs into which individual manifestations of abnormal experience and behaviour (Level A) can be grouped according to their form constitutes the discipline of descriptive psychopathology or psychiatric *phenomenology* (Level B). Formulation of classes of diagnostic syndrome or disease according to phenomenological, aetiological or other criteria is the aim of psychiatric *nosology* (Level C).

Some General Rules about Technique

To categorise the phenomenological features of a patient's mental state (Level B), convincing evidence at Level A is needed, especially where subjective experiences, attitudes and intellectual functions are being assessed. A certain boldness of approach and some direct questioning will be required if the assessment is to be both accurate and adequately comprehensive. Queasiness about asking a patient if he can name the day and date, for example, or whether he has wished for death could have even fatal consequences if it contributed to overlooking, respectively, the temporal disorientation of an organic confusional state or the suicidal intentions of a depressive.

Practice in the detailed assessment of normal and disordered patients and, if possible, comparison of findings with those of a more experienced observer will be needed before a reliable threshold for recognition of abnormality can be established.

Recording Observations

The record of the mental state examination should provide a sufficiently objective account to enable the reader to form his own opinion as to the interpretation of findings. A representative sample of the evidence (Level A) as well as the interviewer's opinions about it (Levels B and C) is needed, so that it will be helpful to record a sample of the patient's talk as well as important questions and answers verbatim. Evidence is best recorded in straightforward descriptive language rather than abstract jargon. Over-used words such as the following, which now convey almost negligible information, are best avoided: disturbed, confused, aggressive, bizarre, regressed, acting-out, attention-seeking, uncooperative, hysterical. It is not enough to record that the patient is 'suicidal' or 'depressed'; evidence of the degree of severity and persistence of such feelings is crucial. A common mistake in recounting a psychiatric assessment is to include the interviewer's opinions and observations while relating the history; they should await the presentation of the mental state.

Signs and Symptoms Elicited by Examination of the Mental State

Appearance and general behaviour

The interviewer's aim should be to record a graphic description of the patient's appearance and his general behaviour in the interview and outside it. His demeanour, comportment, style of dress and attitude towards the interviewer (and towards accompanying relatives or other patients and staff) may convey important clues about his personality, life-style and illness.

Gross abnormalities such as violent, embarrassing, incongruous and disinhibited behaviour will be noted. Other gross evidence of disorder may appear as follows.

Conscious level. The level of consciousness and alertness to external stimuli may be impaired by organic cerebral dysfunction. *Clouding of consciousness* of any degree or duration is a sign of pre-eminent importance; it is the hallmark of acute organic confusional states and an organic cause must be presumed unless it is proved otherwise. Fluctuation of consciousness during the interview or during the day and the occurrence of lucid intervals should be particularly noted; they suggest organic cerebral disease and may be especially striking with subdural haematoma. *Stupor* in psychiatric terminology denotes apparent inaccessibility and lack of spontaneous speech with, however, preservation of conscious alertness. Causes include depression, schizophrenia, hysterical states and organic cerebral dysfunction. *Akinetic mutism* describes stupor (in the psychiatric sense) due to an organic cause.

Facial expression. Many patients with severe psychiatric illness, particularly depression and organic states, look generally unwell. Tension and misery or elation and euphoria are often immediately recognisable, as may be other affective states such as anxiety, perplexity or suspiciousness. In depressive illness there may be a persistent frown. Even the severely depressed patient may smile, but the smile is likely to lack warmth or conviction.

Motor activity. Anxiety may be evident in sweaty palms on hand-shake, fine tremor of hands and motor restlessness and fidgeting. Thyrotoxicosis may need to be included in the differential diagnosis; anxiety states are much commoner.

Severe restlessness is a feature of *agitation*, a term which encompasses motor hyperactivity combined with persistent feelings of inner tension and discomfort. It may be marked in depressive illness, especially in the older patient, in other affective disturbances and in organic psychoses and states of drug intoxication and withdrawal. Increased motor activity is the rule in manic illness. *Psychomotor retardation*, a general slowing of motor activity, speech and cerebration, may occur in severe depression, in schizophrenia and some cases of organic cerebral disease, including myxoedema. Retardation may co-exist with agitation in depressive illness.

Tics (repetitive actions such as blinking or facial grimacing) and other abnormalities of movement, posture and gait should be noted.

Motor abnormalities are prominent in catatonic schizophrenia, which is now seldom seen since the introduction of modern physical treatments. *Catatonic phenomena* include negativism (the patient does the opposite of what he is being asked), waxy flexibility (a characteristic rigidity combined with prolonged holding of abnormal postures in response to passive movement by the examiner), automatic obedience, 'mitgehen' (the patient allows himself to be moved into strange postures by very light pressure), ambitendency (the patient moves as if in response to conflicting impulses e.g. to shake a proffered hand and to withdraw), echopraxia and other echo phenomena, stereotypies (purposeless repetitive movements), mannerisms (odd stylised behaviours with special personal meaning or significance), stupors and excitements. Similar phenomena can be due to organic cerebral disease.

Dress and hygiene. Self-neglect with slovenliness of dress, unkempt hair and neglect of shaving and personal hygiene may be associated with social deprivation, vagrancy, or advanced chronic alcoholism. When occurring in spite of ample opportunities for self-care, it may be indicative of serious illness such as depressive psychosis, schizophrenia and organic dementias. Exhibitionistic and provocative dress, carefully studied for effect, indicate the love of self-display which may be found in histrionic personalities. When of recent onset and grotesquely flamboyant it may result from mania or other states of excitement.

Other visible clues. Non-verbal communications such as eye-contact, facial expression, gestures and posture may convey nuances of attitude and feeling. The interviewer's 'wide-angled lens' will take in such diverse evidence as old scars of self-injury at the wrist and elsewhere, injection marks of 'main-line' drug abuse, tattoos, the reddened abraded hands of the compulsive hand-washer, loosened clothing from recent weight loss.

Observation by others. Observations of the patient's interactions with other people and his way of spending the day may be included under the heading of general behaviour. Behaviour patterns may reflect enduring personality traits, interests or abilities or they may reflect recent illness. The evidence of other witnesses may also be of particular value in recognising psychotic symptoms, suicidal actions, obsessional rituals, phobic avoidance, alcohol or drug abuse, angry outbursts or other antisocial behaviour and evidence suggestive of organic cerebral disease such as impaired consciousness, disorientation, forgetfulness, dysphasia, fits or incontinence.

Speech

In this section the focus is not on what the patient talks about but on formal aspects of his speech including its *flow, speed, quantity, spontaneity, coherence* and *relevance* to the point at issue. Where disorder of the formal organisation of speech is suspected, an illustrative verbal sample is essential.

Increased flow of speech, the rate and quantity being increased as if under pressure, constitutes *pressure of talk*. It is quite likely to occur with manic elevation of mood, in schizophrenia, or in any state of normal or morbid excitement or agitation. Limited or absent flow of spontaneous speech with marked delay, pausing and slowness in response to questions may result from psychomotor retardation. Such slowness of speech should be distinguished from simple restriction of speech without slowness.

The restricted accessibility of vocabulary or of language functions which characterise the *dysphasias* and the paraphasias are important signs of organic cerebral disease or dysfunction. *Perseveration* (persistence or repetition of a response after it has ceased to be relevant) is suggestive of organic disease; *echolalia* (repetition by the patient of the interviewer's words with similar inflection and tone of voice) may occur in schizophrenia and organic states.

Muttering, whispering or other interjections which are not directed to the interviewer should be noted. They may be a response to hallucinations or an expression of internal preoccupations. Mouthing, lip-smacking or other such abnormal movements may be manifestations of *tardive dyskinesia*, a common complication of prolonged treatment with phenothiazines or other neuroleptic drugs. *Dysarthria* may be associated with dementias (e.g. neurosyphilis, arteriosclerosis, Huntington's chorea, multiple sclerosis) or parkinsonism. Slurring of speech may be due to alcohol, barbiturates, or other drug intoxication. In hysterial aphonia, the patient loses his voice and may only whisper: phonation on coughing is normal (unlike aphonia due to laryngeal paralysis).

In many cases of schizophrenia there is impairment of the ability to communicate coherently and, by inference, an underlying disorder of thinking processes. These abnormalities are subsumed under the title *schizophrenic formal thought disorder.*

When mild, schizophrenic thought disorder may be difficult to distinguish from the vaguely allusive and inconsequential speech patterns favoured, for example, by youth-cultures such as the hippie culture. When it is more marked, speech becomes disjointed, with sudden inexplicable 'Knight's Move' changes of topic and increasing obscurity of meaning, though it may still convey a general feeling tone of sometimes strangely poetic quality. The patient introduces ideas without attention to the listener's capacities for comprehension and appears to be unaware of the impaired communication-value of what he says. Gross degrees lead to incoherence of speech. Pitch and tone of voice, grammar and syntax may become irregular and the disorder may also be evident in writings. Formal thought disorder may be a feature of chronic schizophrenia, but it initially appears only during acute exacerbations of illness and then perhaps only when the patient is emotionally aroused (e.g. when talking about abnormal experiences and preoccupations) or when discussing abstract concepts (e.g. when asked to explain the abstract meaning of a proverb or the difference between a child and a dwarf, or a ball and an orange). In some cases there is a striking *poverty* of speech-content; although the patient may talk fairly readily, his content of speech is vague, repetitive and impoverished of meaning or elaboration of ideas. *Neologisms* (entirely new words or familiar words modified in novel ways) or *thought-blocking* (sudden interruption of speech with loss of the thread of conversation) may be associated features.

A single example would be inadequate to convey all the features described as manifestations of schizophrenic thought disorder, but the following illustrates a moderately severe disorder.

CASE HISTORY. The patient was a 29-year-old woman with an illness of 12 years' duration. She was trying to explain her difficulties with acquaintances and with her parents:

'I get morbid thoughts. People don't like me. Sister Brown thought I was a goody goody. The other Sister is like Dame Sheldon. She does not like me. Like Noël. I don't see him now. Like Tess. Tess does not like me. I listen to 'La Boutique Fantasque' — very changeable, makes me worked up, I like ballet. It's very sad. When mother died (the mother was alive), she played Mozart. She might die. Father says she's very frail. She does not stand up to my father. This man in the job — he's a pilot. I suggested to my mother she might marry him — he is married. She's a very capable woman (his wife). He's a bit frightened of her. Do you think he is?'

At this point the interviewer interjected that he did not known whom she was talking about.

'But you might know him. He flies. I've always wanted to fly an aeroplane — float away. Everything is very psychological with my mother. I had drinks because of this boy. I don't think it was the drinks. Do you think it was the drinks?'

Another major type of thought disorder is *flight of ideas*, most characteristically associated with elevation of mood and pressure of talk in mania, but also occasionally observed in schizophrenia or states of excitement from organic causes and intoxications. Speech wanders far from its starting point by jumping from topic to topic, but the connections between one idea and the next are usually discernible rather than obscure as in schizophrenic thought disorder. Elements are introduced because the patient is distracted by stimuli around him. One idea reminds him of another, often according to familiar associations or the sound of words *(clang associations)*. Rhymes and puns are frequent. Flight of ideas may occasionally co-exist with schizophrenic thought disorder; sometimes differentiation of the two may be difficult.

Severe incoherence of speech may result not only from gross degrees of schizophrenic thought disorder or flight of ideas but also from organic cerebral disease.

Hesitation of speech, discursiveness, circumstantiality (taking a long way round to the point, with much unnecessary detail) and prolixity (saying much to mean little) are worth comment. In *talking past the point* the patient answers irrelevantly or inappropriately. In the variety known as 'vorbeireden' or *approximate answers*, the patient gives answers which are absurdly wrong in a way that suggests that he knows the correct answer (e.g. 'How many legs has a dog?' A. 'Five.' Q. 'What do two and two make?' A. 'Three.') It may occur in a variety of conditions including organic and schizophrenic psychoses as well as in hysterical pseudo-dementia and malingering.

Mood (affect)

The patient's mood is inferred from his description of the feeling state of his emotions and from other observations made by the interviewer. The subjective aspect will be elicited by asking him how he feels in himself or in his spirits and by finding out the emotional colouring and content of his preoccupations, his attitudes towards himself, his circumstances and his future, and his reports of his physical sensations and health. Observations will be made of his appearance, general behaviour, social interactions, demeanour, motor activity, posture, cognitive abilities and biological functions such as appetite, sleep and libido.

Assessment should be made not only of the *quality* and severity of the patient's prevailing mood, but also of its *constancy* during the interview and throughout the day, its *reactivity* to influences within the interview and outside it and its *appropriateness* to what is being talked about. Evidence that the patient is under- or over-stating his account of his feelings should be carefully evaluated (e.g. the 'smiling' depressive may deny depressed feelings but the interviewer will be able to elicit plentiful evidence of severe depressive mood, with attendant suicidal risk).

Besides noting the patient's mood in relation to the continuum from the 'high' of extreme elation to the 'low' of extreme depression, the interviewer should record evidence of other aspects of the mood-state, including anxiety, irritability, suspiciousness, resentment, hostility, perplexity.

In *depression*, the subjective mood is usually miserable and despondent, but many variants may occur, which patients differ in their capacity to describe. Feelings of unnameable dysphoria, of not being right, of feeling 'down', despair for the future, desire to cry, resentment, anger directed against the self or others may be accompanying or predominant features. Gloomy or morbid pre-occupations hold sway, with thoughts of suicide or desire for oblivion. In more severe cases persistent feelings of futility, guilt and self-blame become marked. The patient may feel physically unwell with loss of drive, initiative and ability to make decisions. Nothing brings pleasure and every activity becomes an exhausting chore. Social contact is avoided or there may be an increase in dependent and demanding behaviour. Concentration on outside events becomes increasingly difficult as the patient becomes more and more absorbed in an inner state of unrelieved tension, despair and self-recrimination or of feelings of being slowed down, empty of feeling, or even dead inside. There may be unpleasant physical sensations and symptoms such as headache, dryness of the mouth, tinnitus and constipation; concern about physical health commonly increases. In depression of any severity sleep is likely to be disturbed and there may be changes of appetite and libido (see below). Diurnal variation of mood, with depression worst in the morning, is characteristic of severe cases. Retardation or agitation may become marked. Insight may be lost. Depressive delusions or hallucinations may occur. Cognitive impairment may become apparent.

In *elevation of mood* or *elation* the subjective mood is buoyant and euphoric. The patient feels extraordinarily full of well-being, energy and ability. Thinking is experienced as speeded up. There may be initially an increased capacity for pleasure with a hectic abundance of new ideas and new enthusiasms, lavish spending of money, intensified sexual drive and diminished need for sleep or rest. With increasing elation, jocular good-humour gives way to intolerance and the patient becomes more assertive, disinhibited and hostile and irritable if thwarted. Insight is often lacking; the patient denies illness and may strenuously resist efforts to persuade him to accept treatment. Other people find his behaviour increasingly difficult to tolerate. He becomes distractible and unable to sustain attention and concentration. The elation may progress towards restless excitement, flight of ideas and pressure of talk. His self-image becomes more extravagantly self-congratulatory, and there may be grandiose ideas, delusions or hallucinations. In extreme elation, wild excitement occurs with incoherence of speech, gross hyperactivity and risk of ensuing exhaustion and collapse.

Enduring depression may occur in personality disorder, particularly of cyclothymic type in which alternation with elation of varying duration may occur. Apart from its occurrence in depressive illness a marked degree of depressive mood-change may accompany any neurotic or psychotic illness including acute and chronic organic syndromes, other physical illnesses, alcoholism or as a side-effect of medication (e.g. reserpine, methyldopa). Elation of mood may occur in cyclothymic personalities and as a response to alcohol and drugs (amphetamines, corticosteroids, cannabis and other hallucinogens) or it may be a transient sequel to relief of depressive illness following spontaneous remission or treatment with antidepressants or ECT. Marked and persistent degrees characterise hypomania and mania, occurring usually in the course of bipolar affective (manic-depressive) psychosis in which episodes of depressive illness also occur, or more rarely as an isolated or recurrent illness on its own without episodes of depression. Elevated mood may also occur in schizophrenia or schizo-affective psychosis or in organic cerebral disease. It has been regarded as characteristic of GPI and multiple sclerosis, in the former as grandiose delusions and in the latter as a fatuous euphoria, but in both these illnesses dementia is the commonest psychiatric disorder. Mixed-states of elation and depression may be seen in affective psychoses.

Anxiety. Many terms are available to describe nuances of the subjective feeling such as tension, apprehension, nervousness, consternation or, in the more severe cases, fear, panic, dread. Discomforting bodily symptoms, largely of autonomic nervous origin, are usually prominent and the subject may be more aware of these than of his inner feelings. This awareness can induce further alarm so that it may seem as if a vicious circle is established with positive feedback between subjective state and physiological changes rapidly producing a state of panic. Symptoms can include tightness in the chest and throat, a sense of difficulty in breathing, epigastric discomfort, nausea, vomiting, loss of appetite, palpitations (from tachycardia or extrasystoles), blushing, sweating, dizziness, tremor (perhaps with a fear of shaking visibly or of dropping things), weakness in the legs, headache, insomnia, dryness of the mouth, impotence or frigidity, urgency of micturition or defaecation. Overbreathing, by lowering the carbon dioxide content of the blood, can cause dizziness and lightheadedness which can progress to fainting or paraesthesiae and tetany.

Anxiety in response to stress or threat is a normal component of everyday life. Abnormal anxiety is experienced as excessive in degree and persistence, without recognisable cause and inappropriate to any stimuli. Anxiety-proneness may be a personality trait which becomes exaggerated to a degree which the patient feels is abnormal and disabling, perhaps in response to stressful life-events or increased responsibilities. Alternatively a patient who has not previously been anxiety-prone may develop a state of morbid anxiety. In anxiety neurosis anxiety is the predominant symptom, either severe, generalised and 'free-floating' or occurring mainly in the form of acute panic attacks, self-limiting episodes of overwhelming anxiety, often with acute fear of impending death. These are sometimes situation-specific or may be triggered off by incidents or mental imagery of an upsetting kind.

A *phobia* is a morbid fear which is disproportionate to the stimulus feared and leads to avoidance of the fear-inducing situation. Phobic anxiety, therefore, is situational and leads to avoidance, in contrast to non-situational 'free-floating' anxiety. Simple monosymptomatic phobias in adult life usually represent the continuance or recrudescence and exaggeration of normal childhood fears of small animals, heights, etc. Reinforced by the anxiety-reducing effects of avoidance they may become more generalised and handicapping. Social phobias are characterised by anxiety in social situations such as meeting new people or inter-acting with a group; avoidance results. In phobic anxiety state, or agoraphobia (literally 'fear of the market place') there is often a variety of phobias, such as of going out or of being alone in enclosed, open or crowded spaces, and of travelling in lifts, underground or on buses, together with a high level of 'free-floating' anxiety. Panic attacks may be frequent and there may be symptoms of depression, depersonalisation or obsessions. Such patients often have a history of anxious traits of personality but the onset of illness may be relatively acute. Other kinds of situational anxiety can occur or there may be morbid fears of death or disease.

Morbid anxiety may be an accompanying feature of any neurotic or psychotic disturbance, including organic cerebral syndromes, or can result from alcoholism or drug withdrawal. It is very commonly associated with depression and there has been debate whether anxiety states and depressive illness are distinct or whether they lie on a continuum with varying predominance of each.

Lability is the term used to describe exaggerated changeability of mood with marked reactivity to outside events or to the topic of conversation. Emotions are poorly sustained and sadness or tears may quickly change to gaiety and laughter when gloomy topics are changed to cheerful or humorous ones. It is normal at the extremes of life. Lability may be a striking feature of hysterical personality disorder. It is the commonest kind of emotional change seen in dementia when it may be so pronounced as to amount to 'emotional incontinence'. Related to this is the 'catastrophic reaction' which may be seen in dementing conditions whereby the patient reacts to stress such as a failure of a test of knowledge or memory with a sudden breakdown into acute distress, perhaps with tears or anger.

Suspiciousness may be a personality trait, often exaggerated by old age, and may be very marked in paranoid schizophrenia or other paranoid states and sometimes in dementias.

Perplexity may occur in a variety of minor psychiatric disorders but may be particularly evident in acute schizophrenia, organic confusional states or as a premonitory epileptic phenomenon.

Flattening or blunting of affect is a common accompaniment of severe and chronic schizophrenic illnesses. The patient seems to have lost normal emotional responsiveness and there is difficulty in making rapport with him. Since the term may be mistakenly taken as synonymous with a diagnosis of schizophrenia it should be used with extreme caution and then only if the abnormality is very marked and persistent. Milder degrees of apparent blunting may be noted in depression or organic states. A parkinsonian facies should be distinguished.

Incongruity of affect, whereby the patient's emotions seem grossly incongruous or inappropriate to his situation or to the topic of conversation, is also traditionally taken as synonymous with schizophrenia and similar caution is needed. It is most commonly manifest as a silly fatuousness in hebephrenic schizophrenia but other varieties may occur. Since it is an extremely subjective judgement it is of low diagnostic reliability.

Vegetative functions

This includes sleep, appetite, sexual performance and drive, excretion. Although this information strictly belongs to the history rather than to the mental state examination, it is useful to review here as part of the latter, particularly because of the help it may give in the recognition of affective disturbance.

Sleep. Difficulty in going to sleep or interrupted sleep and nightmares can be a product of any psychiatric disorder or states of anxiety and tension, including 'neurotic' depression. The pattern of sleep disturbance characteristic of severe or 'endogenous' depression is early morning waking and being unable to return to sleep. Although very common this pattern is not invariable. Diminished sleeping may also occur in states of excitement and mania. Much of the insomnia associated with demands for hypnotics represents drug withdrawal effect and is iatrogenic; any patients who regularly take a hypnotic for more than a few days will experience several days of increased difficulty in sleeping on withdrawal due to a rebound increase in REM (rapid eye movement) sleep, previously suppressed by the drug. Insomnia is the rule during withdrawal from heavy alcohol indulgence and is extreme in delirium tremens. Caffeine, amphetamine-like substances and monoamine oxidase inhibitors are among drugs which may prevent sleep.

Appetite and weight. Loss of appetite (anorexia) may result from any psychiatric disorder or from normal experiences of mental distress and anxiety. Resulting weight loss, sometimes marked, may occur in depressive illness; its occurrence and degree may be a useful index of the severity and persistence of illness. Some mildly depressed people eat for consolation and gain weight. Severe weight loss occurs in the syndrome of anorexia nervosa, as part of a diagnostic triad of selective refusal of food believed to be fattening, amenorrhoea (or corresponding endocrine changes and loss of sexual drive in males) and abnormal attitudes including fear of fatness, a resolute pursuit of thinness and denial of emaciation or illness. Obesity may reflect long-standing behavioural traits, but as a new development it may result from psychiatric illness, organic cerebral (and particularly hypothalamic) or other physical disease or medication with phenothiazines or tricyclic antidepressants. Compulsive over-eating may also be associated with anorexia nervosa.

Changes in sexual drive or performance. Loss or absence of sexual drive (libido) should be distinguished from failure of sexual performance such as impotence (failure to obtain or sustain an erection), premature ejaculation, frigidity, vaginismus. Both can result from psychiatric disorder. Libido is commonly diminished by depression or other serious disorder. Life-long lack of sexual drive may reflect a gonadal endocrine anomaly or chromosome abnormality. Impotence is most commonly the result of anxiety, but may be due to alcohol or other drug abuse, medication (such as thioridazine), psychiatric or physical illness. It is important to enquire whether the difficulty only occurs with a particular sexual partner. Recent stresses and difficulties in the sexual relationship should be explored as possible precipitants. Premature ejaculation is common in the sexually inexperienced, as is some difficulty in female responsiveness. Long-standing failures of performance may reflect personality problems. Delayed ejaculation or failure to achieve ejaculation may be due to anxiety factors involving fears of 'letting go' or can be caused by drugs (e.g. monoamine oxidase inhibitors). Heightened sexual drive may be a feature of mania. Intense preoccupation with sex and a variety of abnormal sexual sensations or delusions may occur in schizophrenia or less commonly in other psychoses. Sexual deviations such as self-exposure may result from dementing conditions or functional psychosis if they are a new phenomenon; much more usually they are the expression of long-standing personality problems.

Excretory functions. Constipation is a feature of severe depression, when food intake is reduced, but it may also occur or be a source of anxiety in other psychiatric disturbances and may be aggravated by drugs. In depression, the patient's anxiety may reflect heightened concern with bodily functions and in extreme cases there may be nihilistic delusions that the bowel is blocked. Bowel disturbance is frequently due to anxiety which appears to be an important factor in the 'irritable bowel' syndrome. Abnormal indulgence in laxatives may cause persistent diarrhoea and hypokalaemia. Urinary retention can be a hysterical symptom and is a not uncommon side-effect of antidepressant medication. Incontinence can occur in states of stupor (especially if catatonic or organic in origin). Its occurrence must raise the possibility of epilepsy or other organic disease. It may result from excessive night sedation, alcohol or drug abuse.

Preoccupations and content of thought

Here an account is needed of what is on the patient's mind, both in terms of the general focus of his preoccupations and, if possible, in terms of their specific content of ideas, images and fantasies. Preoccupations may be about the past, the present or the future. A depressed patient, for example, may be preoccupied about some long-past peccadillo, about recent loss or current adversity or about a hopeless outlook for the future.

Two brief examples may be given to illustrate the importance of eliciting the exact content of the patient's thoughts. Both concern women whose preoccupations centred on their relationship with their children and whose fears could not be influenced by discussion until their specific fantasies were known:

CASE HISTORIES. A woman of 24 having her first baby became very anxious that the infant would be born with diabetes. Her husband, whose injections of insulin she regularly administered, had been diabetic since his 'teens. Simple reassurance failed to relieve her, until it emerged that she had a horrifying image of having to stick large needles into a tiny, helpless baby.

A housewife aged 31 developed a virilising condition with amenorrhoea, deepening of the voice and growth of facial hair. She became depressed and seriously suicidal. Asked about the content of her thoughts she reluctantly admitted that she had become more irritable and had recently struck her four-year-old son when he was naughty. She had then developed a tormenting fantasy that she might turn into a man like her father, who had beaten her and sexually molested her when she was her son's age.

Much of the patient's fantasies may lie hidden from his full conscious awareness and repeated discussions will then be needed before he can formulate them in words. The content of his dreams and day-dreams may provide valuable pointers.

Suicidal ideas and intentions must be asked about. There is no need to fear putting thoughts into the patient's mind. It is often very helpful for the patient to be able to share ideas which he may be frightened he will put into effect and which he may feel are reprehensible or cowardly. The seriousness of any thoughts of self-injury, and the nature of any plans or preparations, must be carefully enquired about.

Obsessive—compulsive phenomena. Obsessions are a particular form of preoccupation. In psychiatry, the term has a technical meaning more restricted than in common parlance. Obsessions may be defined as: (1) *recurrent* (2) *thoughts, ideas, fears or impulses to action* which the subject (3) *tries to resist:* he experiences them as compelled, (4) as *arising from within his own mind* and as unpleasant, anxiety provoking and (5) *absurd*, i.e. alien to his personality.

If the obsession takes the form of a compulsion to perform actions which have to be done in a particular way or repeated again and again until they are 'right', such as checking or hand-washing, the behaviour is termed an *obsessional ritual.* Alternatively, obsessions may be purely mental phenomena; the term *obsessional rumination* has been used where the patient feels compelled to order his thoughts according to special rules or to solve a difficult mental problem. Several types of obsession may be experienced by one patient. The content is often concerned with fears of contamination (e.g. by dirt, germs, sexual secretions or excreta), fears of harming the self or others (e.g. with knives or scissors either deliberately or by negligence) or other aggressive, sexual or excretory themes.

The development of obsessional symptoms is the predominant change in obsessive—compulsive (or obsessional) neurosis; a variable degree of depression and other neurotic symptoms such as anxiety are common accompaniments. Arising usually before the age of 35, this illness may occur in people of ostensibly normal premorbid personality but often there have been pre-existing *obsessional personality traits*, such as checking tendencies, meticulousness, orderliness, perfectionism, stubbornness and resistance to change and a life-long tendency to indecisiveness. If such traits have caused distress, it is appropriate to diagnose *obsessive—compulsive personality disorder* (also called *anankastic* personality disorder).

The relationship between obsessions and depressive illness is complex. Obsessional symptoms can be a product of depressive illness; this should be suspected particularly if they occur for the first time in a patient past middle age. Patients with obsessional neurosis or obsessional personality may develop a syndrome of depressive illness; this can lead to an exacerbation of previous obsessional symptoms or traits. Obsessions very occasionally occur in schizophrenia. Transition of obsessions to delusions, the abnormal experiences becoming felt as imposed from outside by other agencies, is rare. Compulsive phenomena have been described in organic states, especially following encephalitis, but there are probably differences from neurotic obsessions, particularly in the absence of subjective resistance.

Delusions and misinterpretations. If evidence is obtained that the patient has misinterpreted events or experiences so that he entertains false ideas and beliefs, the interviewer should attempt to ascertain the following: (1) the content of the beliefs; (2) the manner of their development; (3) the degree of conviction with which they are held; (4) whether they are evident only from what the patient says or whether they have led to action; (5) their consistency with the patient's intelligence, education, culture and subculture and his normal beliefs and interests; (6) whether they have arisen as an explanation or elaboration of another abnormality such as a mood-change, hallucinations, etc.; (7) whether they are 'systematised' to the extent of being elaborated into a detailed network of interconnected beliefs.

A *delusion* is a false (and often strange and impossible) belief which is held with total conviction, is not susceptible to rational argument or any sort of disproof and is personal to the patient: it is out of keeping with his intelligence and education and is not shared by other members of his social culture. If the false belief is held with something less than total conviction, in that the patient can admit that other explanations are conceivable but unlikely, it may be appropriate to talk of a *partial delusion*.

A false *idea* can have a powerful hold on the patient but he is able to recognise it as mistaken and originating from within his own imagination. The term *over-valued idea* may be used for an idea which assumes overriding importance and is maintained with fervour, but which lacks the other qualities of a delusion (e.g. hypochondriacal ideas of bodily deformity or illness, political or religious ideas which dominate the patient's life).

In the case of a delusion it is the *form* of belief, that is to say its absolute degree of conviction, its lack of correlation with logical or substantial evidence and its inconsistency with other beliefs and actions of the patient, which make it appear morbid, rather than only its content.

Some idiosyncratic beliefs are normal within certain subcultures in a society (e.g. societies, religious sects, etc.) but are not shared by the society at large. Such beliefs may become delusionally elaborated as a result of psychiatric illness so that even other members of the subculture would regard them as abnormal. Some abnormal beliefs are common expressions of psychiatric disorder specific to certain cultures (e.g. the belief that the penis is being retracted into the abdomen in the syndrome of Koro). These types of belief are rated by Wing et al (1974) as *subculturally influenced delusions*.

Delusions are classified according to their mode of onset as primary or secondary and according to their content, which may relate to the environment, the body or the self. *Primary* delusions arise 'out of the blue' without being understandably derived from some other psychological phenomenon: events or images suddenly acquire a completely new personal significance for the patient. The false belief may arise by the instantaneous crystallisation, as it were, of a preceding *delusional mood*, wherein the patient has a belief that something mysterious is going on which may implicate him but which he cannot exactly pinpoint. Or it may appear suddenly (autochthonously) without preceding delusional mood.

CASE HISTORY. A woman of 61 went to her doctor because she was puzzled that something funny seemed to be happening to the food she was buying and she wondered if it might be poisoning her. When the doctor took her hand to feel her pulse she instantly knew that he was not really her doctor at all but 'Sir Henry Watson, president of the World Police Federation, wearing the mask of an elderly physician.'

Named varieties of primary delusion include *delusional perception* (normally perceived external events suddenly acquire a new significance), *delusional awareness* (a sudden conviction that extraordinary events are taking place somewhere), and *delusional imagination* or *memory* (a sudden new significance is perceived in internal mental images and memories).

Secondary delusions can be understood as explanations of other mental phenomena, as elaborations of primary delusions, or as consistent with an altered mood state. Their diagnostic significance is different from primary delusions. For example a man experiencing auditory hallucinations may develop the secondary delusion that there are hidden loudspeakers in the room; a severely guilt-ridden depressed patient may develop the conviction that he has committed a dreadful crime; a manic patient may believe he is immensely wealthy; a disoriented patient may believe the doctors are policemen.

Ideas of reference are said to exist when a person erroneously feels that other people take notice of him in public places or elsewhere. Such feelings are commonly part of ordinary self-consciousness, but they may occur in more severe form so that the subject feels that others laugh at him or are critical of him in some way. Ideas of reference may be marked in socially phobic and anxious people and in sensitive or paranoid personalities. Accompanied by feelings of guilt and of being blamed by others they occur in depressive illness. In all these instances the subject recognises that the ideas arise from within himself. This awareness is absent in *delusions of reference*; here the patient believes that events seen and heard in his environment, such as other people's actions, gestures, conversations or radio, television, newspapers or advertising hoardings, have a special meaning directed specifically at him. Delusions of reference may be primary or secondary, hostile or benign. A further extension of this kind of delusion is *delusional misinterpretation* or *misidentification* (in the terminology of Wing, Cooper and Sartorius, 1974) when the patient believes that situations have been specially created for the purpose of conveying a particular meaning or message to him.

Delusions are often *paranoid* in content. The word 'paranoid', derived from the Greek 'para nous' (beyond reason), has been used in different senses. In common parlance it has come to refer to unwarranted feelings of being persecuted and 'got at', or to the person who displays them. Such usage is common in psychiatry also, but the term has been used differently to describe delusions and syndromes of disorder (rather than people) in which the patient experiences himself as singled out as the object of special attention from others. The attention is commonly felt to be persecutory and hostile, or the patient may entertain false ideas or beliefs of grandeur or delusions related to litigation, love, hate, envy or the supernatural.

Persecutory ideas are common in a variety of disorders including personality disorders, the 'functional' psychoses, organic cerebral disorders and intoxications. Persecutory *delusions* are common in schizophrenia and other paranoid states, but may also occur in severe affective illness and in organic syndromes. The patient with schizophrenia (or paraphrenia) may believe he is being threatened or pursued, poisoned, subjected to experiments or otherwise victimised by people he knows or by alien forces which he may or may not be able to name. He may describe amazing plots against him whose object is to drive him insane, to kill him or otherwise to harm him. His delusions may implicate science-fiction-like equipment such as transmitters, rays, computers or occult and religious forces; much of this systematisation may be understandable as a secondary phenomenon aimed to explain other abnormal mental experiences. The patient with depressive illness may also experience himself as the object of unpleasant attention from others but here the persecutory ideas or delusions are consistent with the mood-state. The depressed patient is likely to believe that the hostility is justified by his guilt, whereas the patient with schizophrenic illness is likely to resent it as unwarranted and undeserved. The patient with mania may also feel that he is resented or persecuted by others. Persecutory ideas and delusions may be seen also in organic confusional states and other organic illnesses (e.g. hypothyroidism) along with other delusions or, more commonly, misinterpretations of external events. The beliefs are usually fleetingly held and variable and are not systematised or elaborated in detail.

Hypochondriacal delusions of bodily illness and deformity may occur in a similar variety of disorders. Some ideas of bodily deformity or disease are seen in relatively isolated form which may attain delusional intensity in people who often show features of severe personality disorder. Concern is commonly centred on facial features such as size or shape of nose or chin or secondary sexual characteristics such as body proportions, breasts or genitals. Plastic surgery or other operative intervention may be sought with persistence. In depressive illness there may be delusions of malignant or contagious disease or other serious illness. In schizophrenia there may be gross and extraordinary beliefs (for instance, a man insisted that his bones had been injured by radiation beamed on him by his enemies).

The recognition of delusion is always of serious import so that the term should not be used casually to describe all mistaken or over-valued ideas. Some sorts of content are of greater diagnostic significance than others. In schizophrenia for instance a great variety of delusions may be seen, both primary and secondary. Often the content is persecutory, but delusions can also be grandiose, religious, sexual, supernatural, etc; they may be terrifying, perplexing, comforting or apparently a matter for indifference. Apart from the types already mentioned there are some delusions whose occurrence in the absence of gross brain disease are likely to be diagnostic of schizophrenia so the following should be asked about if this diagnosis is suspected: *delusions of passivity* or *influence* (whereby the patient knows that his thoughts, impulses, movements or other actions are directly controlled not by his own will but by outside forces or agents), *thought insertion* (thoughts introduced into his mind which are not his own thoughts), *thought withdrawal* (thoughts are withdrawn from his mind by outside agencies, sometimes a subjective concomitant of thought-blocking), and *thought broadcasting* (an experience that the thoughts are transmitted to others and shared by them).

Delusions in affective illness are secondary to the mood change. In depression they relate to feelings of guilt, unworthiness, hopelessness and worry about health, so that there may be delusions of sin, poverty, physical disease or impending catastrophe. *Nihilistic* delusions in which there are beliefs that the body is dead or rotting in whole or part are included in the so-called Cotard syndrome associated with involutional melancholia, but delusions of nihilistic content can occur in patients at other ages than the involutional period. Belief that the patient has developed an odour offensive to others is also commonly a depressive phenomenon and may accompany other delusions of reference and of being blamed or accused by others.

A variety of false belief which deserves special mention is *morbid jealousy*. This may occur in apparently rather isolated form as an overvalued idea against a personality background with longstanding traits of jealous possessiveness or sexual insecurity. Alcohol indulgence is likely to exacerbate the jealousy. It may become delusional and may accompany other disorders including schizophrenia, affective illness, drug abuse and other organic states. The patient develops the belief that his spouse is unfaithful. He may press for a confession and seek evidence (often absurdly far-fetched) to support his conviction. The spouse's safety and life may be endangered.

Abnormal perceptions and sensations

Assessment of abnormal perceptions should include questions about the *sensory modality* in which they are experienced, their *content*, their *timing, frequency* and *duration*, their *location* (whether inside the mind or referred outside to the environment or the body), their *vividness* and degree of reality, the patient's *emotional response* to them, and the extent to which they are under his voluntary *control*. Any evidence from the patient's behaviour suggesting that he is experiencing abnormal perceptions during the interview should be noted.

Traditional categories probably oversimplify the variety of forms in which abnormal perceptions may occur, but they have been found adequate for ordinary clinical purposes.

Hallucinations and illusions. Hallucinations are false sensory perceptions without an external stimulus. *Illusions* are misperceptions of external stimuli (e.g. mishearing a sudden noise as a voice calling one's name). Both are involuntary. Hallucinations may be auditory, visual, olfactory, gustatory, tactile (haptic) or kinaesthetic, or they may be 'mixed', occurring in more than one modality simultaneously. True hallucinations are experienced as having the substantial external reality and vividness of ordinary perceptions. The term 'pseudohallucination' has been used where the perception is experienced as arising within the subject's mind, so that it lacks external substantiality. Even true hallucinations may in time be recognised by the patient as false perceptions.

Imagery refers to the experiencing of vivid mental images which lack the immediacy or substantiality of perceptions and which are under the conscious control of the will; i.e. the subject can switch them on or off. Eidetic imagery, the capacity to experience a vivid memory of visual scenes, is normal in children and can be strikingly well-developed. Histrionic personalities may recount dramatic descriptions of imagery such as seeing 'black clouds' hanging over them, or hearing 'something inside' that tells them to kill themselves; these experiences should be carefully distinguished from hallucinations.

Hallucinations occurring only when the subject is falling asleep or awaking (hypnagogic and hypnapompic hallucinations, respectively) are of no morbid significance. Normal subjects may possibly also hallucinate under conditions of extreme sensory deprivation.

The significance of morbid hallucinations is quite different according to whether consciousness is clear or clouded. Hallucinations in a setting of clear consciousness occur in schizophrenia, in amphetamine psychosis and alcoholic hallucinosis (rarely in affective illness). Hallucinations in a setting of clouded consciousness occur in the acute organic syndromes due to drug intoxication and other physical causes.

Hallucinations occur at some time in the majority of patients with schizophrenia and are most commonly auditory, though visual and all other kinds may occur. Most often the patient hears voices of one or more members of his family, God, or other people once known to him, and other mystical beings. Their source may not be recognised. Often the voices are persecutory, but they can be benign, helpful or humorous. They most commonly address the patient directly, calling to him, commenting on his actions, instructing, accusing or informing him, but there are three types of auditory hallucination which, although less common, are of much greater diagnostic significance. These are:

1. *Third-party* hallucinations; the patient hears two or more voices talking to each other or arguing, which refer to him in the third person.

2. *Running commentary:* the voice or voices keep up a continuous commentary on his actions.

3. *Thought echo* (écho de pensée, gedankenlautwerden); the patient hears his own thoughts spoken aloud or audibly repeated.

A fourth type of hallucination of diagnostic importance for schizophrenia is the so-called *somatic hallucination*, a kind of somaesthetic experience in which the patient feels sensations in his body which are imposed by some external force or agency (e.g. a man can feel electric rays boring into his skull, a woman complains of feeling a man's penis permanently inside her vagina). These abnormal perceptions, together with delusional perceptions, delusions of influence, thought insertion, thought withdrawal and thought broadcasting have been termed 'first-rank' symptoms of schizophrenia by Schneider.

Hallucinations may rarely occur in severe affective disorder. The content is usually consistent with the mood state. Hallucinations and illusions may be prominent in acute organic delirious illness (e.g. delirium tremens). They are most commonly auditory or visual but tactile and other forms may occur. Visual hallucinations suggest that the possibility of organic disease should be investigated with particular care.

Olfactory and gustatory hallucinations may occur in schizophrenia or organic disorder. Formication, a tactile hallucination of small animals crawling over the body, is particularly associated with cocaine intoxication but may occur in other toxic states. In amphetamine psychosis and alcoholic hallucinosis hallucinations occur in a setting of clear consciousness and are mainly auditory, though visual and other kinds may occur.

Depersonalisation and derealisation. Depersonalisation refers to a state in which the patient feels unreal and detached from himself, from his feelings or from his body. In trying to describe it, he may speak of feelings of artificiality and unnaturalness and of seeing himself as if from a distance. He may feel as if his body is not alive or no longer belongs to him. Derealisation often accompanies depersonalisation; here the patient experiences his surroundings and other people as unreal, artificial and perhaps colourless and lacking in vitality.

Many normal subjects describe having experienced mild transient forms of these symptoms. They can be associated with anxiety or depression and the symptoms may then be intense, persistent and so unpleasant as to lead to thoughts of suicide. They are especially prominent in what has been called the 'phobic-anxiety-depersonalisation' syndrome. They may be marked in some schizophrenic illnesses, particularly at onset, and can also result from intoxication with drugs such as the hallucinogens. They may occur as paroxysmal phenomena in epilepsy.

Other abnormalities of perception and sensation. Episodic abnormalities of perception and sensation are a striking feature of the psychomotor attacks of *temporal lobe epilepsy*. The aura commonly consists of strange visceral sensations, particularly of an uncomfortable feeling in the epigastrium rising upwards into the throat or of odd sensations in the head, the genitals, rectum and other parts of the body. Premonitory feelings of anxiety or irritability may occur, but occasionally the attacks give rise to pleasurable feelings which can be indescribably ecstatic. Depersonalisation or derealisation, changes in the perceived size of objects (macropsia and micropsia) or the loudness of sounds (macrusia or micrusia) may occur and occasionally the patient hallucinates smells or tastes. More complex hallucinatory experiences can occur in several modalities involving previous memories or imagined events. The déjà vu phenomenon, a feeling that the surroundings look familiar, or other feelings of strangeness or familiarity in sights, sounds or events may be intense. The attack may consist of an aura only or there may be observable changes in consciousness varying from fleeting dazedness or a brief 'absence' to more prolonged disturbance of consciousness associated with falling and perhaps a grand mal seizure. Movements such as chewing and lip-smacking, autonomic changes such as flushing or pallor, may be observed. Following the attack there is often a period of confusion, perhaps with dysphasia and sometimes the occurrence of auto-matisms, bits of apparently purposeful behaviour or speech for which the patient is amnesic.

Cognitive functions

Cognitive functions, including (1) *level of consciousness,* (2) *orientation*, (3) *attention and concentration*, (4) *memory*, (5) *language function* and (6) *general intelligence* should be assessed at least briefly in every patient. To acquire familiarity with the normal range of responses to the clinical tests in common use, as well as to avoid overlooking minor degrees of impairment which may be missed by a general appraisal, the interviewer is advised to examine all patients routinely for these functions.

A new development of cognitive impairments is characteristic of organic cerebral disorder, but it is important to be aware of the apparent disturbances of cognition which can result from severe 'functional' illness. In depressive illness, for example, particularly in elderly subjects, cognitive impairment may be severe enough to resemble a syndrome of dementia; this will improve as the patient recovers from his depression.

The patient with impaired intellectual functions is likely to tire quickly so the interviewer should proceed quickly to examining the mental state and cognitive functions. Precious time should not be lost on unfruitful attempts to elicit a detailed history. A friendly encouraging approach, with explanation of the tests and without pressing the patient unduly if he fails an item, will help to gain his co-operation and prevent 'catastrophic' reactions.

The scheme outlined below will serve as a screening guide. Answers to questions are best recorded verbatim.

Level of consciousness: Observe: Is the patient alert, responsive and fully in touch with his surroundings? Any drowsiness? Any fluctuation in consciousness?

Orientation for *time* and *place:* Ask the patient to name time of day, day of week, date, month and year. Ask 'Where are you?' 'Where is that?'

Attention and concentration (and calculating ability): Ask if any subjective difficulties in concentrating have been noted. Can he attend to the tests? Is he distractible? *Serial sevens* — ask the patient to take seven away from 100, again and again; record answers and time taken. Alternatively, ask him to repeat backwards the days of the week or the months of the year or ask him to spell 'world' backwards. *Simple arithmetic* — involving carrying over; e.g. 43 minus 19. *Digit span* — ask patient to repeat after interviewer numbers of increasing length forwards and backwards (normal: 7 forwards, 5 backwards).

Memory: Ask the patient if he has noted increased forgetfulness or any other subjective difficulties. The accuracy of his history should be checked, noting any gaps or inconsistencies. Note confabulation, and whether spontaneous. *Recall of recent events* — Ask patient how long he has been in hospital, how he came to be there, etc. and check from his admission notes. *Learning ability* — Give the patient a fictitious name and address to remember together with a colour and the name of a flower. Ask him to repeat them immediately to check comprehension and registration. If he fails, record number of repetitions necessary before he can accurately repeat them immediately. Test his capacity to memorise by asking him to recall the details after three to five minutes. Test with simpler material, e.g. interviewer's name, if he fails badly.

Language functions: Assess expressive speech and comprehension during interview. *Test for nominal dysphasia* by asking him to name a series of familiar and unfamiliar objects (e.g. parts of wristwatch).

Intelligence: Assess from history of educational attainment and level of occupation achieved and from observation of *verbal fluency* and *understanding of abstract concepts* (e.g. explain common proverbs or difference between dwarf and child). Test *general knowledge* (ask name of the Queen, her husband, children, the Prime Minister and her (or his) predecessor, the President of the USA, the capitals of six countries, the dates of the World Wars).

The tests above overlap to some extent in the functions they sample. Performance on tests of general knowledge, for example, will depend on memory, concentration and general intelligence as well as educational and cultural factors.

Disorientation. Evidence of *disorientation* is a sensitive indicator of organic dysfunction but depressive illness and acute schizophrenia can occasionally give the appearance of some degree of disorientation of time and perhaps place. The patient may be delusionally orientated in an inner world of psychotic fantasy as well as correctly orientated in relation to the external world.

CASE EXAMPLE. A patient with schizophrenia gave his age as 2, and said he had been in hospital for 402 years. Asked to explain this, he replied enigmatically, 'It's too old to talk for those that are elder — and I had apples, walking on the streets of Italy. Intermartial catfish.' Observation of his daily behaviour and further questioning confirmed that he was in fact correctly orientated in time and place.

Attention and concentration. Disturbances of these can result from fatigue, anxiety, depression, excitement, other affective disturbance, schizophrenia or organic disorders. Distractibility may be marked in mania, schizophrenia and organic states.

Memory. Disturbances of *memory* usually indicate an organic disorder though they may occasionally reflect 'functional' illness. Traditionally, memory is described as composed of four processes, perception, registration, retention and recall. Recent research, however, suggests that information is recorded transiently in an ultra-short-term memory store and then has to undergo 'consolidation' if it is to be retained for longer than a few seconds. Impaired perception and registration occurring as part of a confusional state due to cerebral insult such as trauma or intoxication will lead to anterograde or *post-traumatic amnesia* in which new memories cannot be retained. The duration of post-traumatic amnesia is a good measure of the severity of the brain injury. There is also likely to be inability to recall events prior to the insult and this *retrograde amnesia* may extend backwards in time to a variable degree, shrinking with recovery.

Organic cerebral disorder causes marked impairment of the ability to memorise new information as tested by ability to recall a name and address after an interval of a few minutes. Immediate memory, reflected by digit span or the immediate repetition of a given sentence, may be normal. The memorising deficit is seen in relatively specific form, accompanied by disorientation in time, in the dysmnesic syndrome of Korsakoff's psychosis. In the dementia syndromes the memory defects are harder to characterise because they are often overshadowed by the general deterioration of intellectual functions. Besides impairment of memorising ability, recall of previous events will be defective to variable degree, possibly with gaps and patchiness. Although, as in normal ageing, memory for the distant past often seems less impaired than for the more recent past (Ribot's law) there may also be progressive difficulty in recalling remote memories; eventually all memories, even of personal identity, are lost.

Memory is affected by emotional and other psychological factors. Inexplicable forgetting of names and other well-known information is a transient inconvenience of normal life. More disabling 'hysterical' or 'psychogenic' amnesias differ from amnesias due to ascertainable organic pathology in a number of ways, but it is important to note that elements of both can be present together. The memory loss may be selective for events of personal and perhaps embarrassing significance, hence appearing 'motivated'. There may be apparent loss of all memory of the past life or for personal identity in the absence of the gross intellectual deterioration which would accompany such findings in an organic dementia; memorising ability may be normal. There may be other inconsistencies, for example between what the patient can recall spontaneously and his performance on tests of memory whose aim he recognises; in these, he may show total failure even to recall information immediately. Unconscious 'dissociation' of memory is said to characterise hysterical amnesia, but an element of conscious malingering may be suspected. Clinical judgement may be inadequate, as in the case of other hysterical symptoms, to determine the relative preponderance of conscious and unconscious simulation. For example, Gunther Podola, who was accused of murdering a detective, claimed that he could offer no defence because he could recall almost nothing of his life before he was arrested. His plea of unfitness to plead on the grounds of hysterical amnesia was eventually rejected by the court; he was found guilty and hanged. Eminent psychiatrists appeared both for the defence and for the prosecution.

Fugues are states in which the patient wanders or carries on other apparently purposeful behaviour over a period of perhaps hours or days without being able to remember what he was doing or why. To other observers he may have appeared fully conscious during the fugue-state, or perhaps unusually preoccupied, with restricted awareness of his surroundings. Fugues can result from alcohol intoxication, other acute organic states, anxiety, suicidal depression or hysterical neurosis.

False memories. Confabulation denotes the giving of false descriptions of previous events to fill in gaps in memory. It has been regarded as characteristic of Korsakoff's psychosis, but it may also be seen in other organic disorders associated with memory impairment and temporal disorientation. It may be evident spontaneously or may be induced if the interviewer makes false suggestions about previous actions of the patient, upon which he elaborates.

Retrospective falsification of memory may be deliberately done for effect, but it may result involuntarily from emotional factors. In general, pleasant memories may be better recalled than unpleasant ones. The depressed patient may describe himself (falsely) as always inadequate and ineffectual; the patient with paranoid ideas may say that persecution started long before his initial complaints.

Intelligence. Information from the history will be important in forming an approximate clinical estimate of the patient's level of intelligence. Psychometric testing by Raven's Progressive Matrices and the Mill Hill Vocabulary Scale (which can be administered by the doctor) or the Wechsler Adult Intelligence Scale (which requires expert administration and scoring) will be required for more accurate testing and for assessment of recent changes or specific deficits. The results can, however, be vitiated if the patient is unable to co-operate or is in an abnormal mood-state. The tests may nevertheless be useful to provide a baseline for comparison with later testing and to provide at least a minimum estimate of IQ.

It must be remembered that the usual syndromes of psychiatric disorder occur in those with life-long subnormality of intelligence. The clinical picture may at first appear somewhat atypical unless it is recognised that the presentation may be unusually florid, perhaps with marked behavioural disorder and expression of symptoms in more concrete terms than would be found in the intellectually normal.

CASE HISTORY. A 19-year-old girl with an IQ of 67 became depressed after the death of a favourite dog. Besides more typical manifestations of a depressive illness was her repeated insistence that she saw blood and all her 'tubes' floating in her bathwater.

Further cognitive testing. More detailed testing will be indicated if the history suggests the possibility of organic disorder or if the screening tests already listed show abnormal or equivocal results.

Level of conscious awareness should be evaluated with particular care from observations inside and outside the interview. If the patient is seen always at one time of the day, for instance in the morning, he may be in a lucid state at that time and fluctuations of consciousness may be overlooked. *Topographical orientation* and *memorising abilities* may be conveniently tested further once the ambulant patient has adjusted to the new surroundings of a hospital ward by finding out if he knows the location of his bed, the toilet and the dining area and if he has learned the names of doctors and other attendants and can remember when he last saw them. *Memory* functions can be explored in greater detail by asking about past and recent personal and general events. The Gresham Ward Questionnaire (included in the booklet on psychiatric assessment published for the Institute of Psychiatry) provides a scoring method useful in elderly patients in whom the differentiation of organic and 'functional' disorder by clinical means may be especially difficult. Besides testing the patient's ability to learn new verbal material, the interviewer can test visual learning by asking the patient to reproduce drawings of geometrical figures after a few minutes' delay. *Nominal dysphasia* may be the only language disorder; it is tested for by asking the patient to name objects verbally or in writing. Other evidence of dysphasia may emerge from tests of expressive speech, word-finding, repetition and comprehension. The patient should be asked to respond to spoken and written commands (e.g. 'close your eyes') or to explain the point of a simple fable or news item read to him. He should be asked to write spontaneously and to dictation. Reading ability and comprehension of what is read should be tested. *Calculating ability* can be examined using tasks which involve coins and numbers. *Visuospatial and constructional abilities* are tested by getting the patient to draw simple outlines such as a house, a clockface with the hands pointing to specified times, the points of a compass or arrows pointing in specified directions. He should be asked to copy drawings such as a hollow cube or other simple geometrical figures. Tests should be given to detect *apraxias*, which comprise difficulties in performing more or less complex motor tasks in the absence of motor weakness or inco-ordination, and *agnosias*, which are deficits in recognition despite intact vision. The former may be tested by asking the patient to perform movements such as showing how he would comb his hair or shave (or, with female patients, put on lipstick), taking a match from a box and striking it, putting a letter in an envelope, and dressing. The latter can be reviewed by asking him to identify coins, other objects, parts of his body, other people or the meaning of a picture. Ability to discriminate right from left is examined by asking the patient to identify the laterality of parts of his own and the examiner's body. Finger agnosia is detected by asking the patient to name his own and the examiner's fingers.

If the patient is mute and apparently inaccessible, the major differential diagnosis will lie between an organic impairment of consciousness and states of 'stupor' resulting from functional disorder. The patient's alertness, responsiveness to varying degrees of stimulation and capacities for vocalisation should be carefully observed and tested. If the eyes are open, their attentiveness to the surroundings should be noted. If they are shut, the response to passive opening should be observed. Posture, muscular tone and resistance to passive movement should be assessed. The patient's state of hygiene and dress may be informative and his capacities to attend to his own needs should be evaluated. Neurological examination will be especially important.

Insight and appraisal of illness

Under this heading are recorded the patient's views as to the nature and possible origins of his present difficulties and state of mind. According to psychiatric tradition, the patient is said to have insight if he recognises that he is unwell, that his disorder is of mental or nervous origin and that he is in need of treatment. Insight, in this sense, is clearly not an all-or-nothing attribute. Marked lack of insight, the patient insisting perhaps that he is perfectly well and mentally sound, is common in severe psychotic disorders, whether affective, schizophrenic or organic. The depressed patient may believe he is guilty, damned or diseased rather than mentally unwell. Denial of psychological origin for symptoms is common also in hysterical disorders, hypochondriasis and anorexia nervosa. The term 'insight' is also used in another sense in psychiatry to refer to the psychological understanding of symptoms in terms of inner emotions, interpersonal problems and other difficulties in living. The attainment of this kind of insight may be regarded as one of the major aims of psychotherapy.

The patient should be asked what he attributes his difficulties to.

He may ascribe them entirely to the fault of others or he may be able to recognise in some degree the role played by his own behaviour and personality in the generation of symptoms and problems. His views about what can or should be done to help should be elicited, as well as his expectations of its success. Some attempt should also be made to evaluate his motivation to pursue treatment seriously and with persistence and to accept medical recommendations.

FORMULATING PROBLEMS

Under pressure of time, the busy clinician may feel it is impossible to do justice to the multitude of factors which affect a patient's state of mind and which have shaped his personal and medical history. It can be tempting to cut through this complexity by making global diagnostic judgements (e.g. that the patient is 'neurotic' or 'normal' or 'a psychopath') but such judgements must inevitably be highly subjective and over-simple. Even in those cases where evidence points to a major syndrome of disease or mental disorder, plans for further investigation and treatment will need to be geared to the individual patient in a way that is appropriate to his social situation, his personal capacities and his own perceptions and wishes. Some way of focusing attention on particularly important aspects of the patient's predicament is therefore essential.

The traditional way of making a brief summary of the case, as outlined in Chapter 1, is to write a *formulation*; salient points are noted under seven headings as follows: resumé of history, significant findings on examination, descriptive diagnosis (or differential diagnosis), possible aetiological and pathogenic factors, further investigation, plans for management and treatment, likely prognosis. The newer, *problem-orientated* type of formulation may have advantages in favouring a more practical, piecemeal and flexible approach which avoids premature assumptions about the relative importance of different aspects of a patient's difficulties. Each *problem* identified by the doctor or the patient can be explored further with appropriate priority. Equal diagnostic weight can be given to problems in the psychological, social and physical realms. The list of problems can continue to be revised and updated as one learns more about the patient and the factors (and their interrelationship) which affect his well-being. This way, it may be possible to incorporate the psychiatric dimension more easily into general medical assessment, rather than seeing it, mistakenly, as a massive undertaking of time and effort to be reserved only for the psychiatrist or the clerkship in psychiatry.

The general rules of POMR formulation apply: problems are identified which require attention, investigation or treatment in their own right and are named at the highest level of abstraction for which there is definite evidence. Where there is insufficient evidence for a formal medical diagnosis or the problem is of a different kind, simple descriptive language or the patient's own words will be best. Symptoms clearly belonging together as one syndrome do not need to be named separately.

As a guide to the sort of active problems that commonly arise, and which are therefore worth being on the look out for, the list in Table 11.2 may be helpful. Not uncommonly a patient's problems stem from one or more of these problems in a close relative or other

Table 11.2. *Common problems.*

Psychological problems
Subjective complaint(s)
Behavioural problem(s), e.g. as reported by others
Psychiatric symptom(s) or sign(s)
Nameable syndrome of neurosis or psychosis
Personality type or disorder
Intellectual handicap

Social problems
In relationships (e.g. with sexual partner, family members, superiors at work, social milieu)
Occupation (employment or other occupations, including educational and leisure opportunities)
Accommodation and housing
Finance
Conflict with the law

Physical problems
Bodily symptoms
Abnormal physical signs
Abnormal findings on physical tests
Physical disease
Trauma
Drug or alcohol dependence or abuse
Dietary deficiency
Adverse environment (including contact with infection, toxins, etc.)
Adverse effects of physical treatment
Physical disability

important associate (e.g. son with schizophrenia, retirement of supportive GP, alcoholic husband, etc).

Further investigations

In most cases a few minutes in conversation with the patient will be enough to get an idea of the probability of major problems in the areas listed. For each type of problem, as with any physical problem, the interested clinician will develop appropriate sub-routines of enquiry according to his knowledge of important factors which will need further attention. If the possibility emerges, for instance, that the patient is depressed, more detailed enquiries about this will need to be incorporated into the interview, either immediately or at a later time. The interviewer will find that many such avenues will open up. He cannot pursue them all at once, particularly if he wants to avoid subjecting the patient to an exhausting interrogation; but he can bear in mind how far he has got in each of these lines of enquiry so that he can come back to them later. In this way he can allow his time with the patient to range widely over many topics, but he will strive to know at any moment what particular line of interest he is pursuing. Some moments of directionless free-wheeling will be inevitable, but with increasing experience he will learn to cover relevant ground more quickly and comprehensively.

In psychiatry, investigation and treatment are especially closely linked. Very often the patient will help himself over his problems once he has seen more clearly what they are or has identified the forces which thwart the natural drive towards recovery. Interview techniques will be the mainstay of further investigation, but it may be useful to bear in mind a brief summary of some other options, again related to the major headings of psychological, social and physical (Table 11.3).

SOME SPECIAL PROBLEMS IN DIAGNOSIS

Bodily Symptoms of Psychiatric Disorder

A common diagnostic task is to recognise when bodily symptoms are due to psychological disturbance. Many doctors feel more equipped to deal with somatic pathology than with the troubles of the mind. Consequently, if the patient presents with a variety of symptoms the doctor may 'organise' the patient's complaint by responding to the more physical-sounding among them to the neglect of others which might point more directly to a psychological basis (Balint, 1964). Prescription of ineffectual medication, fruitless physical investigations and even repeated surgical exploration may be the result.

Table 11.3. *Options for further investigation.*

Psychological

Further interviews (with definable goals) with the patient
Structured assessment schedules (rating scales, etc.)
Expert psychological investigation (e.g. tests of intellectual functions, evaluation of response contingencies, etc.)
Past records of previous psychiatric treatment (e.g. from GPs, hospitals, other therapists), with the patient's consent as appropriate

Social

Interviews by doctor (or social worker or other member of the therapeutic team) with spouse, other family members or close associates, alone or with the patient also present
Observations by nurses and other staff of patient's behaviour
Domiciliary assessment of home situation
Reports from other social and welfare agencies involved with the patient or his family
Reports from employers, educational establishments, military services, etc.
Occupational assessment (by OTs, DRO, Industrial Rehab. Unit, etc.)

Physical

More detailed neurological and other clinical examinations
Physical investigations — cerebral (e.g. EEG, skull x-ray, CAT scan, etc.) or general (blood, urine, etc.)
Further assessments of physical disability

In many cases the problem can be quickly identified by enquiry into the patient's preoccupations and the reasons for him presenting *now* with the complaint.

CASE HISTORY. A widow aged 43 was admitted to hospital for investigation of severe and persistent but poorly localised chest pain. Extensive investigations brought to light only a small hiatus hernia. Eventually thoracotomy and surgical repair of the hernia were planned, but as a final step before this major procedure was undertaken she was assessed from a psychiatric viewpoint. Invited to talk freely about herself, she recounted a harrowing story of childhood deprivation and family and marital disharmony culminating in a recent breakdown in relations with her only surviving daughter who lived in the flat beneath her own. The pain had started on the day after the final argument. Her mental state showed anxiety and moderate depression. In the course of an hour's interview, during which she wept copiously, the chest pain disappeared. It did not return.

Often, however, the patient himself fails to recognise the source and precipitants of his symptoms. He may be more aware of the physical than of the mental concomitants of emotional distress, as a result perhaps of learning experiences during his upbringing whereby physical ailments were rewarded by his parents' attention and sympathy, or from experiences of physical illness and trauma which he has suffered himself or seen others close to him suffer. Such conditioning may have led to a general tendency to indulge in 'illness behaviour' and to 'somaticise' distress, or it may have provided a focus for hypochondriacal fears or a heightened awareness of certain body areas or functions. He may lack insight into his emotions and may avoid facing the frightening or humiliating possibility that his symptoms stem from a mental disorder.

Sometimes the diagnosis can be difficult. The bodily complaints of psychiatrically disturbed patients are often symptoms which could be due to serious physical disease (e.g. fatigue, malaise, anorexia, weight-loss, headache, backache, or other aches and pains, abdominal discomfort, constipation). The patient, moreover, may insist that he is physically ill and may try to coerce the doctor into providing physical remedies.

The question of whether or not there is underlying physical pathology can be conclusively answered only by physical examination and investigation, but routine tests may fail to detect physical disease even when it is present. The doctor, therefore, faces the dilemma of choosing between the risk on the one hand of overlooking serious disease by inadequate investigation and, on the other, of causing damaging psychological effects by reinforcing the patient's anxiety or hypochondriacal fears. If further investigations are indicated, it is best they are completed quickly rather than allowed to drag on indefinitely with the patient going the rounds of different hospital departments. The physician who 'reassures' the patient that he definitely does not have heart disease but who at the same time orders yet another ECG 'just to be sure' deceives only himself.

There are no infallible rules by which psychiatric causes for bodily symptoms can be recognised. A combination of factors besides negative findings on physical examination or routine investigation need to be taken into account in making the diagnosis. Positive signs of disorder in the physical and mental sphere should be sought, for diagnoses purely by exclusion are likely to be wrong. Disorders in both realms commonly coexist. In the example quoted of the woman with chest pain treatment might well have been required for hiatus hernia *and* depressive neurosis. More widespread adoption of the problem-orientated approach to case taking will make it easier to identify psychological and somatic problems concurrently rather than to make the still frequent mistake of regarding one as precluding the other.

Bodily symptoms associated with psychiatric disorder can be grouped as follows:

Bodily symptoms due to overt neurotic or psychotic illness

Psychiatric history taking and mental state assessment lead to a probable diagnosis by revealing other more clear-cut symptoms and signs of a psychiatric illness which is enough to account for the patient's complaints. The varied bodily symptoms of depressive illness and of morbid anxiety (which may accompany it or occur independently) have already been mentioned. Depression can cause increased preoccupation with physical health and various biological changes. The mainly autonomic symptoms of anxiety reflect exaggerated physiological mechanisms. Hypochondriacal preoccupations may be prominent in other neurotic and psychotic illnesses also. It must be remembered, however, that not only may 'functional' psychiatric syndromes of illness occur coincidentally with physical disease but they may also be directly or indirectly caused by the latter (e.g. carcinoma, myocardial infarction, endocrine disorders, infections, systemic lupus erythematosus, drugs or primarily cerebral disease). Diagnosis of psychiatric illness as sufficient *cause* for the bodily symptoms may, therefore, demand exclusion of physical pathology by further investigation.

Bodily symptoms without other signs of overt psychiatric illness or physical pathology adequate to explain them

Such symptoms are commonly designated 'hysterical', 'functional' or 'psychogenic' when they are presumed to be of primarily psychological origin, but all three terms have been used in a confusing variety of senses. Psychiatrists today tend not to consider hysteria as an illness in itself. The adjective 'hysterical' is still commonly used, however, to refer to certain types of symptoms, a form of neurosis in which they are the major abnormality, the psychological mechanisms believed to be implicated in their production, or the traits of personality and behaviour often found in those predisposed to develop them. Several criteria may be used in diagnosis but each presents dangerous pitfalls if relied on exclusively.

Presence of 'suspect' symptoms. Since the time of Charcot certain pseudoneurological symptoms involving defects of motor, sensory and higher cerebral functions normally mediated through consciousness have been most often quoted as 'hysterical' symptoms (e.g. paralysis, tremors, 'fits', aphonia, blindness, anaesthesia, vomiting, retention of urine, amnesia, fugues). These or other hysterical symptoms do not conform accurately to patterns of symptoms produced by organic disease but are said to represent lay notions about the manifestations of disease. The clinician can elicit evidence that normal function is retained although not apparently accessible to the patient's conscious volition. In hysterical paralysis, for example, neurological examination reveals no abnormality apart from 'loss' of movement. According to the current ICD classification, the somatic pseudoneurological symptoms are called *conversion* symptoms and the mental symptoms are *dissociative* symptoms. Predominance of one or both constitutes hysterical neurosis.

Research studies have demonstrated that isolated conversion symptoms may occur in a wide variety of conditions, including somatic and organic cerebral disease. They are a fairly common acute reaction to overwhelming anxiety and distress (e.g. 'shellshock' cases in World War I) or they may result from depressive illness or may be chronic or recurrent features associated with personality disorder. Long-term follow-up of cases of hysteria diagnosed by neurologists or psychiatrists have shown that a proportion eventually turn out to have serious neurological, other organic or psychiatric illness. The diagnosis of a symptom as purely psychological in origin may be strengthened if typical symptoms have recurred repeatedly in response to stress. Even here, however, there are dangers of missing physical disease.

Mechanisms. The terms 'conversion' and 'dissociation', although used purely descriptively in the ICD classification, derive from theories about underlying psychological mechanisms. Conversion was proposed by Freud as the mechanism by which the anxiety associated with a repressed memory became expressed as a bodily symptom. Janet suggested dissociation was the key to hysteria; due to a 'lowering of the mental level' certain functions become split off from the rest of the personality and are thereby dissociated from conscious awareness and control. Other psychological mechanisms proposed to account for hysterical symptoms have included suggestion and autosuggestion, symbolisation of an underlying conflict, and social psychological mechanisms of using 'body language' or 'illness behaviour' to communicate a need for a helping response from others.

All these accounts of pathogenetic mechanisms may be relevant and valuable, but recognition of their operation is subjective and constitutes a diagnostic method of low reliability.

Relationship in time to psychologically stressful events. If it is found that the onset of symptoms closely follows an event of major psychological significance to the patient or that their severity is clearly influenced by situational factors, a psychological origin may be favoured, but the reservations about such an approach for diagnostic purposes have already been mentioned in the discussion of precipitation of psychiatric illness. Similarly, relief of symptoms following psychological measures such as placebo administration, suggestion or hypnosis or following amelioration of the patient's life situation does not necessarily prove the symptom was psychological in origin. Placebo response or spontaneous remission is common with symptoms of physical disease.

Motivation for symptoms. It is commonly held that hysterical symptoms can be recognised by the fact that they serve a useful function for the patient, helping him to resolve a social, interpersonal or intrapsychic problem. If this aspect is extremely marked it may be of diagnostic value, but it must be noted that there can be an element of 'secondary gain' in all illness, whether or not due to physical pathology. (Freud described 'primary gain' as the relief of otherwise overwhelming anxiety brought about by the mechanism of repression and conversion. 'Secondary gain', an aspect stressed more by later writers, refers to the social advantages and privileges which result from adoption of the sick role.) Effects should not be mistaken for causes.

Motivation for otherwise typical 'hysterical' symptoms is not always discoverable and its attribution must be very subjective. If motivation for symptoms is stressed, hysterical symptoms may be held to be a variety of malingering, the self-aware and deliberate simulation of illness. Many observers have suggested that elements of both conscious and unconscious simulation of illness are likely to be present together in varying proportion. Often no hard and fast distinction can be drawn. Even an admission by the patient later that he was exaggerating or feigning illness may be a rationalisation rather than a true explanation.

Gross simulation of bodily illness, as in the 'Munchausen syndrome' is often associated with severe personality disorder. A diagnosis of 'malingering' is always incomplete, for it states only what the problem is *not*.

The problem of assessing the relative contributions of physical damage and secondary gain is illustrated in cases of what have been loosely called 'compensation neurosis' or 'postconcussional syndrome', when prolonged disability and a multitude of vague complaints, often with accompanying features of depression and anxiety, follow a minor injury to the head, the back or other parts of the body, often in an industrial setting. Psychological factors seem to be of major aetiological importance but their precise nature demands close scrutiny in the individual case. Compensation may or may not relieve the symptoms.

Unusual behavioural reactions. Sometimes the exaggerated way in which patients describe their symptoms may point to the likelihood of a psychological cause. Headaches, for example, become 'screws boring into the head', 'an iron vice', 'red hot nails', etc. The occurrence of emotional over-reaction or apparent under-reaction ('la belle indifférence') is, however, a very doubtful basis for diagnosis. Either may occur in physical disease, since they may reflect cultural factors and upbringing as much as dramatisation or dissociative denial.

CASE HISTORY. An English woman of 33 was brought into Casualty in the early hours of the morning, screaming and writhing in pain which she located vaguely in her abdomen. Her grossly exhibitionistic behaviour continued following admission and to quieten her she was given repeated doses of pethidine. In the absence of physical findings and because her behaviour seemed absurdly over-dramatic the pain was confidently diagnosed as 'hysterical' by the physicians and surgeons who saw her. On the sixth day after admission she said she could now feel a lump in her abdomen. A mass was indeed palpable. At operation the next day a very large chronically infected gall-bladder was removed. The pain did not recur.

Persistently inappropriate anxiety about physical health, failure to be reassured by negative results of examination or investigation, and often multiplicity of symptoms are the features of hypochondriasis. As already mentioned, however, hypochondriacal preoccupations may be prominent in psychiatric illness or physical disease. To diagnose a symptom as hypochondriacal is to describe it rather than to identify its cause.

Hysterical personality traits. Adjectives such as histrionic, immature, egocentric, emotionally shallow and labile, extrovert, suggestible, manipulative and seductive characterise the hysterical personality. People with these traits may have a greater tendency than others to develop conversion and dissociative symptoms but recognition of them does not in itself contribute much to the diagnosis unless there has been a previous history of multiplicity of unexplained physical symptoms or of polysurgery. The current symptoms still warrant assessment on their merits rather than immediate dismissal as yet another psychogenic manifestation.

The problems of diagnosis of bodily symptoms of psychiatric disorder and the need for close collaboration between psychiatrist and physician are particularly illustrated in cases of persistent *pain* which does not appear to be due to organic pathology. Walters has recommended that the terms 'psychogenic regional pain' should be used in order to stress the wide variety of contexts in which pain of primarily psychological origin can be found. Calling a pain 'hysterical' is, as Eliot Slater declared of the concept of hysteria as a whole, a fertile source of clinical error. The causes of the symptom should be sought so that it can be seen in context as a concomitant of physical disease, a manifestation of an anxiety state, depressive illness, organic cerebral disorder, acute psychological stress or long-standing personality disorder. Some of the difficulties are illustrated by the following case history.

CASE HISTORY. A 40-year-old lady had consulted gynaecologists for ten years from the time of her marriage. Her successive complaints were menorrhagia, infertility, abdominal pain, vomiting and dyspareunia. She had a number of surgical operations — a cholecystectomy before her marriage, a myomectomy followed soon by a hysterectomy, and finally a laparotomy to seek out a cause for her persistent abdominal pain. She appeared reluctant to accept having the hysterectomy as this put the seal on her chances of having a family; yet she would not consider adopting a child as she felt not well enough to cope with any added burden. To her husband she gave the appearance of stoicism in the face of adversity. Her sexual life was virtually non-existent, initially because of her complaint of persistent bleeding but when this was dealt with, because of the new symptom of dyspareunia. She had resisted her gynaecologist's advice to seek a psychiatric opinion. When pressure was put on her to acquiesce she reluctantly did so only to remonstrate angrily with her psychiatrist: 'there is nothing wrong with me psychologically'. She even resented being prescribed a tranquilliser (which she identified by consulting a drugs index) on the grounds that she would not accept that her pain was 'imaginary'. On the other hand, she expressed her willingness to have any surgical operation, 'no matter how serious so long as it will bring relief'. Her last operation revealed a postoperative blood cyst in the pelvis, which was considered to be of possible relevance to her symptoms. Postoperatively her pain improved, but she developed a refractory urinary obstruction which was only relieved after a psychiatric interview and the promise of a period of convalescence before returning home. Subsequently, she complained of pain on sexual intercourse, and this effectively deterred her husband from further attempts.

This patient illustrates the diagnostic difficulties. Although there was usually evidence of some pathological changes, they did not fully account for her disabilities. The relevance of psychological mechanisms was suggested by the *life chart* which listed a long series of varied bodily complaints and partially successful operations. One symptom was replaced by another. Her apparent stoicism and eagerness to undergo surgical operations reflected the mechanism of *dissociation* which enabled her to suppress any incipient anxiety. Other evidence of *denial mechanisms* was provided by the angry rejection of the possibility that psychological factors might be relevant. In the course of psychiatric interviews she rapidly swung from a professed hostility to an extreme attachment to her psychiatrist. It seemed likely that one of the motives for her continued semi-invalidism was her wish to avoid a full sexual life.

Psychosomatic disorders

The belief that the pathological changes in certain diseases specifically named as 'psychosomatic', such as asthma, peptic ulcer and ulcerative colitis could be explained by the action of psychological factors in individuals of particular personality type has now been largely discredited and recognised as over-simple. Psychosomatic interactions may, however, play a role in these and many other diseases. In the individual patient it will be important to evaluate evidence that his illness has been precipitated, exacerbated or maintained by psychological stresses. Recent evidence that the functioning of the autonomic nervous system can be instrumentally conditioned provides a possible mechanism by which such stress could lead to specific organ dysfunction, but the relevance of this to known diseases remains conjectural. The word 'psychosomatic' is often used casually to denote any bodily symptoms related to psychological factors, including the exaggerated autonomic responses of anxiety or the common 'tension' headaches which result from contraction of the scalp muscles. Present-day writers tend to emphasise that psychosomatic medicine is concerned with the interplay between mind and body in disease in general rather than being an approach only relevant to certain diseases.

Physical pathology resulting from self-injurious behaviour

Psychological factors are implicated in a wide variety of illnesses which can result directly or indirectly from behaviour which jeopardises health. At one extreme is the deliberately self-inflicted damage of dermatitis factitia. Abuse of alcohol, cigarettes, other drugs and medication such as laxatives, thyroxine etc., constitutes an intermediate group in which damage is not deliberate but can be recognised by the patient as a highly probable outcome. At the other extreme are those illnesses which may be precipitated or aggravated in vulnerable people by bad living habits such as dietary indiscretion or lack of exercise, which are spoken of as the 'diseases of civilisation'. The doctor assessing the individual patient will need to recognise the role of the latter's behaviour in contributing to the causation of bodily symptoms and pathology and also the factors which have led to such behaviour and which may foster its continuation.

Alcohol Problems

Recent surveys have shown in the UK that up to a quarter or more of all medical in-patients may consume alcohol in amounts sufficient to damage health. The problem is likely to present to doctors in some guise years before the classic picture of advanced alcoholism is seen, yet public and medical awareness is still inadequately directed towards the fact that alcohol problems commonly start in the twenties or even adolescence.

Reluctance to identify the problem is likely to exist on the patient's side and perhaps on the doctor's too. The question in diagnosis is not just to decide whether the patient is or is not 'alcoholic' but to assess the role alcohol plays in his life (i.e. the degree of *dependence*) and the extent to which there may be pointers to actual or impending *damage* by alcohol to his physical, mental or social functioning. No single test will answer these questions in all patients and the doctor has to face the unpleasant reality that the patient who is drinking too much on an intermittent or more or less continuous basis is quite likely not to tell the truth. Often in medicine it is customary to take the patient's account on trust until definite evidence emerges that it is misleading or false. In relation to alcohol, however, the fallibility of the patient's capacity to present an accurate picture of his experiences has to be assumed from the start.

A positive interest in the possibility of alcohol abuse and an alertness to any hints of it are likely to be the clinician's most powerful instruments in diagnosis. Many people will be able to talk frankly about their use of alcohol if asked in a detailed and non-judgmental way about alcohol as a factor which might be affecting their health. Sometimes an indirect approach, such as finding out how the patient spends his leisure time, can be more successful. Griffith Edwards' recommendation to 'reconstruct a typical drinking day' will be useful in following up early clues to the possibility of excessive indulgence.

There may be many sorts of hint from the history or examination. Some social groups have a higher risk of alcoholism (e.g. Scots or Irish, single or separated marital status, manual occupation or certain professions such as journalism, liquor trade, military services, doctors). There may be a history of occupational absenteeism, dismissal or decline, marital friction, past history of accidents, suicidal attempts, crime, unexplained illness or injury. Information from relatives can be very revealing. In advanced stages there may be obvious signs of the psychiatric or physical complications of alcoholism. *Physical investigation* may reveal the typical facies and physique of the heavy drinker or there may be an enlarged liver, the stigmata of advanced cirrhosis or peripheral neuropathy. On *mental state examination* there may be signs of alcohol withdrawal, depression or cognitive dysfunction, but often it is 'softer' evidence related to attitude and insight, such as a reluctance to talk about alcohol, denial of the problem or plausible over-optimism about its severity or reversibility, which needs to be noted. Over-indulgence in alcohol is indicated by the finding of macrocytosis in the peripheral blood (a direct toxic effect of alcohol on the bone marrow), raised γ-glutamyl transpeptidase and, if a state of thiamine deficiency has developed, by elevated transketolase levels. The serum alcohol may be raised. *Psychological tests* of intellectual function may confirm memory impairment or dementia.

Patterns of alcohol abuse vary greatly. The patient may drink episodically — perhaps in relation to periods of increased stress or to overcome feelings of social unease and inferiority — or more or less continuously. Episodes of drunkenness may be altogether absent and the problem is detected only when complications or withdrawal symptoms appear, perhaps when abstinence is enforced by hospital admission for treatment of intercurrent illness. An important pointer to developing dependence is *subjective loss of control*: the patient finds it increasingly difficult to stop drinking whenever he takes a drink: one drink leads on to another. Other features which become more evident at this time are increasing preoccupation with drinking and the availability of further supplies, surreptitious drinking, denial of drinking, guilt about indulgence, drinking alone in the morning or at other unusual times of the day, and possibly declining fastidiousness about the quality of alcohol consumed. The patient may become aware of a sense of *craving* for alcohol if opportunities are denied him, but this aspect is not always marked, and its absence does not warrant the conclusion, assumed by many alcoholics, that drinking is not excessive.

Problems of self-control of drinking become more marked as physical dependence rapidly ensues. *Withdrawal symptoms* become troublesome and are usually worst in the early morning after the period of withdrawal during sleep. Relief by further drinking becomes necessary. Tremors ('the shakes'), retching, nausea and vomiting ('dry heaves'), anxiety, insomnia and feelings of general malaise and dysphoria are common symptoms. It is important to enquire about the occurrence of alcoholic *amnesias* ('blackouts') — repeated episodes of amnesia for the events of the night before or other periods of heavy drinking — which may last for a few hours and can be associated with wandering (alcoholic *fugues*). More severe withdrawal symptoms, such as increasing insomnia, severe anxiety, episodes of auditory or visual hallucinations, delirium tremens or fits, appear with further progression of dependence.

The time until onset of social, psychiatric and physical complications of alcoholism varies greatly. Marital difficulties, absenteeism, dismissal from jobs because of repeated late arrival or irresponsible conduct, episodes of violent, disinhibited behaviour and self-injury and repeated driving under the influence of alcohol should be enquired about. The most important general psychiatric complication of alcoholism is *depression*, which occurs both acutely as a stage in intoxication ('maudlin' drunkenness) and more chronically when heavy drinking is continued. *Suicide* is frequent. *Accidents* in the home and on the road are important causes of death in addition to the numerous direct and indirect physical complications. *Impotence* is a common result of heavy drinking and may aggravate marital problems. Eventually alcoholism causes dementia.

Apart from these general complications of alcoholism, more specific complications may be encountered. Some of the more important of these are listed in Table 11.4.

Table 11.4. *Complications of alcohol abuse.*

Withdrawal syndromes
  Delirium tremens
  Epileptic convulsions ('rum fits')
  Alcoholic hallucinations

Thiamine deficiency
  Peripheral neuropathy
  Wernicke's encephalopathy
  Korsakoff's psychosis

Other physical complications
  Dementia
  Alcoholic cerebellar degeneration
  Autonomic neuropathy
  Alcoholic myopathy
  Various forms of liver disease
  Gastritis
  Peptic ulcer
  Pancreatitis
  Porphyria cutanea tarda
  Hypoglycaemia
  Cardiomyopathy
  Oesophageal cancer
  Tuberculosis
  Fetal abnormalities

FURTHER READING

Balint, M. (1964) *The Doctor, his Patient and the Illness.* 2nd edition. London: Pitman Medical.

Hamilton, M. (Ed.) (1974) *Fish's Clinical Psychopathology.* Revised reprint. Bristol: John Wright.

Institute of Psychiatry (1973) *Notes on Eliciting and Recording Clinical Information.* London: Oxford University Press.

Kendell, R. E. (1975) *The Role of Diagnosis in Psychiatry.* Oxford: Blackwell.

Kraüpl Taylor, F. (1979) *Psychopathology.* London: Quartermain House.

Wing, J. K., Cooper, J. E. & Sartorius, N. (1974) *Description and Classification of Psychiatric Symptoms.* London: Cambridge University Press.

Normal Laboratory Values

HAEMATOLOGY VALUES

Haemoglobin

Men	13.5—18.0 g/dl
Women	11.5—16.5 g/dl
Infants (full term, cord blood)	13.6—19.6 g/dl
Infants, 3 months	9.5—12.5 g/dl
Children, 1 year	11.0—13.0 g/dl
Children, 3—6 years	11.5—14.0 g/dl
Children, 10—12 years	11.5—14.8 g/dl

Packed Cell Volume (Haematocrit)

Men	0.40—0.54 l/l
Women	0.35—0.47 l/l
Infants (full term, cord blood)	0.44—0.62 l/l
Infants, 3 months	0.32—0.44 l/l
Children, 1 year	0.36—0.44 l/l
Children, 3—6 years	0.36—0.44 l/l
Children, 10—12 years	0.37—0.45 l/l

Red Cell Count

Men	$4.5—6.5 \times 10^{12}/l$
Women	$3.8—5.8 \times 10^{12}/l$
Infants (full term, cord blood)	$4.0—6.0 \times 10^{12}/l$
Infants, 3 months	$3.2—4.8 \times 10^{12}/l$
Children, 1 year	$3.6—5.2 \times 10^{12}/l$
Children, 3—6 years	$4.0—5.5 \times 10^{12}/l$
Children, 10—12 years	$4.0—5.5 \times 10^{12}/l$

Mean Cell Volume (MCV)

Adults	76—96 fl
Infants (full term, cord blood)	106 fl (mean)
Infants, 3 months	95 fl (mean)
Children, 1 year	70—86 fl
Children, 3—6 years	73—88 fl
Children, 10—12 years	77—91 fl

Mean Cell Haemoglobin (MCH)

Adults	27—32 pg
Infants, 3 months	24—34 pg
Children, 1 year	23—31 pg
Children, 3—6 years	24—30 pg
Children, 10—12 years	24—30 pg

Mean Cell Haemoglobin Concentration (MCHC)

Adults and children	31—35 g/dl

Reticulocytes

Adults and children	0.2—2.0%	$10-100 \times 10^9/l$
Infants (full term, cord blood)	2.0—6.0%	$150 \times 10^9/l$ (mean)

Total Leucocyte Count (WBC)

Adults	$4.0-11.0 \times 10^9/l$
Infants (full term, cord blood)	$10.0-25.0 \times 10^9/l$
Infants, 1 year	$6.0-18.0 \times 10^9/l$
Children, 4—7 years	$6.0-15.0 \times 10^9/l$
Children, 8—12 years	$4.5-13.0 \times 10^9/l$

Differential Leucocyte Count — adults

Neutrophils	$2.5-7.5 \times 10^9/l$
Eosinophils	$0.04-0.4 \times 10^9/l$
Basophils	$0-0.1 \times 10^9/l$
Monocytes	$0.2-0.8 \times 10^9/l$
Lymphocytes	$1.5-3.5 \times 10^9/l$

Platelets

$150-400 \times 10^9/l$

Sedimentation rate (Westergren, 1 h, at $20\pm3°C$)

Men	$0-5$ mm
Women	$0-7$ mm

Coagulation Studies

Bleeding time (Ivy's method)	$3-7$ min
Coagulation time (Lee and White's method, $37°C$)	$5-11$ min
Prothrombin time	$10-14$ s
Activated partial thromboplastin time	$28-35$ s
Plasma fibrinogen	$1.5-4.0$ g/l

MISCELLANEOUS BLOOD PLASMA OR SERUM VALUES

Albumin	$35-48$ g/l
Aldolase	$12-75$ nmol/l
Ascorbic acid	$23-85\,\mu mol/l$
Blood volume	$80-85$ ml/kg
Caeruloplasmin	$1.8-2.5\,\mu mol/l$
Calcium	$2.1-2.6$ mmol/l
Chloride	$100-106$ mmol/l
Cholinesterase (pseudocholinesterase)	0.5 or more arb. unit
Copper	$16-31\,\mu mol/l$
Creatine phosphokinase (CPK)	$0.08-0.58\,\mu mol/l$
Creatinine	$60-130\,\mu mol/l$
Ferritin	$15-300\,\mu g/l$
Folate:	
Red cell	$3-20\,\mu g/l$
Serum	$13-34$ nmol/l
Globulin	$25-32$ g/l
Glucose	$3.9-5.6$ mmol/l
Iron	$13-32\,\mu mol/l$
Iron binding capacity	$45-70\,\mu mol/l$
Lactic acid	$0.6-1.8$ mmol/l
Lactic dehydrogenase	$1.00-2.00\,\mu mol/l$
Lead	Less than $1.0\,\mu mol/l$
Lipids:	
Cholesterol	$3.10-5.69$ mmol/l
Magnesium	$0.8-1.3$ mmol/l

5´-Nucleotidase	30 – 290 nmol/l
Osmolality	285 – 295 mmol/kg
Oxygen saturation (arterial)	96 – 100%
P_{CO_2}	35 – 45 mmHg
pH	7.35 – 7.45
Phosphorus (inorganic)	1.0 – 1.5 mmol/l
Potassium	3.5 – 5.0 mmol/l
Urea nitrogen (BUN)	2.9 – 8.9 mmol/l
Uric acid	0.18 – 0.42 mmol/l
Vitamin B_{12}	160 – 925 ng/l

URINE VALUES

Amylase	24 – 76 U/ml
Calcium	3.8 or less mmol/24 h
Catecholamines:	
Adrenaline	<55 nmol/24h
Noradrenaline	<590 nmol/24h
Copper	0 – 1.6 μmol/24 h
Coproporphyrin	80 – 380 nmol/24 h
Creatine	0.75 mmol/24 h
Creatinine	15.25 mg/kg of body weight/24 h
Creatinine clearance	104 – 125 ml/min
5-Hydroxyindole acetic acid	10 – 45 μmol/24 h
Lead	Less than 0.39 μmol/l
Osmolality	200 – 1200 mmol/kg water
Porphobilinogen	0
Potassium	40 – 120 mmol/24 h
Protein:	
Quantitative	<0.15 g/24 h
Sodium	80 – 250 mmol/24 h
Urea	200 – 600 mmol/24 h

CEREBROSPINAL FLUID VALUES

Albumin	0.3 g/l
Cell count	<5 per μl
Chloride	120 – 130 mmol/l
Glucose	2.8 – 4.2 mmol/l
IgG	0.04 g/l
Pressure (initial)	70 – 180 mm of water
Protein:	
Cisternal	0.15 – 0.25 g/l
Lumbar	0.15 – 0.45 g/l
Ventricular	0.05 – 0.15 g/l

VALUES FOR ENDOCRINE INVESTIGATIONS

Thyroid Function Tests

Total serum thyroxine	58 — 128 nmol/l
Free binding capacity	90 — 105%
Free thyroxine index	53 — 142
Serum T3	1.5 — 3.5 nmol/l
TSH	1 — 5 mU/l

The thyroid hormones circulate in the plasma bound to proteins, particularly thyroxine-binding globulin (TBG). In the interpretation of laboratory results it is important to recognise those factors which may affect the concentration of TBG and thus the assayed hormone concentration, although the actual amount of free hormone may not have changed.

Adrenal Function Tests

	0900 h	*2400 h*
Plasma cortisol	220 — 650 nmol/l	50 — 280 nmol/l
Urinary 17 oxosteroids		
Female		14 — 70 μmol/24 h
Male		17 — 86 μmol/24 h
Urinary 17 oxogenic steroids		
Female		14 — 56 μmol/24 h
Male		21 — 76 μmol/24 h
Urinary free cortisol		
Female		216 — 860 nmol/24 h
Male		300 — 1100 nmol/24 h

There is a variation in the urine excretion of both oxosteroids and oxogenic steroids with age. These steroids are not a reliable index in differentiating Cushing's syndrome from simple obesity. The urinary free cortisol should be preferred.

Dynamic Tests

The estimation of plasma cortisol is of most value when used in conjunction with procedures that directly or indirectly stimulate or suppress the adrenal cortex.

1. The adrenal response to exogenous ACTH: the tetracosactrin test.
2. The ability to produce ACTH in response to hypoglycaemia.
3. The ability to reduce ACTH output in response to a raised plasma cortisol level: the dexamethasone suppression test.

Pituitary Function Tests

Growth Hormone

Basal plasma values of growth hormone are normally low throughout the day, being less than 10 mU/l, and they may often be undetectable. Transient peaks may also occur, which are of a spontaneous nature. It is therefore essential to use provocative tests to demonstrate a deficiency of growth hormone, but the finding of one high value proves that the deficiency does not exist. In cases of suspected hypopituitarism growth hormone values should be followed after insulin-induced hypoglycaemia. If excess growth hormone is suspected, the growth hormone values should be followed during hyperglycaemia after a glucose tolerance test to see if the normal suppression occurs.

FSH and LH

	FSH U/l	*LH U/l*
Females		
Follicular phase	1—10	2.5—14
Mid-cycle phase	6—25	25—70
Luteal phase	1—6	1—10
Post-menopausal	30—120	17—45
Males	1—7	1.5—10
Children: one year to puberty	2.5	—

Serum Prolactin

Females	
Pre-menopausal	40—445 mU/l
Post-menopausal	100—330 mU/l
Males	40—415 mU/l

Ovarian Function Tests

Oestradiol-17-beta:	
Follicular phase	40—60 pmol/l
Peri-ovulatory	350—1500 pmol/l
Luteal phase	180—1000 pmol/l
Post-menopausal	<100 pmol/l
Progesterone:	
Follicular phase	<5 nmol/l
Luteal phase	30—75 nmol/l
Post-menopausal	<5 nmol/l

Testicular Function Tests

1. Semen analysis >80 million per mm^3
2. Plasma testosterone (males) $10.4-38.2$ nmol/l

VALUES IN GASTROINTESTINAL INVESTIGATIONS

Gastric Function Tests

Basal acid output $0-4$ mmol/h
Maximal acid output (pentagastrin) $18-40$ mmol/h
Insulin test (for incomplete vagotomy)   Positive result if increase
                                  >20 mmol/l above basal secretion
                                  (10 mmol/l if basal secretion zero)

Serum gastrin $10-50$ pmol/l

Small Bowel Function

Faecal fat <18 mmol /24 h
Xylose tolerance test   2 h blood level   } $>25\%$ of dose
  (5 g xylose dose)   5 h urinary excretion } $(22-30\%)$
Vitamin B$_{12}$ absorption ^{57}Co B$_{12}>8-30\%$ of the dose/24 h
  (Dicopac test) ^{58}Co B$_{12}>8-30\%$ of the dose/24 h

Pancreatic Function

Lundh test meal $11-20$ I.U. tryptic activity

Liver Studies

Serum bilirubin   Total >19 μmol/l
                          Conjugated >5 μmol/l
Serum alkaline phosphatase $0-35$ I.U./l
Serum γ-glutamyl transpeptidase $0-50$ I.U./l
Serum transaminases:
  SGPT (alanine aminotransferase) $0-40$ I.U./l
  SGOT (aspartate aminotransferase) $0-40$ I.U./l
Immunoglobulins:
  IgA $0.9-4.5$ g/l
  IgG $8-18$ g/l
  IgM $0.6-2.5$ g/l

Index